Techniques in Neuroanatomical Research

Edited by

Ch. Heym and W.-G. Forssmann

With 165 Figures

Springer-Verlag
Berlin Heidelberg New York 1981

Professor Dr. Christine Heym
Anatomisches Institut der Universität
I. Lehrstuhl
Im Neuenheimer Feld 307
6900 Heidelberg
Federal Republic of Germany

Professor Dr. Wolf-Georg Forssmann
Anatomisches Institut der Universität
III. Lehrstuhl
Im Neuenheimer Feld 307
6900 Heidelberg
Federal Republic of Germany

ISBN 3-540-10686-3 Springer-Verlag Berlin Heidelberg New York
ISBN 0-387-10686-3 Springer-Verlag New York Heidelberg Berlin

Library of Congress Cataloging in Publication Data
Main entry under title: Techniques in neuroanatomical research. Bibliography: p. Includes index. 1. Neuroanatomy—Technique. 2. Histology—Technique. I. Heym, Christine. II. Forssmann, W.-G. (Wolf-Georg), 1939– . QM576.T43 599.04′8′028 81-9214
ISBN 0-387-10686-3 (U.S.) AACR2

Typesetting, Printing and Bookbinding: Konrad Triltsch, Graphischer Betrieb, Würzburg
2125/3140-543210

Foreword

"Anatomy is the mother of physiology" – this statement was used to characterize the evolution of physiology from anatomy as an independent science in the late nineteenth century. It had particular truth for neurophysiology, which started as functional neuroanatomy based on the observation of changes in behaviour after lesions of the nervous system both in experimental animals and in human patients. Today, anatomy may again be considered the mother of physiology; however, the meaning of this statement is rather different from that 100 years ago: The modern mother provides a dwelling for an increasing number of children endowed with new functional capabilities. This book provides a good illustration of such semantic metamorphosis in the case of neuroanatomy.

After a long period of little progress in either macroscopic neuroanatomy or neurohistology, during which the heritage of Cajal, Golgi, and others was developed and refined to yield a functional concept of the nervous system, the past two decades have seen tremendous progress in methods applicable to the analysis of the nervous system. The new era was heralded by the introduction of the electron microscope to investigate the nervous system. This book is an impressive witness to the more recent developments. Methods of physics, electrical engineering, chemistry, biochemistry, and immunology and combinations of these govern the approaches of today and have led to a tremendous renaissance of neuroanatomy – the mother of the neurosciences!

These new techniques have yielded some exciting new views with regard to both the structure and function of the nervous system. Thus, even the adult nervous system can no longer be considered a static network of nerve cells, and the electrical nerve impulse is no longer seen as the only carrier of information in the nervous system. The new methods have uncovered numerous new functional aspects, yielding a nervous system which is more dynamic than previously thought. The often exciting beautiful pictures of neuronal elements that can be obtained by these techniques might be symbols for the richness of intrinsic features of this brain world, the basis of the fantasy, culture, and technology of mankind.

Apart from bearing witness to and illustrating these new glimpses of the brain, the book should have a highly practical value. For progress in neurobiological research it is often necessary to apply methods not previously used in the laboratory. There are many examples of such multidisciplinary work providing access to major complementary aspects of a problem and thus leading to progress in the field. I hope that this book will stimulate and help researchers to go beyond their methodological traditionalism and encourage them to try one or more of the methods presented here. I hope that the descriptions given are sufficiently practical to make reproduction of the methods possible. In this way the knowledge of neurophysiologists, neuropharmacologists, neurochemists, and behavioral scientists will be expanded, and they will find themselves in the flourishing house of neuroanatomy!

Heidelberg, September 1981

Manfred Zimmermann
Professor of Physiology

Preface

In the past few decades neuroanatomy has undergone revolutionary advances which are due mainly to newly available research methods such as electron microscopy, histochemistry, immunohistochemistry and various other marker methods. Most of these methods needed technically specialised personnel in order to obtain quality results in routine laboratory procedures relevant to neuroanatomical research. Following a workshop sponsored by the German Research Foundation on "Methods in Neuroanatomy" a decision was made to make available pertinent information of investigators interested in neuroanatomical problems. The editors were delighted with the overwhelming positive response from numerous internationally known researchers and authors who chose to contribute to this "neuroanatomical method book".

We are particularly thankful for the magnitude and explicitness of the authors' description of the basic principles of neuroanatomical methods, their routine application, critical problems in the execution of these techniques as well as examples dealing with personal research projects, thereby indicating their reliability and purpose.

We express our thanks to Springer-Verlag for their excellent cooperation and positive feedback, particularly from Dr. Thiekötter, who has provided continuous encouragement during the preparation of this edition.

Many people have helped us with this book and we acknowledge the work of all, especially, Mrs. H. Ehlers, Mrs. R. Botz, Mrs. Ch. Wedel, J. Greenberg and W. Wyrwas.

We hope that this edition will be of valuable assistance and provides stimulation to those engaged in laboratory work. Critical suggestions from the reader would be highly appreciated for future editions in order to improve the quality of neuroanatomical research in all laboratories.

Heidelberg, September 1981

Christine Heym and Wolf-Georg Forssmann

Contents

List of Contributors

Professor Dr. K. AKERT
Physiologisches Institut der Universität
Rämistraße 69, CH-8001 Zürich
Switzerland

Professor Dr. K. H. ANDRES
Institut für Anatomie II, Ruhruniversität
Universitätsstraße 150, D-4630 Bochum
Federal Republic of Germany

Professor VICTORIA CHAN PALAY, Ph. D., M. D.
Department of Neurobiology
Harvard Medical School
25 Shattuck Street
Boston, Massachusetts 02115, USA

Dr. MONIKA VON DÜRING
Institut für Anatomie II, Ruhruniversität
Universitätsstraße 150, D-4630 Bochum
Federal Republic of Germany

Professor Dr. WOLF-GEORG FORSSMANN
Anatomisches Institut der Universität
Im Neuenheimer Feld 307, D-6900 Heidelberg
Federal Republic of Germany

Professor Dr. HELMUT GRUBER
Anatomisches Institut der Universität Wien
Währingerstraße 13, A-1090 Wien IX
Austria

Dr. KLAUS HAUSEN
Max-Planck-Institut für biologische Kybernetik
Spemannstraße 36, D-7400 Tübingen
Federal Republic of Germany

Professor Dr. CHRISTINE HEYM
Anatomisches Institut der Universität
Im Neuenheimer Feld 307, D-6900 Heidelberg
Federal Republic of Germany

Dipl. Biol. DIETER HOCK
Anatomisches Institut der Universität
Im Neuenheimer Feld 307, D-6900 Heidelberg
Federal Republic of Germany

Professor Dr. GÖSTA JONSSON
Department of Histology, Karolinska Institutet
S-10401 Stockholm
Sweden

Dr. Dr. HUBERT KNORR
Institut für Medizinische Strahlenkunde
Versbacher Straße 5, D-8700 Würzburg
Federal Republic of Germany

Professor Dr. K. MELLER
Institut für Anatomie I, Ruhruniversität
Universitätsstraße 150, D-4630 Bochum
Federal Republic of Germany

Professor Dr. JÜRGEN METZ
Anatomisches Institut der Universität
Im Neuenheimer Feld 307, D-6900 Heidelberg
Federal Republic of Germany

Dr. H. MOOR
Physiologisches Institut der Universität
Rämistraße 69, CH-8001 Zürich
Switzerland

Professor Dr. D. KENT MOREST
Department of Anatomy
The University of Connecticut Health Center
Farmington, Connecticut 06032
USA

Professor Dr. VIRGINIA D. PICKEL
Department of Neurology, Laboratory of Neurobiology
Cornell University, Medical College
525 East 68 Street, New York, N. Y. 10021
USA

Dr. M. REINECKE
Anatomisches Institut der Universität
Im Neuenheimer Feld 307, D-6900 Heidelberg
Federal Republic of Germany

Dr. J. G. RICHARDS
Pharmaceutical Research Department
F. Hoffmann-La Roche & Co., Ltd.
CH-4002 Basel
Switzerland

Dr. C. SANDRI
Physiologisches Institut der Universität
Rämistraße 69, CH-8001 Zürich
Switzerland

MADHABANANDA SAR
The University of North Carolina at Chapel Hill
111 Swing Bldg. 217 H, Chapel Hill, N. C. 27514
USA

Dr. A. SCHILLER
I. Physiologisches Institut der Universität
Im Neuenheimer Feld 326, D-6900 Heidelberg
Federal Republic of Germany

Professor Dr. PETER SCHUBERT
Max-Planck-Institut für Psychiatrie
Kraepelinstraße 2, D-8000 München 40
Federal Republic of Germany

Professor WALTER E. STUMPF, M. D., Ph. D.
Department of Pharmacology
The University of North Carolina at Chapel Hill
111 Swing Bldg. 217 H, Chapel Hill, N. C. 27514
USA

Profesor Dr. R. TAUGNER
I. Physiologisches Institut der Universität
Im Neuenheimer Feld 326, D-6900 Heidelberg
Federal Republic of Germany

Professor Dr. E. THOMAS
Neurologisches Institut der Universität (Edinger Institut)
Deutschordenstraße 46, D-6000 Frankfurt-Niederrad
Federal Republic of Germany

Professor Dr. KLAUS UNSICKER
Anatomisches Institut der Universität
Robert-Koch-Straße 6, D-3505 Marburg
Federal Republic of Germany

Dr. HEINZ WÄSSLE
Max-Planck-Institut für biologische Kybernetik
Spemannstraße 36, D-7400 Tübingen
Federal Republic of Germany

Part I

General Research Methods in Neuroanatomy

Chapter 1

General Methods in Light Microscopy of the Nervous System

Helmut Gruber

1 Introduction

Development and progress in neuroanatomical research largely depend on the methods available to persons studying the nervous system. Much of our knowledge is primarily based on the detailed macroscopic descriptions of the old anatomists. Important impulses to neuroanatomical research emerged with the introduction of microscopic techniques and new staining methods. With the aid of selective myelin stains, nerve cell stains, and silver impregnation methods the basis of our present knowledge on central nervous nuclei and fiber tracts was established. One of the most fundamental steps of this development was Cajals statement of his neuron theory.

With increasing knowledge the disciplines of neuroanatomy and neurophysiology came closer to each other. Today, neuroanatomical techniques are no longer the privileges of anatomists. Experimental work involving the study of the behavior after ablations or focal lesions, tracing studies concerned with the elucidation of fiber tracts and with questions of topical representation, and studies on the effects of damage of toxic or other agents to the central nervous system are all using microscopic techniques for exact localization. In addition, classic light microscopy is a valuable reference method for orientation in electron microscopy, histochemistry, immune fluorescence methods, autoradiography, and peroxidase labeling studies. The following chapter gives a brief survey of the chief light microscopic techniques of neuroanatomy and their applications.

2 Fixation of Nervous Tissue for Light Microscopy

The structure of nervous tissue is rather sensitive to postmortal degradation. For sufficient structural preservation it is essential to bring the tissue into contact with a fixative as soon as possible. The bony coverings of the central nervous system make the quick removal of the tissue difficult. At least slight mechanical damage is inevitable. Since Cammermeyer (1960) demonstrated that a well-fixed brain is much less sensitive to traumatical artifacts, it should generally be recommended to fix the nervous tissue in situ before removal. In small animals the spinal cord and its roots may be fixed by applying the fixative directly to the exposed vertebral canal of the anesthetized animal. However, usually relatively large blocks of nervous tissue or even whole brains are needed in experimental studies and penetration of the fixative would be rather slow. For good tissue preservation in light microscopy, therefore, fixation by vascular perfusion is desirable. This technique has the advantage of optimal and simultaneous penetration of the fixative and also avoids any mechanical traumatization of the tissue prior to fixation.

In human brain, where vascular perfusion immediately after death is impossible, injection of the fixative through the carotid and vertebral arteries is recommended. After cutting the brain into slices, freehand or by means of a macrotome (Jung, Heidelberg; Lipshaw, Detroit Mich.), fixation is continued by immersion in the same fixative for several weeks (Schaltenbrand and Wahren 1977). In case vascular injection is impossible or unwanted, immersion fixation should start with low concentrations ascending during the following weeks. In this way the formation of diffusion barriers is avoided (B. Schlesinger, personal communication). Immersion fixation should start with a formaldehyde concentration of 4% and finally reach 10%.

In most animal experiments it is possible to fix tissue by vascular perfusion. Several technical papers have been published on perfusion fixation (Cammermeyer 1960; Palay et al. 1962; Schultz and Karlsson 1965; Andres 1966; Cammermeyer 1967; Forssmann et al. 1967; Peters 1970; Gil and Weibel 1971; Clark 1978, among others). Most of these publications are concerned with optimal fixation for electron microscopy. However, the information is relevant also for light microscopy. Perfusion fixation reduces to a large extent the incidence of mechanical artifacts, retraction of neurons, and nuclear pyknosis (Cammermeyer 1960). In perfusion-fixed nervous tissue significantly higher numbers of glial mitoses are demonstrable, which indicates that the fixation effect starts immediately, thus preventing mitoses from finishing before the onset of the fixation process (Fleischhauer 1967).

2.1 Perfusion Fixation

2.1.1 Anesthesia

Most authors use barbiturates to anesthetize laboratory animals. In small animals intraperitoneal application is preferred, whereas in larger animals like rabbits, cats, or monkeys intravenous injection is more reliable. Nembutal (sodium pentobarbital, Abbott Laboratories, North Chicago, Ill.) in a dosage of 40 mg/kg body weight is recommended for most species. For guinea pigs, a neurolept analgesia is proposed: Premedication with Ketanest (Parke-Davis) 10 mg/kg i.m.; after 5 min i.m. injection of dihydrobenzperidole (Janssen Pharmaceutica, Belgium) 5 mg/kg and Fentanyl (Janssen) 0.05 mg/kg. A neurolept analgesia can also be applied in dogs and cats: i.m. injection of xylazin hydrochloride (ROMPUN, Bayer-Leverkusen) 0.15 ml/kg and Ketanest 10 mg/kg. Urethane should be avoided due to its vasoconstrictor effect. For additional analgesia, Wacker and Forssmann (1972) use Pentacocine (30 mg/kg, i.m.) as premedication before anesthesia.

2.1.2 Anticoagulant

For achieving optimal results it is necessary to apply an anticoagulant prior to washing-out of the blood. Most authors use heparin preparations (available at various concentrations in every pharmacy). In our laboratory 2000 i.u. (16.8 mg) heparin per kilogram body weight are injected intravenously 5 min prior to opening of the chest. Within this period the agent has time enough to distribute throughout the whole circulatory system. Alternatively, heparin may also be injected after abdominal incision into the spleen (Andres 1966).

2.1.3 Artificial Respiration

Palay et al. (1962) and other authors use artificial respiration with a mixture of 95% O_2 and 5% CO_2 by inserting a tube into the cervical trachea. In this way oxygen deficiency of nervous tissue during the time interval between opening of the chest and effective start of the fixation can be avoided to a large extent. These precautions have to be considered seriously when fixing for electron microscopy, but for light microscopy artificial respiration is dispensible. For the same reason oxygenation of the Ringer solution used for washing-out the blood (Forssmann et al. 1967) is not necessary for light microscopical purposes.

2.1.4 Vasodilatant

Washing out the blood with solutions at body temperature and at a pressure beyond the systolic pressure of the animal usually dilates the vessels sufficiently prior to perfusion of the fixative. As an additional vasodilatant, Palay et al. (1962) and Peters (1970) inject 1% sodium nitrite into the circulatory system. In this laboratory 1 ml 1% sodium nitrite or 1 ml 1% sodium-nitroprusside is injected in rats together with heparin intravenously.

2.1.5 Cannulation

For fixation of the brain the cannula is either introduced through the heart into the ascending aorta or by retrograde insertion of a smaller cannula into the descending aorta. The cannula must always fill the lumen of the aorta and should be fixed with a ligature. In small animals cannulation is best performed by polyethylene or Teflon tubes of adequate size. In larger animals glass or metal cannulae may also be used.

For perfusion through the ascending aorta the sternum is divided in the median line, the chest opened by a retractor, the heart exposed, and the cannula inserted through an incision of the left ventricle into the ascending aorta where it is held by a ligature through the transverse pericardial sinus. Then the right auricle of the heart is opened in order to let the blood escape.

When cannulating the descending (abdominal) aorta, the inferior caval vein is cut for efflux.

2.1.6 Removal of the Blood

For washing out the blood prior to fixation a buffered solution of 0.9% NaCl or modified Ringer solutions may be used (Andres 1966; Forssmann et al. 1967). Other authors prefer a solution of sucrose (e.g., 8.5% sucrose as recommended by Clark 1978). The solution should be warmed to 40 °C, and the perfusion pressure should exceed the systolic blood pressure of the animal. Short (approx. 30 s) washing-out periods were optimal, since prolonged perfusion prior to fixation may cause artifacts of the nervous tissue. Most authors use simple apparatuses working with hydrostatic pressure. When peristaltic pumps are used it is essential to control the pressure (attention must be given to fluids of different viscosity!). An optimal apparatus with automatic pressure control has been described by Gil and Weibel (1971).

2.1.7 Fixation

The fixative should follow immediately without any interruption of the flow. For nearly all staining procedures the optimal perfusion fixative is a solution of 4% formaldehyde buffered by 0.15 M sodium cacodylate or phosphate buffer to a pH of 7.4. In order to avoid widening of the extracellular spaces some authors add 0.9% NaCl or sucrose at concentrations of 5% or even higher (Clark 1978). The fixative should be warmed to 40 °C. At this temperature constriction of blood vessels is minimal (Peters 1970).

The formaldehyde should be prepared freshly from paraformaldehyde by dissolving it in distilled water at 65 °C (Pease 1962) adding a few drops of 1 N NaOH until the solution is clear. For a rat with 300 g body weight we use 800–900 ml, for a rabbit with 2–3 kg a volume of 2 liters of fixative. This volume should perfuse the vascular system within 5 min when introduced via the ascending aorta. After perfusion the tissue should be transferred for immersion fixation into a vessel containing the same fixative. The period of immersion fixation should last at least for 1 week. The volume of the fixative should exceed that of the tissue block 20 times. In order to minimize mechanical artifacts during preparation, Cammermeyer (1960) recommends waiting for several hours before removing the brain from the animal. In any case the tissue has to be removed with great care since the chemical process of fixation is far from being completed after a few hours.

3 Tissue Preparation for Microtomy

After fixation of the tissue the further treatment depends on whether the rapid frozen section method or one of the embedding methods is chosen.

3.1 Preparation for the Frozen Section Method

This method does not require extensive preparation. It has the advantage that the same tissue block may be used also for histochemical procedures.

The mode of freezing of the tissue prior to sectioning is of crucial influence on the quality of the sections. Nervous tissue, and particularly the grey substance, is very sensitive to freezing artifacts due to formation of large ice crystals during a slow freezing process. Cryoprotection by immersion of the tissue block into a 30% sucrose solution prior to freezing has proved to be useful. For optimal results tissue pieces up to about 1×1×1 cm should be frozen rapidly by dipping them into isopentane (2-methyl butane) or freon cooled by dry ice (–78 °C) or by liquid nitrogen (–195 °C). Larger blocks should be frozen within a CO_2 chamber supplied by some factories (e.g., Jung, Heidelberg). Slow freezing by introducing the tissue into the cryostat gives unsatisfactory results. The frozen tissue blocks may be stored up to several weeks at −20 °C or below prior to sectioning, provided they are protected from drying by enclosing them into a small gastight box or envelope.

3.2 Embedding of Tissue

For many years there have been two alternatives, the paraffin and the celloidin method. The paraffin method is a good routine technique which is excellent for nerve cell and nerve fiber studies of the central nervous system. One of its disadvantages is the marked shrinkage of the tissue during the procedure (up to 20% according to Romeis, 1968). As compared with celloidin, paraffin may be cut into thinner sections, thus yielding clear structural details under the microscope. The celloidin method is very seldom used today, although it has some important advantages. The shrinkage of the tissue is less than with paraffin and the embedding procedure is performed entirely at room temperature. The embedding medium is not removed before staining and due to the good consistency the sections are easily handled without mounting on glass slides. The thickness of celloidin sections is in the ranges between 20 and 100 µm or even more. One of the disadvantages is the long time required for the embedding procedure.

With the introduction of electron microscopy embedding in epoxy resins and ultramicrotome sections of about 1–3 µm thickness (thick- or semithin sections) are common and may also be used in light microscopy. The sections are either evaluated by means of phase contrast optics, without staining, or with normal optics after toluidine blue staining. Dry, floating semithin (thick) sections are transferred to a drop of water on a glass slide. After drying on a hot plate (50 °C) to complete evaporation of the water, sections are stained at 50 °C with a few drops of a diluted toluidine blue solution (1 part stock solution of 1% toluidine blue containing 2.5% Na_2CO_3 and 3 parts distilled H_2O). Usually 1–2 min are sufficient. Surplus staining solution is removed with tap water. Stained sections are dried on the hot plate and covered with a drop of mounting medium and a cover glass. The stain fades within several days. Fixation and embedding are identical to the tissue preparation for electron microscopy (see Chap. 2).

3.2.1 Paraffin Method

Since paraffin and related substances are not soluble in water, the tissue must be dehydrated prior to embedding, usually by graded alcohols (ethanol, methanol, isopropanol, or N-butanol). When ethanol or methanol are used the dehydrated block must be treated with an intermedium (benzene, xylene, or methylbenzoate) prior to embedding in paraffin. Tissue dehydrated with isopropanol or butanol may be transferred directly into the paraffin mixture consisting of equal parts of the alcohol and paraffin. The intermedium is followed by a 1:1 mixture of intermedium and paraffin (60 °C), from which the block is transferred to pure paraffin for embedding.

In recent years a modified paraffin, containing plastic polymeres and DMSO, called Paraplast Plus (Fisher, Sherwood) or Histosec (Merck), has been used with much success. Embedding in Paraplast Plus (PPP) has the advantage of better penetration (i.e., shorter embedding periods). The consistency of the material is superior to conventional paraffin, so that thinner sections are achieved. The blocks need not be chilled during microtomy and the sections adhere better to the glass slides during subsequent staining. Table 1 outlines the steps for a conventional procedure of paraffin embedding and for embedding in Paraplast Plus (PPP).

Embedding vessels are: metal angles (Jung, Heidelberg) adjustable to the size of the block, boxes of cardboard or of folded metal foil, or flat glass bowls. Before the

Table 1. Embedding steps for paraffin and Paraplasts Plus

Tissue block of 1 cm diameter, fixed in formaldehyde for 1 week rinsed for 1 day in tap water	
Ethanol 50% 24 h	Ethanol 70% 3 h
Ethanol 70% 24 h	Ethanol 96% 3 h
Ethanol 96% 24 h	N-butanol 15 h
Ethanol absolut 3 × 12 h	N-butanol 8 h
Methylbenzoate 2 × 12 h	Butanol-PPP (1:1) 15 h
Benzene 30 min	PPP 3 × 3 h
Benzene-paraffin (1:1) 12 h	Embedding in PPP
Paraffin (60°) 3 × 12 h	
Embedding in paraffin	

embedding medium solidifies at room temperature one must be sure of the correct orientation of the tissue block. The solid paraffin block is trimmed by means of a hot knife and is attached to a small block of wood with hot paraffin.

3.2.2 Celloidin Method

Celloidin is available as nitrocellulose (Pro-Celloidin Fluka, Cedukol Merck), which is extremely explosive. The substance is dissolved to 8% in a mixture (1:1) of absolute ethanol and dehydrated diethyl-ether. During the dissolving period the bottle must be turned upside down several times a day in order to avoid coalescence to a viscous mass. This stock solution can be stored in well-closed bottles and is diluted for the different steps of the embedding procedure.

For a whole cat brain the following schedule is recommended:

Rinse fixed tissue in tap water for 24 h
70% ethanol 1 week
96% ethanol two steps, 1 week each
Absolute ethanol 2 × 1 week
Ether-alcohol (1:1) 2 × 1 week
2% celloidin (1 part stock solution of 8% celloidin and 3 parts ether-alcohol) 1 week
4% celloidin 1 part stock solution and 1 part ether-alcohol 1 week
8% celloidin 2 weeks.

The embedding vessel must contain as much celloidin as three times the height of the tissue block. The embedding vessel is put into a desiccator containing a petri dish with concentrated H_2SO_4. The ether-alcohol evaporates and the celloidin is concentrated until it is 16%. This is controlled by indicating the level of celloidin at the beginning of the evaporation process. Concentration takes 1–2 weeks time. Then the vessel is transferred to a desiccator with the bottom covered by 70% ethanol. As soon as the surface of the celloidin hardens, the celloidin is covered by 70% ethanol for 4 days, until the whole celloidin is solid. The block is excised by means of a sharp knife and may be stored in 70% ethanol. Before sectioning, the block is attached to a solid base by means of the celloidin solution or by an acrylate cement.

Alternatively, the concentrated celloidin can be solidified by chloroform instead of 70% ethanol until the block becomes quite firm (from one to several days). The block then may be stored in 70% ethanol.

3.2.3 Celloidin-Paraffin Method

This procedure has the advantage of less shrinkage due to penetration of the block with celloidin; it also has the benefits of paraffin, which allows the cutting of sections even thinner than 5 μm. The dehydrated tissue block is treated in the same manner as for regular celloidin embedding. The celloidin (from the 8% step) is then hardened by chloroform and afterwards immersed in dehydrated chloroform, followed by chloroform-paraffin (a saturated solution of paraffin in chloroform at 37 °C) for several days. Three steps of paraffin penetration (1 day each) lead to final embedding in paraffin.

4 Sectioning

Each type of microtome requires a certain degree of experience for achieving satisfactory results. Usually, the instruction manual of the microtome gives exhaustive information about the technical details of sectioning.

4.1 Frozen Sections

Frozen sections may be cut in a wide range of thicknesses: from less than 10 μm up to 100 μm. Satisfactory results are achieved either by a freezing microtome, equipped with cooling devices for the tissue block and the cutting knife (CO_2 gas or electrical cooling aggregate) or more conveniently by a cryostat. The cryostat has the advantage of constant temperature of the tissue block and microtome knife. With cryostats it is possible to cut serial sections. New cryostat types allow separate adjustment of the temperature of the tissue block. Cryostat microtomes usually are also equipped with an anti-roll plate which flattens the section. The sections either are picked up directly by the glass slides or are transferred to a flotation bath by means of a hair brush (see Sect. 5.1).

For very large frozen sections the tetrander microtome (Jung, Heidelberg) eqipped with a freezing device is optimal. By means of this microtome even sections of the whole human brain are possible (Schaltenbrand and Wahren 1977).

4.2 Paraffin Sections

For paraffin blocks any type of universal microtome can be used. The cutting edge of the knife usually is oriented transversely to the cutting direction. The thickness of paraffin sections is within the range of 4–20 μm. For large paraffin blocks the tetrander microtome (Jung, Heidelberg) is used. Large sections cannot be transferred to the flotation bath unless they are attached to a supporting sheet. A thin soaked paper is laid on the paraffin block before a section is cut. The section is transferred together with the paper to a glass slide. Then the paper may be removed by soaking it with surplus water.

Paraffin blocks are optimal for cutting serial sections. If single sections are not transferred separately to the flotation bath, the adjacent sections are connected to each other loosely, forming a ribbon of serial sections. Some types of rotary microtomes are provided with special supporting bands for ribbons of paraffin sections.

4.3 Celloidin Sections

Celloidin sections are cut on sledge microtomes with long plan-concave knives. The knife is set at an angle of 45° to the direction of the movement of the knife. It is essential to dampen the surface of the celloidin block and the knife with 70% ethanol each time a section is cut. Usually celloidin sections are put into vessels of 70% ethanol before staining.

4.4 Thick Sections of Epoxy Resin Embedded Material

Sections about 1 μm thick may be cut with glass knives on the ultramicrotome, then transferred to a drop of water on a glass slide. After drying on a hot plate the sections may be stained with toluidine blue (Sect. 3.2) and covered.

5 Mounting of Sections

Frozen and paraffin sections usually are picked up by glass slides before staining, whereas celloidin sections, in general, are stained and dehydrated before being mounted and covered.

5.1 Frozen Sections

In many cases the sections from a freezing microtome or cryostat are picked up directly from the microtome knife with a warm glass slide. The section thaws and adheres to the glass surface. Then a drying period of about 10 min is necessary. The drying process may be accelerated by using a hair dryer. For some staining procedures the frozen sections are transferred to a flotation bath of 50% or 70% ethanol before being mounted on the glass slides. The sections must be pressed gently to the glass with filter paper. One must carefully avoid complete drying of the sections! For some staining procedures the frozen sections would not stick well enough to the slides unless these have been pretreated with special adhesives (see Sect. 5.4).

5.2 Paraffin Sections

Paraffin sections are transferred with a needle or hair brush to a flotation bath containing distilled water of 40 °C–50 °C (for Paraplast Plus 47 °C–49 °C). The floating sections flatten on the surface of the water and then are picked up by adhesive-treated slides (see Sect. 2.5.4). If Paraplast Plus is used instead of paraffin, the slides need not be pretreated by special adhesives (Arn and Landolt 1975). The mounted sections are dried for several hours at 40 °C and, if necessary, may be stored for several days or weeks before staining. For removal of the paraffin the slides are heated to 60 °C until liquid paraffin runs down the slide and may be removed. For complete removal of paraffin then the slides are placed into xylene benzene of trichlor-ethylene, if necessary at 50 °C–60 °C. Then the sections are "hydrated" by passing through absolute, 96%, 70%, and 50% ethanol into distilled water. The sections are now ready for staining.

5.3 Celloidin Sections

After sectioning the celloidin sections are stored in 70% ethanol. Before being stained, they are transferred to distilled water. Due to their good consistency the unmounted sections are easily carried through the different fluids of the staining, dehydration, and clearing process. Finally, the cleared sections are mounted on the slides: The section is laid on a drop of mounting medium and a second drop is applied between the section and the cover glass. The cover glass should be pressed down for several minutes with a lead cube in order to flatten the section and to let surplus mounting medium escape.

5.4 Adhesives

Adhesives are used to keep the sections firmly attached to the slides during the staining procedures.

5.4.1 Mayer's Albumin

This well-established routine adhesive is commercially available (Mayer's albumin fixative, Fisher), but may be easily prepared by mixing equal parts of egg albumin or standardized albumin preparations (Merck) and glycerol. A few drops of formaldehyde or thymol are added and the mixture is filtered through a coarse filter. The solution remains stable for a long period. The glass slides are coated with a thin film of the fluid and afterwards dried at 40 °C for 1 h. The effect of the adhesive is enhanced when heating the coated slide over a gas flame.

5.4.2 Gelatin

This method is especially useful for large paraffin sections. The sections are transferred to a flotation bath filled with a 0.1%–1% gelatine solution at 40 °C–50 °C. In this bath the flattened sections are floated onto the slides and pressed gently to the glass slide by means of a wet filter paper. If the filter paper adheres to the section, it may be removed by soaking it with surplus distilled water (Adam and Czihak 1964). The slides are then left on a slide warmer at 40 °C for about 12 h.

5.4.3 Chrome Alum Gelatin

Good results are also achieved with chrome alum gelatin-coated slides. The solution is prepared by dissolving gelatin (0.5%) in boiling water and adding 0.5% $CrK(SO_4)_2$ (chrome alum). The slides are coated by dipping them into the warm solution and are then dried at 40 °C for 1 h.

5.4.4 Celloidin Film

In some staining solutions, sections, particularly frozen ones, will not adhere sufficiently by applying one of the above techniques. In these cases the mounted sections should be coated with a film of celloidin. Glass slides bearing the mounted sections are put for a few seconds into a 0.5% solution of celloidin in ether-alcohol (see Sect. 3.2). Then the celloidin is run off, thus forming a thin film on the surface of the slide and the section. Before the ether-alcohol has evaporated completely, the slide is transferred to 70% ethanol for hardening of the celloidin film (5 min). Then the slide is ready for staining.

5.5 Dehydration, Clearing, and Covering

After staining, all types of sections are dehydrated with short steps of 70%, 96%, and absolute ethanol and afterwards treated with a clearing agent like xylene, Origanum oil, or methyl benzoate, terpineol, among others. The sections are blotted with a filter paper and immediately covered by a drop of a conventional mounting medium (Permount Fisher, Entellan Merck, Eukitt Kindler, Caedax, or others) and a cover glass. The cover glass should be pressed down gently for a few minutes and any surplus mounting medium removed. In a good preparation the sections appear transparent and only the stained structures should give contrast in the transmitted light of the microscope.

6 Staining Procedures

Histological stains enhance the contrast of the details within microscopic sections. Microscopy of unstained sections by means of phase contrast, differential interference contrast, or dark-field inspection are of minor importance in light microscopy of the nervous system.

A single dye usually stains only certain tissue components. Therefore combined procedures are common in histology. In the very compact nervous tissue, however, selective stains for nerve cell bodies, nerve fibers, or glial elements are more conclusive than combined stains.

The contrast between the stained structures and the unstained background is further enhanced by clearing the section. After clearing and mounting of the stained sections only stained structures should give contrast, whereas the unstained background appears translucent.

Neuroanatomical stains may be classified into: (1) routine survey stains like hematoxylin eosin, and (2) selective stains for (a) nerve cell bodies, (b) myelin sheaths, (c) nerve fibers (neurofibrils), and (d) glial elements. Special information about structural differences of cortical areas also may be attained by staining of neuronal pigments (Braak 1978).

6.1 Hematoxylin-Eosin

This well known histological routine method is applicable for frozen, paraffin,

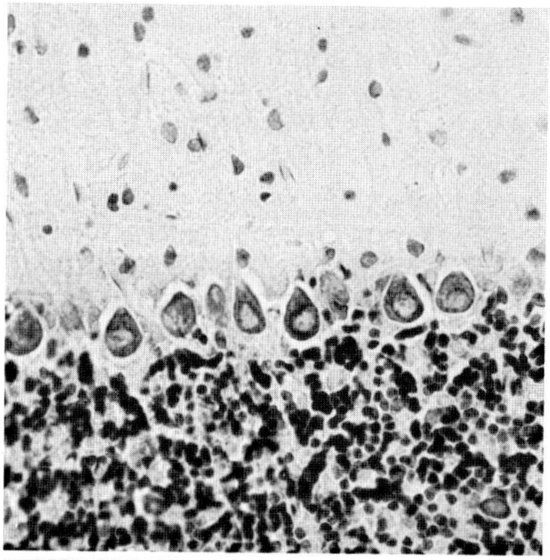

1

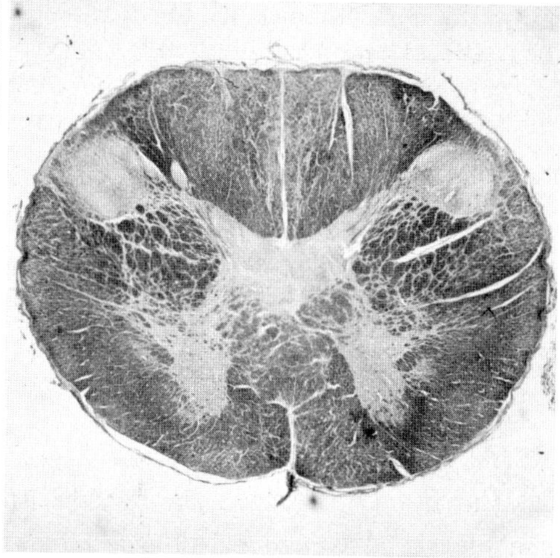

2

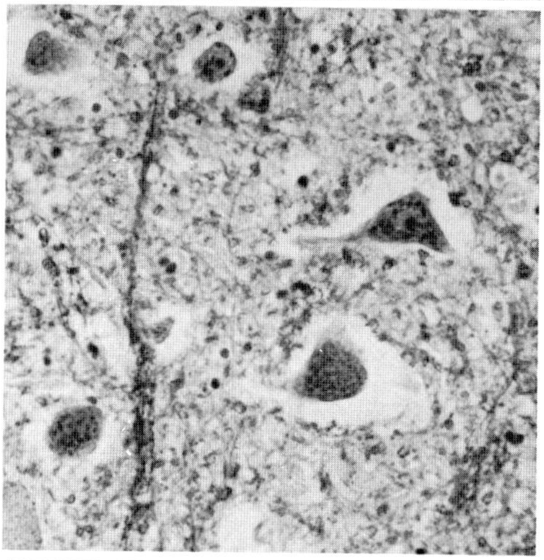

3

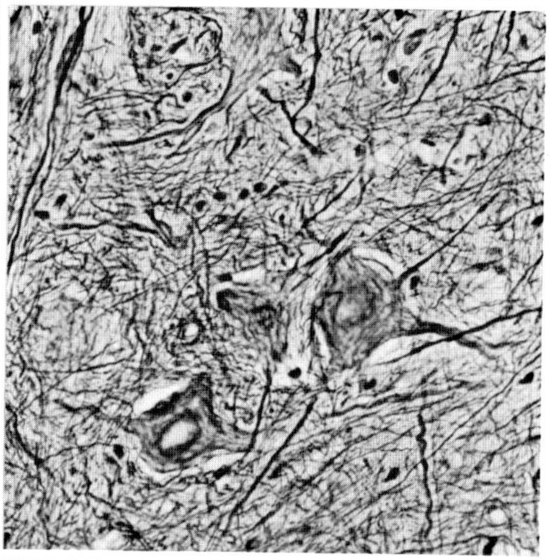

4

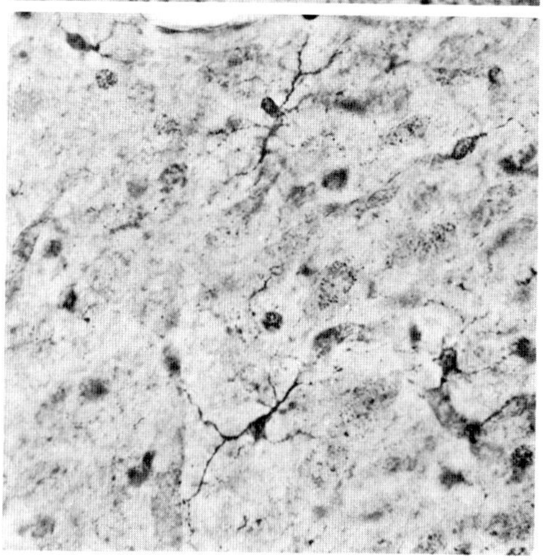

5

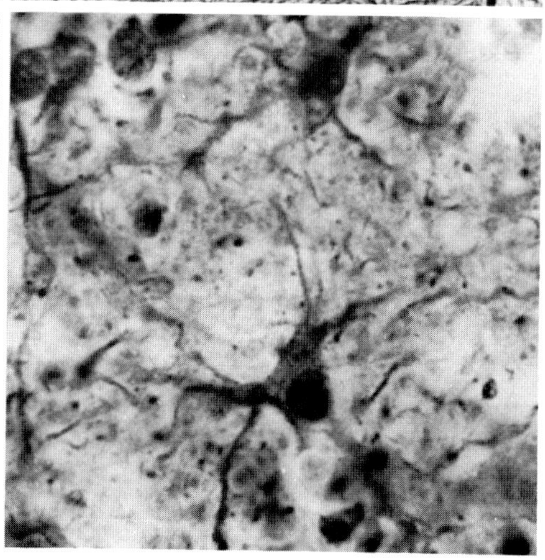

6

and celloidin sections. Since nearly all structures of nervous tissue are stained, the contrast between nerve cell bodies, neuropil, and white matter is less prominent. Therefore this method is not of great importance in neuroanatomical research.

6.1.1 Solutions

1. Alum-hematoxylin after Harris
a) 1 g of hematoxylin is dissolved in 10 ml absolute ethanol;
b) 20 g of $KAl(SO_4)_2$ are dissolved in distilled H_2O. Solutions a and b are heated to boiling temperature in a 500-ml vessel, then 0.5 g MgO (red or yellow mercuric oxide may be used) is added. Cool rapidly and filter. The solution is ready for use and may be stored for at least 1 year.

2. Eosin

10% aqueous eosin solution	0.5 ml
Distilled H_2O	50 ml
Glacial acetic acid	one drop

The solution is stable for at least 1 year.

6.1.2 Staining Procedure for Frozen and Paraffin Sections

1. Mounted frozen or paraffin sections are stained for 2 or 10 min, respectively, in solution 1
2. Rinse in tap water for 10 min
3. Stain for 1 or 10 min, respectively, in solution 2
4. Rinse for 5 min in distilled H_2O
5. Differentiate in 80% ethanol
6. Dehydrate, clear, and mount.

6.1.3 Staining Procedure for Floating Celloidin Sections

1. Stain for 5 min in solution 1
2. Wash with distilled H_2O
3. Differentiate in HCl-alcohol for a few minutes:

96% ethanol	70 ml
H_2O	30 ml
25% HCl	1 ml

4. Rinse in tap water for 10 min (sections turn blue)
5. Stain with solution 2 for 30 s
6. Rinse in distilled H_2O
7. Differentiate with 80% ethanol
8. Dehydrate, clear, and mount.

6.1.4 Results

The nuclei of neurons as well as of glial elements are stained blue, whereas the perikarya and the neuropil appear in different gradations of pink to red. Fiber

Fig. 1. Cerebellar cortex, rat. Perfusion fixation with formaldehyde (4%) in 7.5% sucrose, embedding in Paraplast Plus, section 15 μm thick. Cresyl violet stain, ×310

Fig. 2. Transverse section through the uppermost portion of the human spinal cord at the level of the decussation of the pyramidal tracts. Immersion fixation with 4% paraformaldehyde containing 0.9% NaCl. Embedding in Paraplast Plus, section 15 μm thick. Myelin stain of Heidenhain-Woelcke, ×6

Fig. 3. Transverse section through the ventral horn of a human spinal cord. Fixation and embedding as in Fig. 2. Section 15 μm thick. Staining after Klüver-Barrera. Neurons are stained with cresyl violet, myelinated fibers with Luxol Fast Blue, ×310

Fig. 4. Transverse section through the ventral horn of rat spinal cord. Perfusion fixation with 4% formaldehyde in 7.5% sucrose; cryostat section, 20 μm. Modified Palmgren silver impregnation after Goshgarian, ×340

Fig. 5. Rat brain stem. Perfusion fixation with buffered 4% formaldehyde solution in 4% sucrose and 0.5 mM $CaCl_2$. Cryostat section, 20 μm. Selective staining of microglia after Hortega, ×490

Fig. 6. Human spinal cord white matter, fibrillar astrocytes. Immersion fixation with 4% formaldehyde in 0.9% NaCl. Cryostat section, 20 μm. Gold sublimate staining for astrocytes after Cajal, ×1200

tracts, particularly in transverse sections, are prominent by their marked stain of the axons. This method is mainly a survey stain in neuropathology.

6.2 Nerve Cell Stains

According to the original Nissl stain, the sections of ethanol-fixed tissue were stained in a mixture of methylene blue and Venetian soap. This method had many disadvantages and is now completely out of use. Rapid and permanent cell stains may be achieved in aldehyde-fixed tissue by means of an aqueous solution of cresyl violet, which may also be replaced by thionin or toluidine blue. Most common is the use of cresyl violet, which is applicable for frozen, paraffin, (Fig. 1) and celloidin sections.

6.2.1 Solution

1% cresyl violet acetate (Merck, Fisher) in distilled H_2O or in acetate buffer (0.1 M, pH 4.0). The solution is used many times. If the staining intensity increases the solution may be diluted by adding distilled H_2O.

6.2.2 Staining Procedure for Frozen or Paraffin Sections

1. Cresyl violet, 5 min (dried frozen sections) to 20 min (paraffin sections)
2. Differentiate and dehydrate in 70%, 96%, and two steps of absolute ethanol
3. Clear in xylene (two steps) and mount.

6.2.3 Staining Procedure for Celloidin Sections

1. Cresyl violet, 30 s
2. Differentiate in 70% and 90% ethanol
3. Continue differentiation in a 1 : 1 mixture of origanum oil (Fisher) and absolute alcohol until the background is clear
4. Clear in origanum oil and mount.

6.2.4 Results

The cell nuclei and the Nissl bodies of the neurons are stained red to purple, the nerve cell somata are slightly pink, and the background of the neuropil remains unstained (Fig. 1).

6.3 Myelin Stains

These methods are especially valuable for orientation in the brain stem and spinal cord. In 1885 Weigert published a method of selective staining of myelin sheaths with iron hematoxylin. This rather complicated and time-consuming method yields excellent results, but has the great disadvantage, due to mordanting of the whole tissue block with potassium dichromate before embedding, that other stains cannot be applied on the same tissue block. In the beginning of this century modifications were published which are performed on sections (frozen, paraffin, and celloidin). These methods have the advantage that other stains are applicable to adjacent sections of the same tissue block. Out of a great number some methods are of special importance: Weil (1928), Spielmeyer (1930), Olivecrona (1917) and Heidenhain-Woelcke (Burck 1973; Schaltenbrand and Wahren 1977).

The essential staining agent of these methods is hematoxylin, which must be "ripened" by storing the alcoholic hematoxylin solution in the open bottle for 2–6 months. During this period hematoxylin is mainly converted (oxidized) to hematein (Berube et al. 1965). If a ripened solution is not available, the hematoxylin may be matured artificially in the following way:

8.5% $KMnO_4$ in distilled H_2O	10 ml
10% alcoholic hematoxylin	50 ml.

Mix both solutions and filter the precipitate. This solution may be stored for several weeks.

Another reliable myelin stain is Luxol Fast Blue, which may be combined with cell stains (Klüver and Barrera 1953).

6.3.1 Myelin Stain After Olivecrona

This rapid and reliable single-step procedure for demonstration of myelin sheaths is particularly designed for frozen sections (Olivecrona 1917) but is also applicable for paraffin sections.

6.3.1.1 Solutions

1. 10% alcoholic hematoxylin:
Dissolve 10 g hematoxylin in 1000 ml 96% ethanol. The solution must be well ripened (see Sect. 6.3).
2. Solution of iron(III)chloride:

Iron(III)chloride	1.16 g
Distilled H_2O	98 ml
25% HCl	1 ml

3. Saturated solution of lithium carbonate (Li_2CO_3) in distilled H_2O.

Each of the stock solutions is stable for more than a year.

6.3.1.2 Staining Procedures

1. Pretreatment of frozen sections: 20–30 μm thick frozen sections, mounted on albumin-treated slides and dried for 10 min, are put into 70% ethanol for 10 min
2. The pretreated frozen sections or mounted paraffin sections are stained for 45–60 min in the following solution, which must be freshly prepared:
   30 ml of solution 1
   15 ml of solution 2
3. Rinse in distilled H_2O
4. Differentiate in solution 2 until marked contrast appears between gray and white matter (optical control)
5. Rinse in distilled H_2O
6. "Blue" the stained sections in lithium carbonate solution for 15 min:
   10 ml of solution 3
   40 ml distilled H_2O
7. Dehydrate, clear, and mount.

Optimal results are achieved with frozen sections if the hematoxylin solution is modified:
30 ml of solution 1
15 ml of a 29% $FeCl_3$ solution in distilled H_2O.

6.3.1.3 Results

Myelin sheaths are stained dark blue, gray matter is nearly unstained, and nerve cell somata appear slightly yellow.

6.3.2 Myelin Stain After Heidenhain-Woelcke

This method is applicable to celloidin-coated frozen sections, mounted paraffin sections (Fig. 2), and floating celloidin sections (Burck 1973).

6.3.2.1 Solutions

1. 2.5% solution of ferric alum ($FeNH_4(SO_4)_2$) in distilled H_2O.
2. 10% alcoholic hematoxylin solution: 100 g hematoxylin dissolved in 1000 ml absolute ethanol. The solution must be well ripened!
3. Saturated solution of lithium carbonate (Li_2CO_3) in distilled H_2O.

6.3.2.2 Procedure

1. Sections stay for 2–3 h in distilled H_2O
2. Mordant in solution 1 for 12 h (overnight)
3. Rinse twice in distilled H_2O
4. Stain in the hematoxylin solution for 4–7 h:

10% hematoxylin (solution II)	10 ml
Saturated Li_2CO_3 (solution III)	7 ml
Distilled H_2O	83 ml

5. Rinse twice in distilled H_2O
6. Rinse with 96% ethanol
7. 96% ethanol for 8 h (or overnight)
8. Dehydrate with two steps of absolute alcohol, clear with xylene and mount.

6.3.2.3 Results

This procedure takes much longer than the rapid method of Ovilecrona (Fig. 2). Excellent results are achieved with celloidin sections.

6.3.3 Combined Cell and Myelin Stain After Klüver-Barrera

This is a well-established method for studying the internal structure of brain stem and spinal cord (Fig. 3). Its advantages are the simultaneous display of myelinated fibers and nerve cell groups within the same section. The method is applicable for mounted frozen and paraffin sections.

6.3.3.1 Solutions

1. Luxol Fast Blue (Fisher, Chroma):
   0.1 g Luxol Fast Blue dissolved in 96% ethanol 100 ml
   10% solution of acetic acid 0.5 ml
2. 0.05% aqueous lithium carbonate (Li_2CO_3) solution
3. 1% aqueous solution of cresyl violet.

6.3.3.2 Staining Procedure

1. Stain with Luxol Fast Blue (solution 1) at 60 °C for 3 h
2. Rinse with 96% ethanol
3. Rinse with distilled H_2O
4. Dip into solution 2 for a few seconds
5. Differentiate with 70% ethanol for 20–30 s
6. Rinse in distilled H_2O
7. Treat with solution 2 for 10–25 s
8. Differentiate with 70% ethanol for a few seconds
9. Rinse in distilled H_2O.

Microscopical control. If differentiation is unsatisfactory, repeat steps 7, 8, and 9.

10. Stain cells with cresyl violet (solution 3) for 5 min (frozen sections) or 20 min (paraffin sections)
11. Differentiate with 96% ethanol
12. Dehydrate, clear, and mount.

6.3.3.3 Results

Myelin sheaths appear in intensive blue, nerve cell bodies show typical cresyl violet stain, and the neuropil is nearly unstained (Fig. 3).

6.4 Selective Silver Staining of Nerve Fibers

Most of the silver methods are known to be capricious and unreliable. In many cases failure of adequate impregnation is due to impure chemicals and contaminated glassware. It is essential to clean glassware scrupulously and to avoid metal instruments during the whole staining procedure.

The argyrophilic substrate of nervous tissue are primarily the neurofilaments, the ultrastructural correlates of the neurofibrils of classical histology. According to the content and density of neurofilaments, the silver impregnation methods stain, more or less completely, the axons, nerve cell bodies, and larger dendrites. In this way it is possible with serial sections to trace nerve fibers over longer distances. In some regions of the CNS it is even possible to follow up single axons to their terminals, appearing as neurofibrillar rings or clubs at the surface of nerve cell bodies and dendrites.

Two very reliable impregnation methods are described in this chapter. Bodian's protargol technique is optimal for paraffin sections. The modified Palmgren method by Goshgarian is optimal for frozen sections. The latter method has the great advantage that it can be applied to serial sections, alternating with other stains, including various histochemical procedures.

6.4.1 Protargol Method for Neurofibrils After Bodian (1937)

As a special feature this method uses silver protein (Protargol, Merck) instead of silver nitrate. Silver is precipitated at the nerve fibers provided metallic copper is present in the impregnation fluid. Further processing is similar to other conventional impregnation techniques. The method is especially designed for paraffin sections.

6.4.1.1 Solutions

1. Silver protein solution:
   Distilled H_2O at 37 °C 100 ml
   Dissolve silver protein 1 g
   (Scatter 1 g silver protein in small portions on the water surface. Avoid stirring. The solution must be clear.)
2. Developer
   Hydroquinone 1 g
   Anhydrous Na_2SO_3 5 g
   distilled H_2O to 100 ml
3. 1% gold chloride
   Add glacial acetic acid, three drops per 100 ml
4. 2% oxalic acid
5. Fixative: 5% sodium thiosulfate ($Na_2S_2O_3$)

6.4.1.2 Staining Procedure

1. Impregnate in solution 1 for 12–48 h at 37 °C. Just before the slides are put into the solution add 4 g metallic copper (chips or wire). Copper must be purified with concentrated nitric acid
2. Intensive rinsing with distilled H_2O and drying
3. Reduce in solution 2 for about 10 min. The process is finished when the yellow sections turn brown and no further intensification is observed
4. Rinse three times with distilled H_2O for 3–5 min
5. Tone with solution 3 until the sections turn purple (usually 2–5 min)
6. Rinse three times in distilled H_2O
7. Place in oxalic acid (solution 4) until sections assume a purple tint (usually 2–5 min)
8. Rinse three times carefully in distilled H_2O
9. Fix in solution 5 for 5–10 min
10. Rinse, dehydrate, clear, and mount.

6.4.1.3 Results

Axons appear dark red to black, nerve cell bodies are reddish-purple.

6.4.2 Modified Palmgren Method for Neurofibrils

A rapid and reliable modification of Palmgren's silver impregnation procedure (Palmgren 1960) for central and peripheral nerve fibers has been described by Goshgarian (1977). The advantage of this method is that it can be utilized with both paraffin and mounted frozen sections (Fig. 4).

6.4.2.1 Solutions

1. Pretreatment for better impregnation of terminal axon arborization
   0.15 M 2-amino-2-methyl-1-propanol solution
   Adjust with nitric acid to 5.0 pH.
2. Silver nitrate:
   10% aqueous silver nitrate.
3. 2% sodium borate ($Na_2B_4O_7$)
4. Developer:
   2% fresh sodium borate solution 100 ml
   Add 0.05 g hydroquinone
   Add 5.0 g sodium sulfite (Na_2SO_3)
5. 0.5% gold chloride
6. 0.5% oxalic acid in 50% ethanol
7. 5% sodium thiosulfate ($Na_2S_2O_3$)

6.4.2.2 Staining Procedure

1. Dehydrate frozen sections through graded 70% to absolute ethanol and

rehydrate back to distilled H_2O (essential for uniform staining)
2. Treat sections with solution 1 for 5 min
3. Wash in three changes of distilled H_2O, each 1.5 min
4. Impregnate in solution 2 for 30 min at 37 °C
5. Transfer slides without rinsing to freshly prepared solution 3 for 3–5 s and agitate
6. Rinse in distilled H_2O until the precipitate is removed
7. Develop for 10 min at 37 °C in solution 4
8. Rinse three times in 50% ethanol (each step 1.5 min)
9. Tone with solution 5 for 3 min
10. Rinse with distilled H_2O
11. Intensify with solution 6 for 1 min at 37 °C
12. Rinse in distilled H_2O
13. Fix in solution 7 for 10 s
14. Rinse, dehydrate, clear, and cover.

6.4.2.3 Results

Nerve fibers are black to dark purple, nerve cell bodies and neuropil appear faintly red (Fig. 4).

6.5 Staining of Neuroglia

Cell stains like cresyl violet or hematoxylin-eosin do not differentiate satisfactorily between small granular neurons and glial elements. Most glia stains stain all types of glia equally. Only two methods may be regarded as selective methods for certain types of glial elements: (1) The weak silver carbonate method of Hortega for microglia and (2) the gold sublimate method of Cajal for demonstration of astrocytes.

In general, glial element stains are of relevance for the neuropathologist. In normal tissue these methods are less specific. Exact glial element studies should reasonably include epon embedding and toluidine blue staining of thick sections as well as electron microscopy.

The metal solutions of the following two methods require special precautions: All glassware used must be cleaned scrupulously and metal tools should be avoided.

6.5.1 Silver-Carbonate Stain for Microglia

This method of Hortega (1921) is more or less specific for microglia. Although some authors modified the technique for paraffin and even celloidin sections, the stain usually is performed on frozen sections (Fig. 5).

Perfusion-fixed tissue is postfixed by immersion in a solution of 5% formaldehyde and 2% ammonium bromide. 3 mm thick slices should be immersed for 1–2 days. Just prior to freezing the slices are put into a solution of the same composition at 50 °C for 10 min.

6.5.1.1 Solutions

1. Weak silver carbonate solution:
   10% aqueous solution of $AgNO_3$ 5 ml
   5% aqueous Na_2CO_3 anhydrous 20 ml
   Add concentrated ammonium hydroxide, drop by drop, while shaking until the solution starts to clear. The solution should remain slightly turbid. Filter just before using. Add distilled H_2O to total volume of 75 ml.
2. 0.4% formaldehyde solution
3. 0.5% aqueous gold chloride solution
4. 5% aqueous solution of sodium thiosulfate ($Na_2S_2O_3$).

6.5.1.2 Staining Procedure

1. Transfer 20–30 μm thick frozen sections of brom-formaldehyde-fixed tissue to distilled H_2O
2. Pass the sections through three baths of distilled H_2O; the second of these three baths should contain 4–5 drops of ammonium hydroxide
3. Impregnate in solution 1 for 2 min

4. Reduce in 0.4% formaldehyde (solution 2) for 1 min (agitate!)
5. Rinse in distilled H_2O
6. Tone the sections with solution III until they appear gray. Avoid long periods of gold chloride! Sections should not turn purple
7. Fix in sodium thiosulfate (solution 4)
8. Rinse in distilled H_2O
9. Mount sections on albumin-treated slides, dehydrate, clear with xylene, and mount.

6.5.1.3 Results

Neurons and blood vessels appear gray, microglia, dark gray to black (Fig. 5). Prolongation of the treatment with silver carbonate and with gold chloride accentuates staining of astrocytes.

6.5.2 Gold Sublimate Stain for Astrocytes

Cajal's method for astrocytes is applicable only to frozen sections of fixed nervous tissue (Fig. 6). The sections are transferred from the microtome to distilled water and are stained floating within a transporting sieve.

6.5.2.1 Solutions

1. Gold sublimate

1% aqueous gold chloride (yellow)	5 ml
5% aqueous $HgCl_2$	5 ml
Distilled water	30 ml

2. Fixing solution
   5% aqueous sodium thiosulfate ($Na_2S_2O_3$).

6.5.2.2 Staining Procedure

1. Impregnate floating sections in solution 1 for 2–3 h
2. Rinse in distilled H_2O
3. Fix in solution 2 for 5 min
4. Mount on albumin-treated slides and press the sections gently with a filter paper
5. dehydrate, clear in xylene, and mount.

6.5.2.3 Results

Neurons are nearly unstained, axons and fiber tracts are red, and astrocytes stained in purple. The method is very reliable, particularly in the human central nervous system (Fig. 6).

Romeis (1968) recommends fixation in a mixture of formaldehyde (5%) and ammonium bromide (2%).

References

Adam H, Czihak G (1964) Arbeitsmethoden der makroskopischen und mikroskopischen Anatomie. Fischer, Stuttgart

Andres KH (1966) Zur Methodik der Perfusionsfixierung des Zentralnervensystems von Säugern. Mikroskopie 21:129

Arn D, Landolt R (1975) Direkte Fixierungsmöglichkeit von Schnitten auf Objektträgern durch Verwendung des Einbettungsmediums Paraplast-Plus. Mikroskopie 31:99–106

Berube GR, Powers MM, Clark G (1965) Iron hematoxylin chelates. I. The Weil staining bath. Stain Technol 40:53–62

Bodian D (1937) The staining of paraffin section of nervous tissues with activated protargol. The role of fixatives. Anat Rec 69:153–162

Braak H (1978) Eine ausführliche Beschreibung pigmentarchitektonischer Arbeitsverfahren. Mikroskopie 34:215–223

Burck H-C (1973) Histologische Technik. Leitfaden für die Herstellung mikroskopischer Präparate in Unterricht und Praxis, 3rd ed. Thieme, Stuttgart

Cammermeyer J (1960) The post-mortem origin and mechanism of neuronal hyperchromatosis and nuclear pyknosis. Exp Neurol 2:379–405

Cammermeyer J (1967) Submerged heart method to prevent intracardial influx of air prior to perfusion fixation of the brain. Acta Anat 67:321–337

Clark G (1978) Tissue preparation and basic staining techniques. In: Robertson RT (ed) Neuroanatomical research techniques. Academic Press, New York San Francisco London, pp 26–44

Fleischhauer K (1967) Postnatale Entwicklung der Neuroglia. Zentralbl Neurol 188:385–386

Forssmann WG, Siegrist G, Orci L, Giradier L, Pictet R, Roullier C (1967) Fixation par perfusion pour la microscopie électronique. Essai de généralisation. J Microsc (Paris) 6:279–304

Gil J, Weibel ER (1971) An improved apparatus for perfusion fixation with automatic pressure control. J Microsc 94:241–244

Goshgarian HG (1977) A rapid silver impregnation for central and peripheral nerve fibers in paraffin and frozen sections. Exp Neurol 57:296–301

Hortega P (1921) El tercer elemento de los centros nerviosos: histogenesis y evolucion normal; exodo y distribucion regional de la microglia. Mem R Soc Esp Hist Nat 11: 213–268

Klüver H, Barrera E (1953) A method for the combined staining of cells and fibers in the nervous system. J Neuropathol Exp Neurol 12:400–403

Olivecrona H (1971) Eine vereinfachte Methode zur Darstellung der Markscheiden an Gefrierschnitten. Centralbl Allg Pathol 28/21: 521–523

Palay SL, McGee-Russel S, Gordon S, Grillo M (1962) Fixation of neural tissues for electron microscopy by perfusion with solutions of osmium tetroxide. J Cell Biol 12:385–410

Palmgren A (1960) Specific silver staining of nerve fibers I. Technique for vertebrates. Acta Zool 41:239–265

Pease DC (1962) Buffered formaldehyde as a killing agent and primary fixative for electron microscopy. Anat Rec 142:342

Peters A (1970) The fixation of central nervous tissue and the analysis of electron micrographs of the neuropil, with special reference to the cerebral cortex. In: Nauta WJH, Ebbesson SOE (eds) Contemporary research methods in neuroanatomy. Springer, Berlin Heidelberg New York, pp 56–76

Romeis B (1968) Mikroskopische Technik, 16th ed. Oldenburg, München Wien

Schaltenbrand G, Wahren W (1977) Atlas for stereotaxy of the human brain, 2nd ed. Thieme, Stuttgart

Schultz RL, Karlsson U (1965) Fixation of the central nervous system for electron microscopy by aldehyde perfusion. II. Effect of osmolarity, pH of perfusate, and fixative concentration. J Ultrastruct Res 12:187–206

Spielmeyer W (1930) Technik der mikroskopischen Untersuchung des Nervensystems, 4th ed. Springer, Berlin

Wacker Ph, Forssmann WG (1972) Immersion and perfusion fixed rat adrenal medulla: The problem of mixed cells, clear cells, and the mode of secretion. Z Zellforsch 126:261–277

Weigert C (1885) Über Schnittserien von Celloidinpräparaten des Zentralnervensystems zum Zwecke der Markscheidenfärbung. Z Wiss Mikrosk 2:490–495

Weil A (1928) A rapid method for staining myelin sheats. Arch Neurol Psychiatr 20: 392–393

Chapter 2

General Methods in Transmission Electron Microscopy of the Nervous System

Wolf-Georg Forssmann

1 Introduction

The application of electron microscopy to morphological, neuroanatomical research resulted in the development of more refined methods of obtaining reliable electron micrographs in an attempt to show the corresponding counterparts of living structures. In comparison to other organs, the preparation of specimens from the nervous system requires careful attention due to the particularities of the soft nervous tissue. The central nervous system is quite fragile with regard to mechanical stress and sensitive to lack of oxygen. Thus, the use of immersion fixation results in many artifacts which can be caused by mechanical damage and slow penetration of fixatives.

The method of choice for the fixation of the central nervous system tissue is, therefore, that of vascular perfusion (Koenig et al. 1945; Palay et al. 1962). Many authors have attempted to introduce and improve the general immersion fixation with osmium-containing solutions (Palade 1952; Bahr 1955; Caulfield 1957; Millonig 1961) and aldehyde-containing solutions (Sabatini et al. 1963; Fahimi and Drochmans 1965; Karnovsky 1965; Karlsson and Schultz 1965 a, b, 1966; Maunsbach 1966; Ito and Karnovsky 1968). In this chapter attention will be primarily given to the perfusion fixation method since other techniques such as embedding and staining have become more routine and are easy to employ. Although used in many variations in different research laboratories, the perfusion technique still requires accurate technical knowledge.

2 General Problems of Fixation for Electron Microscopy

The general problems in fixation discussed in this chapter will be the basis for a consideration of future progress towards improving and introducing new methods of tissue preparation. The thermodynamic parameters involved in fixation are the groundwork for understanding errors and performing necessary corrections of the fixation technique.

2.1 Chemical and Physical Methods of Fixation

Fixation is defined as a means of interrupting the dynamic chemical life processes of tissue or cells and conserving the structures in a state which is as similar as possible to reality, such that the final electron micrograph obtained corresponds to the actual state of living tissue. Preventing alterations in fluid movement, molecular shifts, or compartment deteriorations are among the factors involved in preserving a living structure.

2.1.1 Chemical Fixation

This method utilizes the principle of binding or precipitating larger molecules of cells and tissue together so that the network of a cytoskeleton is preserved. The tissue is then embedded or frozen, subsequently sectioned and stained, and thereafter observed in the transmission electron microscope. The most common chemical fixatives are osmium tetroxide (Palade 1952), aldehydes (Sabatini et al. 1963), and permanganates (Luft 1956).

2.1.2 Physical Methods

These methods include the use of frozen tissue which is either sectioned immediately, or the aqueous phase of the tissue is evaporated before embedding or further preparation. The investigation of natural surfaces after physical fixation or of freeze-fractured surfaces by replication is also useful (see chapters on scanning microscopy and freeze-etching, Chaps. 3, 4).

2.1.3 Chemical-Physical Methods

Both chemical fixation and physical treatment methods may be combined, such as in freeze-substitution, freeze-fracturing of aldehyde-fixed tissue, or vapor phase fixation of the frozen sections. The freeze-substitution method may be of special interest in the future, especially when combined with ultrarapid freezing (see Chap. 15).

The most common and reliable fixation for routine investigations, however, is chemical fixation with aldehydes and subsequent postfixation treatment with osmium tetroxide. Only these methods will be treated in detail in this chapter.

2.2 Application of Fixatives

In chemical fixation there are three methods of obtaining a certain degree of rapid fixation:

2.2.1 Immersion Fixation

This is carried out using small tissue blocks which are introduced into the fixation solution after dissection. This method is accompanied by an interruption of the living state, which usually produces mechanical damage during dissection and hypoxia due to the slow penetration of the fixatives.

2.2.2 Dripping Method

Introduction of chemical fixatives to living tissue is also possible by dripping the fixative onto exposed surfaces of organs. This type of application is seldom used although it could be advantageous in fixation of the outer surface of the central nervous system or of structures lining the ventricles, particularly the ependyma. Similarly, the application of fixatives by injection, which would be of possible use for preserving nervous tissue of hollow organs, is of theoretical interest. The above-mentioned disadvantages could be circumvented by systemic vascular perfusion.

2.2.3 Perfusion Fixation

This most common and reliable method is widely used for fixation of central nervous system tissue as well as of nerves in all peripheral systems. The fixation solution is applied through the blood vessels, generally after introduction of a cannula into the heart, the aorta, or an arterial vessel such as the carotid artery. The fixative is rapidly flushed through the whole organism providing complete and homogeneous tissue preservation. Since the fixative passes through the natural pathway of the blood circulation, the disadvantages of this method are negligable when compared to the numerous alterations due to immersion or dripping fixation.

3 Thermodynamic Parameters in (Perfusion) Fixation

The parameters influencing fixation are common to all fixation methods and will be discussed with respect to the perfusion method which is considered the method of choice.

3.1 Diffusion

Diffusion of soluble phases is a rather slow process and can be defined according to the law of Fick:

$$\frac{\Delta N}{\Delta t} = D \cdot q \cdot \Delta C.$$

From this, the vectorial penetration can be mathematically derived as a relation of the C/C_s (Concentration of fixative in phase 1 C_s, i.e., the fixative solution and the concentration C in the tissue):

$$C = C_s \cdot \left(1 - \frac{2}{\sqrt{\pi}} \cdot \int_0^{\frac{X}{2\sqrt{D \cdot X}}} e^{-y^2 \cdot dy}\right).$$

Schematically the time dependence of this relation is seen in the schematic drawing (Fig. 1) of various time lapses (t_1–t_4).

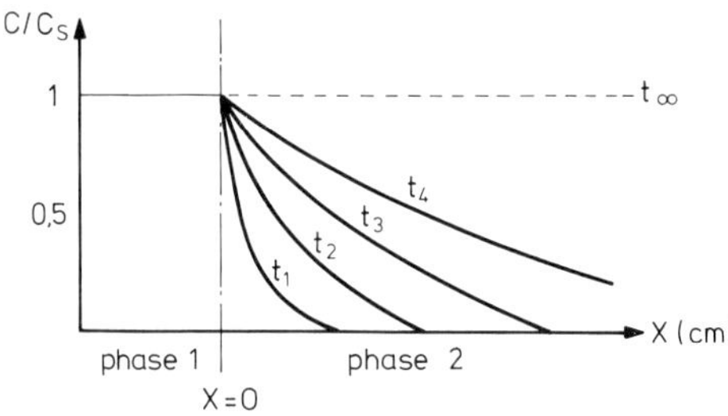

Fig. 1. The time dependence of the penetration of the fixative (phase 1) into the tissue (phase 2)

Fig. 1 illustrates that the highest concentration of fixative and the smallest possible bloc size would be an adequate way of satisfying these parameters. It can also be concluded that complete penetration or equal distribution of the fixative can theoretically not be achieved in larger blocs. As the distance between capillaries in the central nervous system is rather large compared with the heart and liver, fixation of brain tissue is still more problematic than in these other organs. Many authors have therefore used higher aldehyde concentrations for central nervous system fixation.

3.2 Repartition and Distribution

The final distribution of the fixative is also dependent upon the solubility of the fixing component according to Nernst's law:

$$\frac{C\ \text{phase 1}}{C\ \text{phase 2}} = K$$

where K is the coefficient of solubility. This parameter is primarily important for the effective osmotic pressure in the system to be fixed (see below).

3.3 Hemodynamic, Mechanical Pressure

It should be briefly mentioned here that the intravital tissue pressure is sustained by certain techniques such as retrograde perfusion. This may be of importance when considering morphometric studies of tissue which is highly vascularized (for example the liver) and when vascular structures are investigated. The exact hemodynamic properties are controlled by either the perfusion pressure or the perfusion volume/time ratio. Capillaries are generally occluded and shrunken after immersion fixation and relations of extracellular space are altered as a rule when the perfusion pressure is not exact (edema, etc.). The range of perfusion pressure between 50 and 200 mm Hg, however, may be of minor importance for the fixation of brain. In experiments with variable perfusion pressures we could not observe significant differences in brain fixation, although in these same studies other organs were dramatically altered. The important prerequisite for brain fixation is a patent vasculature. Decarries and Schröder (1968) have therefore recommended a perfusion with high volume rate which decreases the incidence of unperfused tissue.

3.4 Temperature and pH

Numerous researchers have tested the effect of temperature and pH on fixation. It was shown that the introduction of adequate buffer systems for osmium tetroxide and the adaptation to the natural pH resulted in a tremendous improvement in fixation. Also, aldehyde fixation with various buffer systems (compared with solutions for light microscopy) resulted in a reduction of fixation artifacts such as cell swelling, dark and clear cells, and swelling of mitochondria and rough endoplasmic reticulum.

The effects of temperature have been claimed to be important for fixation. However, no concrete data have been published so far demonstrating a temperature-dependent alteration in fixation. As a rule in immersion fixation with osmium and aldehyde a temperature of 0 °C to +4 °C should be used while in perfusion fixation temperatures of up to body temperature give satisfactory results.

3.5 Concentration of Vehicle Components in Fixation

The concentrations of both the fixative and the vehicle (i.e., buffer, additional salts, and sucrose) is of importance for proper fixation. Higher concentrations of the fixative will create not only increased penetration into the tissue, but also an increase in the concentration of the fixative in the tissue blocs. This principle is realized in Karnovsky's (1965) high osmolarity fixation. In perfusion fixation and when isolated cells are investigated, this principle is limited due to the osmotic effects, i.e.,

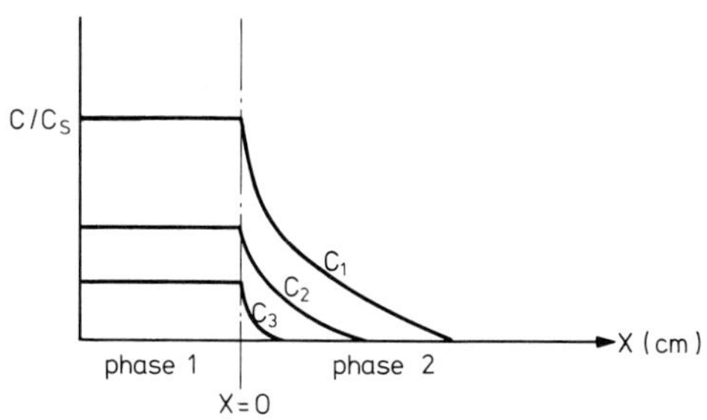

Fig. 2. The concentration (C_1–C_3) dependence of the penetration of fixative (phase 1) into tissue (phase 2) for a constant time lapse of incubation

osmotic pressure changes which result in artificial water fluxes. The theoretical effect of variable concentrations of fixative is seen in the schematic drawing (Fig. 2).

Varying the concentration of the fixative and/or the vehicle could result in important parameters affecting the fixation such as osmotic pressure, and colloid osmotic pressure which are dependent on the respective permeabilities through cell and tissue membranes (see below).

3.5.1 Osmotic Pressure and Reflection Coefficient

Most of the biological systems contain membranes which are only partially permeable for the molecules in a fixation solution. Thus, an osmotic gradient is produced which is proportional to the particle concentration in the fixation solution:

$$P = \frac{nRT}{V}.$$

The osmotic pressure P is variable for each particle and each membrane type and dependent on the relation of the concentration gradient and the permeability (Fig. 3).

It has been observed by use of isolated cell systems that application of various substances in the same osmotic concentration gives different results (Fig. 4).

This demonstrates the difficulty in using a stable fixation solution:

$$P = l_n \frac{C_e - C_i}{C_e} \cdot \frac{V}{A} \cdot \frac{1}{t}.$$

The permeability is a variable function of time due to the equilibration phenomena during the application of a solution resulting from changes in the external concentration (C_e) and the internal concentration (C_i) after exposure to fixatives or other solutions.

This indicates that the osmotic pressure is continuously changing during the process of fixation and, additionally, that the changing membrane properties between unfixed and fixed state produce a factor which is difficult to control during the fixation process. It is well known that the aldehyde fixatives commonly used are hyperosmotic compared with blood plasma. Another factor which affects the osmotic pressure is the solubility coefficient of the fixative and vehicle. This can be measured by an osmometer based on the freezing point decrease or the increase in the vapor pressure. Aldehydes in general have a low effective osmotic pressure on all membranes. The effective osmotic pressure exerted by a given number of molecules on a certain membrane depends essentially on

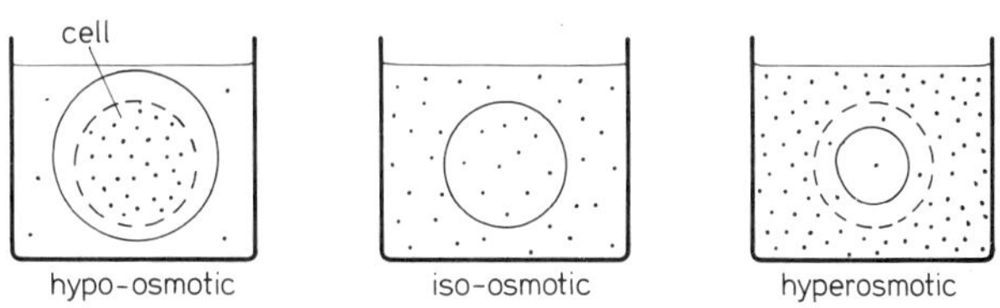

Fig. 3. Osmotic effect on cells or tissue components exhibiting a semipermeable membrane. Note that the osmotic effect is dependent on the difference of osmotically active particles

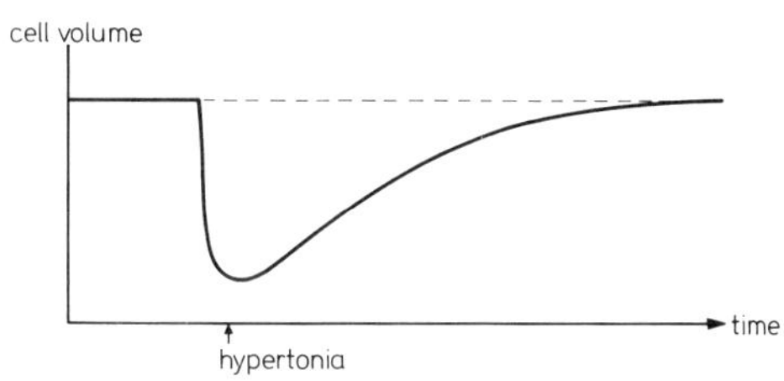

Fig. 4. Varying osmotic effect exerted on cell volume by hypertonia during an equilibration period

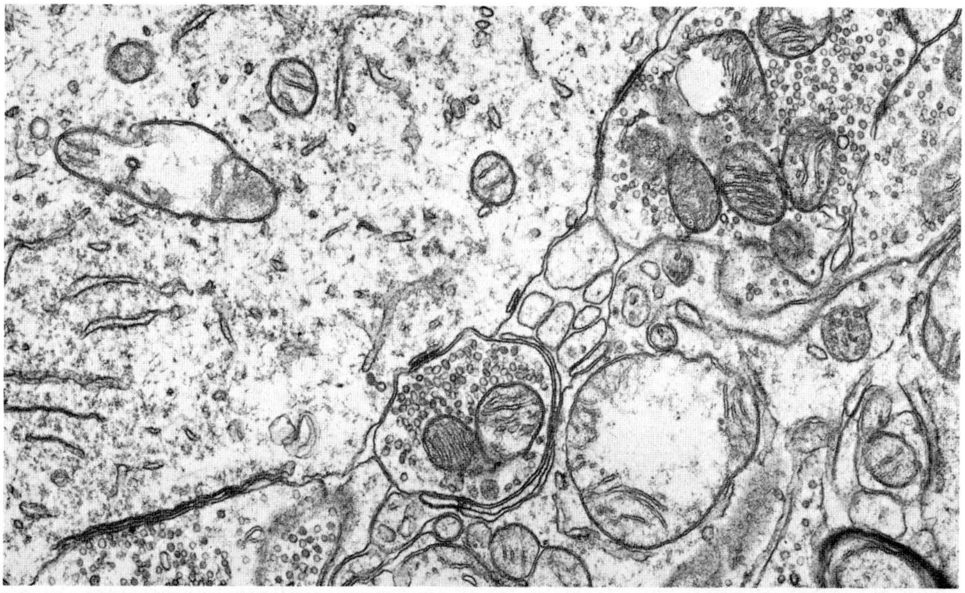

a

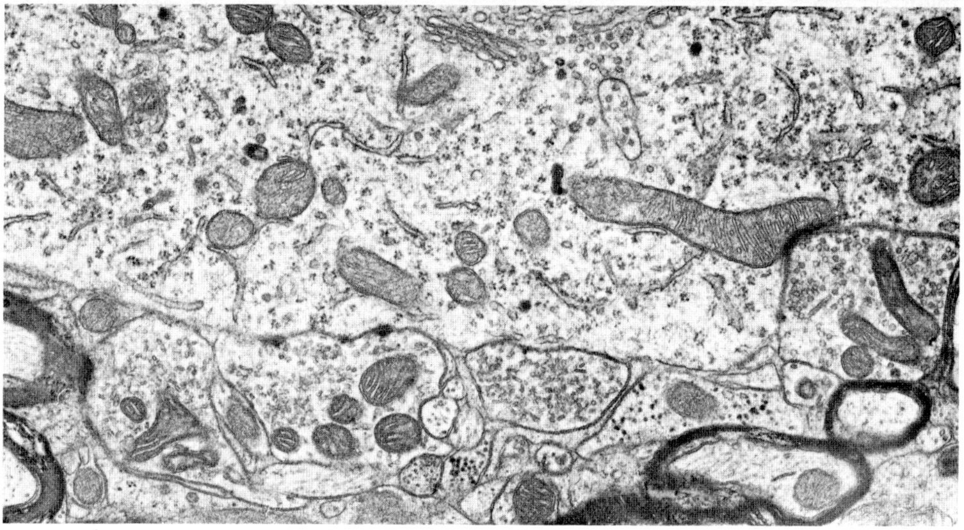

b

Fig. 5 a, b. Perfusion-fixed central nervous system with variable aldehyde concentration. **a** Low aldehyde concentration: 0.75% formaldehyde and 0.75% glutaraldehyde. Note the mitochondrial swelling. ×75,000 **b** 3% formaldehyde and 3% glutaraldehyde. The tissue is well preserved. Rinsing solution and vehicle of the fixative see routine fixation in the text. ×50,000

the reflection coefficients (r):

$$r = \frac{m_r}{m_a}$$

which means that the number of reflected molecules (m_r) on the membrane surface is, as a rule, low compared to the number of molecules which penetrate the membrane (m_a). The reflection coefficient of the common vehicles (buffers, etc.) approximates 1, while it is quite low for aldehydes. This implies that slight changes in buffer concentration result in more hypo- or hyperosmotic effects than drastic changes

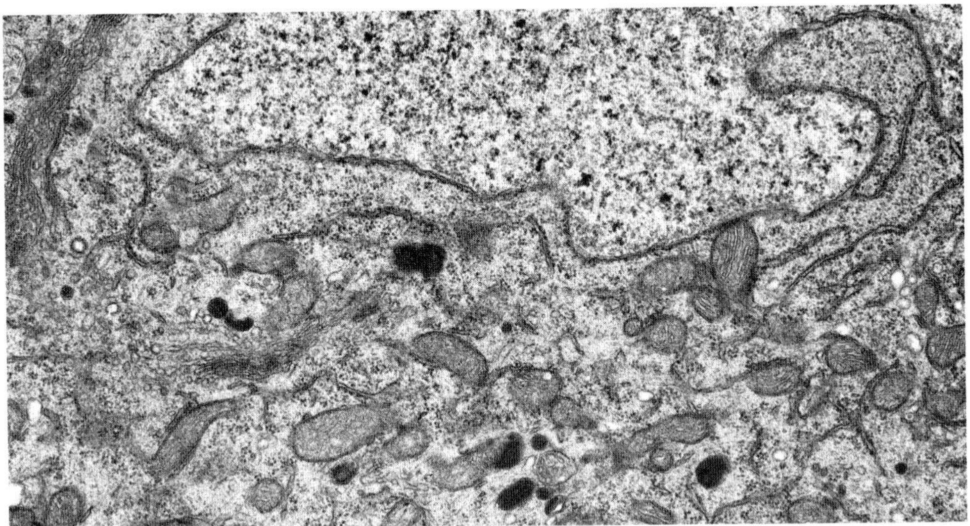

a

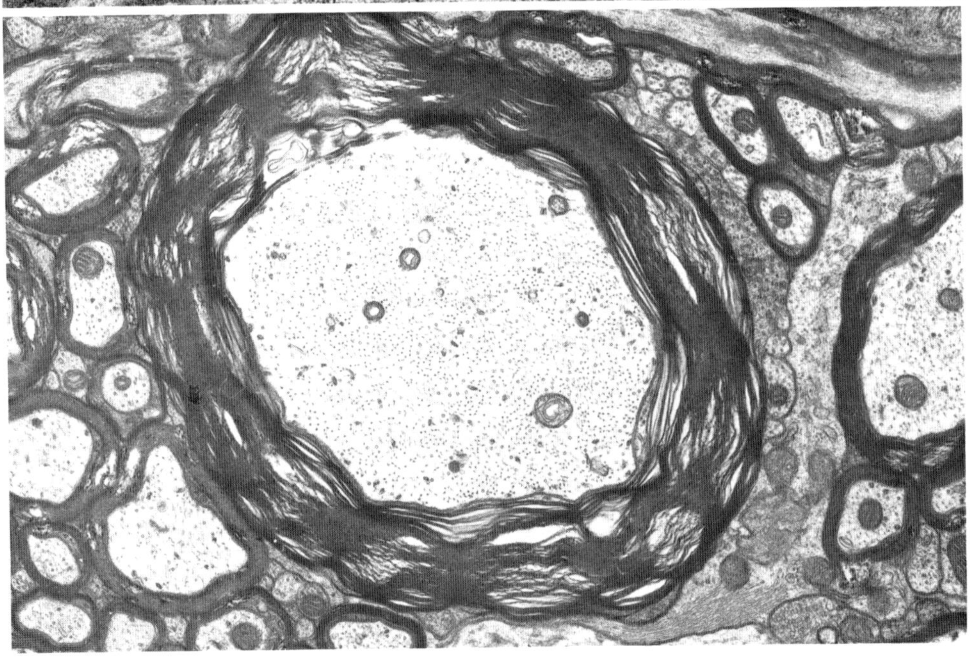

b

Fig. 6 a, b. Effect of vehicle concentration of the routine fixation of central nervous system (see text). **a** Addition of 300 mM sucrose results in a denser cytoplasm and darker mitochondria. The nuclear membrane of the neuron is undulated. ×52,000 **b** No positive effect of an increase of polyvinyl-pyrrolidine to 7.5%. Note the defective myelin sheath. ×35,000

in the aldehyde concentrations in the fixative (Fig. 5).

3.5.2 Colloid-Osmotic Pressure

The same properties of molecules producing an osmotic pressure are valid in the special cases of small particles, molecular aggregates, or macromolecules. These colloidal particles produce the colloid-osmotic pressure which is of importance for the regulation of intra- and extravascular spaces. The colloid-osmotic pressure is defined as the osmotic pressure exerted by large molecules through the membranous vascular wall. The colloid-osmotic pressure considerably influences the amount of net flux of water through the endothelium. It corresponds to a filtration pressure of about 18 mm Hg. Therefore, in tissues having a vascular wall with a low permeability for these particles (tissues with continuous capillaries) the perfusion fluids must be adjusted to an appropriate colloid-osmotic pressure by use of macromolecules such as dextrans or polyvinylpyrrolidone (Fig. 6). It has been observed that in tissues with continuous capillaries, the excessive addition of these macromolecules may produce a fluid withdrawal from the tissue and a reduction of the interstitial space. In tissues containing open capillaries (liver), the colloid-osmotic pressure is directly exerted on the parenchymal cells. Excessive colloid-osmotic pressure in these organs produces shrinkage of the cells. In the central nervous system little effect is observed from substances which in other tissues are necessary to maintain normal colloid-osmotic pressure (Fig. 6).

4 Practical Methods of Fixation

4.1 Immersion Fixation

Immersion fixation may be carried out for human biopsies of nervous system or organs including peripheral nerves or ganglia. For immersion, the high osmolarity fixative of Karnovsky (1965) is recommended as well as all other mentioned methods of postfixation, embedding, sectioning, and staining (see below).

4.2 Operation Methods for Perfusion Fixation

Vascular perfusion may be carried out as a general whole body perfusion or in special cases for single organs. The latter implies the cannulation of an organ artery and perfusion at the measured pressure of the respective artery. Systemic vascular perfusion is carried out through the left ventricle and the ascending aorta or retrograde through the abdominal aorta.

4.2.1 Transcardial Perfusion

This method has been widely used for brain or central nervous system fixation (Palay et al. 1962; Andres 1967; Descarries and Schröder 1968; Langford and Coggeshall 1980) and for the peripheral nervous system (Webster and Collins 1964; Forssmann et al. 1967).

The animals must be anesthetized and artifical respiration employed. The thoracic cage is opened widely and a thread for ligature is passed around the ascending

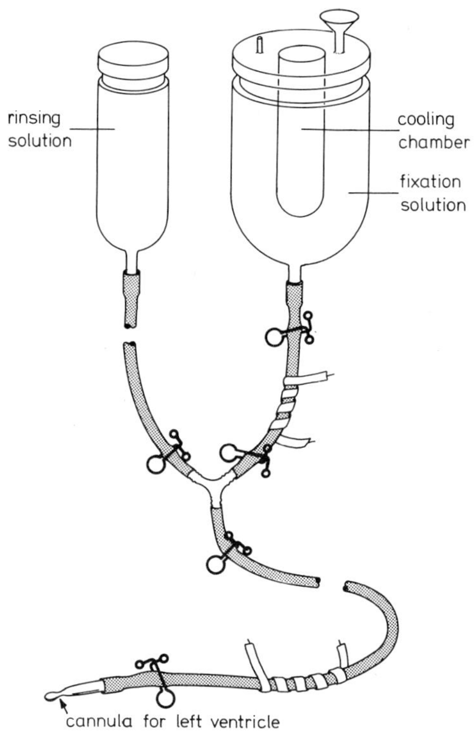

Fig. 7. Perfusion device for a transcardial perfusion according to Palay et al. (1962). Redrawn and modified from Journal of Cell Biology

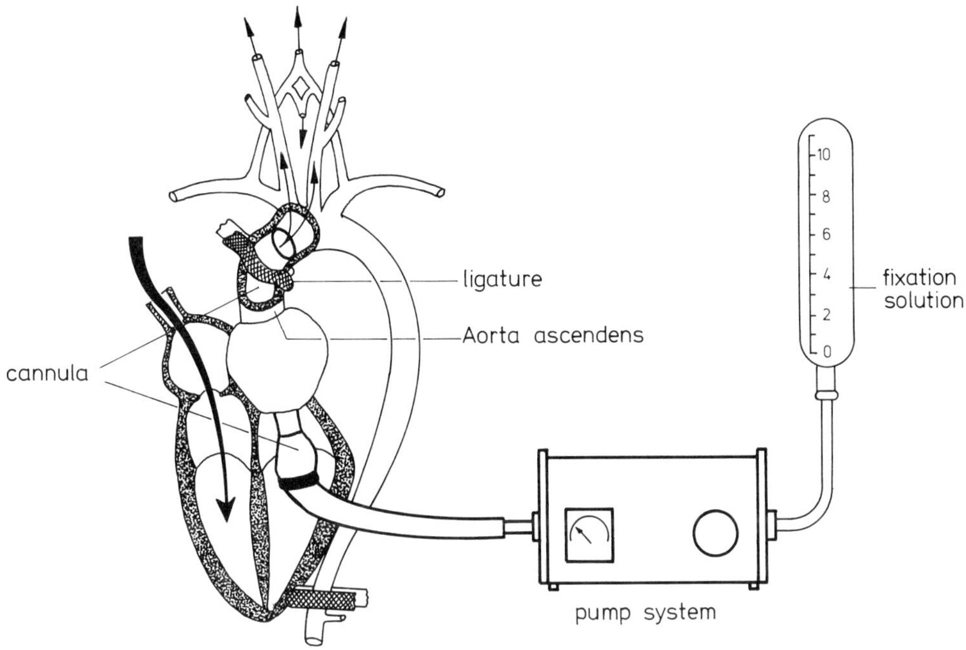

Fig. 8. High volume rate perfusion according to Descarries and Schröder (1968) using a pump system and transcardial pathway. Redrawn and modified from Journal de Microscopie

aorta. The left ventricle is then incised and a cannula is inserted into the ascending aorta. The cannula is fixed by a special clamp or the ligature around the ascending aorta, and the right ventricle is opened widely to allow an easy flow of the fixative. The perfusion solutions are immediately flushed through the entire body. All tissues excluding the heart and the lung will be fixed. For brain fixation a ligature may be placed around the aorta descendens below the branching of the left subclavian artery in order to prevent the fixative from flushing through the lower parts of the body.

4.2.2 Retrograde Perfusion

Retrograde perfusion has been introduced (1) to omit thoracotomy and the need for artificial respiration, (2) to provide perfusion of the heart in situ, and (3) to maintain the systemic blood pressure (Forssmann et al. 1967, 1977). The anesthetized animal is laparotomized and the abdominal aorta cannulated (Fig. 10). The cannula may be inserted without producing a change in the blood pressure as is the case for a short time when the left ventricle is incised in transcardial perfusion.

4.3 Application of Fixatives

4.3.1 Rinsing Solution

To prevent blood clotting, a rinsing solution is flushed as a rule before the application of the final fixative. Various rinsing solutions such as pure saline or complete electrolyte solution have been used. To prevent a drop in the colloid-osmotic pressure certain macromolecules, such as polyvinylpyrrolidone or rheomacrodex, are added to the saline. Furthermore, vasodilating agents are added to prevent a reduction of blood flow through the vasculature.

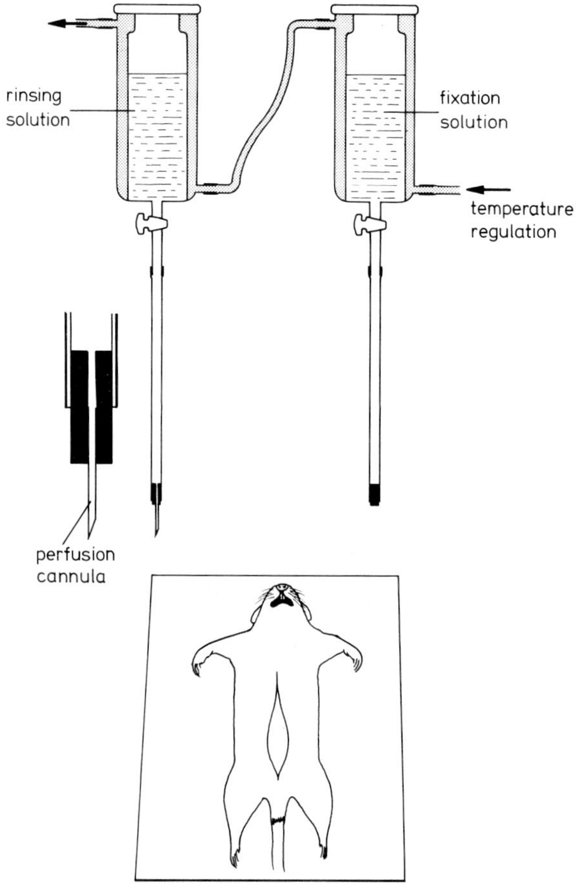

Fig. 9. Perfusion system according to Forssmann et al. (1967) for retrograde perfusion fixation. Redrawn and modified from Journal de Microscopie

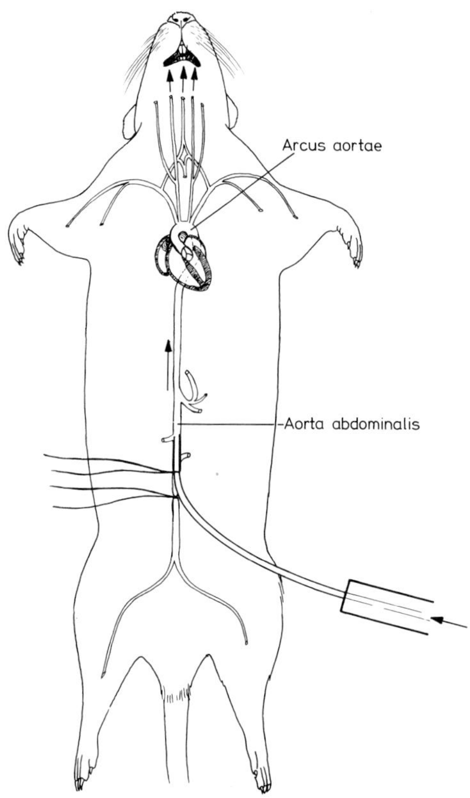

Fig. 10. Schematic drawing of the pathway used in the retrograde perfusion system according to Forssmann et al. (1967, 1977). Note the cannula is introduced into the aorta abdominalis. During perfusion the aortic valves are closed and the entire body is fixed, except for the lower extremities

The rinsing solution according to Forssmann et al. (1977) is prepared as follows:

9.0 g NaCl
25.0 g polyvinylpyrrolidone (PVP M.W. 40,000, Sigma, PVP-40)
0.25 g heparin (Sigma, H 3250)
5.0 g procain-HCl (Merck, Art. 7467).

These are dissolved in distilled water to obtain a final volume of 1 liter. The powdery substances are first thoroughly stirred in approximately 800 ml of distilled water. As the solution becomes clear and faintly yellow, the remaining water is added and the pH is adjusted to 7.3–7.4. The solution is then carefully filtered twice through 3.0 μm pore size filter and 0.6 μm pore size filter (Millipore, Sartorius). This rinsing solution is applied for 30 s to 2 min and then directly followed by the fixation perfusion. Another rinsing solution was proposed by Langford and Coggeshall (1980) which gives similarly reliable results: to 500 ml of distilled water 0.1% NaCl, 1000 I.U. of heparin, and 1 g sodium nitrate is added.

4.3.2 Fixation Solution

The fixation solution we routinely use is a phosphate buffered formaldehyde-glutaraldehyde solution made from the following stock solutions and substances:

45 ml 0.2 m monosodium phosphate (NaH_2PO_4)
405 ml 0.2 m disodium phosphate (Na_2HPO_4)
60 ml 25% formaldehyde (made from paraformaldehyde powder dissolved in hot water according to Karnovsky 1965)
60 ml 25% glutaraldehyde (electron microscopic grade)
25 mg polyvinylpyrrolidone (PVP M.W. 40,000).

The mixture is produced by adding the substances in the following sequence: first, the phosphate buffer is made, then PVP is added and stirred until dissolved. Formaldehyde and glutaraldehyde are then added as the solution is stirred. The solution is completed to 1 liter with distilled water, the pH is adjusted to 7.35, and the solution is filtered as well as the rinsing solution. This fixative is perfused for at least 10 min. Thereafter, the desired nervous tissue can be removed and either stored in fixative solution or immediately processed for postfixation and embedding. Some authors (Peters 1970) allow the brain to be left in situ for several hours or overnight before the tissue is dissected.

Langford and Coggeshall (1980) have proposed an adequate alternative using a 3% glutaraldehyde, 3% paraformaldehyde, and 0.1% picric acid solution in a 0.1% molar cacodylate buffer at pH 7.4. The use of a high osmolarity fixative is not adequate for peripheral nervous system or the vasculature of the central nervous system. Another reliable method is the use of a low osmolarity fixative followed by a high osmolarity fixative (see Reese and Brightman, personal communication 1968, see Peters 1970; Forssmann et al. 1977). However, no important advantages in the application of this method for the nervous system have been found in our laboratory.

4.4 Postfixation and En Bloc Staining

For postfixation two types of osmium tetroxide solutions are routinely used: (1) phosphate buffered 1% OsO_4 (Millonig 1961) or (2) ferrocyanide-reduced OsO_4 (Karnovsky 1971). Small tissue blocs or slices of less than 1 mm in one dimension are rinsed twice in the buffer used for fixation, e.g., 0.2 M sodium phosphate buffer or 0.2 M sodium cacodylate buffer, for at least 1 h. The postfixation is then carried out at room temperature for 1 h during ferrocyanide-OsO_4 treatment or 1–2 h when phosphate buffered OsO_4 is used.

Recently Langford and Coggeshall (1980) have claimed that a 1.5% ferricyanide, 1% OsO_4, 0.2 M cacodylate buffered (pH 7.4) solution for a 2h postfixation should be routinely used, especially for good preservation of myelin sheaths.

After postfixation, the tissue blocs are rinsed 3 times (10–30 min) in 0.2 M cacodylate buffer or 0.2 M sodium phosphate buffer and then dehydrated and embedded. If "en bloc staining" with uranyl acetate is employed, the rinsing is carried out with 0.2 M sodium maleate buffer at pH 5.6 for at least 1 h with three solution changes. The en bloc staining with 1% uranyl acetate in 0.2 M sodium maleate buffer at pH 5.6 for 1–2 h is in fact a procedure comparable to an additional postfixation which we routinely apply. The 3 h rinsing with maleate buffer after the en bloc staining is performed by carefully changing the buffer at least three times. The changes of buffer are important in order to prevent overstaining and precipitation deposits in the outer part of the blocs.

4.5 Dehydration and Embedding

Among the numerous variations of dehydration and embedding the Epon method of Luft (1961, 1974) has been employed with reliable and constant results. Further methods with Araldite-Epon mixtures, the ERL-4206 method, Vestopal W, or Maraglas are of varying advantages.

In our laboratory Epon, Araldite-Epon, or ERL-4206 are used. The following schedule for dehydration is common for all these methods.

4.5.1 Dehydration

Increasing series of ethanol are applied according to the following schedule:

5 min	ethanol 30%	cold or room temperature
5 min	ethanol 50%	
5 min	ethanol 70%	
5 min	ethanol 96%	
2×5 min	ethanol 100%	
45 min	ethanol 100%	
20 min	ethanol 100%	room temperature
20 min	ethanol 100%	

The Epon, Epon-Araldite, or ERL embedding is then carried out as described in the following sections.

4.5.2 Epon Embedding

For Epon embedding, the tissue blocs must be immersed in propylene oxide before they are transferred into the final Epon-mixture. From the last ethanol step the tissue is placed directly into 100% propylene oxide:

10 min 100% propylene oxide
10 min 100% propylene oxide
1 h 1 : 1 mixture of 100 propylene oxide and Epon (see below)
12 h Epon.

Change into new Epon and introduce the blocs into the beem capsules and polymerize for 24–72 h at +60 °C.

We use the following chemical products:

ethanol (Merck, Art. 972)
propylene oxide (Merck, Art. 12492).

100 g Epon mixture contains: 46.2 g Epikot (Epon 812, Serva 21045), 28.5 g DDSA (dodecenyl succinic anhydride, Serva 29452), 25.1 g MNA (methylnadic anhydride, Serva 20755), 1.5 g DMP-30 (2,4,6-tri(dimethyl-aminomethyl)phenol, Serva 36975).

4.5.3 Epon-Araldite Embedding

For Epon-Araldite the schedule is similar to that above. However, the passage through the final mixture is short and carried out in a warm embedding mixture:

10 min 100% propylene oxide
10 min 100% propylene oxide
3–12 h 1 : 1 mixture 100% propylene oxide, and Epon-Araldite mixture.

After 15 min or less the specimen blocs are transferred into new tubes containing

100% Epon-Araldite mixture with DMP-30 and immediately embedded in beem capsules or flat embedding wells.

12–24 h polymerization at +64 °C.

Epon-Araldite mixture is made up as follows:

10 ml Epon 812
10 ml Araldite 6005 (Serva 13828)
24 ml DDSA.

This mixture is routinely stored cold (below 0 °C) in amounts of 10 or 20 mg using glass scintillation counting vials. Immediately before use, the individual portions are warmed to 60 °C and we add two drops of DMP-30 per 1 ml Epon-Araldite mixture by use of a pasteur pipette. It is suggested that the embedding medium be thoroughly mixed and a constant warm temperature be maintained. Once prepared, this medium can only be used within the next few minutes, due to its rapid polymerization.

4.5.4 ERL Mixture

In this embedding method (see Spurr 1969) the steps through propylene oxide are not necessary. The mixture has a rather low viscosity. The schedule after ethanol dehydration was as follows:

30 min ERL and 100% ethanol 1 : 1
30 min ERL and 100% ethanol 2 : 1
2–6 h 100% ERL mixture
6–12 h 100% ERL mixture (if very small tissue blocs are used this step can be omitted).

The blocs are then introduced into beem capsules filled with ERL mixture and the polymerization is carried out for 8–16 h at +70 °C.

ERL mixture:

10.0 g ERL-4206 (vinylcyclohexen dioxid, Serva 38216)
6.0 g DER 736 (diepoxid, Serva 18247)
26.0 g NSA (nonenyl succinic acid anhydride, Serva 30812)
0.4 g S-1 (2-dimethylaminoethanol, Serva 20130).

4.5.5 Comments on Embedding Methods

Most of the embedding media are resins or polyesters. The penetration and osmotic effects vary according to the viscosity of the monomeric compound. Although Epon is rather viscous it is the preferred embedding medium. ERL or other low viscosity embedding methods (Luft 1974) which have been proposed, however, include substances which are expensive and toxic (carcinogenic). The main basis for the choice of an embedding medium may be summarized as follows: the reliability of the polymerization, the low degree of shrinking or swelling during polymerization, the advantages in staining properties of the semithin and thin sections, the stability of the sections in the electron beam, and the possibility for redissolving the polymerized embedding medium (see immunocytochemistry). The main properties of the proposed media are summarized in Table 1.

Further embedding media such as Araldite (Glauert and Glauert 1958),

Table 1. Main properties of various proposed embedding media.

	Shrinkage	Miscible with ethanol	Viscosity	Stainability
Epon	Variable	–	Medium	+ +
Araldite-Epon	+	–	Medium-high	+
Araldite	+	+	High	Difficult
ERL	–	+	Low	+

Maraglas (Spurlock et al. 1963), and Vestopal (Ryter and Kellenberger 1958) are widely used with varying advantages (for details see Luft 1974).

4.6 Sectioning and Microscopic Evaluation

Sectioning and microscopic evaluation are general methods described in numerous editions on electron microscopy (see Koehler 1974, 1978) and will therefore not be extensively described here. Stereological evaluation (Weibel et al. 1966; Haug 1970, 1972, 1976; Anker and Cragg 1974; Reinecke and Walther 1980), computer processing of electron micrographs (Frank 1974), or high voltage electron microscopy (Hama 1974) are recommended in the relevant literature.

4.7 Thin Section Staining

For staining of thin sections we routinely use uranyl acetate followed by lead citrate. The staining procedure is carried out in a Petri dish with a 6 cm diameter. The cover is used as the bottom and covered with clean dental wax. The bottom must completely close the staining chamber on the dental wax to prevent evaporation or CO_2 penetration. A small dish filled with fresh pellets of sodium hydroxide is placed in the chamber to reduce the amount of CO_2 present.

4.7.1 Uranyl Acetate Staining

This staining (Watson 1958) is done with a 5% aqueous solution of $UO_2\ (CH_3COO)_2 \cdot 2\ H_2O$ (Merck, Art. 8473). The stock solution is prepared and filtered on standing. Before use, the solution is centrifuged and small drops are placed on the dental wax bottom of the chamber. The grids containing sections are then placed on the drops and staining is carried out for 10–20 min. Staining of sections on uncoated grids can also be carried out by immersing the grid in uranyl acetate solutions with has been diluted with an adequot of methanol, and centrifuged for 30–40 s. The sections are carefully washed by flushing distilled water through a grid flask and are then dried on a filter paper.

4.7.2 Lead Citrate Staining

This follows in the same manner as the uranyl acetate staining, however for only 3–5 min. Here the close contact of the lid with the dental wax is essential to prevent the formation of lead carbonate from atmospheric CO_2. A solution of lead citrate is prepared according to Reynolds (1963) or Venable and Coggeshall (1965). For this, 100 ml lead citrate solution are made up from 0.1–0.4 g lead citrate (Merck, Art. 12438) is distilled water to which 0.1 ml of 10 N sodium hydroxide is added. The solution is made up in a flask by vigorous shaking. The staining solution may be kept in a refrigerator as stock for several months. Small portions are centrifuged before use in an Eppendorf centrifuge for 1 min using 2-ml plastic vials. The centrifuged solution can also be kept in a syringe. Before the drops for staining are ejected a small portion is discarded.

This staining method has become so routine and easy that, for routine electron microscopy, no further improvement has been necessary in the past few years.

5 Concluding Remarks

This chapter has dealt mainly with general methods of transmission electron microscopy for nervous tissue. The technique of fixation as a crucial problem is stressed here in some detail. It is recommended that further editions be consulted for techniques such as embedding, sectioning, and electron microscopy (Reimer 1967;

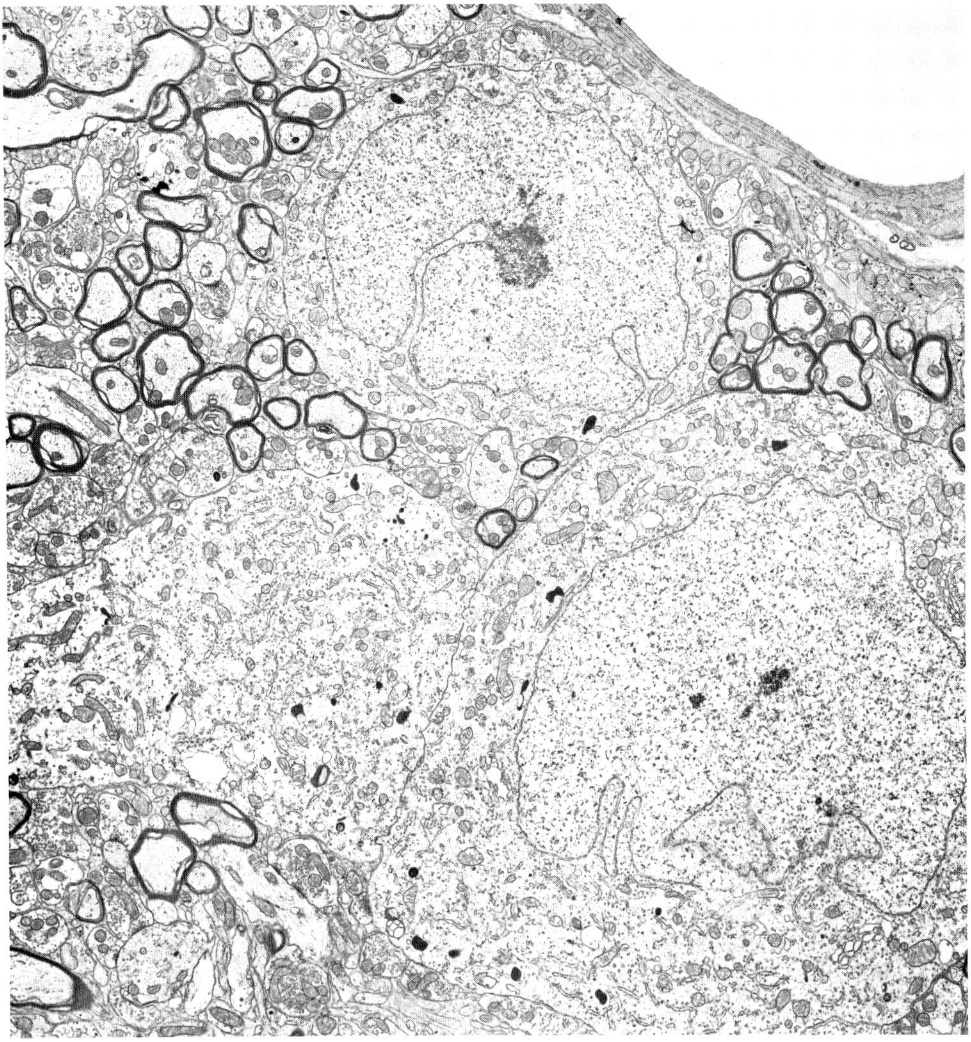

Fig. 11. Routine fixation (see text) of the cerebral cortex (Tupaias). Note the good overall preservation of neurons and neuropil. ×12,500

Goodhew 1973; Beeston et al. 1973; Koehler 1974, 1978; Agar et al. 1974; Alderson 1975; Glauert 1975; Reid 1975; Lewis and Knight 1977). The fixation methods described here may also be adequate for other applications such as immunocytochemistry, cytochemistry (e.g., retrograde peroxidase transport), autoradiography, and particularly for high voltage electron microscopy, which has scarely been used for nervous tissue. The methods described here are the methods of choice (for scanning electron microscopy and morphometric evaluation) in our laboratory (Metz and Bressler 1979; Nimmrich et al. 1980), for both peripheral and central nervous tissue as well as for most of the tissues in mammals and certain other vertebrates.

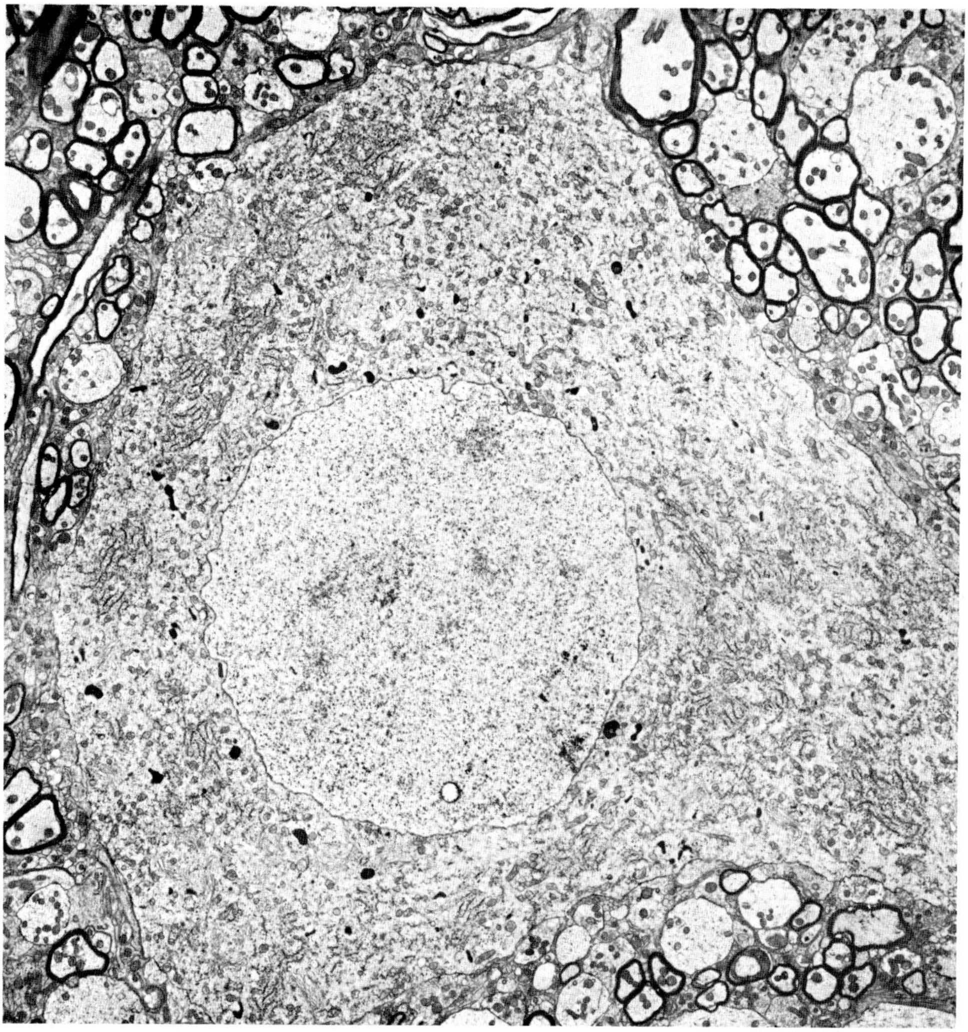

Fig. 12. Routine fixation (see text) of the spinal cord anterior horn. Note the good preservation of the motor neuron in Tupaia. ×9200

Fig. 13 a, b. Fixation of the peripheral nervous system (routine method, see text). A neuron of duodenal plexus submucosus of the monkey is seen. × 14,000 and 36,000

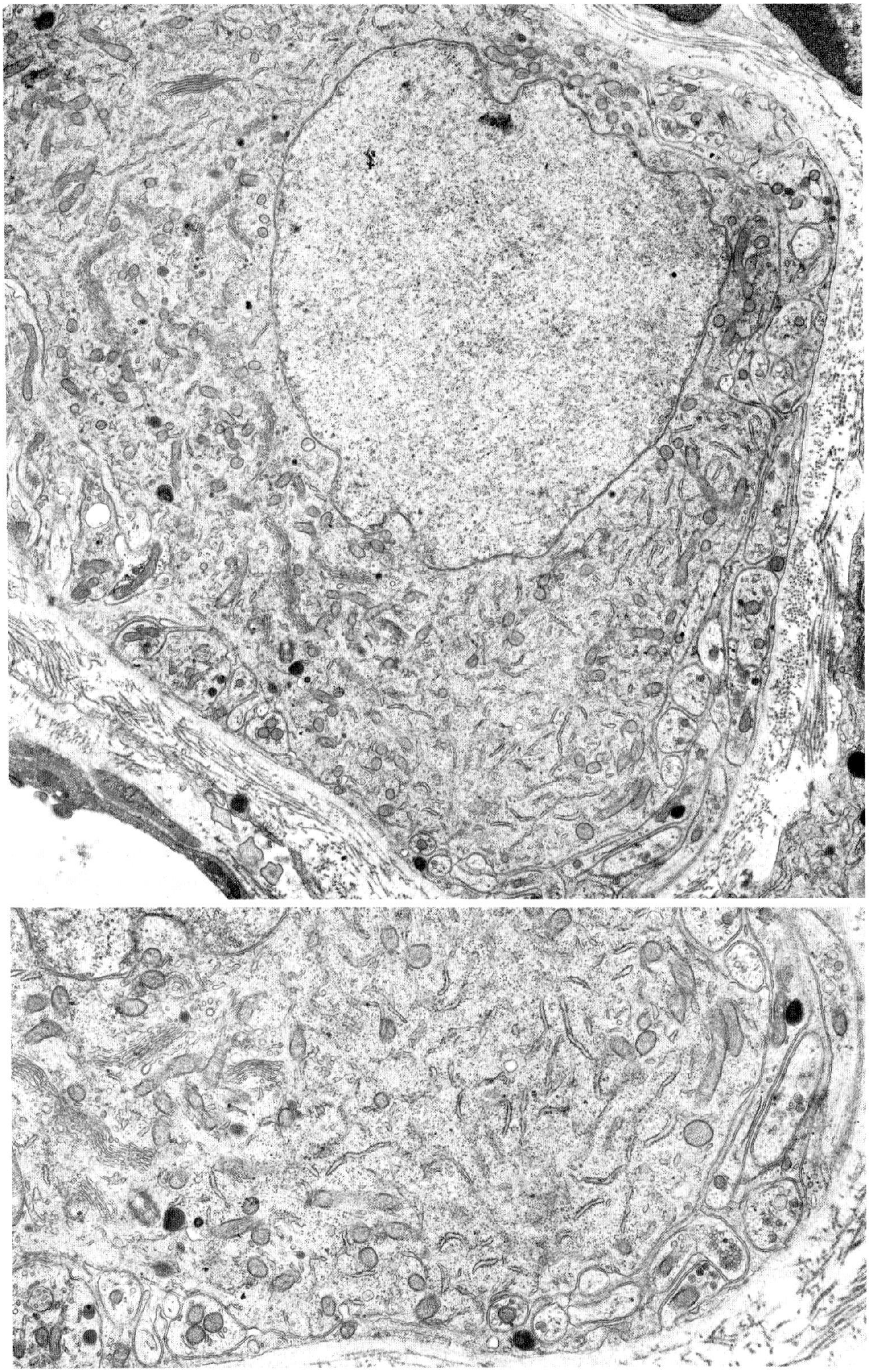

a

b

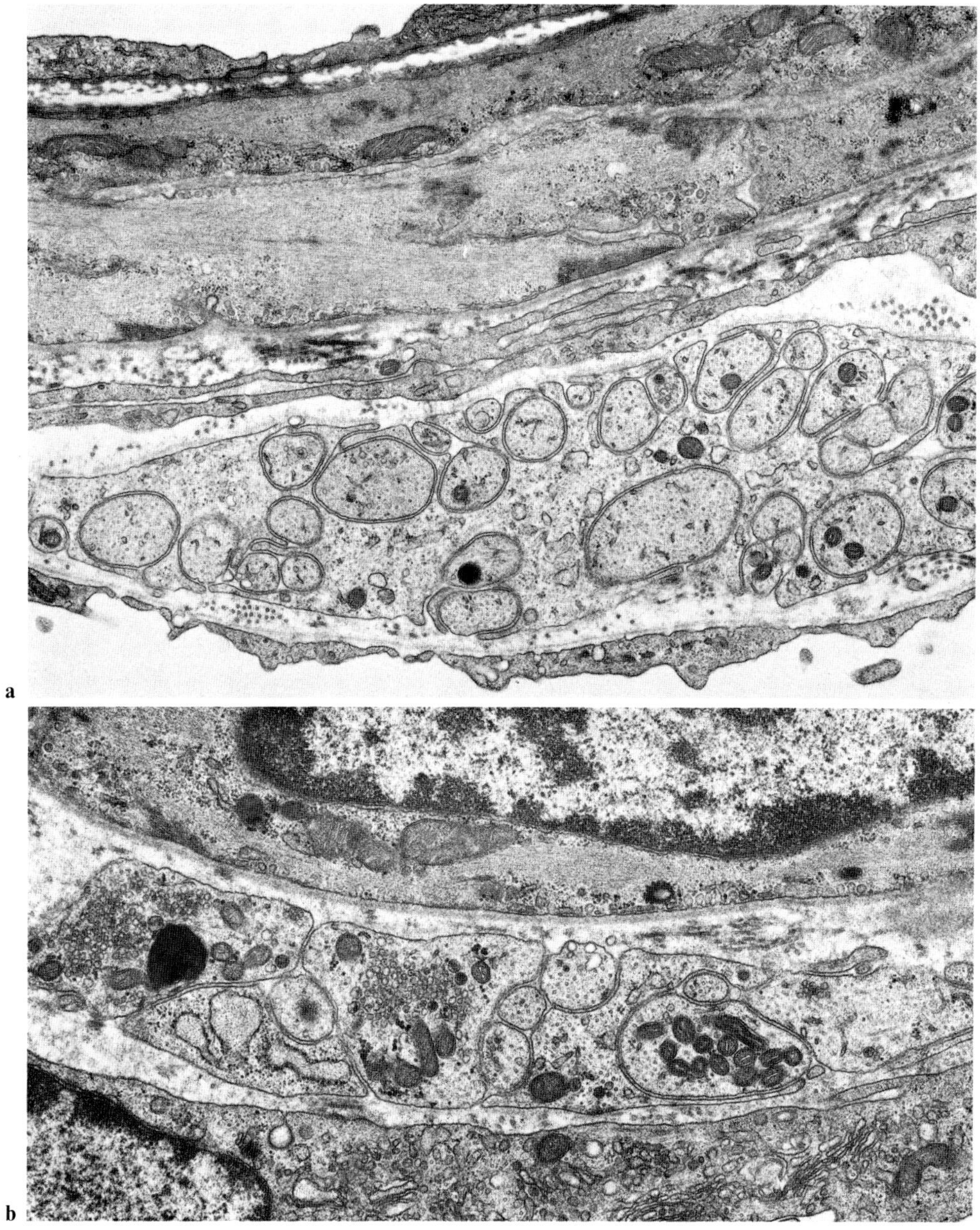

Fig. 14 a, b. Routine fixation of vascular nerves from **a** guinea pig and **b** tupaia kidney. These micrographs show that the fixation of peripheral autonomic nervous system is carried out without any problems. ×45,000

Acknowledgements. I wish to acknowledge the technical help of Mathias Ehrbar, Wolf Wyrwas, and Heidrun Kosubek, as well as the help in preparing the manuscript by Rosa Botz, Anita Miehle, Alan Shakelford, and Jon Greenberg.

6 References

Agar AW, Alderson RH, Chescoe D (1974) Principles and practice of electron microscope operation. In: Glauert AM (ed) Practical methods in electron microscopy. Elsevier, Amsterdam

Alderson RH (1975) Design of the electron microscope laboratory. In: Glauert AM (ed) Practical methods in electron microscopy. Elsevier, Amsterdam

Andres KH (1967) Zur Methodik der Perfusionsfixierung des Zentralnervensystems von Säugern. Mikroskopie 21:169

Anker RL, Cragg BC (1974) Estimation of the number of synapses in a volume of nervous tissue from counts in thin sections by electron microscopy. J Neurocytol 3:725–735

Bahr GF (1955) Continued studies about the fixation with osmium tetroxide. Electron stains IV. Exp Cell Res 9:277–285

Beeston BEP, Horne RW, Markham R (1973) Electron diffraction and optical diffraction techniques. In: Glauert AM (ed) Practical methods in electron microscopy. Elsevier, Amsterdam

Caulfield JB (1957) Effects of varying the vehicle for OsO_4 in tissue fixation. J Biophys Biochem Cytol 3:827–830

Descarries L, Schröder JM (1968) Fixation du tissu nerveux par perfusion à grand débit. J Microscopie 7:281–286

Fahimi HD, Drochmans P (1965) Essais de standardisation de la fixation au glutaraldéhyde. II. Influence des concentrations en aldéhyde et de l'osmocalité. J Microscopie 4:737–748

Forssmann WG, Ito S, Weihe E, Aoki A, Dym M, Fawcett DW (1977) An improved perfusion fixation method for the testis. Anat Rec 188:307–314

Forssmann WG, Siegrist G, Orci L, Girardier L, Pictet R, Rouiller Ch (1967) Fixation par perfusion pour la microscopie électronique. Essai de généralisation. J Microscopie 6: 279–304

Frank J (1974) Computer processing of electron micrographs. In: Koehler JK (ed) Advanced techniques in biological electron microscopy. Springer, Berlin Heidelberg New York, pp 215–274

Glauert AM (1975) Fixation, dehydration, and embedding of biological specimens. In: Glauert AM (ed) Practical methods in electron microscopy. Elsevier, Amsterdam

Glauert AM, Glauert RH (1958) Araldite as an embedding medium for electron microscopy. J Biophys Biochem Cytol 4:191–194

Goodhew PJ (1973) Specimen preparation in materials science. In: Glauert AM (ed) Practical methods in electron microscopy. Elsevier, Amsterdam

Hama K (1974) High voltage electron microscopy. In: Koehler JK (ed) Advanced techniques in biological electron microscopy. Springer, Berlin Heidelberg New York, pp 275–297

Haug H (1970) Quantitative data in neuroanatomy. Prog Brain Res 33:113–127

Haug H (1972) Stereological methods in the analysis of neuronal parameters in the central nervous system. J Microsc 95:165–180

Haug H (1976) Die verschiedenen Verfahren zur Werteerfassung in der biologischen Morphometrie und Stereologie. Microsc Acta 78:197–220

Ito S, Karnovsky MJ (1968) Formaldehyde-glutaraldehyde fixatives containing trinitro compounds. J Cell Biol 39:168a–169a

Karlsson U, Schultz RL (1965a) Fixation of the central nervous system for electron microscopy by aldehyde perfusion. I. Preservation with aldehyde perfusates versus direct perfusion with osmium tetroxide with special reference to membranes and the extracellular space. J Ultrastruct Res 12:160–186

Karlsson U, Schultz RL (1965b) Fixation of the central nervous system for electron microscopy by aldehyde perfusion. II. Effect of osmolarity, pH of perfusate, and fixative concentration. J Ultrastruct Res 12:187–206

Karlsson U, Schultz RL (1966) Fixation of the central nervous system for electron microscopy by aldehyde perfusion. III. Structural changes after exsanguination and delayed perfusion. J Ultrastruct Res 14:47–63

Karnovsky MJ (1965) A formaldehyde-glutaraldehyde fixative of high osmolality for use in electron microscopy. J Cell Biol 27:137A–138A

Karnovsky MJ (1971) Use of ferrocyanide-reduced osmium tetroxide in electron microscopy (abstr.). J Cell Biol 51, ASCB-Meeting, 146

Koehler JK (ed) (1974) Advanced techniques in biological electron microscopy. Springer, Berlin Heidelberg New York

Koehler JK (ed) (1978) Advanced techniques in biological electron microscopy II. Specific ultrastructural probes. Springer, Berlin Heidelberg New York

Koenig H, Groat RA, Windle WF (1945) A physiological approach to perfusion-fixation of tissues with formalin. Stain Technol 20: 13–24

Langford LA, Coggeshall RE (1980) The use of potassium ferricyanide in neural fixation. Anat Rec 197:297–303

Lewis PR, Knight DP (1977) Staining methods of sectioned material. In: Glauert AM (ed) Practical methods in electron microscopy. Elsevier, Amsterdam

Luft JH (1956) Permanganate – a new fixative for electron microscopy. J Biophys Biochem Cytol 2:799–802

Luft JH (1961) Improvements in epoxy resin embedding methods. J Biophys Biochem Cytol 9:409–414

Luft JH (1974) Embedding media – old and new. In: Koehler JK (ed) Advanced techniques in biological electron microscopy. Springer, Berlin Heidelberg New York, pp 1–34

Maunsbach AB (1966) The influence of different fixatives and fixation methods on the ultrastructure of rat kidney proximal tubule cells. I. Comparison of different perfusion fixation methods and of glutaraldehyde, formaldehyde, and osmium tetroxide fixatives. J Ultrastruct Res 15:242–282

Metz J, Bressler D (1979) Reformation of gap and tight junctions in regenerating liver after cholestasis. Cell Tissue Res 199:257–270

Millonig G (1961) Advantages of a phosphate buffer for OsO_4 solutions in fixation. J Appl Physiol 32:1637

Nimmrich H, Meairs S, Forssmann WG, Weihe E (1980) Scanning electron microscopy of endothelium. In: Motta P (ed) Three-dimensional anatomy of cell and tissue surfaces. Elsevier, New York, pp 311–330

Palade GE (1952) A study of fixation for electron microscopy. J Exp Med 95:285–297

Palay SL, McGee-Russell SM, Gordon S, Grillo MA (1962) Fixation of neural tissues for electron microscopy by perfusion with solutions of osmium tetroxide. J Cell Biol 12:385–410

Peters A (1970) The fixation of central nervous tissue and the analysis of electron micrographs of the neurophil, with special reference to the cerebral cortex. In: Nauta WJH, Ebbesson SOE (ed) Contemporary research methods in neuroanatomy. Springer, Berlin Heidelberg New York

Reid N (1975) Ultramicrotomy. In: Glauert AM (ed) Practical methods in electron microscopy. Elsevier, Amsterdam

Reimer L (1967) Elektronenmikroskopische Untersuchungs- und Präparationsmethoden, 2. Aufl. Springer, Berlin Heidelberg New York

Reinecke M, Walther Ch (1981) Ultrastructural changes with high activity and subsequent recovery at locust motor nerve terminals. A stereological analysis. Neuroscience 6:489–503

Reynolds ES (1963) The use of lead citrate at high pH as an electron-opaque stain in electron microscopy. J Cell Biol 17:208–212

Ryter A, Kellenberger E (1958) L'inclusion au polyester pour l'ultramicrotomie. J Ultrastruct Res 2:200–214

Sabatini DD, Bensch K, Barnett RJ (1963) Cytochemistry and electron microscopy. The preservation of cellular ultrastructure and enzymatic activity by aldehyde fixation. J Cell Biol 17:19–58

Spurlock BO, Kattine VC, Freeman JA (1963) Technical modifications in Maraglas embedding. J Cell Biol 17:203–207

Spurr AR (1969) A low-viscosity epoxy resin embedding medium for electron microscopy. J Ultrastruct Res 26:31–43

Venable JH, Coggeshall R (1965) A simplified lead citrate stain for use in electron microscopy. J Cell Biol 25:407–408

Watson ML (1958) Staining of tissue sections for electron microscopy with heavy metals. J Biophys Biochem Cytol 4:475–478

Webster HF de, Collins GH (1964) Comparison of osmium tetroxide and glutaraldehyde perfusion fixation for the electron microscopic study on the normal rat peripheral nervous system. J Neuropathol Exp Neurol 1:109–126

Weibel ER, Kistler GS, Scherle WF (1966) Practical stereological methods for morphometric cytology. J Cell Biol 30:23–38

Chapter 3

Freeze-Etching in Neuroanatomy

K. Akert, C. Sandri, and H. Moor

1 Introduction

The application of the freeze-etching technique as described by Moor and Mühlethaler (1963) to neural tissue was introduced by Bischoff (Bischoff and Moor 1967 a, b) for the study of myelin and by Akert et al. (1969) in an attempt to visualize the active sites of the presynaptic membrane. It turned out in subsequent systematic studies (Orci and Perrelet 1975; Peters et al. 1976; Sandri et al. 1977) that the freeze-etching method is uniquely suitable in describing specialized cell contacts in the nervous system. Especially the quantitative investigations of vesicle-to-membrane and particle-to-membrane relationships turned out to be useful in the evaluation of functional states of chemically and electrically excitable membranes (Streit et al. 1972; Venzin et al. 1977; Tokunaga et al. 1979 a, b, c).

The following is a brief description of the principles and the major practical steps in the application of freeze-fracturing and freeze-etching to the peripheral and central nervous systems. The theoretical aspects as well as the history of the development of the method have been dealt with in more detail in several previous publications (Moor 1971, 1973; Benedetti and Favard 1973; Mühlethaler 1973; Bullivant 1973, 1974).

It should be also mentioned that alternative procedures for the preparation of freeze-etched replicas of nerve tissue exist today. For instance the so-called double-replica technique (Chalcroft and Bullivant 1970; Steere 1973; Mühlethaler et al. 1973), the spray-freezing technique (Bachmann and Schmitt 1971), the quick freezing technique (Heuser et al. 1976, 1979) and the high pressure freezing method (Moor 1977). Pfenninger and Rinderer (1975) succeeded to adapt the freeze-etching technique to thin layers of cells or cellular processes. These alternative approaches have their advantages and disadvantages. Their common goal is to obtain an uncontaminated artifact-free and high-fidelity replica of living cells. Although, physical and chemical alterations of the tissue could be reduced to a minimum, this goal, in its ideal form, has thus far not been reached. Nevertheless, a powerful tool and an effective alternative to conventional thin sectioning techniques has been attained.

This chapter is restricted to the now "conventional" application of freeze-etching nerve tissue in situ or in vitro according to the Zürich School.

2 Principles of Freeze-Etching

2.1 Freezing

The aim of freezing is to solidify a specimen in the natural state without any changes in structure and chemistry. This can be achieved by vitrification, a process in which heat is extracted faster than it can be produced by crystallization. Under these conditions, crystallization occurs with a vast increase of the number of crystals and a reduction in size to about 10 nm. The transition from heterogeneous to homogeneous nucleation takes place at the "critical freezing rate" which for water amounts to a temperature loss of about 10^6 K/s^{-1}. For tissue the critical freezing state is reduced to 10^4 K/s^{-1}. At this rate the cells probably suffer no damage from crystals and are not altered morphologically. If the object is cooled from one side only, the low thermal conductivity of water reduces the zone on which the critical freezing rate can be achieved to a superficial layer of only a few μm. The layer of vitrified tissue can be enlarged four times when thin platelets are used and 6–7 times when cylindrical or spherical specimens are applied respectively (Riehle 1968).

Good results have been obtained by the spray-freezing technique of Bachmann and Schmitt (1971). According to this method cells are suspended in a suitable medium and sprayed into liquid propane at –180 °C resulting in a vitrification of droplets up to 20 μm in diameter.

Heuser et al. (1979) have built a new apparatus using liquid helium for rapid freezing of tissues. They claim to be able to vitrify tissue blocks within 100 μm from the surface.

Moor and his collaborators tried to approach the problem from still another side (Moor 1977). Under very high pressure (2100 bar) the freezing point of water is lowered to –22 °C. The cooling by liquid nitrogen jet comes from two sides to the preparation. Fresh tissue slices, 0.5 mm in thickness may be vitrified without fixation and cryoprotection. The cut surfaces are etchable and real membrane surfaces may be visualized.

2.2 Fracturing

The ultrastructural details of a vitrified tissue block are revealed by cleaving it at a temperature below –100 °C. At this temperature the specimens are brittle and therefore fracturing takes place instead of cutting. Fracturing is advantageous because in contrast to cutting it avoids friction heating. The fracturing is performed under high vacuum in order to avoid the condensation of moisture.

2.3 Etching

When cold specimen surfaces are exposed under high vacuum, either sublimation or condensation may occur. Sublimation of a substance takes place if its saturation vapor pressure at specimen temperature is higher than its partial pressure in the vacuum. Thus, both object temperature and vacuum conditions determine whether the specimen may be kept at −100 °C. The etching conditions are altered drastically by a temperature shift from −100° to −120 °C: the saturation vapor pressure of specimen water is lowered below its partial pressure in the vacuum and thus water becomes a contaminant at 10^{-6} Torr (Moor 1971). In order to freeze-fracture samples at liquid nitrogen temperature (etching is impossible) a reduction of the water partial pressure to about 10^{-9} Torr is required. To attain such conditions an ultra high vacuum system must be used. Under these conditions a monomolecular layer of condensed water is formed on the specimen surface in about 1000 s. Contamination can be avoided if the time interval between cleaving and coating is restricted to about 10 s.

Although simple cleaving of frozen specimens reveals main ultrastructural details, etching may expose supplementary elements by a superficial sublimation of the surrounding ice. The etching does not only depend on temperature and vacuum conditions but also on the water content of the specimen: if no free water is available no etching will occur. When anti-freeze agents are used in high concentrations (30%–40%) the etchability is reduced to a negligible amount. At lower concentrations of anti-freeze it is possible that the solved substances may produce a non-etchable coat on top of structural surfaces hiding essential details. Thus, in order to "deep-etch" and expose structures like membrane surfaces, the surrounding medium must be pure water (Pinto da Silva and Branton 1970).

2.4 Replication

The evaporation of high melting point substances onto a deep-frozen specimen may elevate its surface temperature to the point of inducing ultrastructural damage. Heat radiation from the evaporator can be tolerated if the source diameter is reduced to about 2 mm, the source to sample distance is about 15 cm and total evaporation time is about 10 s. Briefer evaporation times resulting from higher coating rates increase condensation heating considerably. Some of the problems of evaporating have been solved with electron guns which confine the hot elements of the evaporator and eliminate electron bombardment onto the specimen (Moor 1971).

During heating of the evaporation source not only are coating materials emitted but gases are also expelled from hot elements of the gun. Such gases (H_2, H_2O, N_2, CO, O_2, and CO_2) reduce the vacuum and may condense on the specimen surface. Such contaminants can only be eliminated by discharging all gases from the evaporator prior to cleaving and etching (that is, by "baking-out" of the guns).

Evaporated heavy metal atoms do not condense on the specimen surface at the point of collision, but they are rearranged producing small crystallites which impart a granularity to the replica. The coarseness of this granularities depends on the vapor pressure of the condensing material. Thus, only the highest melting point metals are used for shadow casting in order to reduce the granularity and thereby improve the resolving power of the replica. The formation of crystallites may be attenuated by the evaporation of alloys such as platinum-carbon or tantalum-tungsten rather than pure metals. In addition, the condensation of evaporated material is influenced by the profile of the specimen and by its physicochemical properties which offer nuclei for crystallization, that is, crystallites may serve as markers for certain fine structures. Therefore, maximum information can be obtained by the use of shadow casting techniques either with highly resolving low granularity or by decoration with crystallites.

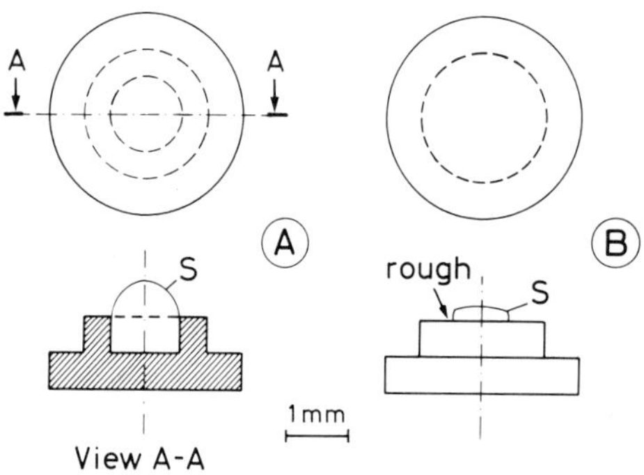

Fig. 1 A, B. Specimen holders made of a gold-nickel alloy which fit the receptacles of the object support on the cooling table (Fig. 3 A). **A** Specimen holder with central depression which provides a solid base for the specimen during sectioning. **B** Specimen holder with flat top and rough surface; this type is needed for the sectioning of extremely thin and/or small specimen (*s*)

For stability reasons the fragile heavy metal coat (2–3 nm) must be reinforced by a low density carbon backing film (20–30 nm). If needed, additional reinforcement is attained by backing the carbon with a coat of evaporated naphthaline which can be removed by evaporation after the replica has been cleaned and mounted on a grid.

3 Preparation of the Tissue

3.1 Fixation

Although it is possible to work with unfixed tissue, we have found that in most cases fixation of tissue with aldehydes may give more satisfactory results. For this, the various modifications of perfusion and immersion fixation that are used in conventional electronmicroscopy are recommended. Immersion fixation is applied to acutely excised tissue and to fractionated tissue components, e.g., synaptosomes and tissue cultures.

3.2 Freezing

Blocks trimmed to 1 mm or less to a side are transferred to the same buffer employed for fixation made isotonic with sucrose and held at 4 °C for 30 min or longer. The specimens are transferred to the cryoprotectant (25% glycerol in Ringer solution) for 30 min while the freezing equipment is being set up.

Under a dissecting stereomicroscope the tissue samples are carried to gold-nickel specimen holders (Fig. 1), i.e., 3 mm discs designed to fit the object support of the cooling table of the cryotome. Two types of specimen holders are currently in use. The tissue should remain in proper contact with the metal of the specimen holder. Therefore, it is more convenient to use a support with a hole for large specimens and a flat support with scratched surface for smaller objects (Fig. 1).

The transfer of the specimen to the holder is accomplished in a drop of glycerol-Ringer solution and the tissue orientated to the plane desired for sectioning. The holder held between the dried tips of a watchmaker (Nr. 4–5) Dumont forceps is then dipped into Freon 22 for 10–15 s and transferred immediately into liquid nitrogen in a small specimen container where it can be stored until ready for freeze-fracture and etching (Fig. 2 D).

The most convenient equipment for this procedure is shown in Fig. 2: A small Dewar flask serving for the rapid freezing in Freon 22 (Fig. 2 A) and a second Dewar flask for the long term storage of the specimens (Fig. 2 B).

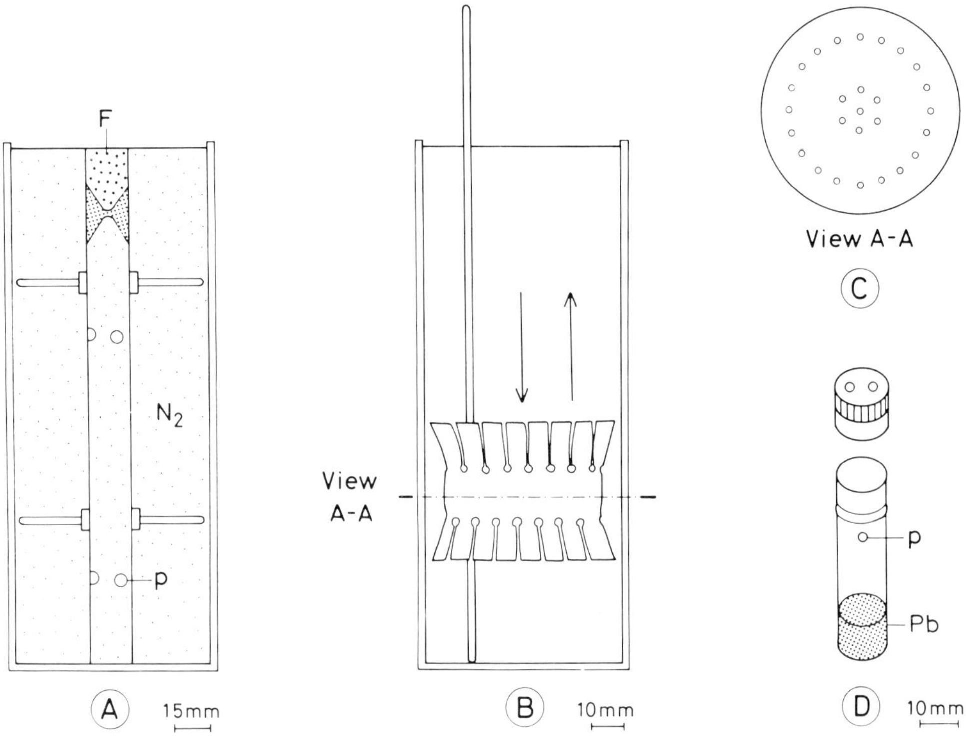

Fig. 2. A Dewar flask filled with liquid nitrogen (N_2). Small freon container (*F*) which is supported by an aluminum stage. **B** Dewar flask filled with liquid nitrogen. Stainless steel basket mounted to a rod for handling. Position of basket can be changed in vertical direction (*arrows*). This basket can be loaded with up to 8 specimen containers (D). **C** Equatorial view A–A of basket (Fig. 2 B) with 2 mm perforations. **D** Specimen container with cap. Perforations (*p*) allow liquid N_2 to enter. Lead weight at the bottom of the container (*Pb*) prevents floating

Both Dewar flasks are filled with liquid nitrogen (LN_2). The Freon 22 container in the first flask (Fig. 2A) consists of a small cup which is supported by an aluminum stage. The Freon has a freezing point of –150 °C while the temperature of the surrounding liquid nitrogen is at –196 °C. Therefore, before dipping the specimen holder into the Freon 22 chamber, one has to melt the frozen Freon by means of a warm (held by hand) metal rod.

3.3 Fracturing, Etching, and Replication

Fracturing and replication are accomplished according to standard Moor-Balzer's technique using a cooling table and a microtome. The cooling table includes an exchangeable object support (Fig. 3) with three receptacles for the specimen holders. These are held in position by means of a cover which is tightly clamped to the object support (Figs. 3 B, 3 C). The transfer of the specimen holders to the object support and the cooling of both is carried out with special equipment kept in a Dewar flask completely filled with LN_2. The object support is positioned in the teflon container resting on a fine iron mesh (Fig. 4). The transfer of the specimen holders from the long term storage Dewar flask (Fig. 2 B) to the receptacles in the object support follows only after most careful elimination of ice crystals from the bottom

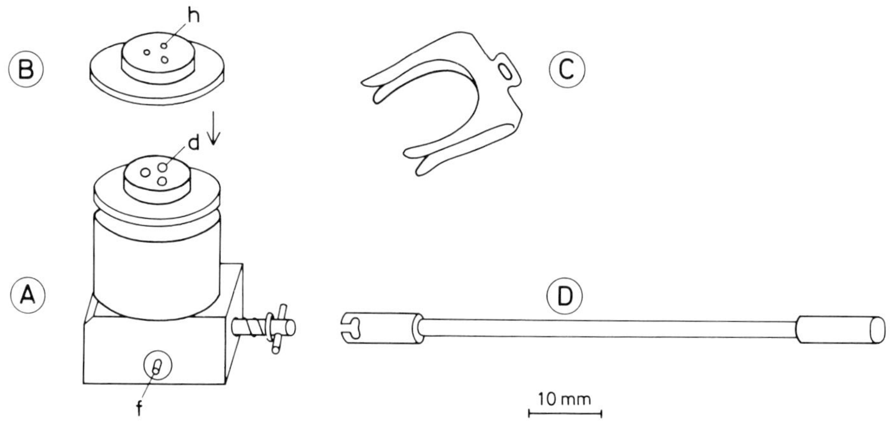

Fig. 3. **A** Object support of the Balzers BAF 300 cooling table (*not illustrated*) modified for freeze-fracturing of tissue blocks. On top three receptacles (Φ 3 mm) for three golden specimen holders. **B** Cover with three holes (Φ 2 mm) (*h*) which are positioned corresponding to the receptacles in Fig. 3 A in order to keep specimen holders in place during sectioning. **C** Clamp to fix the cover tightly to object support. **D** Manipulator for mounting the object support on the cooling table in the vacuum chamber

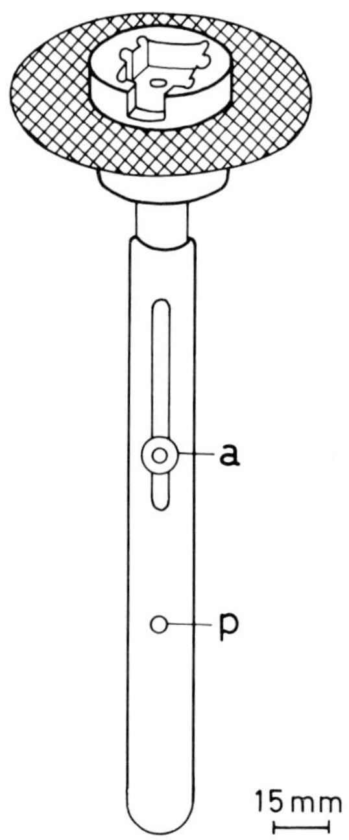

Fig. 4. Equipment for cooling of object support during the loading with frozen specimens. Teflon container is surrounded by a fine metal net which prevents specimens from dropping to the bottom of the flask. The profile of the teflon container provides better contact with liquid N_2 with the specimen support. The container is mounted on a supporting stage similar to that in Fig. 2 A. *a*, vertical adjustment; *p*, perforation

surface and the upper border of the golden discs. This is necessary in order to ensure the firm contact of the discs to the receptacles and the cover (Fig. 3 B) of the object support.

With the precooled manipulator (Fig. 3 D) the loaded specimen support can now be introduced through a small door into the vacuum chamber and fixed on the cooling table (–150 °C). It should be emphasized that handling of the specimen holders, i.e., the transfer from the Dewar flask to the cooling table should be done as quickly as possible in order to prevent frozen specimens from warming up.

Fracturing of the tissue is usually performed in several steps in a vacuum more than 2×10^{-6} Torr. Rough cutting to approach the desired plane of sectioning is made at a temperature of cryotome table and knife (a very strong razor blade) below –160 °C. Then the table is warmed up to –110 °C and the final 2–3 fine cuts are made as slowly as possible so that the removed material forms a fine powder. At this moment and during the period of etching and coating the vacuum should be 10^{-6} Torr or more.

After the final cut the LN_2-cooled knifeholder is kept for 5 min over the surface of the specimen; in this position, the holder acts as a shroud. During etching the evaporation equipment is prepared for the replication. Following this the Pt-C film (2.5–3 nm in thickness) and the carbon backing (25–30 nm) are formed and the specimens removed after about 5 min which are needed to cool down the hot guns. During this period the specimen temperature is lowered to −150 °C. Then, the vacuum chamber is vented with dry nitrogen gas, which prevents ice formation at cold surfaces inside the chamber.

3.4 Removal and Cleaning of Replica

The object support is removed from the apparatus and the specimen holders are transferred to methanol (extracting lipids from the tissue) where the specimens are carefully removed from the holders. The specimens are further processed after at least 4 h. The replicas with attached tissue are passed successfully through a series of solvents. It is convenient to handle these small blocks by aspirating them into the tip of a Pasteur pipette. From 100% methanol, the specimens are passed through 50% methanol to double-distilled water which is exchanged 4 times. Then, the specimens are transferred through 10% into a 35% filtered solution of chromic acid anhydride which is subsequently warmed to 40°–50 °C in a thermostat. The dissolution at this temperature is completed in about 1–3 h (first control after 1 h). The replicas are then passed with the pipette through at least five changes of distilled water in order to remove any residual chromic acid crystals. For most tissues a subsequent treatment with chlorox for about 30 min can be recommended. The metallic replicas sink to the bottom as they are clean. After another careful washing in double-distilled water they are mounted on coarse meshed copper grids coated with a formvar film.

4 Interpretation

In the early days of freeze-etching it was generally assumed that the fracture plane would follow the surface between cell membrane and the cytoplasm or between the cell membrane and the extracellular space. However, Branton (1966) pointed out that the membrane fracture faces are non-etchable and that a small ridge can be observed, representing the second half of membrane which has been partially removed by cleaving. In addition, it became possible to expose the true surfaces of cells in aqueous media by etching and to distinguish between membrane surface and fracture face of erythrocyte ghosts by the help of ferritin labelling (Pinto da Silva and Branton 1970). An excellent review of the subject has been provided by Bullivant (1973), who has studied the complementary fracture faces of membranes by means of the double-replica technique. Today, membrane surfaces (S) and membrane fracture faces (F) can be clearly differentiated, and the nomenclature established by Branton et al. (1975) has become generally accepted (Fig. 5).

The membrane fracture face through which one's view is directed towards the cytoplasm is labelled P face (PF).

This holds true whether the outer leaflet of the cytolemma or the inner leaflet of an intracytoplasmic organelle is removed. In both instances, we are looking towards the cytoplasm and thus the membrane face is a P face.

The true membrane surface adjacent to the cytoplasm is the P surface (PS), that bounding the extracellular space is the E surface (ES). The membrane leaflet which is closest to the extracellular space exposes a fracture face which is designated as E face (EF). This also holds true for the removal of the external leaflet of an intracellular organelle.

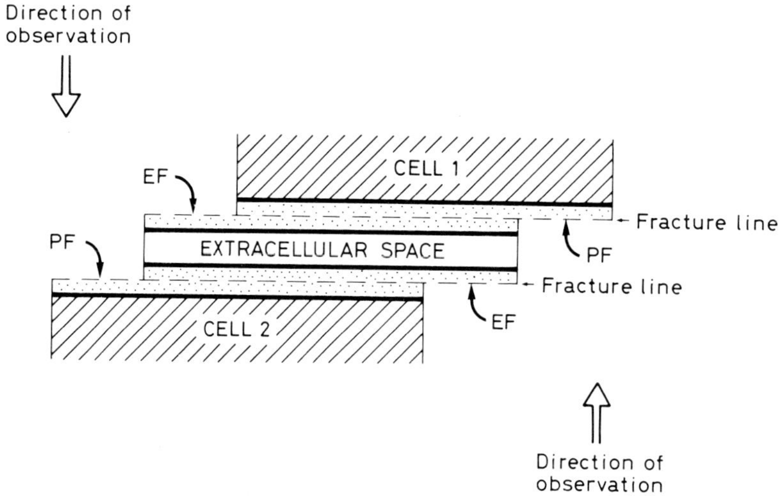

Fig. 5. Nomenclature of membrane fracture faces according to Branton et al. (1975). *PF,* Plasmatic face; *EF,* External face

5 Artifacts

Artifacts can occur in each of the preparational steps in the freeze-etching technique. A most helpful analysis and documentation of the major sources of failures is given by Böhler (1975). According to our experience with nerve tissue we would like to emphasize the following types of artifacts:

5.1 Artifacts Caused by Cryoprotectants

The most frequent effects of glycerol are the swelling of mitochondria, the vesiculation of the membranes of the endoplasmic reticulum, the aggregation of intramembranous particles into clusters (Fig. 6), and the formation of blisters at the cytolemma (McIntyre et al. 1974). These artifacts can be prevented by tissue fixation with aldehydes.

5.2 Artifacts Arising During Freezing

If the freezing rate is very slow, the cells are dehydrated by extracellular ice formation. The result is a general deformation by considerable shrinkage of the cells (Figs. 7, 11). Cells frozen at an average speed (less than 100 °C/s) do not change their shape. However, intracellular freezing of the cell water destroys the cytoplasmic membrane systems. The higher the water content of the cell, the greater is the danger of ice crystal formation (Moor 1964); it can be minimized only by the use of cryoprotectants.

Recrystallization is due to the warming of the specimen above the recrystallization point. It may occur during slow transfer of the specimen to the object support or when transporting the specimen with a warm forceps, or it may be due to covering the object support of the cooling table with the warm metal cover etc. Freezing damage due to recrystallization is caused by careless work or insufficient equipment (Fig. 8).

5.3 Artifacts Arising During Fracturing

Relatively deep fracture steps may arise primarily when fracturing the frozen tissue with a large knife advance. Less trivial is the displacement of tissue fragments on the fractured surface of the specimen, e.g., occasional remains of material sticking to

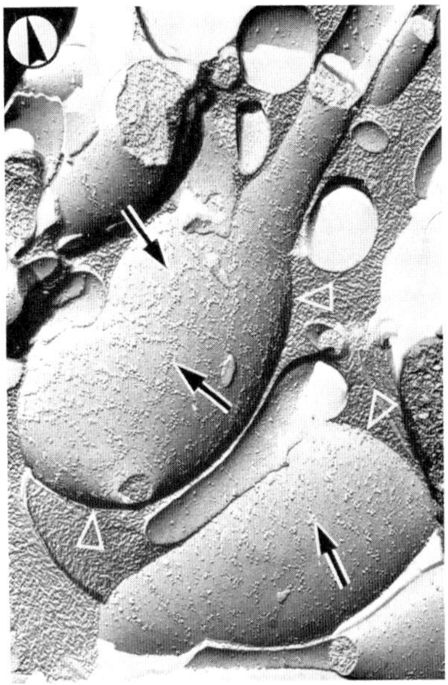

6

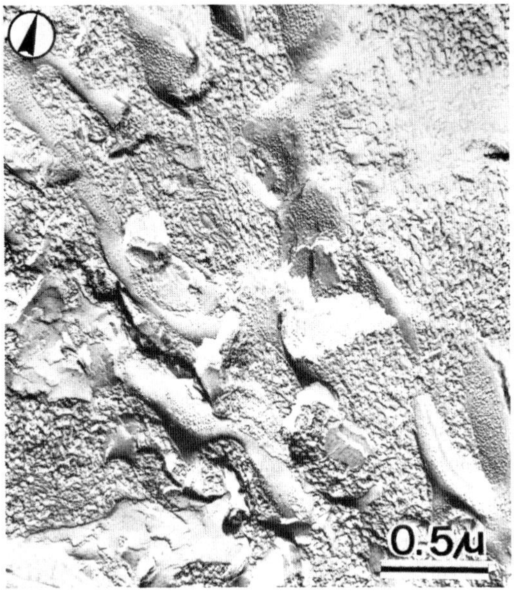

7

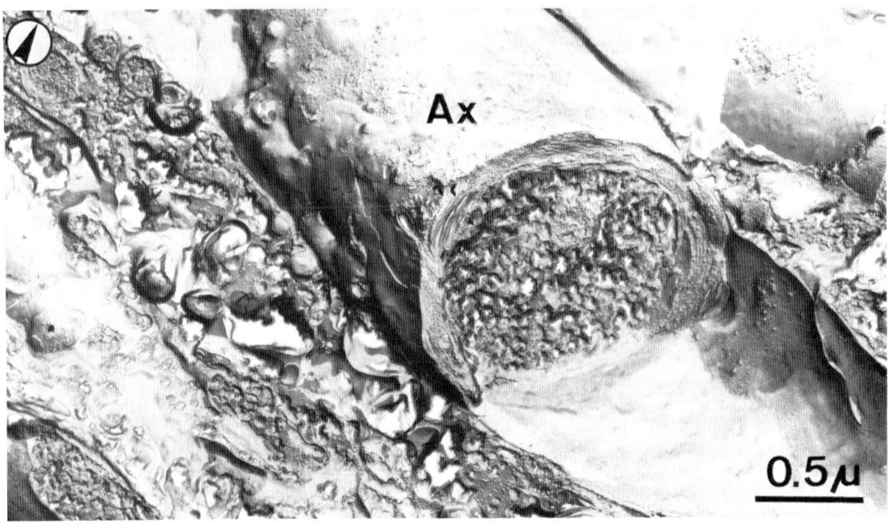

8

Fig. 6. Artifactual aggregation of membrane particles (*arrows*) under the influence of cryoprotectant (glycerol 25%). This effect is usually observed in unfixed tissue. Aldehyde fixation is known to prevent this effect. The swelling of dendrites or glial processes (*arrow-head*) may also be due to cryoprotectant. Pigeon tectum opticum, unfixed tissues. (*Encircled arrows* in this and the following electronmicrographs indicate the angle of shadow casting)

Fig. 7. Extracellular ice crystal formation due to slow freezing rate in the frog neuromuscular endplate. The remaining membrane fragments represent junctional folds

Fig. 8. The product of recrystallization caused by a brief raising of the temperature above −110 °C during transfer of frozen tissue to the cryotome or due to insufficient thermal contact between object support and specimen holder. The ice crystals have lead to the partial destruction of the axon (*Ax*). Cat, spinal cord

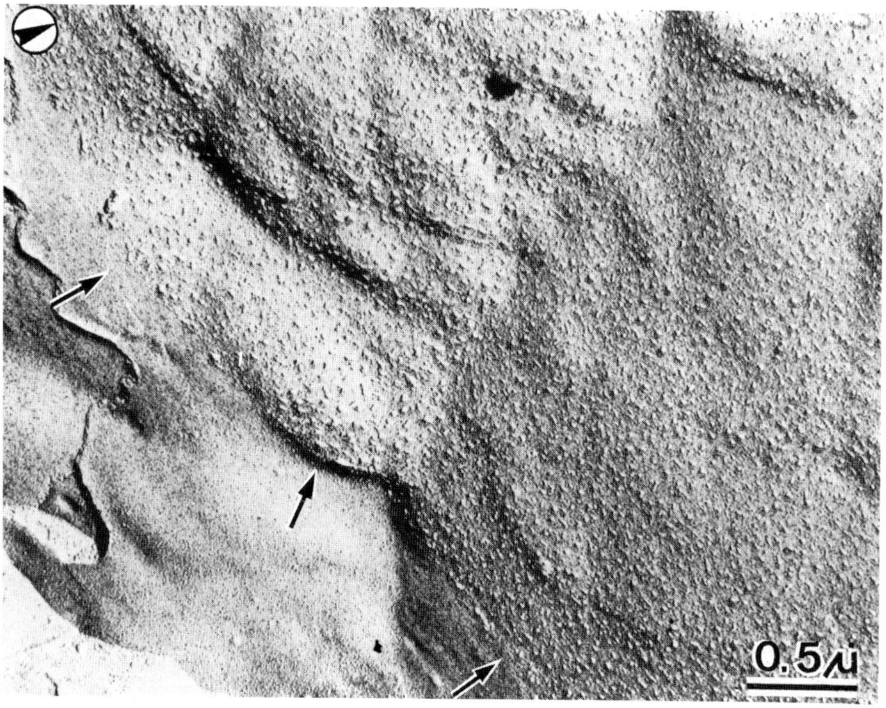

9

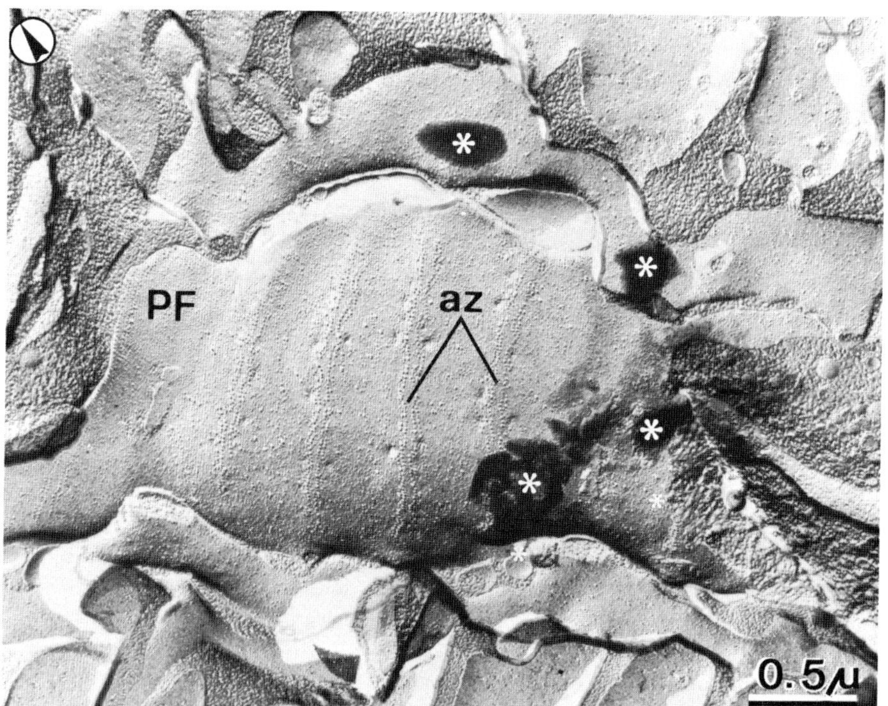

10

the knife are swept across the specimen surface and accumulate at an edge of the fractured tissue. The displaced material is etched and replicated and appears as flakes and tiny chips on the membrane faces. Unfortunately, this type of artifact can hardly be avoided.

In addition, such material has lost the thermal contact with the cooled specimen and therefore will rewarm and expel gases which my condense on fracture faces (Fig. 9) and produce particle-like artifacts.

5.4 Artifacts Caused by Sublimation and Condensation

The lack of temperature control during freeze-etching procedures may lead to high temperatures of the specimen during etching. As a consequence very deep cavities may arise which are "decorated" with remaining glycerol. Such artifacts can only be prevented by applying adequate temperature control equipment.

Deep etching may cause dark borders of organelles. The formation of dark borders can be prevented by shortening the etching time and lowering the specimen temperature.

Condensation of water vapor on the specimen surface: The main residual gas in high vacuum systems is water. An object temperature colder than $-110\,°C$ or a vacuum pressure lower than 10^{-6} Torr provide condensation during the etching procedure. At places with reduced saturation pressure (e.g., small holes), condensation may take place while etching conditions are maintained. The product of water condensation may be particles resembling membrane structures.

The condensation of water vapor on the specimen can be reduced by selecting a suitable specimen temperature in relation to the attainable vacuum, by carefully protecting the specimen with the knife-holder, used as a shroud during etching, or by immediate coating of the freshly prepared freeze-fractured surface.

5.5 Artifacts Arising During Replication

Insufficient shadowing: Contrast and resolving power of a replica can be noteably increased by shadow casting. Conveniently, a platinum-carbon mixture is applied. If the ratio of platinum to carbon in the shadowing film is too low, the picture will exhibit poor contrast and fine structural details will be lost.

Too heavy shadowing: in order to achieve optimal results with platinum-carbon shadowing, not only the ratio of platinum and carbon but also the thickness of the coat must be carefully balanced. If the platinum electrode is exhausted the carbon predominates in the film giving rise to black specks (Fig. 11). If the shadowing film is too thick, fine specimen details are masked.

Shadowing angle: The correct angle of shadowing is of great importance. If the shadowing angle is too steep small structural details may be completely submerged by the evaporated film and no longer be identified. On the other hand, low shadowing angles may blur the fracture lines

Fig. 9. Contamination which originates from tissue debris produced during cutting. Such debris have lost thermal contact with the specimen; they consequently warm up and evaporate water and other constituents which eventually condense on fracture faces. The contaminated area is clearly limited (*arrows*). The clean area exhibits fine electron dense grains which are due to recrystallization of platinum. Sternarchus, electric organ

Fig. 10. Insufficient cleaning of replica: Electron dense areas (*asterisks*) are produced by undissolved tissue remnants adhering to the replica. Frog neuromuscular endplate. Note the P-face with linearly arranged active zones (*az*)

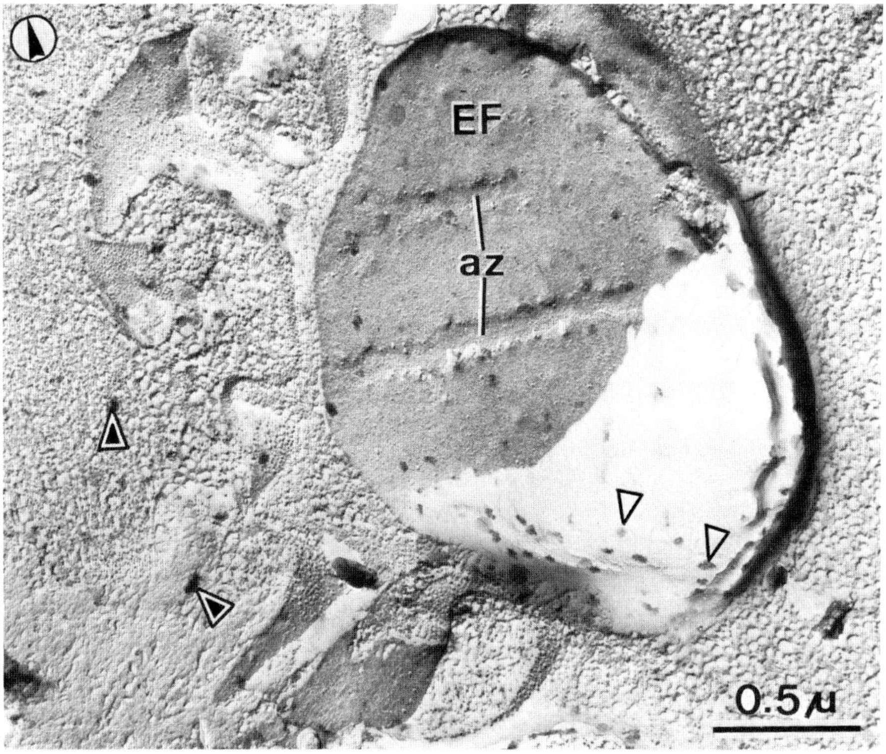

11

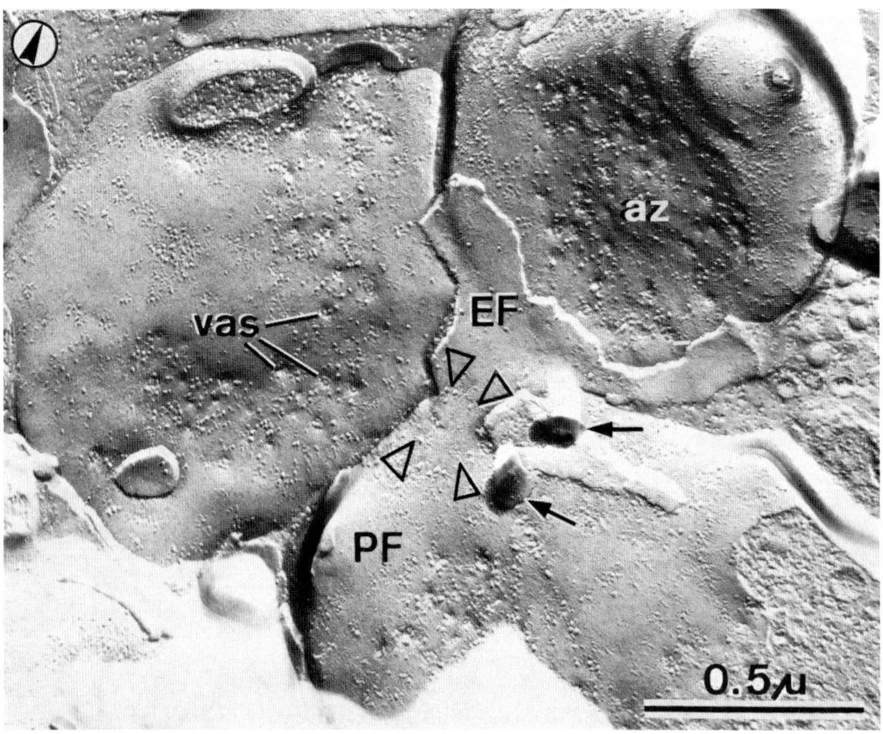

12

across membrane leaflets (Fig. 12). The optimum shadowing angle may vary considerably from specimen to specimen.

Recrystallization of the shadowing film: If a specimen replica which has been shadowed with platinum-carbon is examined in the electron microscope at an excessive beam intensity it may warm up so much that the platinum recrystallizes. Thus, platinum crystals may be seen in the micrograph as small black grains (Fig. 9). The formation of platinum crystals can be avoided by reducing the beam intensity.

5.6 Artifacts Arising From Insufficient Cleaning of the Replica

Residues of the specimen on the replica may occur as a consequence of insufficient cleaning. These residues appear as black spots on the photograph (Fig. 10).

Acknowledgments. This work was supported by grants of the Swiss National Foundation for Scientific Research Nr. 3.611.75 and 3.636.75, the Dr. Eric Slack-Gyr Foundation, The Hartmann-Müller Foundation, and the EMDO Stiftung in Zürich.

Addendum. The freeze-etching procedure described in this chapter has recently been significantly advanced by a new technique which is based on high pressure (2100 bars) freezing. This procedure obviates the use of aldehyde fixatives and cryoprotectants and facilitates deep etching. The formation of large ice crystals is prevented in tissue blocks up to 0.5 mm in thickness. The reader is referred to Moor, H, et al., Cell Tiss. Res. 209:201–216 (1980).

6 References

Akert K, Moor H, Pfenninger K, Sandri C (1969) Contributions of new impregnation methods and freeze-etching to the problems of synaptic fine structure. Prog Brain Res 31:223–240

Bachmann L, Schmitt WW (1971) Improved cryofixation applicable to freeze-etching. Proc Natl Acad Sci USA 68:2149–2152

Benedetti EL, Favard P (eds) (1973) Freeze-etching techniques and applications. Société Française de Microscopie Electronique, Paris

Bischoff A, Moor H (1967 a) Ultrastructural differences between the myelin sheaths of peripheral nerve fibres and CNS white matter. Z Zellforsch 81:303–310

Bischoff A, Moor H (1967 b) The ultrastructure of the "difference factor" in the myelin. Z Zellforsch 81:571–580

Böhler S (1975) Artifacts and specimen preparation faults in freeze-etch technology. Balzers Aktiengesellschaft für Hochvakuumtechnik und Dünne Schichten, Liechtenstein, pp 1–37

Branton D (1966) Fracture faces of frozen membranes. Proc Natl Acad Sci USA 55:1048–1056

Branton D, Bullivant S, Gilula NB, Karnovsky MJ, Moor H, Mühlethaler K, Northcote DH, Packer L, Satir B, Satir P, Speth V, Staehelin LA, Steere RL, Weinstein RS (1975) Freeze-etching nomenclature. Science 190:54–56

Bullivant S (1973) Freeze-etching and freeze-fracturing. In: Koehler JK (ed) Advanced techniques in biological electron microscopy. Springer, New York Heidelberg Berlin, pp 67–112

Bullivant S (1974) Freeze-etching techniques applied to biological membranes. Philos Trans R Soc Lond [Biol] 268:5–14

Chalcroft JP, Bullivant S (1970) An interpretation of liver cell membrane and junction structure based on observation of freeze-fracture replicas of both sides of the fracture. J Cell Biol 47:49–60

Fig. 11. Replica contaminated with dark spots (*arrowheads*) which are the product of an exhausted platinum carbon electrode. Note also the extracellular ice crystal formation due to slow freezing (cf. Fig. 6). Frog neuromuscular endplate; E-face with active zones (*az*)

Fig. 12. Blurring of fracture lines (*between arrowheads*). The normal rim representing the fracture step between inner and outer membrane leaflet has disappeared. Instead there is a smooth transition between E- and P-faces. Possibly, inadequate fixation may also contribute to this effect. Note the contamination by two tiny tissue remnants (*arrows*). Rat, spinal cord; Presynaptic terminals with active zones (*az*). *vas*, vesicle attachment sites

Heuser JE, Reese TS, Landis DMD (1976) Preservation of synaptic structure by rapid freezing. Cold Spring Harbor Symp Quant Biol 40: 17–24

Heuser JE, Reese TS, Dennis MJ, Jan Y, Jan L, Evans L (1979) Synaptic vesicle exocytosis captured by quick-freezing and correlated with quantal transmitter release. J Cell Biol 81: 275–300

McIntyre JA, Gilula NB, Karnovsky MJ (1974) Cryoprotectant-induced redistribution of intramembranous particles in mouse lymphocytes. J Cell Biol 60: 192–203

Moor H (1964) Die Gefrierfixation lebender Zellen und ihre Anwendung in der Elektronenmikroskopie. Z Zellforsch 62: 546–580

Moor H (1971) Recent progress in the freeze-etching technique. Philos Trans Soc Lond [Biol] 261: 121–131

Moor H (1973) Cryotechnology for the structural analysis of biological material. In: Benedetti EL, Favard P (eds) Freeze etching-techniques and applications. Société Française de Microscopie Electronique, Paris, pp 11–19

Moor H (1977) Limitations and prospects of freeze-fixation and freeze-etching. Thirty-Fifth Annual EMSA Meeting, pp 334–337

Moor H, Mühlethaler K (1963) Fine structure in frozen-etched yeast cells. J Cell Biol 17: 609–628

Mühlethaler K (1973) History of freeze-etching. In: Benedetti EL, Favard P (eds) Freeze-etching techniques and applications. Société Française de Microscopie Electronique, Paris, pp 1–10

Mühlethaler K, Hauenstein W, Moor H (1973) Double fracturing method for freeze-etching. In: Benedetti EL, Favard P (eds) Freeze-etching techniques and applications. Société Française de Microscopie Electronique, Paris, pp 101–106

Orci L, Perrelet A (1975) Freeze-etch histology. A comparison between thin sections and freeze-etch replicas. Springer, Berlin Heidelberg New York, p 168

Peters A, Palay S, de Webster HF (1976) The fine structure of the nervous system: The neurons and supporting cells. Saunders, Philadelphia London Toronto, p 406

Pfenninger KH, Rinderer ER (1975) Methods for the freeze-fracturing of nerve tissue cultures and cell monolayers. J Cell Biol 65: 15–28

Pinto da Silva P, Branton D (1970) Membrane splitting in freeze-etching. J Cell Biol 45: 598–605

Riehle U (1968) Über die Vitrifizierung verdünnter wäßriger Lösungen. Dissertation, ETH Zürich

Sandri C, Van Buren JM, Akert K (1977) Membrane morphology of the vertebrate nervous system. A study with freeze-etch technique. Prog Brain Res 46, p 384

Steere RL (1973) Preparation of high-resolution freeze-etch, freeze-fracture, frozen-surface, and freeze-dried replicas in a single freeze-etch module, and the use of stereo electron microscopy to obtain maximum information from them. In: Benedetti EL, Favard P (eds) Freeze-etching techniques and applications. Société Française de Microscopie Electronique, Paris, pp 223–255

Streit P, Akert K, Sandri C, Livingston RB, Moor H (1972) Dynamic ultrastructure of presynaptic membranes at nerve terminals in the spinal cord of rats. Anesthetized and unanesthetized preparations compared. Brain Res 48: 11–26

Tokunaga A, Sandri C, Akert K (1979 a) Ultrastructural effects of 4-aminopyridine on the presynaptic membrane in the rat spinal cord. Brain Res 163: 1–8

Tokunaga A, Sandri C, Akert K (1979 b) Increase of large intermembranous particles in the presynaptic active zone after administration of 4-aminopyridine. Brain Res 174: 207–219

Tokunaga A, Akert K, Sandri C (1979 c) Three types of membrane modulations during transmitter release in rat spinal cord synapses. Neurosci Lett 12: 147–152

Venzin M, Sandri C, Akert K, Wyss UR (1977) Membrane associated particles of the presynaptic active zone in rat spinal cord. A morphometric analysis. Brain Res 130: 393–404

Chapter 4

General Methods in Scanning Electron Microscopy of the Nervous System

K. Meller

1 Introduction

The scanning electron microscope (SEM) allows one to obtain a three-dimensional representation of biological structures. In this way the SEM study of nervous structures may have filled the gap between the information provided by the classic Golgi-technique and the fine structural data supplied by transmission electron microscopy. One drawback of the SEM is that it provides most information about free surfaces; these surfaces however, such as the ventricular surface, cover only a small portion of nervous tissue. The achievement of optimal preserved internal regions of the nervous system and the observation of not naturally occurring surfaces is still the object of SEM methodological efforts. The present accomplishments of the SEM technique are not restricted by the resolution power of the microscope but rather by the unsolved problems concerning the preparation of specimens.

As pointed out by Boyde and Wood (1969) three important points must be considered when preparing biological specimens: (1) the necessity of preparing all surfaces to be observed free of contamination with extraneous matter, (2) the problems inherent in obtaining surfaces that reveal the internal organization and (3) the problems of dehydrating the tissues but avoiding significant shrinkage.

Furthermore, good topographic pictures of specimen surfaces can be obtained only if the surface to be examined conducts electricity and is homogeneous in regard to secondary electron emission.

These problems are also characteristic of the preparation procedures for nervous tissues. Despite the existence of the "free surfaces" of the ventricular system and of many sensory organs (olfactory mucosa, retina, cochlea, etc.), creating surfaces by means of blunt dissection, freeze-fracturing or sectioning allows only a limited preservation of cell structures. All methods directed toward examining the nervous system in situ have encountered serious technical difficulties. The complicated organization of neuropil with long cell prolongations and the characteristic cell arborizations of neural elements easily become distorted. Consequently, one often encounters a disparity of results upon examination of SEM reports dealing with the structure of ventricular walls and other regions of the nervous system (Seymour and Berry 1979) (see Tables 1–4).

2 Methods

2.1 Fixation

In general the fixation procedure for SEM requires the same quality of tissue preservation as for the transmission electron microscopy (TEM). For this reason the fixation methods utilized for SEM are essentially the same as those employed for TEM, and the wealth of experience gathered during two decades of TEM procedures has been very useful. The fixed specimens are often submitted to both procedures for comparative studies (Scott et al. 1973 b; Scott and Paull 1978). In order to localize a given structure accurately it is necessary to examine the same specimen using the SEM first and then embed it in resin for thin sectioning for TEM study. Glutaraldehyde or glutaraldehyde-paraformaldehyde mixtures (frequently the Karnovsky method) are usually utilized for all types of specimens. Glutaraldehyde is used at concentrations of 1%–3% followed by a postfixation in 1%–2% osmium tetroxide. Thin specimens as in the case of tissue cultures, can be fixed with osmium vapours (Boyde et al. 1968). The best results are obtained when fixation is accomplished by vascular perfusion of the experimental animals, whereas embryological specimens are currently fixed by immersion. Many authors (Borit and Sidman 1972; Peters 1974; Phillips et al. 1974, Scott et al. 1976; Coates 1977; Paull et al. 1977; Walsh et al. 1978) extend the fixation time to overnight or to even longer to make the tissue more stable for subsequent procedures (dehydration, critical point drying).

2.2 Dehydration

The first SEM reports dealing with biological material described a dehydration procedure involving successive series of concentrations of alcohols or acetone and finally air or vacuum drying (see Tables 1–4). This procedure produces major changes in the three-dimensional arrangement of the specimens due to the forces exerted by the surface tension at the interface between liquid and gas. The critical point drying technique as described by Anderson (1966) avoids damaging the specimens and the formation of surface artifacts by drying them. The critical point drying technique entails substituting tissue water by a dehydrating liquid and then by a gas under pressure in the liquid phase. At a specific pressure and temperature a liquid exists only in the fluid phase the surface tension of which is zero. When the pressure and the temperature of the critical point drying are biologically acceptable (as in the case of carbon dioxide), the specimens can dry without appreciable distortion. Since the water in the specimens is not miscible with carbon dioxide (or Freon/Frigen) the specimens must be passed through a series of miscible liquids. The procedure consists of the following steps (Anderson 1966):

1. Dehydration of specimens in a series of alcohols.
2. Substitution of the 100% alcohol by ascending mixtures of alcohol-amyl acetate (3 : 1, 1 : 1, 1 : 3, 0 : 1).
3. Placement of the specimens in a critical point bomb completely filled with amyl acetate.

4. Substitution of the amyl acetate by carbon dioxide in the liquid state. The temperature in the pressure vessel is approximately 25 °C or lower.
5. After complete substitution, the temperature in the bomb is raised to 45 °C (the pressure inside reaches 130 atm.). The gaseous CO_2 is then allowed to escape slowly from the pressure vessel (this prevents cooling by expansion) until the pressure in the bomb decreases to 1 atm.

The critical point method recommended by Fromme et al. (1972) is similar to that of Anderson:

1. Dehydration of specimens in a graded series of acetones (also methanol)
2. Substitution of acetone by ascending mixtures of acetone-Frigen 11.
3. Substitution of Frigen 11 by Frigen 13 in the pressure vessel.

After critical point drying the specimens are extremely fragile and hygroscopic. For observation in the microscope they must be mounted on a specimen holder with double-faced adhesive tape. The specimens then are coated with a conductive layer by means of evaporation or by the more recent sputtering method. In a recent paper Cohen (1979) gives a detailed description of the critical point drying method that should be consulted. An alternative to critical point drying of biological specimens is freeze-drying, especially indispensable when analytical methods are employed in SEM studies. This procedure, as thoroughly described by Anderson (1966) and Boyde and Wood (1969), is not yet widely used by neurobiologists (see Tables 1–4) and can only be recommended for the study of small specimens. The use of large specimens as is usually the case in SEM studies, makes it difficult to avoid the formation of large ice crystals with subsequent changes in the structure of specimens.

2.3 Examination of Not Naturally Occurring Surfaces

The study of the parenchyma of the nervous system with the SEM is still plagued by many unsolved methodological problems. One easy procedure is fracturing or dissecting the specimens after fixation. Applying this method, good results are obtained only with embryological material and then only in restricted regions of the nervous system, such as the retina, the cerebral hemispheres, and the medulla. Greater difficulties are encountered in the dissection of cell- and fiber-rich zones, such as in the cerebellum or in the olfactory bulb. The retina can be rent between two fine forceps and the cerebral hemisphere can be cut into sections with a blunt rasor blade. The results are not reproducible and of varying quality. The desired plane of section may be obtained only after many patient and diligent attempts. Fracturing should be performed after fixation when the specimens have been placed in 70% alcohol. Fractures performed after critical point drying become very irregular and the cell prolongations are often amputated.

Despite all mechanical techniques available, the adult nervous system presents the investigator with a considerable number of troublesome handicaps. It is not surprising, therefore, that methods have not yet been adopted for routine analysis. The lack of reproducibility in fracturing, the consequent damage of tissue and the disturbed intercellular relations are not conducive to the fruitful study of neuroanatomical problems.

2.4 Sectioning and Embedding Methods

Brown et al. (1976), in an attempt to avoid the mechanical distortion caused by dissection techniques, proposed sectioning tissue with a Sorvall TC-2 "Smith & Farquhar" tissue sectioner subsequent to fixation with glutaraldehyde and postfixation. During sectioning the dessication of the specimens must be prevented. The sections were treated according to the technique of Kelley et al. (1973) and conventionally dehydrated (critical point drying). Paraffin sections (Faltin et al. 1974) whose wax has been removed and which have been coated with metal and observed in the scanning electron microscope provide only a rough overview of topographical cell relations. The amount of new information obtained from such sections is rather limited.

Other embedding techniques seem more promising for the future. Mestres and Rascher (1977) proposed the immersion of specimens (e.g., rat brains) after fixation in a mixture of 3% glutaraldehyde and 2% paraformaldehyde (solution satured with O_2). After an inclusion in agar-agar sectioning was accomplished with a tissue sectioner. Cell fragments and debris were removed from sections with a delicate paintbrush. Following the usual dehydration in methanol, the critical point drying method with Freon 13 was applied.

Alexander et al. (1973) following studies of Barber and Boyde (1968) and Cleveland and Schneider (1969) propose embedding in plastics to maintain the cytoarchitecture of tissues and then eroding the surface. This method, also used in our laboratory, provided optimal conservation of topographical relationships in neuropil zones of the nervous system in young animals. This procedure is not complicated and makes critical point drying unnecessary. The following important steps must be observed: 1) After fixation in glutaraldehyde and osmium postfixation the specimens are dehydrated through graded alcohols and become impregnated in a mixture of araldite-epoxypropane overnight. 2) After a short polymerisation at 60 °C, the specimens are broken between two forceps or cut with a blunt rasor blade in the desired plane. The resin is then removed from the surface with acetone and subsequently returned to the incubator at 60 °C for 48 h.

The use of resins for the SEM study of vascular relationships has produced satisfactory results in the laboratory of Miodonski et al. (1979). This author studied the vascularization of the choroid plexus using low viscosity resins. After the vascular system has been flushed with a saline solution and the injected resin has polymerized, the tissues are digested with an 18%–20% sodium oxide solution.

Tanaka (1972) proposed a method for observing the inner structures of cells. After glutaraldehyde fixation, postosmication, the specimens are dehydrated in a series of alcohols and propylenoxide and placed in gelatin capsules containing an epoxy resin (Cemedine) without addition of a catalyst. After hardening of the resin at 30 °C for 1–2 h, the capsules are cracked open with a hammer and chisel. The resin is removed with propylene from the free surfaces of the tissues. The specimens are then critical point dried and the broken surfaces coated.

3 Applications

3.1 The Study of the Ependymal Surface

Table 1 shows that most of the authors who have studied the ependymal surface with SEM employed the fixation, perfusion, and the critical point drying methods described above. Despite this, a considerable number of authors simultaneously

Fig. 1. A Surface view of the choroid plexus (20-day-old chick embryo) (courtesy of S. el Gammal). The *arrow* shows an epiplexus cell, critical point drying with Frigen 13. ×6500 **B** Portion of the cortex plate of a mouse embryo, 12.5 days old, obtained by blunt dissection after fixation in glutaraldehyde, critical point drying with Frigen 13. ×9000

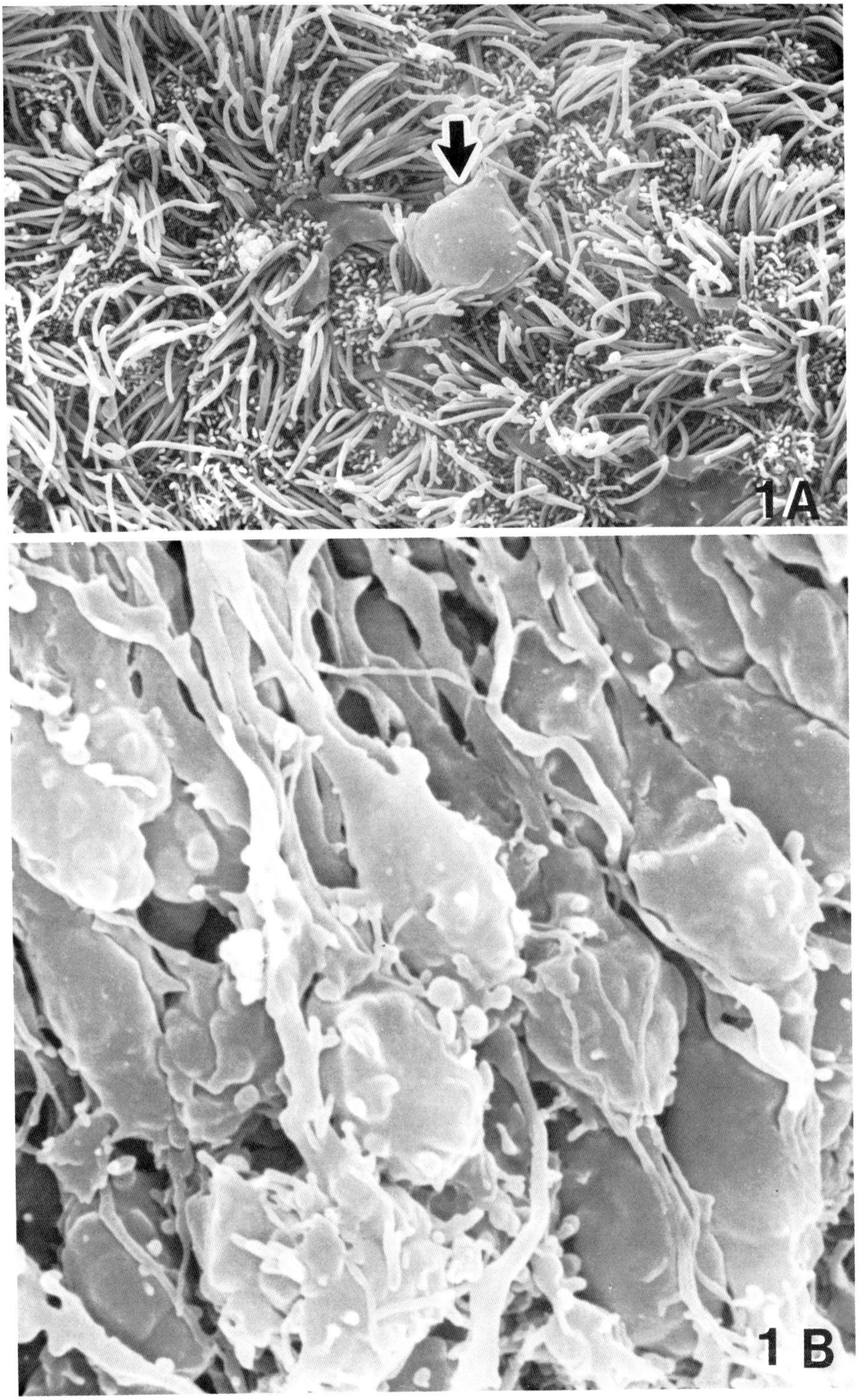
1A
1 B

Table 1. Studies on ependymal surface

Author	Fixation	Postfixation
Allen and Low (1973)	Perfusion Karnovsky	2% Os 30′
Azzam and Trow (1976)	G	
Bleier (1975)	Immersion 2% G, 2% para F 1 h	Os
Borit and Sidman (1972)	Perfusion Karnovsky – 10% F (overnight)	
Bruni et al. (1977)	Perfusion 1.3% F/2.5% G – immersion 2 h	1% Os
Clementi and Marini (1972)	Perfusion 2% F – 2% G 1 h	
Coates (1977)	4% para F/0.5% G (overnight)	
Collins and Morriss (1975)	Perfusion 1% para F + 1% G/1% Karnovsky 2 h overnight	1% Os 2 h
Cupedo (1977)	Perfusion 2% G (overnight)	Os vapour 3 days
Dellmann and Simpson (1976)	Perfusion 5% G 2 h	1% Os
Dellmann (1978)	Immersion/perfusion 2 h 5% G	1% Os 1 h
Dempsey (1973)	Immersion 3% G	Os
De Waele et al. (1974)	Immersion 3.9% G (4 days)	
Dierickx et al. (1972)	Immersion G 1 h 3′	
Hannah and Geber (1977)	Immersion 3% para F, 0.5% G, 2.5% dimethylsulfoxide or: 3% G	16% glycerin 24 h
Hetzel (1978)	Immersion/perfusion 2.5% G/Karnovsky 4 h/several days	2% Os 2 h
Hirunagi and Yasuda (1979)	Perfusion 1% para F/0.5% G/4% para F	1% Os
Jacobs and Monroe (1977)	Perfusion Karnovsky 6 h	–
Klara and Brizzee (1977)	Perfusion 1% G – 1% para F 24 h	Os
Kozlowski et al. (1972)	Ventricular perfusion Karnovsky 4 h	1% Os 3 – 4 h
Kozlowski et al. (1973)	Ventricular perfusion Karnovsky 4 h	1% Os 3 – 4 h
Krisch et al. (1978)	Perfusion 3.5% G	
Leonhardt and Lindemann (1973a)	Perfusion 3.5% G	
Leonhardt and Lindemann (1973b)	Perfusion 3.5% G 20′	
Leslie et al. (1978)	Perfusion 0.5% G – 4% F 2 – 24 h	Os
Lindberg and Talanti (1975)	Immersion 2.5% G 1 h	1% Os 2 h
Lindberg et al. (1977)	Immersion 2.5% G 3 h	1% Os 2 h
Mikami and Asari (1978)	Perfusion Karnovsky – immersion 6 h	1% Os 4 h
Nelson and Wright (1974)	G 1 – 3%	1% Os
Noack et al. (1972)	Perfusion 2.3% G 30′	
Paull et al. (1977)	Perfusion 2% G + 2% para F (overnight)	Os
Peters (1974)	Perfusion 1.25% G/1% para F – 5% G/ 4% para F overnight	1% Os
Phillips et al. (1974)	Perfusion – ventricular perfusion 25% G (overnight)	0.1% Os 4 – 8 h
Ribas (1977)	Perfusion Karnovsky	
Scott and Paull (1978)	Perfusion Karnovsky	Os
Scott et al. (1972)	Karnovsky	1% Os 4 h
Scott et al. (1973a)	Karnovsky 36 h	1% Os
Scott et al. (1974)	Ventricular perfusion Karnovsky 48 h	
Scott et al. (1976)	Perfusion Karnovsky/ventricular perfusion	Os
Scott et al. (1977)	Perfusion Karnovsky/ventricular perfusion (overnight)	Os
Takei et al. (1978)	Immersion G/perfusion Karnovsky/ventricular perfus.	1% Os
Vigh et al. (1977)	Perfusion 5/6% G 15 – 20′	
Walsh et al. (1978)	Perfusion 3% G (overnight)	2% Os 2 h
Weindl and Schinko (1975)	Perfusion Karnovsky	Os THC
Weindl et al. (1975)	Perfusion Karnovsky	1% Os 2 h

Abbreviations: G, glutaraldehyde; F, formaldehyde; CP, critical point; Os, osmium tetroxide.

Preparation for SEM		Material	Animal
Drying	Coating		
Ethanol amyl-acetate CP CO_2	C-Au-Pd	Lateral ventricle	Dog
		Lateral ventricle	Rat
Ethanol amyl-acetate CP CO_2	Au-Pd	IIIrd ventricle	Mouse
Freeze-dried	Au	Ependymal surface	Mouse
Alcohol CP CO_2	Au	Ependymal surface	Rabbit
Alcohol, vacuum dried	Au-Pt	Ependymal surface	Cat
CP Freon/CO_2	C-Au-Pd/Au	IIIrd ventricle	Monkey
Acetone CP CO_2	C-Au-Pd	Choroid plexus	Rat
Acetone CP Freon 13	Au	Ependymal surface	Rat
Ethanol amyl-acetate CP	Au-Pd/Cr	Subfornical organ	Rat
CP	C-Au	Subfornical organ	Frog
Freeze-dried	Au-Pd	Area postrema	Rat
Acetone CP CO_2	Pd	IIIrd ventricle	Frog
Ethanol air dried		Tuber cinereum	Frog
Ethanol CP CO_2	Au-Pd	IIIrd ventricle	Hamster
Ethanol CP	Au	Ependymal surface	Rabbit
Ethanol CP CO_2	Au	IVth ventricle	Domestic fowl
Acetone CP CO_2	Au-Pd	Ependymal surface	Armadillo
Ethanol CP CO_2	Au/Au-Pd	Area postrema	Cat
Ethanol air dried	C/Au-Pd	Lateral ventricle	Sheep
Ethanol air dried	C/Au-Pd	IIIrd ventricle	Sheep
Ethanol CP Frigen 13		IVth ventricle	Rat
Alcohol Frigen 11 CP Frigen 13	C-Au	Subfornical organ	Rabbit
Alcohol CP Frigen 13	C-Au	Ependymal surface	Rabbit
Acetone CP	Au-Pd	Area postrema	Cat
Aethyl-alcohol CP	C-Au	Subfornical organ	Cow
Ethanol CP	C-Au	Lateral ventricle	Rat
Ethanol CP CO_2	C/Au/Pd	Subfornical organ	Japanese quail
Ethanol CP CO_2	C-Au	Ependyma – choroid plexus	Frog
Acetone – air dried	Au	Lateral ventricle	Cat
Alcohol CP Freon 113	Au	IIIrd ventricle	Rat
Acetone CP CO_2	Au-Pd	Choroid plexus	Rat
Alcohol CP	Au-Pd	Subfornical organ	Rat
Acetone CP		Ventricular system	Rat
CP		IIIrd ventricle	Rat
Alcohol air dried	C-Pd-Au	IIIrd ventricle	Human
Acetone CP CO_2	Au	IVth ventricle	Human
CP		Choroid plexus	Human
Acetone CP		Ependymal surface	Rh. monkey
Acetone CP Freon 113	Au	Ependymal surface	Rh. monkey
Ethanol CP CO_2	Au	Subfornical organ	Japanese quail
Ethanol CP CO_2	C-Au	Spinal cord	Submammalian vertebrates
Ethanol CP CO_2	Au-Pd	IIIrd ventricle	Rat
CP Frigen 13	C-Au	Subcommissural organ	Cat, rabbit, guinea pig, hamster
Ethanol CP Frigen 13	C-Au	Ependymal surface	Rat, cat, guinea pig, hamster, rabbit

Table 2. Studies on embryological development

Author	Fixation	Postfixation
Backhouse (1974)	3% G 24 h	
Bancroft and Bellairs (1975)	3% G 4 – 24 h/1/2 Karnovsky	1% Os
Breipohl and Fernandez (1977)	3% G overnight	1% Os
England and Cowper (1976)	Karnovsky 12 h	
Mak (1978)	2% para F, 2% G, 0.5% acrolein 48 h	1% Os
Meller and Tetzlaff (1975)	2.5% G overnight	Methanol
Meller and Tetzlaff (1976)	2.5% G overnight	Methanol
Mestres and Rascher (1977)	Immersion/perfusion 3% G, 2% para F/ agar-agar-embedding	2% Os
Olson (1977)	Aldehydefixation 1 – 3 h	2% Os 30′
Portch and Barson (1974)	2.5% G 1 h	1% Os
Seymour and Berry (1975 a)	G/Karnovsky	Os + $HgCl_2$
Seymour and Berry (1975 b)	0.5 – 12.5% G 3 h – 7 days	Parducz's fixative
Waterman (1972)	1 – 7 h Karnovsky	Os
Waterman (1975)	Immersion 2% para F, 2% G, 0.01% trinitro-phenol 3 h – 3 days	

Abbreviations: G, glutaraldehyde; F formaldehyde; CP, critical point; Os, osmium tetroxide

perfused through the ventricular system and the heart. Ventricular perfusion is also utilized by Phillips et al. (1974) and Kozlowski et al. (1972, 1973) (see Table 1). Leonhardt and Lindemann (1973 a, b) propose washing the ventricular surfaces with a saline solution to avoid contamination. Peters (1974), Paull et al. (1977), and Collins and Morriss (1975), propose that perfusion be followed by prolonged post-fixation in a fresh fixative for as long as overnight. Furthermore, Hetzel (1978) extends the fixation time to 4 days or more in his study of the structure of the lateral ventricles. Hannah and Geber (1977) studied the structure of the third ventricle of the hamster using a 16% solution of glycerine in 0.1 M cacodylate buffer to prevent shrinkage caused by dehydration (Fig. 1 A).

Table 3. Studies on nervous system cell cultures

Author	Fixation	Postfixation
Ben-Shaul and Moscona (1975)	Karnovsky	1% Os
Blood (1975)	3% G	
Boyde et al. (1968)	Os vapour 10′	
Dalen et al. (1971)	Os vapour 10′ – 2% G 3 h	1% Os 1 h
Ebendal (1974)	1.5% G – 3% G 1 – 3 days	1% Os 1 h
Faltin et al. (1974)	Karnovsky – paraffin sections	1% Os
Hill et al. (1974)	5% G	
Lodin et al. (1973)	4% G 1 h – 4 weeks	1% Os
Privat et al. (1972)	2.5% G 24 h – 6% glycerine 48 h	
Sheffield et al. (1971)	2.5% G	
Shimada and Fischman (1972)		
Shimada and Fischman (1975)	1/2 Karnovsky	Os

Abbreviations: G, glutaraldehyde; F, formaldehyde; CP, critical point; Os, osmium tetroxide

Preparation for SEM		Material	Animal
Drying	Coating		
Ethanol CP CO_2	C-Au	Neural plate	Chick embryo
Ethanol CP CO_2	C-Au	Neural plate	Chick embryo
Alcohol CP Freon 13	Au	Olfactory epithelium	Chick embryo
Acetone CP CO_2	Au	Neural plate	Chick embryo
Ethanol CP Freon 13	Au-Pd	Neural plate	Amphibian
CP Frigen 13	Au	Cortex	Mouse
CP Frigen 13	Au	Retina	Chick embryo
Methanol CP Freon 13	Au	Hypothalamus	Rat/rat embryo
Acetone CP CO_2	Au-Pd	Retina	Chick embryo
Alcohol-fluoracil, air dried	Au-Pd	Neural tube	Chick embryo
CP CO_2	Au-Pd	Cortex	Rat embryo
Ethanol – amyl acetate CP CO_2	Au-Pd	Cortex	Rat
Acetone – isoamyl acetate	C-Pd-Au		Rat, mouse, hamster, chick
Ethanol CP CO_2	Au-Pd	Neural tube	Hamster, mouse

3.2 The Study of Embryological Specimens

Immersion in glutaraldehyde or glutaraldehyde-paraformaldehyde for 4 h appears to be sufficient to obtain hardened specimens appropriate for blunt dissection as described above (Meller and Tetzlaff 1975, 1976). Backhouse (1974) proposed a fixation time of 24 h and Seymour and Berry (1975 b) from 3 h to 7 days with post-fixation in Parducz's fixative. Thorough osmication of embryological specimens is recommended. This can be achieved with good results according to the procedure of Kelley et al. (1973) modified by Malick et al. (1975) using the ligand thiocarbohydrazide (TCH) to link additional layers of osmium to the tissues. The principal steps are the following: (1) After fixa-

Preparation for SEM		Material	Animal
Drying	Coating		
Ethanol CP CO_2	Au-Pd	Nervous cells	Chick embryo
Ethanol – air dried	Au	Spinal ganglia	Chick embryo
Air dried	C-Au	Spinal cord	Chick embryo
Ethanol – air dried	Au	Cerebellum	Rat
Ethanol CP CO_2	C-Au-Pd	Spinal ganglia	Chick embryo
Ethanol – air dried	Al-Au	Nervous cells	Rabbit
Araldite embedding	Au	Sympathetic ganglia	Rat/guinea pig
Ethanol – air dried	Al	Spinal ganglia	Chick embryo
Ethanol – air dried	Au-Pd	Cerebellum	Rat
Freeze-dried	Au	Retina	Chick embryo
CP	Au	Spinal cord	Chick embryo
CP Freon CO_2	C-Au	Spinal cord	Chick embryo

tion and washing of the specimens they are placed in a freshly prepared 1% solution of TCH for 20–30 min at room temperature. (2) Following renewed washing (H_2O), the samples are placed in 1% osmium for 2–3 h. (3) Steps 1 and 2 are repeated two more times if necessary before dehydration and critical point drying.

Our experiences with this method in embryological material of the nervous system shows that in this case the thickness of the metal coating of tissues can be considerably reduced so that fine structural details of the cell surface are not masked and the artifact problems caused by the heat involved in the shadowing procedure are reduced (see Table 2 and Figs. 1 B, 2 A).

3.3 The Study of Cell Cultures

SEM of cell cultures requires for certain purposes a determined number of precautions (see Table 3).

It is necessary to remove medium and solid contaminants with saline solution from the cultures (Fig. 2 B). Furthermore, the adhesion of cells to the substrate can cause cracking of the cell prolongations on account of shrinkage during dehydration and the critical point drying procedure. To avoid this it is convenient to utilize a collagen substrate (Ebendal 1974) which prevents heat cracking during sputtering. Hill et al. (1974) impregnated cultures of sympathetic ganglia with araldite and then removed the excess resin prior to polymerization. Isolated cells or cell cultures of aggregates of dissociated nervous tissues are difficult to prepare for SEM observations. Mazia et al. (1975) utilized preheated glass or plastic surfaces coated with 0.1% aqueous solution of poly-L-lysine to firmly adhere cells to the substrate. These cells are not detached by treatment with the fixative or the critical point drying procedure. Isolated nuclei and other intracellular structures also attach to the poly-L-lysine-coated surfaces and can subsequently be examined by SEM.

Gopalakrishnan and Thompson (1975) prepare the cover slips as described by Edelman et al. (1971) with concanavalinA [1.5 ml of WSC (1-cyclohexyl-3-(2-morpholinoethyl)-carbodiimide metho-p-toluenesulphonate)] in 0.15 M NaCl and 1.5 ml concanavalinA and also in 0.15 M NaCl. The cells adhere firmly to the surface and can be enucleated with cytochalasin B as described by Prescott et al. (1972). This procedure is applicable to nerve cell cultures (Fig. 2 C) and is especially advantageous for the study of the effects of enucleation on the process of cell differentiation (Meller, unpublished).

3.4 The Study of Sensory Organs

Breipohl et al. (1973) studied different types of sensory cells with SEM. When sensory cells have accessible cell surfaces such as in the olfactory mucosa, the retinal receptors or the taste buds, the technical procedure does not differ greatly from the general methods described for the natural surfaces. These authors recommended a careful washing in physiological saline in order to remove the superficial mucus of the olfactory mucosa or to study the retinal receptors in adult animals in which fixation must be instituted for a few minutes before dissection to avoid the damage caused by removing the pigment epithe-

Fig. 2. A Portion of the ventricular matrix of the cerebral vesicles of a 12.5-day-old mouse embryo. *VS*, ventricular surface. Blunt dissection, critical point drying with Frigen 13. ×5000 **B** Overview of a cell culture of rat brain, 13 days old in vitro, 2.5% glutaraldehyde fixation. Critical point drying with Frigen 13. ×4000 **C** Enucleated nerve cell from a spinal ganglion with cytochalasin B. The *arrow* shows the broken cytoplasmic stalk between cytoplast and caryoplast. The slides were coated with concanavalin A. 2.5% glutaraldehyde fixation, critical point drying with Frigen 13. ×6000

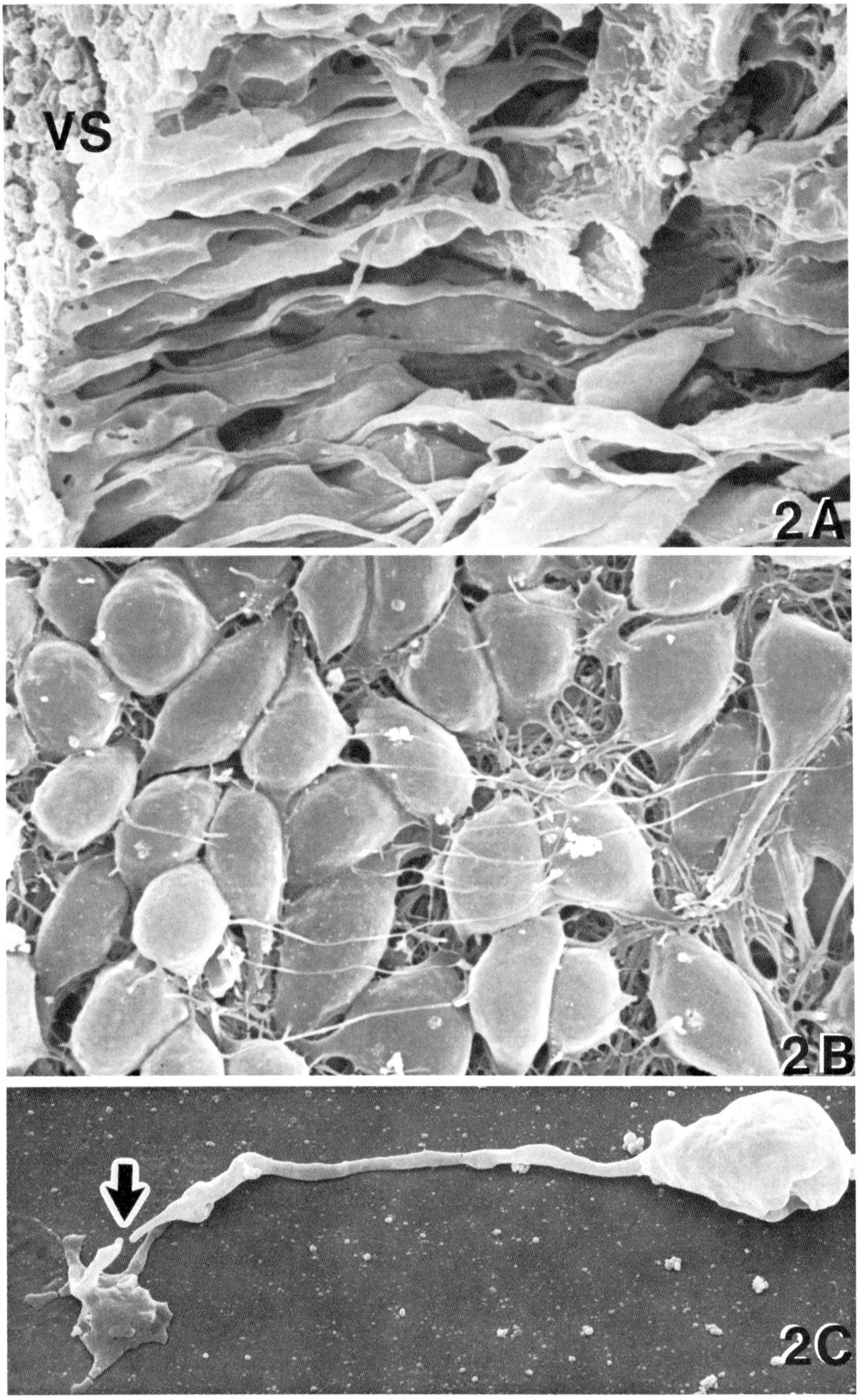
VS
2A
2B
2C

Table 4. Studies on sensory organs

Author	Fixation	Postfixation
Bagger-Sjöbäck and Wersäll (1973)	Os – 3% G	
Breipohl et al. (1973)	Karnovsky 3 – 4 h	1% Os 8 – 16 h
Breipohl et al. (1974)	G	1% Os
Hillman and Lewis (1971)	Os	
Kawabata and Ishii (1971)	10% formalin 5 – 24 h	
Kosaka et al. (1971)	Immersion 2% Os – 2.5% G	
Landolt et al. (1975)		
Lindeman and Bredberg (1972)		
Maeda et al. (1974)	Immersion 2.5% G	1% Os 2 h
Miller (1973a)	In situ fixation 3% G; 3 – 10 days trimming before drying	
Miller (1973b)	Immersion 3% G	
Rivera-Dominguez et al. (1974)	Perfusion 10% formalin	
Ross (1974)	Perfusion 3% G, 4% para F, immersion Held's solution	1% Os
Tanaka and Smith (1978)	Perfusion of labyrinth-Karnovsky 3 – 24 h	1.5% Os 1 h
von Düring et al. (1974)	Immersion perfusion 2.5% G, 1.6% F 24 h	4% Os
Wersäll et al. (1971)	1% Os	

Abbreviations: G, glutaraldehyde; F, formaldehyde; CP, critical point; Os, osmium tetroxide

lium. Kawabata and Ishii (1971), studying the tympanic membranes of guinea pigs, incubated the dissected specimens in 1% trypsin or 0.1% pronase at 37 °C for 3–48 h to remove the mucous and cutaneous layer.

In any case the study of the inner ear structures requires particular dissection and preparation procedures before the specimens are ready to be studied by SEM. The specific literature should be consulted in each case (see Table 4).

Acknowledgments. A part of this work was supported by a grant from the Ministerium für Wissenschaft und Forschung des Landes Nordrhein-Westfalen (Az. IIB5-FA7470). I gratefully acknowledge K. Donberg for preparing the photographs, K. Rascher and H. C. Kondo for their help with the English translation, and C. Bloch for typing the chapter.

4 References

Alexander IGS, Capicchiano PM, Ritchie BC, Maloney JE (1973) Plastic embedding and surface erosion technique in soft tissue scanning electron microscopy. J Microsc 99: 69–74

Allen DJ, Low FN (1973) The ependymal surface of the lateral ventricle of the dog as revealed by scanning electron microscopy (1). Am J Anat 137:483–489

Anderson TF (1966) Electron microscopy of microorganisms. In: Pollister AW (ed) Physical techniques in biological research, 2nd ed, vol III/A. Academic Press, New York and London, p 319

Azzam NA, Trow LJ (1976) A scanning electron microscopic observation of the phagocytic activity of the rat ependymal cells. Anat Rec 184:348–349

Backhouse M (1974) Observations on the development of the early chick embryo. In: Johari O (ed) Scanning electron microscopy 1974, part III. IIT Research Institute, Chicago, Ill., p 525

Bagger-Sjöbäck D, Wersäll J (1973) The sensory hairs and tectorial membrane of the basilar

Preparation for SEM		Material	Animal
Drying	Coating		
		Basilar papillae	Lizard
Alcohol CP	Au-C-Au	Olfactory epithelium	Fish
Alcohol – CP Freon 13		Olfactory epithelium	Goldfish, chick, mouse
Alcohol	Au		Frog
Acetone – air dried	C-Au	Tympanic membrane	Guinea pig
Alcohol-acetone – air dried	C-Au	Organ of Corti	Guinea pig
Freeze-dried 40 h	Au	Vestibular apparatus	Pigeons
Sections freeze-dried		Organ of Corti	Cat, guinea pig, chinchilla
Ethanol CP CO_2	C-Au	Middle ear	Rat
Alcohol ethanol CP CO_2	Au	Basilar papillae	Lizard
Alcohol CP CO_2	Au	Ductus cochlearis	Lizard
Freeze-dried	Au-Pd	Organ of Corti	Rh. monkey
Alcohol freeze-dried CP	Au	Tectorial membrane	Rat
Ethanol – CP Freon 13	Au-Pd	Inner ear	Chick
Alcohol CP CO_2	Au	Inner ear	Caiman crocodilus
Alcohol freeze-drying	Au	Crista ampullaris	Guinea pig

papilla in the lizard calotes versicolor. J Neurocytol 2:329–350

Bancroft M, Bellairs R (1975) Differentiation of the neural plate and neural tube in the young chick embryo. Anat Embryol 147:309–335

Barber VC, Boyde A (1968) Scanning electron microscopic studies of cilia. Z Zellforsch 84: 269–284

Ben-Shaul Y, Moscona AA (1975) Scanning electron microscopy of embryonic neural retina cell surfaces. Dev Biol 44:386–393

Bleier R (1975) Surface fine structure of supraependymal elements and ependyma of hypothalamic third ventricle of mouse. J Comp Neurol 161:555–568

Blood LA (1975) Scanning electron microscopic observations of the outgrowth from embryonic chick dorsal root ganglia in culture. Neurobiol 5:75–83

Borit A, Sidman RL (1972) New mutant mouse with communicating hydrocephalus and secondary aqueductal stenosis. Acta Neuropathol 21:316–331

Boyde A, Wood C (1969) Preparation of animal tissues for surface-scanning electron microscopy. J Microsc 90:221–249

Boyde A, James DW, Tresman RL, Willis RA (1968) Outgrowth from chick embryo spinal cord in vitro, studied with the scanning electron microscope. Z Zellforsch 90: 1–18

Breipohl W, Bijvank GJ (1974) Scanning electron microscopy of various sensory receptor cells in different vertebrates. In: Johari O (ed) Scanning electron microscopy/1974, part III. IIT Research Institute, Chicago, Ill., p 557

Breipohl W, Bijvank GJ, Zippel HP (1973) Rastermikroskopische Untersuchungen der olfaktorischen Rezeptoren im Riechepithel des Goldfisches (carassius auratus). Z Zellforsch 138:439–454

Breipohl W, Fernandez M (1977) Scanning electron microscopic investigations of olfactory epithelium in the chick embryo. Cell Tissue Res 183:105–114

Brown MF, Brotzman HG, Kinden DA (1976) Use of a tissue sectioner to expose internal structures of biological samples for scanning electron microscopy. Stain Technol 51: 267–270

Bruni JE, Montemurro DG, Clattenburg RE (1977) Morphology of the ependymal lining of the rabbit third ventricle following intraventricular administration of synthetic luteinizing hormone-releasing hormone (LH-RH): A scanning electron microscopic investigation. Am J Anat 150:411–426

Clementi F, Marini D (1972) The surface fine structure of the walls of cerebral ventricles and of choroid plexus in cat. Z Zellforsch 123:82–95

Cleveland PH, Schneider CW (1969) A simple method of preserving ocular tissue for scanning electron microscopy. Vision Res 9:1401

Coates PW (1977) The third ventricle of monkeys. Scanning electron microscopy of surface features in mature males and females. Cell Tissue Res 177:307–316

Cohen AL (1979) Critical point drying – Principles and procedures. In: Johari O, Becker RP (eds) Scanning electron microscopy/1979, part II. SEM, AMF O'Hare, Ill., p 303

Collins P, Morriss GM (1975) Changes in the surface features of choroid plexus of the rat following the administration of acetazolamide and other drugs which affect CSF secretion. J Anat 120:571–579

Cupedo RNJ (1977) The surface ultrastructure of the habenular complex of the rat. Anat Embryol 152:43–64

Dalen H, Schlapfer WT, Mamoon A (1971) Cilia on cultured ependymal cells examined by scanning electron microscopy. Exp Cell Res 67:375–379

Dellmann H-D (1978) Scanning and transmission electron microscopy of the subfornical organ of the frog (rana pipiens). Cell Tissue Res 186:361–374

Dellmann H-D, Simpson JB (1976) Regional Differences in the morphology of the rat subfornical organ. Brain Res 116:389–400

Dempsey EW (1973) Neural and vascular ultrastructure of the area postrema in the rat. J Comp Neurol 150:177–200

De Waele G, Dierickx K, Goossens N (1974) Scanning electron microscopy of the wall of the third ventricle of the brain of rana temporaria. Cell Tissue Res 154:511–518

Dierickx K, Druyts A, Vandenberghe MP, Goossens N (1972) Identification of adenohypophysiotropic neurohormone producing neurosecretory cells in rana temporaria. I. Ultrastructural evidence for the presence of neurosecretory cells in the tuber cinereum. Z Zellforsch 134:459–504

Düring v. M, Karduck A, Richter H-G (1974) The fine structure of the inner ear in caiman crocodilus. Z Anat Entwicklungsgesch 145:41–65

Ebendal T (1974) Scanning electron microscopy of chick embryo nerve fibres and heart fibroblasts on collagen substrata in vitro. Zoon 2:99–104

Edelman GM, Rutishauser U, Millette CF (1971) Cell fractionation and arrangement on fibers, beads, and surfaces. Proc Natl Acad Sci USA 68:2153–2157

England MA, Cowper SV (1976) A transmission and scanning electron microscope study of primary neural induction. Experientia 32: 1578–1580

Faltin J, Lodin Z, Booher J (1974) The surface of dissected neurons, neurons in smears, cultivated cells and sections as studied by means of scanning electron microscopy. Acta Histochem 50:187–199

Fromme HG, Pfautsch M, Pfefferkorn G, Bystricky V (1972) Die „Kritische Punkt"-Trocknung als Präparationsmethode für die Raster-Elektronenmikroskopie. Microsc Acta 73:29–37

Gopalakrishnan TV, Thompson EB (1975) A method for enucleating cultured mammalian cells. Exp Cell Res 96:435–439

Hannah RS, Geber W (1977) Specializations of the ependyma in the third ventricle of the developing hamster. Am J Anat 149:597–603

Hetzel W (1978) Ependyma and ependymal protrusions of the lateral ventricles of the rabbit brain. Cell Tissue Res 192:475–488

Hill CE, Chamley JH, Burnstock G (1974) Cell surfaces and fiber relationships in sympathetic ganglion cultures: A scanning electron-microscopic study. J Cell Sci 14:657–669

Hillman DE, Lewis ER (1971) Morphological basis for a mechanical linkage in otolithic receptor transduction in the frog. Science 174:416–419

Hirunagi K, Yasuda M (1979) Scanning electron microscopic analysis of the linings of the fourth ventricle in the domestic fowl. Cell Tissue Res 197:169–173

Jacobs JJ, Monroe KD (1977) A scanning electron microscopic survey of the brain ventricular system of the female armadillo. Cell Tissue Res 183:531–539

Kawabata I, Ishii H (1971) Fiber arrangement in the tympanic membrane. Scanning electron microscope observations. Acta Otolaryngol 72:243–254

Kelley RO, Dekker RAF, Bluemink JG (1973) Ligand-mediated osmium binding: Its application in coating biological specimens for scanning electron microscopy. J Ultrastruct Res 45:254–258

Klara PM, Brizzee KR (1977) Ultrastructure of the feline area postrema. J Comp Neurol 171: 409–432

Kosaka N, Tanaka T, Takiguchi T, Ozeki Y, Takahara S (1971) Observation on the organ of Corti with scanning electron microscope. Acta Otolaryngol 72:377–384

Kozlowski GP, Scott DE, Murphy JA (1972) Scanning electron microscopy of the lateral ventricle of sheep. Am J Anat 135:561–566

Kozlowski GP, Scott DE, Krobisch-Dudley GK (1973) Scanning electron microscopy of the third ventricle of sheep. Z Zellforsch 136: 169–176

Krisch B, Leonhardt H, Desaga U (1978) The rhombencephalic recess in the rat. A light and electron microscopic study. Cell Tissue Res 189:479–495

Landolt JP, Correia MJ, Young ER, Cardin RPS, Sweet RC (1975) A scanning electron microscopic study of the morphology and geometry of neural surfaces and structures associated with the vestibular apparatus of the pigeon. J Comp Neurol 159:257–288

Leonhardt H, Lindemann B (1973 a) Surface morphology of the subfornical organ in the rabbit's brain. Z Zellforsch 146:243–260

Leonhardt H, Lindemann B (1973 b) Über ein supraependymales Nervenzell-, Axon-, und Gliazellsystem. Eine raster- und transmissionselektronenmikroskopische Untersuchung am IV. Ventrikel (Apertura lateralis) des Kaninchengehirns. Z Zellforsch 139:285–302

Leslie RA, Gwyn DG, Morrison CM (1978) The fine structure of the ventricular surface of the area postrema of the cat, with particular reference to supraependymal structures. Am J Anat 153:273–290

Lindberg L-A, Talanti S (1975) The surface fine structure of the bovine subcommissural organ. Cell Tissue Res 163:125–132

Lindberg L-A, Vasenius L, Talanti S (1977) The surface fine structure of the ependymal lining of the lateral ventricle in rats with hereditary hydrocephalus. Cell Tissue Res 179:121–129

Lindeman HH, Bredberg G (1972) Scanning electron microscopy of the organ of corti after intense auditory stimulation: Effects on stereocilia and cuticular surface of hair cells. Arch Klin Exp Ohren Nasen Kehlkopfheilkd 203:1–15

Lodin Z, Faltin J, Booher J, Hartman J, Sensenbrenner M (1973) Formation of intercellular contacts in cultures of dissociated neurons from embryonic chicken dorsal root ganglia. An electron microscopic and scanning electron microscopic study. Neurobiology 3: 376–390

Maeda S, Honjo S, Mogi G (1974) Surface structures of the normal mucosa in developing rat middle ear. In: Johari O (ed) Scanning electron microscopy/1974, part III. IIT Research Institute, Chicago, Ill., p 565

Mak LL (1978) Ultrastructural studies of amphibian neural fold fusion. Dev Biol 65: 435–446

Malick LE, Wilson RB, Stetson D (1975) Modified thiocarbohydrazide procedure for scanning electron microscopy: Routine use for normal, pathological, or experimental tissues. Stain Technol 50:265–269

Mazia D, Schatten G, Sale W (1975) Adhesion of cells to surfaces coated with polylysine. Applications to electron microscopy. J Cell Biol 66:198–200

Meller K, Tetzlaff W (1975) Neuronal migration during the early development of the cerebral cortex. A scanning electron microscopic study. Cell Tissue Res 163:313–325

Meller K, Tetzlaff W (1976) Scanning electron microscopic studies on the development of the chick retina. Cell Tissue Res 170:145–159

Mestres P, Rascher K (1977) Some aspects of the early development of the rat hypothalamus: A scanning electron microscopic (SEM) study. In: Johari O (ed) Scanning electron microscopy/1977, vol II. IIT Research Institute, Chicago, Ill., p 381

Mikami S-I, Asari M (1978) Ultrastructure of the subfornical organ of the japanese quail, coturnix coturnix. Cell Tissue Res 188:19–33

Miller MR (1973 a) Scanning electron microscope studies of some lizard basilar papillae. Am J Anat 138:301–330

Miller MR (1973 b) A scanning electron microscope study of the papilla basilaris of gekko gecko. Z Zellforsch 136:307–328

Miodonski A, Poborowska J, De Grubenthal F (1979) Scanning electron microscopic study of the choroid plexus of the lateral ventricle in the cat. Anat Embryol 155:323–331

Nelson DJ, Wright EM (1974) The distribution, activity, and function of the cilia in the frog brain. J Physiol 243:63–78

Noack W, Dumitrescu L, Schweichel JU (1972) Scanning and electron microscopical investigations of the surface structures of the lateral ventricles in the cat. Brain Res 46:121–129

Olson MD (1977) The development of photoreceptor inner and outer segments in the retina of the chick as observed by scanning electron microscopy. In: Johari O (ed) Scanning electron microscopy/1977, vol II. IIT Research Institute, Chicago, Ill., p 453

Paull WK, Martin H, Scott DE (1977) Scanning electron microscopy of the third ventricular floor of the rat. J Comp Neurol 175: 301–310

Peters A (1974) The surface fine structure of the choroid plexus and ependymal lining of the rat lateral ventricle. J Neurocytol 3: 99–108

Phillips MI, Balhorn L, Leavitt M, Hoffman W (1974) Scanning electron microscope study of the rat subfornical organ. Brain Res 80: 95–110

Portch PA, Barson AJ (1974) Scanning electron microscopy of neurulation in the chick. J Anat 117:341–350

Prescott DM, Myerson D, Wallace J (1972) Enucleation of mammalian cells with cytochalasin B. Exp Cell Res 71:480–485

Privat A, Mandon P, Drian MJ (1972) Contribution de la microscopie électronique à balayage pour l'étude du tissu nerveux en culture organisée. Exp Cell Res 71:232–235

Ribas JL (1977) The rat epithalamus. I. Correlative scanning-transmission electron microscopy of supraependymal nerves. Cell Tissue Res 182:1–16

Rivera-Dominguez M, Agate JR. FJ, Noback CR (1974) Scanning electron microscopic observations of the organ of corti of the rhesus monkey. Brain Res 65:159–164

Ross MD (1974) The tectorial membrane of the rat. Am J Anat 139:449–482

Scott DE, Paull WK (1978) Correlative scanning-transmission electron microscopic examination of the perinatal rat brain. Cell Tissue Res 190:317–336

Scott DE, Paull WK, Krobisch Dudley G (1972) A comparative scanning electron microscopic analysis of the human cerebral ventricular system. I. The third ventricle. Z Zellforsch 132:203–215

Scott DE, Kozlowski GP, Paull WK, Ramalingam S, Krobisch-Dudley G (1973 a) Scanning electron microscopy of the human cerebral ventricular system. II. The fourth ventricle. Z Zellforsch 139:61–68

Scott DE, Kozlowski GP, Krobisch-Dudley G (1973 b) A comparative ultrastructural analysis of the third cerebral ventricle of the North American Mink (mustela vison). Anat Rec 175:155–168

Scott DE, Van Dyke DH, Paull WK, Kozlowski GP (1974) Ultrastructural analysis of the human cerebral ventricular system. III. The choroid plexus. Cell Tissue Res 150:389–397

Scott DE, Krobisch-Dudley G, Paull WK, Kozlowski GP, Ribas J (1975) The primate median eminence. I. Correlative scanning-transmission electron microscopy. Cell Tissue Res 162:61–73

Scott DE, Paull WK, Steger RW, Mestres P, Mitchell JA, Hafez ESE (1976) The primate hypothalamus: Correlative scanning-transmission electron microscopy (SEM/TEM). In: Johari O (ed) Scanning electron microscopy/1976, part VI. IIT Research Institute, Chicago, Ill., p 431

Scott DE, Krobisch-Dudley G, Paull WK, Kozlowski GP (1977) The ventricular system in neuroendocrine mechanisms. III. Supraependymal neuronal networks in the primate brain. Cell Tissue Res 179:235–254

Seymour R, Berry M (1975 a) Surface changes in epithelial cells during mitosis in vivo. J Anat 120:401–402

Seymour RM, Berry M (1975 b) Scanning transmission electron microscope studies of interkinetic nuclear migration in the cerebral vesicles of the rat. J Comp Neurol 160:105–126

Seymour RM, Berry M (1979) The nervous system. In: Hodges GM, Hallowes RC (eds) Biomedical research applications of scanning electron microscopy. Vol I. p 127

Sheffield JB, Isaacson M, Johnson D (1971) Visualization of surface structures on embryonic cells with a simple electron gun scanning microscope. Exp Cell Res 64:49–56

Shimada Y, Fischman DA (1972) Scanning electron microscopy of neuromuscular junctions in cell culture. J Cell Biol 55:237 a

Shimada Y, Fischman DA (1975) Scanning electron microscopy of nerve-muscle contacts in embryonic cell culture. Dev Biol 43:42–61

Takei Y, Tsuneki K, Kobayashi H (1978) Surface fine structure of the subfornical organ in the japanese quail, coturnix coturnix japonica. Cell Tissue Res 191:389–404

Tanaka K (1972) Freezed resin cracking method for scanning electron microscopy of biological materials. Naturwiss 59:77

Tanaka K, Smith CA (1978) Structure of the chicken's inner ear: SEM and TEM study. Am J Anat 153:251–272

Vigh B, Vigh-Teichmann I, Aros B (1977) Special dendritic and axonal endings formed by the cerebrospinal fluid contacting neurons of the spinal cord. Cell Tissue Res 183:541–552

Walsh RJ, Brawer JR, Lin PS (1978) Early postnatal development of ependyma in the third ventricle of male and female rats. Am J Anat 151:377–408

Waterman RE (1972) Use of the scanning electron microscope for observation of vertebrate embryos. Dev Biol 27:276–281

Waterman RE (1975) SEM observations of surface alterations associated with neural tube closure in the mouse and hamster. Anat Rec 183:95–98

Weindl A, Schinko I (1975) Evidence by scanning electron microscopy for ependymal secretion into the cerebrospinal fluid and formation of Reissner's fiber by the subcommissural organ. Brain Res 88:319–324

Weindl A, Schinko I, Wetzstein R (1975) Rasterelektronenmikroskopische Untersuchungen am Ventrikelependym. Verh Anat Ges 69: 463–471

Wersäll J, Björkroth B, Flock A, Lundquist P-G (1971) Sensory hair fusion in vestibular sensory cells after gentamycin exposure. A transmission and scanning electron microscope study. Arch Klin Exp Ohren Nasen Kehlkopfheilkd 200:1–14

Chapter 5

Lesion Methods in Neurobiology

G. Jonsson

1 Introduction

Different types of lesion techniques have for many years been extensively used to analyze neuronal circuitry and function and they represent fundamental tools for the experimental neurobiologist. Lesion techniques have also come to be of ever increasing interest for studies on the biochemical properties of neurons as well as on the action of psychoactive drugs on neurons and associated effector cells. The basis for employing the lesion approach to these kinds of studies is related to the fact that the neuron, which is a highly differentiated cell, undergoes very particular reactions following a separation of the axon from the soma. The various types of alterations that can take place in a neuron after a lesion are schematically depicted in a simplified manner in Fig. 1. An axotomy will invariably (in vertebrates) lead to a degeneration of the separated distal part of the axon (*anterograde degeneration, Wallerian degeneration*) and a denervation of previously innervated elements (target or effector cells). Furthermore, in many cases the axotomy will be followed by a series of morphological changes in the soma (perikaryon), which collectively are called the *axon reaction,* involving chromatolysis, nuclear eccentricity, and soma swelling (see Lieberman 1971). In some instances, particularly when the axotomy is close to the soma and there are no sustaining collateral branches proximal to the lesion, the cell body can ultimately undergo cell death and completely disappear (*retrograde degeneration*), a reaction which is particularly pronounced in young animals. The retrograde degeneration is generally limited to the most distal end of the proximal axon stump. It is furthermore known that the degenerative changes are not always

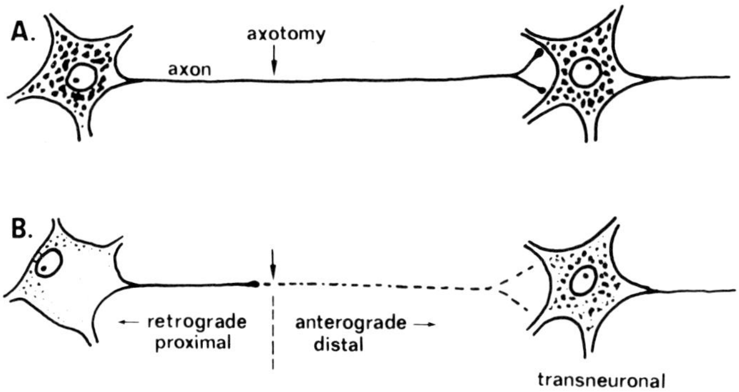

Fig. 1 A, B. Schematic representation of the alterations which can occur in neurons following a transection of the axon (axotomy). **A** the normal state; **B** after axotomy (↓). The degenerative changes are gradual with great differences in time-course between different categories of neurons. Proximal to the axotomy most neurons undergo a limited *retrograde degeneration* with axon reaction, which in certain cases can be severe, leading to cell death. Distal to the transection there will always occur an *anterograde degeneration* of the entire axon stump divided from the soma. In some neuronal systems *transneuronal degeneration* can also occur, which can be either retrograde or enterograde. The latter type is depicted here

restricted to the severed neuron, but an axotomy can in addition in certain neuronal systems lead to an atrophy or degeneration of neurons that are in direct or indirect synaptic contact with the damaged neuron in the same circuit. This phenomenon is called *transneuronal degeneration* (see Smith and Kreutzberg 1976) which can be either of retrograde or anterograde type (see Fig. 1). All these different types of reactions can be used for neuronal pathway mapping using different staining methods, mainly silver impregnation techniques. Although we have in recent years seen a tremendous development where the more conventional degeneration methods to a large extent have been replaced by axonal transport techniques for tracing neuronal connections (see Jones and Hartman 1978), recent observations have, however, demonstrated that degeneration methods may still be very useful, particularly for the study of human brain (Leonard 1979). For obvious reasons it is clear that the combination of degeneration and axonal transport techniques is a particularly powerful approach for the mapping of neuronal pathways.

For many years the most frequently used lesion techniques have been surgical and electrolytical and thus nonselective with respect to their effects on neuronal elements as well as on nonneuronal structures. Several selective lesioning techniques based on different principles have been developed during the last twenty years of which the chemical neurotoxin approach has come to be the most extensively used, mainly due to the ease by which it can be employed from an experimental viewpoint. During the last decade various types of chemical neurotoxins have been discovered which have a site- or target-directed neurodegenerative action making it possible to induce degeneration of particular classes of neurons. Two principal types of neurotoxins are at present available which can be used to achieve selective lesions, namely the monoamine neurotoxins and the excitotoxins (excitotoxic amino acids) (see Jonsson 1980). Both types have target-directed action, although the neurotoxic action is mediated via recognition sites which have different localization and properties. The monoamine neurotoxins thus affect a given neuron type defined with respect to its neurotransmitter, while the excitotoxins can affect most neurons. However, when the excitotoxins are injected locally in the CNS, there will be a degeneration of neuronal structures with their somata within the infusion site while afferents and fibers *en passant* are spared (Coyle and Schwarcz 1976; McGeer and McGeer 1976). The chemical neurotoxins have received great attention in recent years and have provided the neurobiologist with unique possibilities of attacking numerous neurobiological problems of a basic nature and have in addition made it possible to develop animal models for certain human diseases (e.g., Parkinson's disease, Huntington's chorea).

The purpose of this chapter is to briefly review nonselective and selective lesioning techniques with emphasis on the use of chemical neurotoxins. Specificity aspects, limitations, and pitfalls connected with these techniques, as well as some interpretation problems associated with effects seen following degeneration of neuronal systems will also be dealt with. Although the stereotaxic technique (Horsley and Clarke 1908) is generally the basis for the production of localized lesions of any type in the CNS, it is however beyond the scope of this review to deal with this technique. For a description of the stereotaxic technique and references on stereotaxic atlases see Moore (1978).

2 Nonselective Lesion Techniques

The most frequently used techniques over the years are different mechanical or surgical and electrolytic methods of which the former include aspiration and knife methods.

2.1 Aspiration Technique

The CNS tissue is soft enough to be able to be removed by aspiration under vacuum. This is a very simple technique which only requires a suitable tubing (glass or metal) connected to a vacuum device and the head of the animal suitably fixed. The aspiration technique is best suited for lesions of external CNS structures. This approach has been used extensively in studies on, for example, thalamocortical relationships (Rose and Woolsey 1943, 1949), hippocampus and septum (Moore 1964; Moore et al. 1971), superior colliculus (Schneider 1970), and corpus callosum (Meyers 1956). Although the technique must be considered crude, it can with proper application and with the use of an operation microscope be employed to produce precise and reproducible lesions, particularly of cortical structures as well as some subcortical structures. In the latter case it will for obvious reasons be necessary to damage part of the cerebral cortex. Therefore, if the cortical damage is considered to be undesirable, other types of lesions should be chosen where this can be avoided. For further details on the aspiration technique see Moore (1978).

2.2 Knife Methods

The knife methods also represent relatively simple and inexpensive procedures for obtaining lesions and have their main application for transection of fiber bundles. The main consideration when using this type of lesion in experimental work is of course the anatomical organisation of the structure(s) to be lesioned. In certain situations it may be possibe to transect relatively selectively a fiber bundle, e.g., the lateral lemniscus and pathways of the spinal cord, whereas in most other situations it will be a compromise leading to more or less extensive damage of structures in addition to the particular fiber bundle at which the lesion is aimed. More controlled and reproducible lesions can be obtained when the knife method is combined with stereotoxic technique. Among the first to use this approach was Halasz and Pupp (1965) who used a thin knife with two 90° bends making it possible to deafferentate the hypothalamus completely, a lesion which subsequently has been shown to be very useful for studies on neuroendocrine functions (Halasz 1969). The use of bent or differently oriented parts of the lesion knife is very valuable and makes it possible in many situations to avoid undesired lesions. In order to reduce the incidental damage caused by the Halasz-type of knifes, there has been developed various modifications where the lesion-knife is kept within a carrier (Voloschin et al. 1968; Sclafini and Grossman 1969; Gold et al. 1975). For obvious reasons and in spite of all the care and precautions undertaken, the knife lesions will cause more or less massive incidental damage, in particular in the diencephalon and brain stem, which limits their usefulness. The knife lesions are usually used when the intention is to completely lesion a certain fiber system without paying attention to effects on adjacent systems.

2.3 Electrolytic Methods

The most frequently used technique for producing localized lesions within the CNS are the electrolytic methods, which involve passage of an electrical current from the tip of an insulated metal electrode (see Rowland 1966; Gold 1973). The lesion can be produced by applying either anodal or cathodal current. The lesion is a result of the ionic flow inducing irreversible changes in cell metabolism leading to tissue damage and degeneration. The ionic flow is measured in coulomb units, the product of the current in amperes applied multiplied by its duration in seconds. There is in general a direct relation between the size of the lesion and coulombs applied, although this relationship may vary considerably due to the type of metal used for the electrode and if anodal or cathodal current is employed.

The anodal current procedure is the most frequently used and produces more reproducible lesions in terms of size and shape than those seen after application of cathodal current. Anodal lesions lead, however, to a deposition of metal at the lesion site, which varies greatly depending on the metal used as electrode material. The deposition of metal is generally neglected, but is in certain cases considered to be of importance for the functional consequences observed following the lesion. It is therefore important for the investigator to be aquainted with the properties of the electrode used. Stainless steel and "nichrome" electrodes are the most commonly used. For further information on this point the reader is referred to the work of Gold (1973).

As for the cathodal current procedure, which releases gas during the passage of current, the lesions tend to vary considerably in size with constant lesioning parameters which has led to its limited use.

An important aspect for the evaluation of the electrolytic lesion is that its size can change markedly with time after its production, which has to be considered when checking the lesion histologically. The progressive histological changes after placing small electrolytical (anodal) lesions in the caudate nucleus and the hypothalamus have been reported by Wolf and DiChiara (1969). The authors have shown that during the first day after the lesion there is a marked increase in the apparent size of the lesion (100%–400%), which most likely reflects difficulties in determining the exact extension of the lesion and the appearance of edema in the lesion area. After the first postoperative week there is a progressive shrinkage of the lesion which may also involve a marked tissue distortion (see also Moore 1978). The studies of Wolf and DiChiara (1969) have clearly documented two important characteristics of the electrolytic lesions; the size and shape of the lesion vary in different areas with constant lesion parameters and the postoperative shrinkage is different from area to area. These are certainly very important factors when evaluating the lesions for functional correlations.

2.4 Radiofrequency Lesion Method

A lesion technique which has received an increasing popularity is the *radiofrequency lesion method*, which is adapted to produce localized destruction of neuronal tissue by converting electrical energy into heat in the tissue (see Arnow 1960). The current is passed through an insulated electrode with a small uninsulated tip that is stereotaxically placed in the region where the lesion is intended to be produced. In this technique a low-power, continuous-wave radiofrequency current is passed between the brain electrode and an indifferent electrode which is placed at some remote point of high conductivity (e.g., muscles of the neck). The size of the lesion is within limits roughly a linear function of the radiofrequency current (mA) applied. This technique has the advantage of giving rather reproducible lesions and does not deposit metal or release gas during the lesion procedure as is the case with electrolytic lesions. However, the lesion parameters have to be tested out carefully for each area and type of lesion desired, as with electrolytic lesions. The histological alterations seen after a radiofrequency lesion are very much the same as those seen after electrolytic lesions, i.e., progressive changes in size with time and distortion of the lesion within the neuronal tissue.

2.5 Miscellaneous Nonselective Lesion Techniques

Apart from the lesioning techniques described, there are also types employing different principles to obtain localized lesions, e.g., cryogenic, ultrasound, and radioisotopic lesions. Most of these techniques are generally, however, relatively complicated, require expensive and specialized equipment, and do not in most situations offer any substantial advantages compared to the more conventional techniques. Another approach that has been used for many years involves local application by microinjection of non-selective toxic substances such as $CuSO_4$, AgCl, and other tissue-damaging compounds. The greatest problem associated with these latter techniques is that they produce lesions of unpredictable size, shape, and histological characteristics (Carpenter and Whittier 1952; Routtenberg 1972). There is in addition very little known about the mechanism of toxicity and these procedures have by many authors been considered unsatisfactory for producing localized lesions in the CNS. The problems associated with local microinjections are also of relevance when using selective neurotoxins (see p. 80).

3 Selective Lesion Techniques

These techniques involve procedures which possess a target- or site-directed cytotoxic action leading to degeneration of a particular class of neurons. In view of the heterogeneity of the nervous tissue, these lesion techniques have received a great deal of attention in recent years and have been used frequently. They have undoubtedly opened up quite unique possibilities for the morphological, pharmacological, and functional studies of certain defined neuron systems both in the central and peripheral nervous system. The selective lesion methods are of two types, chemical and immunochemical, and are carried out by the administration of specific chemical neurotoxins and antisera, respectively. There are at present two principal types of selective chemical neurotoxins available, namely the *monoamine neurotoxins* and the so called *'excitotoxic' amino acids*.

3.1 Monoamine Neurotoxins

The breakthrough for the use of chemical neurotoxins as denervation tools in experimental work came from the discovery of Tranzer and Thoenen (1967 a) that the noradrenaline (NA) analogue 6-hydroxydopamine (6-OH-DA; 2,4,5-trihydroxyphenylethylamine, Fig. 2) can induce an acute and selective degeneration of sympathetic adrenergic nerves. The basis for this target-directed neurotoxic action is due to 6-OH-DA being a generally cytotoxic agent which is selectively taken up and accumulated by neurons using catecholamines as neurotransmitters. This principle could later be applied to 5-hydroxytryptamine (5-HT) neurons where it could be shown that 5,6- or 5,7-dihydroxytryptamine (5,6-HT, 5,7-HT, Fig. 3) act on 5-HT neurons very much in the same manner as 6-OH-DA on catecholamine neurons (Baumgarten et al. 1971; Baumgarten and Lachenmeyer 1972). In addition several other compounds have been discovered which are structurally different from 6-OH-DA and the dihydroxytryptamines, which possess a more or less selective neurotoxic action on monoamine neurons. Although these latter compounds often have limitations in their use, they can in certain situations have some advantages and therefore be the neurotoxin of choice.

3.1.1 Catecholamine Neurotoxins

3.1.1.1 6-Hydroxydopamine

The most frequently used and best characterized neurotoxin for denervation of catecholamine neurons is 6-hydroxydopamine (6-OH-DA). In view of the extensive information available on the use of 6-OH-DA as a denervation tool, here it will only be possible to give some general guidelines on its use and discuss some general points. For particular applications and problems the reader is recommended to consult other review articles and symposium books (Malmfors and Thoenen 1971; Kostrzewa and Jacobowitz 1974; Breese 1975; Jonsson et al. 1975; Sachs and Jonsson 1975 a; Jonsson 1980).

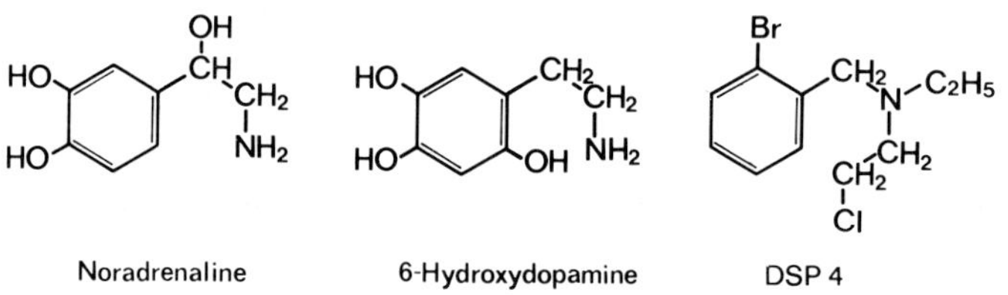

Fig. 2. Structural formulae of NA, 6-OH-DA and DSP4

For the proper use of monoamine neurotoxins as denervation tools it is of great importance to have some general knowledge as to their mode of action. This is especially important when applying this technique to species, regions, or systems that have not been studied before. It is generally agreed that there are two features which are of fundamental importance for the degenerative action of 6-OH-DA on catecholamine neurons. First, 6-OH-DA is efficiently taken up and accumulated intraneuronally due to its affinity to the transport mechanism localized at the axonal membrane of catecholamine neurons. Second, 6-OH-DA is very susceptible to non-enzymatic oxidation with formation of reactive molecular species. The former property accounts for the *specificity* and the latter for *cytotoxic action* of 6-OH-DA (see Jonsson and Sachs 1971; Jonsson 1980). The degenerative effects are initiated when 6-OH-DA reaches a threshold concentration intraneuronally (Thoenen and Tranzer 1968; Jonsson and Sachs 1970). Consonantly, the general experience is also that 6-OH-DA acts very much in an 'all-or-none' fashion with a complete destruction of catecholamine uptake-storage mechanisms and functional properties in a proportion of adrenergic nerves related to the dose of 6-OH-DA administered (Jonsson and Sachs 1972).

6-OH-DA can be taken up in the amine storage granules acting as a "false transmitter," although this is seen only at very low, non-degenerative doses. The relatively high affinity of 6-OH-DA to the storage-granules can be used to identify these structures at the ultrastructural level, very early after the 6-OH-DA administration (1 h or less; Bennett et al. 1970; Cobb and Bennett 1971), although 5-hydroxydopamine is generally the compound of choice for this purpose (Tranzer and Thoenen 1967 b). So far, very little evidence has appeared suggesting that 6-OH-DA can produce a transient damage of functional significance not associated with degeneration from a structural and biochemical viewpoint, although this can not always be excluded. The neurotoxic action of 6-OH-DA has a very rapid onset with an almost complete disappearance of the catecholamine stores within 30 min–1 h after the 6-OH-DA administration. The neurotoxicity is also reflected by a similarly rapid loss of catecholamine uptake functions ('membrane pump') (Thoenen and Tranzer 1968; Jonsson and Sachs 1970) and a disappearance of the ability to generate and conduct action potentials (Haeusler 1971; Furness et al. 1970). The first signs of degeneration at the ultrastructural level can already be observed 1–4 h after the administration of 6-OH-DA (Furness et al. 1970; Hökfelt et al. 1972). The degenerative changes are very similar to those seen after surgical axotomy, although they appear generally much faster due to a direct action of 6-OH-DA on the nerve terminals. The very rapid neurodegenerative effects of 6-OH-DA is an important factor to consider when sampling tissue for ultrastructural identification of degeneration, since in many situations the degenerating structures will soon disappear and are not detectable after a few days. Using fluorescence histochemistry for the demonstration of catecholamine neurons, the neurotoxic actions of 6-OH-DA are, in addition to the disappearance of transmitter from the nerve terminals, seen as massive accumulations of catecholamines in non-terminal axons due to a disruption of the axoplasma flow. This is a relatively sensitive index, although not always exclusively related to a degenerative damage of a nerve terminal field. As a consequence of the degeneration there will also be a disappearance of the transmitter synthesizing enzymes, e.g., tyrosine hydroxylase and dopamine-β-hydroxylase.

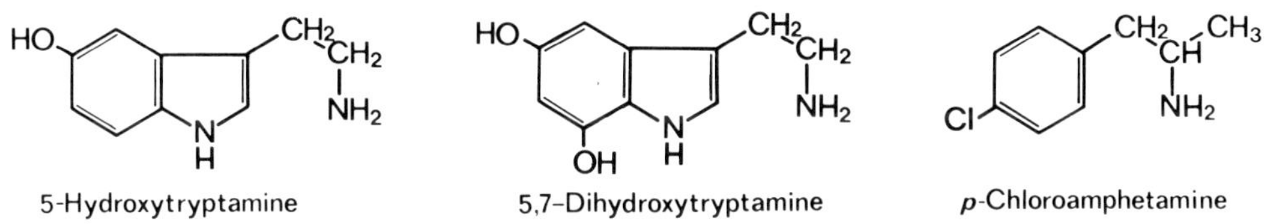

Fig. 3. Structural formulae of 5-HT, 5,7-HT and pCAM

Although a great deal of work has been undertaken to elucidate the *molecular mechanism(s) of the neurodegenerative actions* of 6-OH-DA, it still remains somewhat unclear. It is generally accepted that the cytotoxic actions are associated with the ease of auto-oxidation of 6-OH-DA, which, however, involves a series of complex reactions with simultaneous formation of several potentially cytotoxic agents, such as quinones (Saner and Thoenen 1971; Jonsson 1976 a), hydrogen peroxide (Heikkila and Cohen 1972), 5,6-dihydroxyindole (Blank et al. 1972), superoxide, and hydroxy radicals (Heikkila and Cohen 1973; Cohen and Heikkila 1974). There are two molecular theories proposed to explain the cytotoxic effects, both based on the fact that 6-OH-DA is very easily oxidized. The first suggested theory postulates that quinoid-like oxidation products of 6-OH-DA may act as alkylating agents on i.a. SH groups (Saner and Thoenen 1971; Jonsson 1976 a) while the other theory postulates that reactive oxygen oxidation products (hydrogen peroxide and radicals) are the causative molecular species (Heikkila and Cohen 1975). It is conceivable that both mechanisms could cause changes of the structural and functional properties of important neuronal proteins and lipids leading to irreversible damage and initiating degeneration. There is experimental evidence corroborating both theories, although the relative importance of the two proposed mechanisms is less clear. Recent investigations carried out to resolve this question have provided results suggesting that both processes are operating simultaneously (Borchardt et al. 1977; Graham et al. 1978). Therefore, it appears as the neurodegeneration is the result of complex chemical reactions involving both alkylation by electrophiles (6-OH-DA, quinone, aminochromes) and oxygen oxidation products.

Concerning the *practical use* of 6-OH-DA as a denervation tool, it is a well known fact that there is a considerable heterogeneity in the response to 6-OH-DA in the various central and peripheral catecholamine neuron systems. Certain systems have thus been found to be very sensitive while others are almost completely resistant to the neurotoxic action of 6-OH-DA. There is, in addition, a variable sensitivity in different parts of the single catecholamine neuron and between different species. It has generally been found that the nerve terminals (varicosities) are the most sensitive structures, the axons less so, while the cell bodies in most cases are very resistant to the neurodegenerative actions of 6-OH-DA. The reasons for this are not fully understood, although it is reasonable to assume that differences in local circulation, diffusion conditions, uptake-accumulation properties, surface-volume relationships of the neuronal structures, and certain intraneuronal factors are responsible for the heterogenous effects of 6-OH-DA (see Jonsson 1980). This makes it necessary to empirically work out optimal conditions for each given system that the investigator wishes to denervate. There is, however, a considerable amount of information on this point which has been summarized in papers by Kostrzewa and Jacobowitz (1974) and Breese (1975).

When using 6-OH-DA experimentally, it is important to use it freshly prepared in physiological saline or artificial cerebrospinal fluid (for intracerebral or intraventricular injections) containing an antioxidant (e.g., 0.2 mg/ml ascorbic acid). It is recommended that the 6-OH-DA substance should be stored under dark and dry conditions to minimize spontaneous break-down. Ascorbic acid is used in the injection solutions to prevent oxidation. High concentrations of ascorbic acid itself can have general cytotoxic effects (see Waddington and Crow 1979), which is especially important when performing intracerebral injections. In many species (rat, mouse, guinea-pig, rabbit) an intravenous injection of 50 mg/kg 6-OH-DA (free base) will produce an efficient sympathectomy which is almost complete in, for example, iris, heart, salivary glands. In order to obtain more consistent results, it may be recommended to inject the same dose once more one day after the first injection. In the mouse an almost complete sympathectomy can be achieved even with a dose of 20 mg/kg (i.v.) in the mentioned organs. For a complete denervation of sympathetic adrenergic nerves in the vas deferens very high doses are needed (100–500 mg/kg i.v.) which must be injected slowly in order to avoid lethal effects (see Malmfors 1971). When administering these high doses of 6-

OH-DA there are signs of non-specific cytotoxic effects (hemolysis, damage to tubules of the kidney). With doses up to 50 mg/kg very little cytotoxic effects have been observed on the cell-bodies in sympathetic ganglia, while after high doses (250–500 mg/kg) a certain decrease in the number of cell bodies has been observed (Malmfors 1971). Although 6-OH-DA administered to adult animals does not easily pass the blood-brain barrier, it is known that this barrier does not protect the brain completely from the neurotoxic actions of 6-OH-DA. It has thus been observed that there is a permanent NA depletion of about 25% in the rat cerebral cortex and spinal cord after 100 mg/kg 6-OH-DA, i.v. (Sachs and Jonsson 1973).

Since 6-OH-DA, as mentioned, does not easily enter the brain after systemic administration, this has to be circumvented when employing 6-OH-DA for denervation of neurons in the CNS. This can be achieved by intraventricular, intracisternal, or intracerebral injections of 6-OH-DA. Since the route of administration and the injection technique are crucial factors for the outcome, it is very difficult to state anything definite as to the sensitivity of the various catecholamine neuron systems in the CNS. The general experience is, however, that the terminal projections of the locus coeruleus NA system appear to be the most sensitive structures to 6-OH-DA, while the adrenaline (A) neuron systems are the most resistant (Jonsson 1980). It is unclear at present whether 6-OH-DA can induce a degeneration of A neurons at all, although there are data suggesting that they can be at least partially affected after large doses (Fuxe et al. 1975). The *dopamine* (DA) systems exhibit a differential sensitivity, from being relatively sensitive (the *nigrostriatal* DA system) to almost completely resistant to the cytotoxic action of 6-OH-DA (the *tubero-infundibular* DA system). In most situations the catecholamine perikarya will survive, although it is known that the DA cell bodies in the *substantia nigra* are relatively sensitive and can disappear completely after 6-OH-DA. Intracisternal or intraventricular injections of very large doses of 6-OH-DA (500–1000 μg in 25–50 μl) have generally been found to cause remarkably little non-specific cytotoxic effects. An intraventricular injection of 2×400 μg of 6-OH-DA has thus been found to produce a very selective effect on catecholamine neurons from a biochemical viewpoint (Jacks et al. 1972). Certain unspecific damage of ependymal cells have been noted after such high doses which may lead to hydrocephalus (Descarrier and Saucier 1972; Poirier et al. 1972). However, these modes of administration will lead to a very heterogenous denervation pattern, from complete denervations in, for example, the cerebral cortex, to very marginal effects in, for example, the hypothalamus. The degenerative effect is generally more pronounced on NA than on DA neuronal systems. These types of injections can also lead to differential denervation patterns, depending on whether the effect of 6-OH-DA is directly on the nerve terminals with a rapid denervation (within one day) or whether it is on the axons, resulting in an anterograde degeneration which will take several days before reaching its maximal denervation state. Another drawback with intraventricular injections is that in order to avoid asymmetrical effects, the neurotoxin has to be administered bilaterally (see Gershanik et al. 1979).

Although the intraventricular route of administration can be regarded as producing rather selective effects on catecholamine neurons, it is obvious that the heterogenous denervation pattern will considerably limit its use, especially in functional studies (see Ungerstedt 1968, 1971; Gershanik et al. 1979). Therefore, local intracerebral injections of 6-OH-DA were introduced with the intention of selectively denervating one principal catecholamine system (Ungerstedt 1971). This procedure involves stereotaxic placing of an injection cannula in a brain region where cell bodies or axons are localized. The cannula is connected to an injection device making it possible to infuse microliter quantities of the 6-OH-DA solution. The amounts of 6-OH-DA generally injected have been in the order of 1–10 μg in 1–10 μl solvent. This technique has been extensively used for the analysis of various aspects of catecholamine transmitter functions (see Jonsson et al. 1975). Although theoretically very attractive, this denervation method has been subjected to a great deal of controversy. While Ungerstedt (1971) in his early publications stated that the technique produced very selective lesions, Poirier et al. (1972) and Butcher et al. (1974; Butcher 1975) have concluded that 6-OH-DA injected locally in the brain does not produce any more selective lesions than those observed after using conventionally non-selective lesioning techniques. As in many situations of controversy, the sound judgment of the situation is also in this case somewhere in between the extreme positions. In view of the fact that 6-OH-DA is a generally cytotoxic agent and its specificity solely dependent on its selective accumulation, it is obvious that any tissue element can be damaged if it is exposed to high enough concentrations of 6-OH-DA. Such a situation can of course, be easily reached when high concentrations are infused locally at a relatively rapid speed.

The general experience is that concentrations not higher than 2 μg/μl of 6-OH-DA infused at a rate of 1–5 μl/min should be used in order to minimize the non-specific effects. There will always be mechanical damage due to the introduction of the injection cannula and this first zone will in older lesions be surrounded by a reactive gliosis (second zone) which is a general response in the CNS after mechanical damage. Further out from the infusion point there will appear a third zone where all structures seem to be affected and the size of this zone is most likely mainly related to the 6-OH-DA concentration used for infusion. The third zone gradually passes over to a fourth zone where only certain structures are affected. This fourth zone is considered to be the zone of specific action of 6-OH-DA and its extent is mainly a function of the volume and the rate at which the 6-OH-DA solution is infused. This is a simplified description of the consequences following a local 6-OH-DA infusion from a structural viewpoint and it has to be pointed out that there can be a considerable variation from this general picture in various CNS regions and depending on the injection technique used. Although there is a great deal of information on dose, volume, and injection conditions for the selective denervation on various catecholamine neuron system in rat brain (see Agid et al. 1973; Hökfelt and Ungerstedt 1973; Ungerstedt 1973; Lidbrink 1974; Lidbrink and Jonsson 1974; Koda et al. 1978), it has to be emphasized that the specificity and extent of the lesion in each particular case has to be evaluated by morphological, biochemical, and physiological indices related to the purpose of the denervation.

In recent years a new technique for local denervation of catecholamine nerves using 6-OH-DA has been introduced making use of osmotic minipumps (Kasamatsu and Pettigrew 1976; Kasamatsu et al. 1981). This technique is based on local infusion of a 6-OH-DA solution (4 mM) via a small cannula placed in the cerebral cortex. The continuous infusion of 1 μl/h over 1 week is obtained by connecting the cannula to an osmotic minipump (Alzet). With this technique it is possible to obtain an almost complete NA denervation in the cortex about 5 mm around the infusion cannula with limited non-specific damage.

In spite of the fact that it is impossible to obtain a completely specific catecholamine denervation with 6-OH-DA using the local microinjection technique, it is obvious that it is possible to obtain reasonably selective catecholamine denervation if properly used, both from a structural and biochemical as well as a functional viewpoint. There are also several experimental possibilities of modifying the neurotoxic action and potency of 6-OH-DA, to be used in an advantageous way to improve the lesion, both from a quantitive and specificity viewpoint (see Jonsson 1980).

Since 6-OH-DA can affect both NA and DA neurons, a specificity problem can arise if only one of the neuron types is to be denervated in an area with a mixed NA and DA innervation. For the selective denervation of DA neurons it is possible to use a potent NA uptake inhibitor such as desipramine or protriptyline (25 mg/kg i.p.). Treatment of the animal with the uptake inhibitor 30 min before the 6-OH-DA administration will protect the NA neurons but not DA neurons from undergoing degeneration, thereby providing a procedure for the selective denervation of DA neurons. There has so far not been reported any similar approach for the selective denervation of NA neurons, mainly because of lack of a potent, selective DA uptake inhibitor, although benztropine has been used in this respect with limited success. The use of selective uptake inhibitors can, in many situations, be very valuable in order to control for nonspecific cytotoxic effects in functional studies (see Lidbrink and Jonsson 1975). The newly discovered neurotoxin DSP4 (Fig. 2), which has been found to possess a remarkable selectivity for NA neurons, might be the neurotoxin of choice for the selective NA denervation in regions with a mixed NA/DA innervation (see below). The specificity of 6-OH-DA for catecholamine neurons can vary between different species. Although 6-OH-DA is very selective for catecholamine neurons in rat and mouse, it has been observed that 5-HT neurons are also affected by 6-OH-DA in cat (Laguzzi et al. 1971). This problem can be overcome by pretreatment with the preferential 5-HT uptake blocker chlorimipramine.

For studies on the *developmental aspects* of catecholamine neurons, 6-OH-DA is the most frequently and extensively used neurotoxin, administered either systemically or intracisternally (intracranially). Developing rats and mice tolerate 6-OH-DA very well, and doses of 100 mg/kg can be administered systemically (i.p. or s.c.) and up to 100 μg intracisternally (in 10 μl), from the day of birth. This treatment can be repeated over several days without any marked increase in mortality, according to the author's experience. Systemic 6-OH-DA administration can only be used after birth since it does not pass the blood-placenta barrier.

Although 6-OH-DA has been shown to possess a selective neurotoxic effect on developing catecholamine neurons, several studies have disclosed that the neurons react quite differently to the neurotoxin during the development compared to the adult stage. Angeletti and Levi-Montalchini (1970) have thus reported that systemic injection of 6-OH-DA in the neonatal stage causes a selective and permanent destruction of the perikarya in sympathetic ganglia, leading to a permanent sympathectomy. This finding has been confirmed several times, although it has generally been observed that the sympathectomy is not as complete as originally reported. Systemic administration of 6-OH-DA to newborn rats also causes effects in the CNS due to a not fully developed blood-brain barrier, which for 6-OH-DA matures around 7–10 days after birth (Sachs 1973). Systemic 6-OH-DA (1–3 × 100 mg/kg s.c.) administration during the first postnatal week produces selective and permanent alterations of the postnatal development of central NA neurons (Clark et al. 1972; Sachs and Jonsson 1972; Singh and de Champlain 1972; Jonsson et al. 1974). The data available point to a preferential effect on the terminal projections of the locus coeruleus NA system while the NA perikarya are apparently unaffected (Jonsson and Sachs 1976; Jonsson et al. 1979). The 6-OH-DA-induced changes are characterized by striking regional variations, with pronounced and permanent NA denervations in distant projections, e.g., cerebral cortex, hippocampus, and spinal cord, and a marked increase in the NA nerve terminal density near the NA cell bodies, e.g., in the cerebellum and pons-medulla. The altered development of the central NA neurons are most likely due to a "pruning effect" (see Fig. 5). Similar alterations in the development of NA neurons can also be seen after intracisternal administration of 6-OH-DA (up to 50 μg) (Zieher and Jaim-Etcheverry 1973, 1975; Kostrzewa and Harper 1974; Sachs and Jonsson 1975 c; Kostrzewa and Garey 1977). However, injection of larger doses of 6-OH-DA (100 μg) intracisternally will mainly produce permanent denervations, although rather heterogenously, and will in addition produce permanent DA denervations (Breese 1975; Sachs and Jonsson 1975 c). While systemically administered 6-OH-DA has very little effect on the growth and general development of the rats (Sachs et al. 1974), it has been found that a intracisternal 6-OH-DA injection leading to a DA denervation also causes growth deficits (Breese et al. 1973).

For prenatal studies, it is possible to use 6-OH-DA by directly administering the neurotoxin into the fetus (see Thierry et al. 1975). This is, however, generally a difficult approach experimentally with high mortality rate among the fetuses. On the whole very little has been published on the use of catecholamine neurotoxins as denervation tools in the prenatal stage and more work is needed for the evaluation of their usefulness for such studies.

A considerable number of 6-OH-DA derivatives and related polyphenols have been synthetized and tested, over the years, but none of them has been found to be superior to 6-OH-DA as a tool for inducing degeneration of catecholamine neurons. Of all the compounds developed, only 6-OH-DOPA and 6-amino-DA have come to be used to a certain extent (see Kostrzewa and Jacobowitz 1974; Sachs and Jonsson 1975 a).

3.1.1.2 6-Hydroxy-DOPA

The amino acid 6-OH-DOPA has the advantage of passing the blood-brain barrier and can therefore be administered systemically. Alterations in the development of NA-neurons has been observed after systematic administration of 6-OH-DOPA (100 mg/kg s.c.) to newborn rats. Pregnant rats can also be injected with 6-OH-DOPA in doses of 100 mg/kg i.v. with rather selective actions on catecholamine neurons of the offspring (Jaim-Etcheverry and Zieher 1975). However, the compound is not so well tolerated by the animals and relatively large doses must be used to obtain a substantial catecholamine denervation in the CNS, which in addition is very heterogeneous with respect to various catecholamine neuron systems.

3.1.1.3 6-Aminodopamine

This neurotoxin acts very much like 6-OH-DA on catecholamine neurons, although it is more generally cytotoxic than 6-OH-DA which makes its use as a denervation tool less attractive (Jonsson and Sachs 1973).

3.1.1.4 DSP4

Recently a new interesting catecholamine neurotoxin has been discovered, namely *N*-(2-chloroethyl)-*N*-ethyl-2-bromobenzylamine (DSP4, see Fig. 2). This compound which is structurally different from 6-OH-DA has been found to produce in mice an acute and selective degeneration of both central and peripheral NA nerve terminals (Ross 1976 a; Jonsson et al. 1978 b; Hallman and Jonsson 1980), without any apparent neurotoxic effect on DA, A, and 5-HT neurons. The data so far obtained have disclosed that DSP4 acts on the NA nerve terminals very much in the same manner as 6-OH-DA, as monitored by histochemical and neurochemical techniques, although very little is known at present as to the exact molecular mechanism of action. It is likely that DSP4 which is unstable and very reactive produces its neurotoxic effects via an alkylation reaction. The neurodegenerative effects can be completely prevented by pretreatment with the NA uptake inhibitor desipramine (25 mg/kg i.p., 30 min before DSP4 administration) indicating that DSP4 acts directly on NA neurons, although it is unclear whether it has to be accumulated intraneuronally like 6-OH-DA or mediates the neurotoxicity via interaction with receptor or uptake sites on the external membrane surface of the NA nerve terminals. DSP4 easily passes the blood-brain barrier unlike 6-OH-DA and can therefore be administered systemically (i.v. or i.p.). An i.p. injection of DSP4 (50 mg/kg) produces a preferential neurodegenerative effect on nerve terminal projections (in, for example, cerebral cortex, cerebellum, spinal cord) originating from the locus coeruleus NA perikarya. The degenerative effect is relatively rapid, within 4–6 h, without any substantial recovery in most regions of the CNS after 2–3 months (Jonsson, unpublished observations). DSP4 is well tolerated by newborn rats (50 mg/kg s.c.) and passes the blood-placenta barrier when injected to pregnant rats in doses up to 25–50 mg/kg i.v. (Hallman and Jonsson 1980; Jaim-Etcheverry and Zieher 1980). It may therefore be employed as a NA degenerative agent in developmental work.

In the mouse the selectivity of DSP4 for NA neurons seems to be very high from a histochemical and biochemical viewpoint, but it has been noted in the rat that DSP4 can have a small degenerative effect on 5-HT nerve terminals. However, this specificity problem can be overcome by pretreatment with a preferential 5-HT uptake blocker (zimelidin, 25 mg/kg i.p., 30 min before DSP4) which results in a protection of 5-HT neurons without diminishing the neurotoxic potency on NA nerves. In view of the fact that DSP4 can pass the blood-brain barrier and appears to have a rather selective neurodegenerative effect on NA neurons, it may prove to be a neurotoxin of choice in many situations for studies of various aspects of NA transmitter functions in the CNS. However, more work with this compound is needed to substantiate this view.

3.1.1.5 Guanethidine

Another selective neurotoxin that ought to be mentioned in this context is guanethidine, an adrenergic neuron blocking agent, which has been used for many years in the treatment of hypertension. Chronic treatment with this compound has been observed to cause a very marked and selective degeneration of sympathetic adrenergic neurons (Burnstock et al. 1971; Eränkö and Eränkö 1971; Jensen-Holm and Juul 1971; Heath et al. 1972). There is a different sensitivity towards the neurotoxic action of guanethidine between different sympathetically innervated organs; the short adrenergic neurons innervating the vas deferens appears to be the most sensitive (Gannon et al. 1971; Evans et al. 1972; Bittiger et al. 1977). The reason for this is not clearly understood, although differences in neuronal activity could partly contribute to this (Evans 1979). The selectivity in neurotoxic effect of guanethidine is most likely due to its accumulation in adrenergic neurons, whereas the cytotoxic action is believed to be associated with the ability of guanethidine to inhibit oxidative phosphorylation. Although guanethidine has so far had only limited use as a denervation tool, it has been claimed that this compound may have some advantages over 6-OH-DA for obtaining sympathectomy, especially in developing animals (Johnson et al. 1975).

3.1.2 Serotonin Neurotoxins

The discovery of 6-OH-DA as a tool for selective degeneration of catecholamine neurons provided the impetus to search for compounds with similar neurodegenerative effects specific for 5-HT neurons. These attempts led to the successful discovery by Baumgarten and co-workers of the dihydroxy indoles 5,6-HT and 5,7-HT which can be used to produce reasonably selective denervations of 5-HT neurons (Baumgarten et al. 1971, 1972, 1973; Baumgarten and Lachenmeyer 1972).

3.1.2.1 Dihydroxytryptamines

The specificity of these compounds is like 6-OH-DA related to a selective uptake-accumulation and the neurodegenerative action elicited by formation of highly cytotoxic molecular species intraneuronally. The exact mode of action at the molecular level is not known, although the cytotoxic action appears in certain respects to be similar to that of 6-OH-DA. It is clear, however, that there are distinct differences between the neurotoxic tryptamines and 6-OH-DA as well as differences in the action between the dihydroxytryptamines themselves (see Jonsson 1980). Since their discovery the neurotoxic dihydroxytryptamines have been extensively used as denervation tools for studies on various aspects of structure and function of 5-HT neurons (see Baumgarten and Björklund 1976; Baumgarten et al. 1977; Jacoby and Lytle 1978). Of the large number of hydroxylated indole derivatives that have been tested for neurotoxic potency and specificity on 5-HT neurons, 5,6-HT and 5,7-HT appear the most suitable compounds to be used as experimental denervation tools (Baumgarten et al. 1975 a). Although both 5,6-HT and 5,7-HT have efficient neurotoxic action on 5-HT neurons, there are clear differences between the properties of the two compounds which are important when considering employing them in experimental work. 5,6-HT has thus been found to have a high degree of specificity for 5-HT neurons among the various monoamine neurons, but due to its instability and high reactivity can cause marked nonspecific cytotoxic effects on non-monoamine neurons, especially after administration of large doses. 5,7-HT, which is more stable and has a high neurotoxic potency on 5-HT neurons, produces clearly less damage to non-monoamine-containing structures and is therefore more attractive as a denervation tool for 5-HT neurons. It has been found, however, that 5,7-HT, apart from neurotoxic effects on 5-HT neurons, can also affect the catecholamine neurons, in particular the NA neurons. This drawback can, however, to a large extent be circumvented by various pharmacological treatments (see below), making it possible to obtain rather selective 5-HT denervations. Therefore, 5,7-HT is the serotonin neurotoxin of choice in most situations, particularly in functional studies when the specificity is a critical issue.

The main application for the serotonin neurotoxins is as a denervation tool of central 5-HT neurons, although both 5,6-HT and 5,7-HT can induce a degeneration of sympathetic adrenergic nerves. However, 6-OH-DA is preferable for inducing a chemical sympathectomy.

Neither 5,6-HT nor 5,7-HT pass the blood-brain barrier. In experimental work they have to be introduced directly into the brain by intraventricular or intracisternal administration or by local intracerebral microinjections. Using the intraventricular or intracisternal modes of administration it is possible to achieve quite marked 5-HT denervations, although there will be a very heterogeneous denervation pattern with marked regional variations; from very marked denervations, e.g., in the spinal cord, to relatively minor effects, e.g., in the pons-medulla (Baumgarten et al. 1971, 1973). The 5-HT nerve terminals are the most sensitive structures while the cell bodies are to a large extent unaffected by such injections. In certain cases, however, marked and permanent cell body losses have been observed (Nygren and Olson 1977). The highest dose of 5,6-HT that rats can tolerate is generally 75 μg (in 20 μl), whereas 5,7-HT can be injected in doses up to 200 μg intracisternally or intraventricularly. In order to avoid asymmetrical effects after a unilateral injection of 5,7-HT intraventricularly, it has been recommended to administer the neurotoxin as a pulse injection (Jenner and Baumgarten 1980). These authors also noted a more pronounced effect by 5,7-HT on 5-HT neurons if the injection was performed in ether- as compared to nembutal-anaesthetized animals. After administration of large doses of 5,7-HT there will in addition to the effects on 5-HT neurons also be substantial neurodegenerative effects on NA neurons as well as DA neurons, though to a lesser degree. The nonselective effect with respect to NA neurons can be largely overcome by pretreatment with the NA uptake blocker desipramine 25 mg/kg i.p. (Björklund et al. 1975; Gershon and Baldessarini 1975; Sachs and Jonsson 1975 b). It has recently been proposed that pretreatment with nomifensine (25 mg/kg i.p.) gives a better and more complete protection towards the neurotoxic action of 5,7-HT on both NA and DA neurons after an intraventricular injection (Baumgarten et al. 1980).

The limitations and drawbacks associated with the use of the intraventricular or intracisternal injection technique for denervation of catecholamine neuron systems using 6-OH-DA are for obvious reasons also of relevance when employing these modes of administration of 5,6-HT or 5,7-HT for denervation of 5-HT neurons. In order to obtain a more selective and a better defined denervation of a particular or principal 5-HT neuron system, the local intracerebral injection technique has to be applied (Daly et al. 1973, 1974; Björklund et al. 1973; Fuxe and Jonsson 1974; Hole et al. 1976; Fuxe et al. 1978). For this purpose 5,7-HT is the neurotoxin of choice and similar considerations as those pointed out when using 6-OH-DA (neurotoxin concentration, volume infused, and speed of infusion) are of importance when administering 5,7-HT intracerebrally. A concentration of 1 μg/μl of 5,7-HT and a total dose of 4 μg is generally used in the rat. In order to increase the specificity of 5,7-HT the same pharmacological approach can be used as that described for intraventricular injection of 5,7-HT. It should be emphasized that the optimal conditions have to be tested out empirically for the particular 5-HT neuronal system that is intended to be lesioned. As with 6-OH-DA, it is very difficult to avoid nonspecific cytotoxic effects completely after an intracerebral injection. The lesions after 5,7-HT are, however, small compared to lesions produced by electrolysis (Lorens et al. 1976).

Concerning the use of serotonin neurotoxins for studies on developing 5-HT neurons, only data for the postnatal development have been published. 5,7-HT appears to be the neurotoxin of choice, since developing rats do not tolerate 5,6-HT very well (Sachs and Jonsson 1975 b). The nonselective effects of 5,7-HT on NA neurons can be counteracted by pretreatment with desipramine (Jonsson and Sachs 1975 b; Breese et al. 1978). For intracisternal injections doses up to 100 μg in 10 μl can be injected with marked neurodegenerative effects on 5-HT neurons (Lytle et al. 1974; Baumgarten et al., 1975 b; Breese and Cooper 1975; Breese et al. 1978). 5,7-HT can also be injected systemically in doses up to 100 mg/kg s.c. leading to an altered development of central 5-HT neurons (Sachs and Jonsson 1975 b; Jonsson 1976 b; Jonsson et al. 1978 a) in an analogous manner as that seen after neonatal 6-OH-DA treatment on NA neurons (Jonsson et al. 1974). The blood-brain barrier for 5,7-HT matures about 1 week after birth in rats (Jonsson et al. 1978 a).

3.1.2.2 Halogenated Amphetamines

The halogenated amphetamines, which are structurally different from the dihydroxytryptamines, constitute another class of compounds with a selective neurotoxic action on 5-HT neurons. The first discovered and apparently most potent of these neurotoxic compounds is *p*- or 4-chloroamphetamine (*p*CAM, Fig. 3; Sanders-Bush et al. 1972) which has been used to a certain extent as a denervation tool. *p*CAM can be administered systemically and produces a selective long-lasting depletion of 5-HT in the rat brain. The dose of *p*CAM for the rat is generally 10–20 mg/kg i.p., whereas higher doses are needed for mice (50 mg/kg). The effect can be abolished by 5-HT uptake blockers like zimelidine (Ross 1976 b), indicating that the neurotoxic action is mediated by a direct action on 5-HT neurons, possibly via an intraneuronal uptake and accumulation. The molecular mechanisms of the neurotoxic action of these compounds is largely unknown. There is some controversy as to which 5-HT neuronal systems are preferentially affected by *p*CAM and related compounds. However, on the basis of histochemical and fluorescence histochemical data it appears that *p*CAM mainly induces a degeneration of ascending but not descending 5-HT nerve terminal projections (see Köhler et al. 1978 a). There is thus a very marked variability in the sensitivity of 5-HT nerve terminals in different CNS regions, from an almost complete 5-HT denervation (cerebral cortex) to practically no effects (spinal cord). Moreover, *p*CAM has been found ineffective in the neonatal stage, even after large doses (Clemens et al. 1978). The reason for this variable sensitivity is not known, but this emphasizes the opinion that *p*CAM is not generally applicable as a denervation tool for denervation of 5-HT neurons. The halogenated amphetamines can, however, in situations where it is possible to obtain almost complete 5-HT denervations have clear advantages compared to 5,6-HT and 5,7-HT due to less specificity problems, which is particularly important in functional studies (see Fuller 1978; Ögren et al. 1980).

3.2 Excitotoxic Amino Acids

During the last decade it has become increasingly clear that the putative neurotransmitter glutamate (Fig. 4) and certain of its structural analogues have potent neurotoxic actions in the CNS. The first evidence for this came from studies showing that glutamate administration to neonate mice led to a degeneration of certain retinal neurons (Lucas and Newhouse 1957). Later Olney et al. (1971) could demonstrate that glutamate and certain analogues could all induce neuronal degeneration in the brain and the common feature of these compounds is their excitatory effect on most CNS neurons (Curtis et al. 1972) and the neurotoxic potency correlates very well with their neuroexcitatory activity. These compounds have therefore been called excitotoxic amino acids, the most powerful of which is kainic acid (Fig. 4), a conformationally restricted analogue of glutamic acid (Olney et al. 1974).

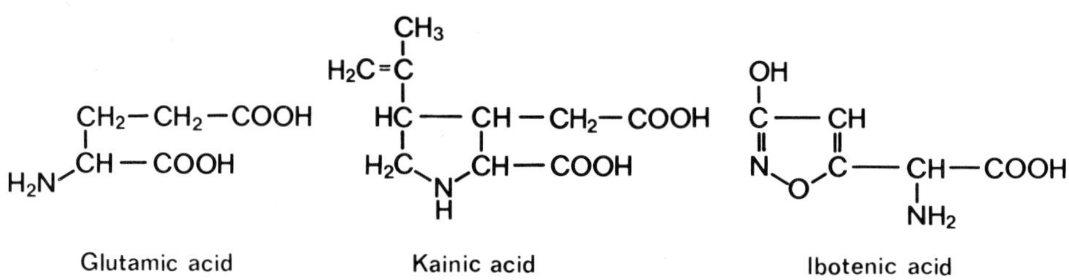

Fig. 4. Structural analogues of glutamic acid

3.2.1 Kainic Acid

The breakthrough for the use of the excitotoxic amino acids as denervation tools came from studies demonstrating that local intracerebral injection of kainic acid produces a rapid degeneration of neurons with cell bodies near the site of infusion sparing the axons of passage and afferent nerve terminals (Coyle and Schwarcz 1976; McGeer and McGeer 1976). These findings opened up new possibilities for neurobiologists to use kainic acid for the exploration and analysis of complex neuroanatomical circuitries and in the localization of various biochemical markers to specific types of structures. It has in addition opened up possibilities to develop animal models of diseases involving general loss of neurons in specific brain loci (e.g., Huntington's chorea, epilepsy). During the last couple of years we have seen an enormous activity in this field with a steady increase in the number of studies published (see McGeer et al. 1978 a, b; Coyle 1979; Nadler 1979).

It was initially proposed that the neurotoxic action of kainic acid and related compounds is produced by prolonged depolarization and that this effect is mediated through direct activation of glutamate receptors that are concentrated in the dendritic and somatic region of the neuron but largely absent from axons (Olney et al. 1974; Coyle and Schwarcz 1976). Recent observations have, however, indicated that the neurotoxic action of kainic acid most probably involves an indirect process, possibly by a cooperative interaction between kainic acid at specific receptors on vulnerable neurons and synaptically released endogenous neurotransmitters, in particular glutamic acid (McGeer and McGeer 1978; Biziere and Coyle 1979).

The applicability of kainic acid and related excitotoxins is much broader with respect to neuron types compared with the monoamine neurotoxins, since most perikarya and dendrites are considered to have receptors or recognition sites through which the neurotoxic action is mediated (Curtis and Watkins 1963; Curtis and Johnston 1974; Buu et al. 1976). This is the basis for the use of these compounds as denervation tools by local intracerebral injection for ablation neuronal cell populations localized in specific brain loci. For this purpose a generally used procedure in the rat is to inject intracerebrally 1–2 μg kainic acid in 0.5–1 μl artificial CSF solution of 1-min duration. The greatest experience from the use of kainic acid comes from studies of the rat striatum. It has been found that injection of 2 μg kainic acid into rat striatum leads to a rapid degeneration (within 48 h) of intrinsic neurons (cholinergic, GABAergic) within a radius of about 1.5 mm while afferents (DA and 5-HT nerve terminals) and fibers of passage are left apparently unaffected (Coyle and Schwarcz 1976; McGeer and McGeer 1976). The initial degeneration phase is followed by a marked proliferation of astrocytes in the gray matter (formerly populated by neurons) over a couple of weeks after the neurotoxin administration (Coyle et al. 1978). There is a marked atrophy in the chronically lesioned striatum (Zaczek et al. 1978) which must be considered when interpreting the effects of the lesion. The neuronal degeneration seen after intrastriatal injection of kainic acid in the rat resembles that of Huntington's disease (see Coyle 1979).

Although simple in theory, it is clear that the experimental use of kainic acid as a selective denervation tool is complicated by several factors. There is a considerable variation in vulnerability of different neuron types to the neurotoxic action of kainic acid which appears to depend at least partly on the synaptic input to the neurons. Lesions of the cerebral cortex have thus been observed to abolish the neurotoxic action of kainic acid injected into the striatum, indicating that neurotoxicity is dependent on an intact corticostriatal glutaminergic pathway (McGeer et al. 1978 a, b; Biziere and Coyle 1979). Another example of the synaptic input affecting the neurotoxicity of kainic acid is the observation that combined transections of perforant path and commissural fibers prior to the injection of kainic acid into hippocampus prevented the degeneration of hippocampal granule cells (Köhler et al. 1978 b). The neuronal vulnerability has been observed to vary considerably from region to region and within the same region. An illustrative example of this is the finding that intraventricularly administered kainic acid preferentially destroys hippocampal pyramidal cells (Nadler et al. 1978). The doses of kainic acid that are needed to induce degeneration of the most resistant neurons often approach lethal doses ($LD_{50} = 1–5$ μg, depending on the area). Brain maturity has also been shown to be an important factor affecting the neurotoxic potency of kainic acid. Campochiaro and Coyle (1978) have found that striatal neurons are almost insensitive to kainic acid at day 7 postnatally and that their vulnerability increases with age. The sensitivity to the neurotoxic action develops between the 2nd and 3rd week after birth. Another problem of kainic acid is its rapid diffusion rate that can lead to an undesirable degeneration of highly sensitive cells distant from the injection site (Wuerthele et al. 1978). Although many studies have demonstrated that kainic acid destroys intrinsic neurons with reasonable selectivity, it has been reported that kainic acid can cause damage to ascending NA fibers when injected into the mesencephalon where they constitute fibers of passage (Mason and Fibiger 1979). All of these findings strongly emphasize the importance of a careful analysis of the specificity and extent of kainic acid-induced lesions.

3.2.2 Ibotenic Acid

It has recently been observed that ibotenic acid, also a conformationally restricted glutamic acid analogue, can produce lesions after local intracerebral injection which in many respects are similar to those seen after kainic acid (Schwarcz et al. 1979). For the striatum a dose of 10 μg/1 μl is used. The exact mode of action of ibotenic acid as in the case of kainic acid, is not known, although there are indications that they may act by somewhat different mechanisms. It is notable, however, that some of the drawbacks of kainic acid are not so pronounced for ibotenic acid, which has been found to be less generally toxic and to produce more discrete lesions than kainic acid (Schwarcz et al. 1979). Ibotenic acid may, therefore, in many situations be the neurotoxin of choice for the morphological and functional analysis of central neuronal systems.

During the last couple of years there has been an ever-increasing use of conformationally restricted analogues of glutamic acid as denervation tools. These studies have demonstrated that with appropriate attention paid to the analysis of the extent and specificity of the lesions, the technique of local injection of these neurotoxins constitutes a powerful denervation tool for neurobiologists for selectively ablating neuronal cell groups in the brain.

3.3 Immunological Lesions

3.3.1 Antiserum to Nerve Growth Factor

One of the first lesion procedures of the selective type was introduced by Levi-Montalchini and co-workers who found that administration of antiserum to nerve growth factor (NGF) to newborn animals leads to an extensive destruction of the peripheral sympathetic neuron system and the term *"immunosympathectomy"* was coined (Cohen 1960; Levi-Montalchini and Booker 1960; Levi-Montalchini and Cohen 1960). NGF is an essential protein for the development of sympathetic and sensory ganglia and administration of antibodies to NGF will lead to an interference with the supply of NGF to the dependent neurons and consequently cause degeneration. The antiserum to NGF is most effective when administered to newborn animals and the sympathetic ganglia of several species (mouse, rat, cat, rabbit) have been shown to be sensitive (Levi-Montalchini and Angeletti 1966, 1968). A limitation of the procedure is, however, that all sympathetic ganglia are not affected to the same extent. The paravertebral ganglia have thus been shown to be most sensitive, while prevertebral ganglia are less so and the short postganglionic sympathetic neurons appear to be unaffected by anti-NGF, which is also the case for central catecholamine neurons. Although the "immunosympathectomy" technique has in recent years largely been replaced by the use of 6-OH-DA neurotoxin (*"chemical sympathectomy"*), which has a more general applicability and is available to most investigators (see Thoenen 1972), the interest in NGF as a factor participating in controlling differentiation and growth of neurons as well as neuron-target cell interactions continues to be an active field of research (see Smith and Kreutzberg 1976; Varon and Somjen 1979).

3.3.2 Antibody to Dopamine-β-hydroxylase

Another interesting type of immune lesion that has been reported in recent years originates from the observations that an i.v. administration of antibodies to the enzyme dopamine-β-hydroxylase (DBH, a vesicle-bound enzyme catalyzing the conversion of DA to NA) in guinea-pigs leads to a marked degeneration of post-ganglionic sympathetic nerves in the heart and intestine (Costa et al. 1976). Subsequent studies have disclosed that this lesion procedure involves a complement-mediated lysis and can be used to produce selective denervations of both central and peripheral NA neurons (Furness et al. 1977; Lewis et al. 1977; Costa et al. 1979). In the rat it has been shown that DBH-antibodies bind to NA nerves without causing any harmful effects (Jacobowitz et al. 1975). However, coadministration of an adequate complement system also induces degeneration in the rat (see Costa et al. 1979). The theoretical basis for this type of lesion is considered to be related to a binding and uptake of DBH antibody when the DBH present in synaptic vesicle membranes is exposed to the extracellular space during exocytototic release of NA. Although the immune lesion technique making use of antibodies to DBH does not at present have any advantages over 6-OH-DA for producing NA denervation, it is obvious that this approach is of utmost interest in view of the possibilities of extending it to a more general technique for selective lesioning of transmitter identified neuronal systems.

3.4 Miscellaneous Selective Lesion Techniques

Apart from the lesion methods described there are some other techniques of interest which are based on different principles and which can be used to produce selective lesions. It has been reported that *capsaicin*, the pungent element in fruits of various species, can be used as a chemical neurotoxin for inducing degeneration of certain primary sensory neurons (Jancsó et al. 1977). Administration of capsaicin (50 mg/kg s.c.) to newborn rats has thus been found to produce a selective degeneration of a distinct population of primary sensory neurons involved in mediation of chemogenic pain, as revealed by both functional and ultrastructural analyses. *Colchicine* and *vinca alkaloids* (vinblastine and vincristine), which are well-known inhibitors of mitosis and axoplasmic transport, can also be used for inducing degeneration of neurons (Dahlström 1971; Bennett et al. 1973, 1976; Hanbauer et al. 1973, 1974). The neurodegenerative action of these compounds is most likely related to their property of interfering with the structural integrity of microtubules leading to a blockade of axoplasmic transport. The vinca alkaloids and colchicine do not possess any absolute specificity per se, but can with an appropriate administration technique be employed for the selective degeneration of certain neuron systems (see Dahlström 1971; Bennett et al. 1976). Finally, it ought to be mentioned that techniques for the selective destruction of single neurons have been reported where the degeneration is induced by intracellular injection of proteolytic enzymes (Pronase; Miller and Silverston 1979) or by injection of fluorescent dye (Lucifer Yellow CH) followed by irradiation with blue light (Parnas and Bowling 1978). These techniques involve the use of microelectrodes where the injections are produced by pressure or iontophoresis into electrophysiologically identified neurons (see Chap. 19).

4 General Considerations

The methodological development over the years have resulted in a large number of lesion techniques based on different chemical-physical principles with variable applicability. The choice of lesion technique will for obvious reasons largely depend on the purpose of the lesion. Apart from the lesion technique per se, there are also other factors that have to be considered such as anesthesia (short- or long-acting) and the general effects that the operation or injection procedure used to obtain the lesion may cause in the acute phase, e.g., blood loss, pain, hydrocephalus, intracerebral hemorrhage, and edema. Depending on the parameters recorded in order to evaluate the effects of the lesion, the interpretation can be made within different reference frames (structural, biochemical, physiological) and the ultimate goal is generally to integrate this information to obtain structure-function relationships. In view of the very complex organization and the large number of functions in which the nervous system is involved, it is obvious that the use of the lesion approach to establish structure-function relationships is associated with major interpretion problems, which are not only of technical nature and related to imperfections of the lesion procedure used (see Moore 1978). Nevertheless, there will in most situations be great demands made upon precise information as to specificity and extent of the lesion. The situation in this respect is generally much more favorable when using the selective lesioning techniques as compared with the nonselective ones. Although several of the former techniques can be considered to produce reasonably selective denervations when properly used, it must be kept in mind that none of them possess absolute specificity at present. Experience has clearly demonstrated that the blind acceptance of the selective lesioning procedures causing only degeneration of neuronal elements in accord with the theoretical basis for the technique is unwarranted (see Bloom 1975; Mason and Fibiger 1979). A very important aspect of the lesion approach used to study structure and function is, therefore, *a careful evaluation of the specificity and extent of the lesion,* a view that is equally important irrespective of whether selective or nonselective lesioning techniques are employed. In this context it is of course very important that this evaluation be carried out by using adequate morphological, biochemical, and physiological indices, preferrably in quantitative terms.

The lesion approach has traditionally been used with a relatively static view as to the structural organization of the brain and its changes following a lesion The postlesion state is, however, by no means a static situation and there can be substantial changes with time from a structural viewpoint (see Fig. 5), which may have important functional implications. These changes display a considerable variation and have to be considered in all types of lesion procedures for an adequate interpretation of the consequences following a lesion. The acute degeneration phase is followed by reparative processes which start relatively early after the lesion and continue over months. In the CNS the processes involve both glia and nerve cells. Apart from the degenerative changes that occur in the lesioned neurons, transneuronal degeneration of anterograde or retrograde type can also occur in certain systems (see Fig. 1). The reaction of the glia cells involve scarring (gliosis) and phagocytotis to remove degenerated material, which in certain cases can be very pronounced and lead to tissue distortion. Although the regenerative capacity of peripheral nerves has been known for a long time, it is only in recent years that it has been realized that the central neurons can also demonstrate a remarkable growth capacity with considerable remodelling of the neuronal organization after a lesion (see Fig. 5, also Eidelberg and Stein 1974; Stein et al. 1974; Björklund and Stenevi 1979).

The reaction to injury differs remarkably between different classes of neurons as well as between various maturity states of the same neuron type. Lesioned central axons, in particular nonmyelinated axons, have been shown to undergo a considerable regenerative sprouting from the proximal stump leading in most cases to an abberant innervation of regions relatively close to the lesion, although in certain cases as with 5-HT neurons of the spinal cord both a structural and functional regeneration has

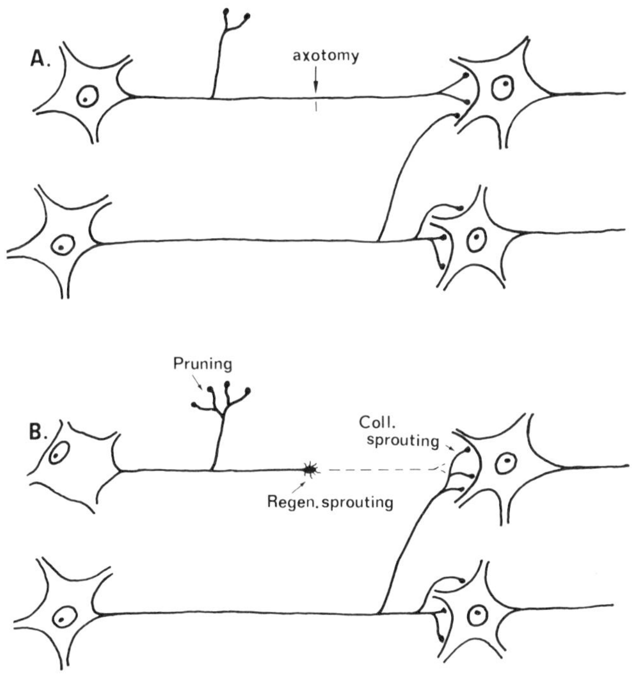

Fig. 5 A, B. Schematic illustration of various growth responses that can occur in the CNS after a lesion. **A** the normal state; **B** after axotomy (↓). There are three main types of growth responses: (1) *Regenerative sprouting* from the cut axon and regrowth to restore the normal situation. This is very seldom seen in the CNS. (2) *Collateral sprouting.* Intact collaterals near the degenerating nerve terminals will be activated and grow to replace vacated synaptic sites. (3) *Pruning effect,* intact collaterals will be activated and extend their terminal network, most frequently seen during the development

been observed after a 5,6-HT-induced lesion (Nygren et al. 1974). However, the end result of an axonal lesion of most long pathways in the brain will be a permanent degeneration of the distal part of the axon, a situation that has been called abortive regeneration (see Björklund and Stenevi 1979). Although structural regeneration to restore the original neuronal organization is a seldom seen event in the CNS, collateral sprouting (see Fig. 5) is a growth response to damage that has been observed in many regions and is a well-established phenomenon in both developing and mature CNS (see Björklund and Stenevi 1979). This growth response is considered to be of great importance in determining the chronic effects of a lesion. In some instances collateral sprouting has been ascribed to the functional recovery seen after a lesion, although in other cases it has not been possible to determine whether it is a compensatory mechanism or aggravates the consequences of a lesion leading to "neuronal confusion."

Finally, it ought to be mentioned that another type of growth response has also been seen, especially in the developing CNS, where the damaged neuron undergoes a "pruning effect" following a lesion of an axonal branch of a collateralized neuron (see Jonsson et al. 1979). All of these growth responses seen after lesions of CNS neurons emphasize the importance of the morphological analysis of the effects of a lesion both in the acute and chronic state. Other complicating factors for an adequate interpretation of the functional outcome of a lesion are various types of compensatory mechanisms that come into play after a lesion, such as changes in transmitter release and turnover of neurons spared by the lesion, readjustments in the functional balance between interacting neuronal systems, and receptor supersensitivity (see de Champlain et al. 1975; Zigmond and Stricker 1975).

Acknowledgments. Part of the studies reviewed have been supported by grants from the Swedish MRC (04X-2295), Bergvalls Stiftelse and Expressens prenatalfond. The author is very grateful to Mrs Birgit Frideen for typing the manuscript.

5 References

Agid Y, Javoy F, Glowinski J, Bouvet D, Sotelo C (1973) Injection of 6-hydroxy-dopamine into the substantia nigra of the rat. II. Diffusion and specificity. Brain Res 58:291–301

Angeletti PU, Levi-Montalcini R (1970) Sympathetic nerve cell destruction in newborn mammals by 6-hydroxydopamine. Proc Natl Acad Sci USA 65:114–121

Arnow S (1960) The use of radiofrequency power making lesions in the brain. J Neurosurg 17:431–438

Baumgarten HG, Björklund A (1976) Neurotoxic indoleamines and monoamine neurons Ann Rev Pharmacol Toxicol 16:101–111

Baumgarten HG, Björklund A, Lachenmayer L, Nobin A (1973) Evaluation of the effects of 5,7-dihydroxytryptamine on serotonin and catecholamine neurons in rat CNS. Acta Physiol Scand [Suppl] 391

Baumgarten HG, Björklund A, Lachenmayer L, Nobin A, Stenevi U (1971) Long-lasting selective depletion of brain serotonin by 5,6-dihydroxytryptamine. Acta Physiol Scand [Suppl] 373

Baumgarten HG, Björklund A, Nobin A, Rosengren E, Schlossberger HG (1975 a) Neurotoxicity of hydroxylated tryptamines: structure-activity relationship. Acta Physiol Scand [Suppl] 429

Baumgarten HG, Jenner S, Schlossberger HG (1979) Serotonin neurotoxins: Effects of drugs on the destruction of brain serotonergic, noradrenergic, and dopaminergic axons in adult rat by intraventricularly, intracisternally, or intracerebral administered 5,7-dihydroxytryptamine and related compounds. In: Chubb W, Geffen L (eds) Neurotoxins, Fundamental and Clinical Advances. Adelaide University Union Press, Adelaide, pp 221–226

Baumgarten HG, Lachenmayer L (1972) 5,7-dihydroxytryptamine: Improvement in chemical lesioning of indoleamine neurons in mammalian brain. Z Zellforsch 135:399–414

Baumgarten HG, Lachenmayer L, Björklund A (1977) Chemical lesioning of indoleamine pathways. In: Myers RD (ed) Methods in psychobiology, vol 3. Academic Press, New York, pp 47–98

Baumgarten HG, Lachenmayer L, Schlossberger HG (1972) Evidence for a degeneration of indolamine-containing nerve terminals in rat brain induced by 5,6-dihydroxytryptamine. Z Zellforsch 125:553–569

Baumgarten HG, Viktor SJ, Lovenberg W (1975 b) A developmental study of the effects of 5,7-dihydroxytryptamine on regional tryptophan hydroxylase in rat brain. Psychopharmacol Commun 1:75–88

Bennett T, Burnstock G, Cobb JLS, Malmfors T (1970) An ultrastructural and histochemical study of the short-term effects of 6-hydroxydopamine on adrenergic nerves in the domestic fowl. Br J Pharmacol 38:802–809

Bennett T, Cobb JL, Malmfors T (1973) Fluorescence histochemical and ultrastructural observations on the effects of intravenous injections of vinblastine on noradrenergic nerves. Z Zellforsch 141:517–527

Bennett T, Gardiner SM, Tomlinson DR (1976) Selective noradrenergic denervation of the heart following intravenous injections of vinblastine and vincristine. Naunyn Schmiedeberg's Arch Pharmacol 293:175–182

Bittiger H, Maître L, Krinke G, Schnider K, Hess R (1977) A study of long-term effects of guanethidine on peripheral noradrenergic neurons of the rat. Toxicology 8:63–78

Biziere K, Coyle JT (1979) Effects of cortical ablation on the neurotoxicity and receptor binding of kainic acid in striatum. J Neurosci Res 4:383–398

Björklund A, Baumgarten HG, Rensch A (1975) 5,7-Dihydroxytryptamine: Improvement of its selectivity for serotonin neurons in the CNS by pretreatment with desipramine. J Neurochem 24:833–835

Björklund A, Nobin A, Stenevi U (1973) The use of neurotoxic dihydroxytryptamines as tools for morphological studies and localized lesioning of central indolamine neurons. Z Zellforsch 145:479–501

Björklund A, Stenevi U (1979) Regeneration of monoaminergic and cholinergic neurons in the mammalian central nervous system. Physiol Rev 59:62–100

Blank CL, Kissinger PT, Adams RN (1972) 5,6-Dihydroxyindole formation from oxidized 6-hydroxydopamine. Eur J Pharmacol 19: 391–394

Bloom FE (1975) Monoaminergic neurotoxins: Are they selective? J Neural Transm 37: 183–187

Borchardt RT, Burgess SK, Reid JR, Liang YO, Adams RN (1977) Effects of 2- and/or 5-methylated analogues of 6-hydroxydopamine on norepinephrine- and dopamine-containing neurons. Mol Pharmacol 13:805–818

Breese GR (1975) Chemical and immunochemical lesions by specific neurotoxic substances and antisera. In: Iversen LL, Iversen SD, Snyder SH (eds) Handbook of psychopharmacology, vol 1. Plenum Press, New York, pp 137–189

Breese GR, Cooper BR (1975) Behavioral and biochemical interactions of 5,7-dihydroxytryptamine with various drugs when administered intracisternally to adult and developing rats. Brain Res 98:517–527

Breese G, Cooper BR, Smith RD (1973) Biochemical and behavioral alterations following 6-hydroxydopamine administration into brain. In: Usdin E, Snyder SH (eds) Frontiers in catecholamine research. Pergamon Press, New York, pp 701–706

Breese GR, Vogel RA, Mueller RA (1978) Biochemical and behavioral alterations in developing rats treated with 5,7-dihydroxytryptamine. J Pharmacol 205:587–595

Burnstock G, Evans B, Gannon BJ, Heath JW, James V (1971) A new method of destroying adrenergic nerves in adult animals using guanethidine. Br J Pharmacol 43:295–301

Butcher LL (1975) Degenerative processes after punctuate intracerebral administration of 6-hydroxydopamine. J Neural Transm 37: 189–208

Butcher LL, Eastgate SM, Hodge GK (1974) Evidence that punctuate intracerebral administration of 6-hydroxydopamine fails to produce selective neuronal degeneration: Comparison with copper sulphate and factors govering the deportment of fluids injected into brain. Naunyn Schmiedeberg's Arch Pharmacol 285:31–70

Buu NT, Puil E, van Gelder NM (1976) Receptors of amino acids in excitable tissues. Gen Pharmacol 7:5–14

Campochiaro P, Coyle JT (1978) Ontogenetic development of kainate neurotoxicity: Correlates with glutamatergic innervation. Proc Natl Acad Sci USA 75:2025–2029

Carpenter MB, Whittier JR (1952) Study of methods for producing experimental lesions in the central nervous system with special reference to stereotaxic technique. J Comp Neurol 97:73–132

Clark DW, Laverty R, Phelan EL (1972) Long-lasting peripheral and central effects of 6-hydroxydopamine in rats. Br J Pharmacol 44: 233–243

Clemens JA, Fuller RW, Berry KW, Sawyer BD (1978) Effect of *p*-chloroamphetamine on brain serotonin in immature rats. Commun Psychopharmacol 2:11–16

Cobb JLS, Bennett T (1971) An electron microscopic examination of the short term effects of 6-hydroxydopamine on the peripheral adrenergic nervous system. In: Malmfors T, Thoenen H (eds) 6-Hydroxydopamine and catecholamine neurons. North Holland, Amsterdam, pp 33–45

Cohen S (1960) Purification of a nerve growth promoting protein from the mouse salivary gland and its neurotoxic antiserum. Proc Natl Acad Sci USA 46:302–311

Cohen G, Heikkila RE (1974) The generation of hydrogen peroxide, superoxide radical, and hydroxyl radical by 6-hydroxydopamine, dialuric acid, and related cytotoxic agents. J Biol Chem 249:2447–2452

Costa M, Geffen LB, Rush RA, Bridges D, Blessing WW, Heath JW (1979) Immune lesions of central noradrenergic neurons produced by antibodies to dopamine-β-hydroxylase. Brain Res 173:65–78

Costa M, Rush RA, Furness JB, Geffen LB (1976) Histochemical evidence for the degeneration of peripheral noradrenergic axons following intravenous injection of antibodies to dopamine-β-hydroxylase. Neurosci Lett 3:201–207

Coyle JT (1979) An animal model for Huntington's disease. Biol Psychiatry 14:251–176

Coyle JT, Molliver ME, Kuhar MJ (1978) In situ injection of kainic acid: A new method for selectively lesioning neuronal cell bodies while sparing axons of passage. J Comp Neurol 180:301–324

Coyle JT, Schwarcz R (1976) Lesions of striatal neurons with kainic acid provide a model for Huntington's chorea. Nature 263:244–246

Curtis DR, Duggan AW, Felix D, Johnston GAR, Tebécis AK, Watkins JC (1972) Excitation of mammalian central neurons by acidic amino acids. Brain Res 41:283–301

Curtis DR, Johnston G (1974) Amino acid transmitters in the mammalian central nervous system. Rev Physiol Biochem Pharmacol 69:97–188

Curtis DR, Watkins JC (1963) Acidic amino acids with strong excitatory actions on mammalian neurons. J Physiol 166:1–14

Dahlström A (1971) Effects of vinblastine and colchicine on monoamine-containing neurons of the rat, with special regard to axoplasma transport of amine granules. Acta Neuropathol [Suppl] (Berl) 5:226–237

Daly J, Fuxe K, Jonsson G (1973) Effects of intracerebral injections of 5,6-dihydroxytryptamine on central monoamine neurons: Evidence for selective degeneration of central 5-hydroxytryptamine neurons. Brain Res 49: 476–482

Daly J, Fuxe K, Jonsson G (1974) 5,7-Dihydroxytryptamine as a tool for the morphological and functional analysis of central 5-hydroxytryptamine neurons Res Commun Chem Pathol Pharmacol 1:175–187

de Champlain J, Gauthier P, Porlier G, van Ameringen MR, Nadeau RA (1975) Compensatory mechanisms following peripheral chemical sympathectomy. In: Jonsson G, Malmfors T, Sachs Ch (eds) Chemical tools in catecholamine research, vol I. North Holland, Amsterdam, pp 231–238

Descarrier L, Saucier G (1972) Disappearance of the locus coeruleus in the rat after intraventricular 6-hydroxydopamine. Brain Res 37: 310–316

Eidelberg E, Stein DG (1974) Functional recovery after lesions of the nervous system. Neurosci Res Program Bull 12:2

Eränkö L, Eränkö O (1971) Effect of guanethidine on nerve cells and small intensely fluorescent cells in sympathetic ganglia of newborn and adult rats. Acta Pharmacol Toxicol (Copenh) 30:403–416

Evans BK (1979) Influence of neuronal activity levels on the cytotoxic effects of guanathidine. J Pharmacol 209:205–214

Evans B, Gannon BJ, Heath JW, Burnstock G (1972) Long-lasting damage to the internal male genital organs and their adrenergic innervation following chronic treatment with the antihypertensive drug guanethidine. Fertil Steril 23:657–667

Fuller RW (1978) Neurochemical effects of serotonin neurotoxins. Ann NY Acad Sci 305: 178–181

Furness JB, Campbell GR, Gillard SM, Malmfors T, Cobb JLS, Burnstock G (1970) Cellular studies of sympathetic denervation produced by 6-hydroxydopamine in the vas deferens. J Pharmacol 174:111–122

Furness JB, Lewis SY, Rush R, Costa M, Geffen LB (1977) Involvement of complement in degeneration of sympathetic nerves after administration of dopamine-β-hydroxylase antibodies. Brain Res 134:67–75

Fuxe K, Eneroth P, Gustavsson JÅ, Hökfelt T, Jonsson G, Löfström A, Skett P (1975) Effects of 6-OH-DA-induced lesions of the ascending noradrenaline and adrenaline pathways to the tel- and diencephalon on FSH, LH, and prolactin secretion in the ovariectomized female rat. In: Jonsson G, Malmfors T, Sachs Ch (eds) Chemical tools in catecholamine research, vol I. North Holland, Amsterdam, pp 273–283

Fuxe K, Jonsson G (1974) Further mapping of central 5-hydroxytryptamine neurons: Studies with neurotoxic dihydroxytryptamines. Adv Biochem Psychopharmacol 10:1–12

Fuxe K, Ögren SO, Agnati LF, Jonsson G, Gustavsson JÅ (1978) 5,7-dihydroxytryptamine as a tool to study the functional role of central 5-hydroxytryptamine neurons. Ann NY Acad Sci 305:346–369

Gannon BJ, Iwayama T, Burnstock G, Gerkens J, Mashford M (1971) Prolonged effects of chronic guanethidine treatment on the sympathetic innervation of the genitalia of male rats. Med J Aust 2:207–208

Gershanik OS, Heikkila RE, Duvoisin EC (1979) Asymmetric action of intraventricular monoamine neurotoxins. Brain Res 174:345–350

Gershon S, Baldessarini RJ (1975) Selective destruction of serotonin terminals in rat forebrain by high doses of 5,7-dihydroxytryptamine. Brain Res 85:140–145

Gold EM (1973) Anodal electrolytic brain lesions: How current and electrode material influence lesion size and hyperphagosity. Physiol Behav 10:813–815

Gold RM, Kapatos G, Carey RJ (1975) A retracting wire knife for stereotaxic brain surgery made from a microliter syringe. Physiol Behav 14:624–632

Graham DG, Tiffany SM, Bell WR Jr, Gutknecht WF (1978) Autoxidation versus covalent binding of quinones as the mechanism of toxicity of dopamine, 6-hydroxydopamine, and related compounds toward C1300 neuroblastoma cell in vitro. Mol Pharmacol 14: 644–653

Haeusler G (1971) Early pre- and postjunctional effects of 6-hydroxydopamine. J Pharmacol 178:49–62

Halasz B (1969) The endocrine effects of isolation of the hypothalamus from the rest of the brain. In: Ganong WF, Martini L (eds) Frontiers in neuroendocrinology. Oxford University Press, New York London Toronto, pp 307–342

Halasz B, Pupp L (1965) Hormone secretion of the anterior pituitary gland after physical interruption of all nervous pathways to the hypophysiotrophic area. Endocrinology 77: 553–562

Hallman H, Jonsson G (1980) DSP4 (*N*-2-chloroethyl-*N*-ethyl-bromobenzylamine) – a useful noradrenaline denervation tool in adult and developing rats. Neurosci Lett [Suppl] 5:S365

Hanbauer I, Jacobowitz D, Kopin IJ (1974) Effect of vinblastine on noradrenergic axons. Br J Pharmacol 50:219–224

Hanbauer I, Kopin IJ, Naengwyn-Davies GD, Thoa NB, Weise DK (1973) Effect of vinblastine on catecholamine biosynthetic enzymes in heart, sympathetic ganglia, and adrenal glands of rats. Br J Pharmacol 48: 106–112

Heath JW, Evans BK, Gannon BJ, Burnstock G, James VB (1972) Degeneration of adrenergic neurons following guanethidine treatment: an ultrastructural study. Virchows Arch [Cell Pathol] 11:182–197

Heikkila R, Cohen G (1972) Further studies on the generation of hydrogen peroxide by 6-hydroxydopamine. Mol Pharmacol 8:241–248

Heikkila RE, Cohen G (1973) 6-Hydroxydopamine; evidence for superoxide radical as an oxidative intermediate. Science 181:456–457

Heikkila RE, Cohen G (1975) Prevention of 6-OH-DA-induced neurotoxicity. In: Jonsson G, Malmfors T, Sachs Ch (eds) Chemical tools in catecholamine research vol I. North Holland, Amsterdam, pp 7–14

Hökfelt T, Jonsson G, Sachs Ch (1972) Fine structure and fluorescence morphology of adrenergic nerves after 6-hydroxydopamine in vivo and in vitro. Z Zellforsch 131:529–543

Hökfelt T, Ungerstedt U (1973) Specificity of 6-hydroxydopamine-induced degeneration of central monoamine neurons. An electron and fluorescence microscopic study with special reference to intracerebral injection on the nigrostriatal dopamine system. Brain Res 60: 269–297

Hole K, Fuxe K, Jonsson G (1976) Behavioural effects of 5,7-dihydroxytryptamine lesions of ascending 5-hydroxytryptamine pathways. Brain Res 107:385–399

Horsley V, Clarke RH (1908) The structure and functions of the cerebellum examined by a new method. Brain 31:45–124

Jacks BR, de Champlain J, Cordeau JP (1972) Effects of 6-hydroxydopamine on putative transmitter substances in the central nervous system. Eur J Pharmacol 18:353–360

Jacobowitz DM, Ziegler MG, Thomas JA (1975) In vivo uptake of antibody to dopamine-β-hydroxylase into sympathetic elements. Brain Res 91:165–170

Jacoby J, Lytle L (1978) (eds) Serotonin neurotoxins. Ann NY Acad Sci 305

Jaim-Etcheverry G, Zieher LM (1975) Alteration of the development of central adrenergic neurons produced by 6-hydroxydopa. In: Jonsson G, Malmfors T, Sachs Ch (eds) Chemical tools in catecholamine research, vol I. North Holland, Amsterdam, pp 173–180

Jaim-Etcheverry G, Zieher LM (1980) DSP4: A novel compound with neurotoxic effects on noradrenergic neurons of adult and developing rats. Brain Res 188:513–523

Jancsó G, Kiraly E, Jancsó-Gábor A (1977) Pharmacologically-induced selective degeneration of chemosensitive primary sensory neurons. Nature 270:741–743

Jenner S, Baumgarten HG (1980) Regional depletion of monoamines and distribution of radioactivity in the rat brain following slow or fast injection of 5,7-dihydroxytryptamine or ^{14}C-5,7-DHT into the left lateral ventricle and the effects of anaesthesia on these parameters. Neurosci Lett [Suppl] 5: S449

Jensen-Holm J, Juul P (1971) Ultrastructural changes in the rat superior ganglion following prolonged guanethidine administration. Acta Pharmacol Toxicol 30: 308–320

Johnson EM, Cantor E, Douglas JR (1975) Biochemical and functional evaluation of the sympathectomy produced by the administration of guanethidine to newborn rats. J Pharmacol 193: 503–512

Jones EG, Hartman BK (1978) Recent advances in neuroanatomical methodology. Annu Rev Neurosci 1: 215–296

Jonsson G (1976 a) Studies on the mechanisms of 6-hydroxydopamine cytotoxicity. Med Biol 54: 406–420

Jonsson G (1976 b) Developmental characteristic of central monoamine neurons and their reciprocal relations. Exp Neurol 53: 801–814

Jonsson G (1980) Chemical neurotoxins as denervation tools in neurobiology. Annu Rev Neurosci 3: 169–187

Jonsson G, Fuxe K, Hökfelt T (1976) Resistance of central phenylethanolamin-N-methyl transferase-containing neurons to 6-hydroxydopamine. Med Biol 54: 421–426

Jonsson G, Malmfors T, Sachs Ch (1975) (eds) Chemical tools in catecholamine research, vol I. North Holland, Amsterdam

Jonsson G, Pollare T, Hallman H, Sachs Ch (1978 a) Developmental plasticity of central serotonin neurons after 5,7-dihydroxytryptamine treatment. Ann NY Acad Sci 305: 328–345

Jonsson G, Ponzio F, Ross S (1978 b) A new neurotoxic compound as denervation tool for noradrenaline neurons (abstract). 7th Int Congr Pharmacol, Paris

Jonsson G, Pycock Ch, Fuxe K, Sachs Ch (1974) Changes in the development of central noradrenaline neurons following neonatal administration of 6-hydroxydopamine. J Neurochem 22: 621–626

Jonsson G, Sachs Ch (1970) Effects of 6-hydroxydopamine on the uptake and storage of noradrenaline in sympathetic adrenergic neurons. Eur J Pharmacol 9: 141–155

Jonsson G, Sachs Ch (1971) Uptake and accumulation of ^{3}H-6-hydroxydopamine in adrenergic nerves. Eur J Pharmacol 16: 55–62

Jonsson G, Sachs Ch (1972) Degenerative and nondegenerative effects of 6-hydroxydopamine on adrenergic nerves. J Pharmacol 180: 625–635

Jonsson G, Sachs Ch (1973) 6-Aminodopamine-induced degeneration of catecholamine neurons. J Neurochem 21: 117–124

Jonsson G, Sachs Ch (1976) Regional changes in ^{3}H-noradrenaline uptake, catecholamine synthetic and catabolic enzymes in rat brain following neonatal 6-hydroxydopamine treatment. Med Biol 54: 286–297

Jonsson G, Wiesel FA, Hallman H (1979) Developmental plasticity of central noradrenaline neurons – Changes in transmitter functions. J Neurobiol 10: 337–353

Kasamatsu T, Itakura T, Jonsson G (in press) Intracortical spread of exogenous catecholamines: Effective concentration for modifying cortical plasticity. J Pharmacol

Kasamatsu T, Pettigrew JD (1976) Depletion of brain catecholamines: Failure of ocular dominance shift after monocular occlusion in kittens. Science 194: 206–209

Koda LY, Schulman JA, Bloom FE (1978) Ultrastructural identification of noradrenergic terminals in rat hippocampus: unilateral destruction of the locus coeruleus with 6-hydroxydopamine. Brain Res 145: 190–195

Köhler C, Ross SB, Srebro B, Ögren SO (1978 a) Long-term biochemical and behavioral effects of *p*-chloroamphetamine in the rat. Ann NY Acad Sci 305: 645–663

Köhler C, Schwarcz R, Fuxe K (1978 b) Perforant path transections protect hippocampal granule cells from kainate lesion. Neurosci Lett 10: 241–246

Kostrzewa RM, Garey RE (1977) Sprouting of noradrenergic terminals in rat cerebellum following neonatal treatment with 6-hydroxydopa. Brain Res 124: 385–391

Kostrzewa RM, Harper JW (1974) Effect of 6-hydroxydopa on catecholamine-containing neurons in brains of newborn rats. Brain Res 69: 174–181

Kostrzewa RM, Jacobowitz DM (1974) Pharmacological actions of 6-hydroxydopamine. Pharmacol Rev 26: 199–288

Laguzzi L, Petitjean F, Pujol JF, Jouvet M (1971) Effets de l'injection intraventriculaire de 6-hydroxydopamine sur les états de sommeil et les monoamines cérébrales du chat. CR Soc Biol (Paris) 165: 1649–1653

Leonard CM (1979) Degeneration methods in neurobiology. TINS 2: 156–159

Levi-Montalcini R, Angeletti PU (1966) Immunosympathectomy. Pharmacol Rev 18: 619–628

Levi-Montalcini R, Angeletti PU (1968) Nerve growth factor. Physiol Rev 48: 534–569

Levi-Montalcini R, Booker B (1960) Destruction of the sympathetic ganglia in mammals by an antiserum to the nerve growth promoting factor. Proc Natl Acad Sci USA 42: 384–391

Levi-Montalcini R, Cohen S (1960) Effects of the extract of the mouse submaxillary salivary glands on the sympathetic system of mammals. Ann NY Acad Sci 85:324–341

Lewis SY, Rush RA, Geffen LB (1977) Biochemical effects on guinea-pig iris of local injection of dopamine-β-hydroxylase antibodies and $F(ab')_2$ fragments. Brain Res 134:173–179

Lidbrink P (1974) The effect of lesions of ascending noradrenaline pathways on sleep and waking in the rat. Brain Res 74:19–40

Lidbrink P, Jonsson G (1974) Noradrenaline nerve terminals in the cerebral cortex – Effects on noradrenaline uptake and storage following axonal lesion with 6-hydroxydopamine. J Neurochem 22:617–626

Lidbrink P, Jonsson G (1975) On the specificity of 6-hydroxydopamine-induced degeneration of central noradrenaline neurons after intracerebral injection. Neurosci Lett 1:35–39

Lieberman AR (1971) The axon reaction: A review of the principal features of perikaryal responses to axon injury. Int Rev Neurobiol 14:49–124

Lorens SA, Guldberg HC, Hole K, Köhler C, Srebro B (1976) Activity, avoidance, learning, and regional 5-hydroxytryptamine following intra-brain stem 5,7-dihydroxytryptamine and electrolytic midbrain raphé lesions in the rat. Brain Res 108:97–113

Lucas DR, Newhouse JP (1957) The toxic effect of sodium L-glutamate on inner layers of the retina. AMA Arch Ophthalmol 58:193–201

Lytle LO, Jacoby JH, Nelson MF, Baumgarten HG (1974) Long-term effects of 5,7-dihydroxytryptamine administered at birth on the development of brain monoamines. Life Sci 15:1203–1217

Malmfors T (1971) The effects of 6-hydroxydopamine on the adrenergic nerves as revealed by the fluorescence histochemical method. In: Malmfors T, Thoenen H (eds) 6-Hydroxydopamine and catecholamine neurons. North Holland, Amsterdam, pp 47–58

Malmfors T, Thoenen H (eds) (1971) 6-Hydroxydopamine and catecholamine neurons. North Holland, Amsterdam

Mason ST, Fibiger HG (1979) On the specificity of kainic acid. Science 204:1339–1341

McGeer EG, McGeer PL (1976) Duplication of biochemical changes of Huntington's chorea by intrastriatal injection of glutamic and kainic acid. Nature 263:517–519

McGeer EG, McGeer PL (1978) Some factors influencing the neurotoxicity of intrastriatal injections of kainic acid. Neurochem Res 3: 501–517

McGeer EG, Olney JW, McGeer PL (eds) (1978 a) Kainic acid as a tool in neurobiology. Raven Press, New York

McGeer EG, McGeer PL, Singh K (1978 b) Kainate-induced degeneration of neostriatal neurons: dependency upon corticostriatal tract. Brain Res 139:381–383

Meyers RE (1956) Function of the corpus callosum in intraocular transfer. Brain 79: 358–363

Miller JP, Silverston AI (1979) Rapid killing of single neurons by irradiation of intracellularly-injected dye. Science 206:702–704

Moore RY (1964) The effect of some rhinencephalic lesions on the retention of a conditioned avoidance response in the cat. J Comp Physiol Psychol 57:65–71

Moore RY (1978) Surgical and chemical lesion techniques. In: Iversen LL, Iversen SD, Snyder SH (eds) Handbook of psychopharmacology, vol 9. Plenum Press, New York, pp 1–39

Moore RY, Björklund A, Stenevi U (1971) Plastic changes in the adrenergic innervation of the rat septal area in response to denervation. Brain Res 33:13–35

Nadler JV (1979) Kainic acid: neurophysiological and neurotoxic actions. Life Sci 24: 289–300

Nadler JV, Perry BW, Cotman CW (1978) Intraventricular kainic acid preferentially destroys hippocampal pyramidal cells. Nature 271: 676–677

Nygren LG, Fuxe K, Jonsson G, Olson L (1974) Functional regeneration of 5-hydroxytryptamine nerve terminals in the rat spinal cord following 5,6-dihydroxytryptamine-induced degeneration. Brain Res 78:377–394

Nygren LG, Olson L (1977) Intracisternal neurotoxins and monoamine neurons innervating the spinal cord: Acute and chronic effects on cell and axon counts and nerve terminal densities. Histochemistry 52:281–306

Ögren SO, Fuxe K, Archer T, Hall H, Holm AC, Köhler C (1980) Studies on the role of central 5-HT neurons in avoidance learning; A behavioral and biochemical analysis. In: Haber B (ed) Serotonin. Current aspects of neurochemistry and function. Plenum Press, New York

Olney JW, Ho OL, Rhee V (1971) Cytotoxic effects of acidic and sulphur-containing amino acids on the infant mouse central nervous system. Exp Brain Res 14:61–76

Olney JW, Rhee V, Ho OL (1974) Kainic acid: A powerful neurotoxic analogue of glutamate. Brain Res 77:507–512

Parnas I, Bowling D (1978) Killing of single neurons by intracellular injection of proteolytic enzymes. Nature 270:626–628

Poirier LY, Langelier P, Roberge A, Boucher R, Kitsikis A (1972) Non-specific histopathological changes induced by the intracerebral injection of 6-hydroxydopamine (6-OH-DA). J Neurol Sci 16:401–416

Rose FE, Woolsey CN (1943) A study of the thalamocortical connections in the rabbit. Bull Johns Hopkins Hosp 73:65–128

Rose FE, Woolsey CN (1949) The relations of thalamic connections, cellular structure, and evocable electrical activity in the auditory region of the cat. J Comp Neurol 91:441–466

Ross SB (1976 a) Long-term effects of *N*-2-chloroethyl-*N*-ethyl-bromobenzylamine hydrochloride on noradrenergic neurons in the rat brain and heart. Br J Pharmacol 58: 521–527

Ross SB (1976 b) Antagonism of the acute and long-term biochemical effects of 4-chloroamphetamine on the 5-HT neurons in the rat brain by inhibitors of the 5-hydroxytryptamine uptake. Acta Pharmacol Toxicol 39:456

Routtenberg A (1972) Intracranial injection and behaviour: A critical review. Behav Biol 7: 601–641

Rowland V (1966) Stereotaxic techniques and the production of lesions. In: Martini L, Ganong WF (eds) Neuroendocrinology, vol I. Academic Press, New York

Sachs Ch (1973) Development of the blood-brain barrier for 6-hydroxydopamine. J Neurochem 20:1753–1760

Sachs Ch, Jonsson G (1972) Degeneration of central noradrenaline neurons after 6-hydroxydopamine in newborn animals. Res Commun Chem Pathol Pharmacol 4:203–220

Sachs Ch, Jonsson G (1973) Changes in central noradrenaline neurons after systemic 6-hydroxydopamine administration. J Neurochem 21:1517–1524

Sachs Ch, Jonsson G (1975 a) Mechanisms of action of 6-hydroxydopamine. Biochem Pharmacol 24:1–8

Sachs Ch, Jonsson G (1975 b) 5,7-Dihydroxytryptamine-induced changes in the postnatal development of central 5-hydroxytryptamine neurons. Med Biol 53:156–164

Sachs Ch, Jonsson G (1975 c) Changes in the development of central noradrenaline neurons following neonatal 6-OH-DA administration. In: Jonsson G, Malmfors T, Sachs Ch (eds) Chemical tools in catecholamine research, vol I. North Holland, Amsterdam, pp 163–171

Sachs Ch, Pycock Ch, Jonsson G (1974) Altered development of central noradrenaline neurons during ontogeny by 6-hydroxydopamine. Med Biol 52:55–65

Sanders-Bush E, Bushing JA, Sulser F (1972) Long-term effects of *p*-chloroamphetamine on tryptophan hydroxylase activity and on the levels of 5-hydroxytryptamine and 5-hydroxyindoleacetic acid in brain. Eur J Pharmacol 20:385–388

Saner A, Thoenen H (1971) Model experiments on the molecular mechanisms of action of 6-hydroxydopamine. Mol Pharmacol 7:147–157

Scalafini A, Grossman SP (1969) Hyperphagia produced by knife-cuts between the medial and lateral hypothalamus in the rat. Physiol Behav 4:533–539

Schneider GE (1970) Mechanisms of functional recovery following lesions of visual cortex and superior colliculus in neonate and adult hamster. Brain Behav Evol 3:295–323

Schwarcz R, Hökfelt T, Fuxe K, Jonsson G, Goldstein M, Terenius L (1979) Ibotenic acid-induced neuronal degeneration: A morphological and neurochemical study. Prog Brain Res 37:199–216

Singh B, de Champlain J (1972) Altered ontogenesis of central noradrenergic neurons following neonatal treatment with 6-hydroxydopamine. Brain Res 48:432–437

Smith BH, Kreutzberg GW (1976) Neuron-target cell interactions. Neurosci Res Program Bull 14:3

Stein DG, Rosen JJ, Butter N (1974) Plasticity and recovery of function in the central nervous system. Academic Press, New York

Thierry AM, Velley L, Stinus L, Tassin JP, Blaue G, Glowinski J (1975) Development of the mesocortical and nigrostriatal dopaminergic systems following various 6-hydroxydopamine treatments. In: Jonsson G, Malmfors T, Sachs Ch (eds) Chemical tools in catecholamine research, vol I. North Holland, Amsterdam, pp 205–210

Thoenen H (1972) Surgical, immunological, and chemical sympathectomy. Their application in the investigation of the physiology and pharmacology of the sympathetic nervous system. In: Blaschko H, Muscholl E (eds) Catecholamines. Springer, Berlin Heidelberg New York, pp 813–844

Thoenen H, Tranzer JP (1968) Chemical sympathectomy by selective destruction of adrenergic nerve endings with 6-hydroxydopamine. Naunyn Schmiedeberg's Arch Pharmacol 261: 271–288

Tranzer JP, Thoenen H (1967 a) Ultramorphologische Veränderungen der sympathischen Nervenendigungen der Katze nach Vorbehandlung mit 5- und 6-Hydroxy-Dopamine. Naunyn-Schmiedeberg's Arch Pharmacol 257:357

Tranzer JP, Thoenen H (1967 b) Electronmicroscopic localization of 5-hydroxydopamine (3,4,5-trihydroxyphenylethylamine), a new "false" sympathetic transmitter. Experientia 23:743–745

Ungerstedt U (1968) 6-Hydroxydopamine-induced degeneration of central monoamine neurons. Eur J Pharmacol 5:107–110

Ungerstedt U (1971) Use of intracerebral injections of 6-hydroxydopamine as a tool for morphological and functional studies on central catecholamine neurons. In: Malmfors T, Thoenen H (eds) 6-Hydroxydopamine and catecholamine neurons. North Holland, Amsterdam, pp 315–332

Ungerstedt U (1973) Selective lesions of central catecholamine pathways. Application in functional studies. In: Ehrenpreis S, Kopin IJ (eds) Chemical approaches to brain function. Academic Press, New York, pp 73–96

Varon SS, Somjen GG (1979) Neuron-glia interactions. Neurosci Res Program Bull 17:1

Voloschin L, Joseph SA, Knigge KM (1968) Endocrine function in male rats following complete and partial isolations of the hypothalamo-pituitary unit. Neuroendocrinology 387–397

Waddington JL, Crow TJ (1979) Drug-induced rotational behavior following unilateral intracerebral injection of saline-ascorbate solution: neurotoxicity of ascorbic acid and monoamine-independent circling. Brain Res 161:371–376

Wolf G, DiChiara LV (1969) Progressive morphological changes in electrolytic brain lesions. Exp Neurol 23:529–536

Wuerthele SM, Lovell KL, Jones MZ, Moore KE (1978) A histological study of kainic acid-induced lesions in the rat brain. Brain Res 149:489–497

Zaczek R, Schwarcz R, Coyle JT (1978) Long-term sequele of striatal kainate lesions. Brain Res 152:626–632

Zieher LM, Jaim-Etcheverry G (1973) Regional differences in the long-term effect of neonatal 6-hydroxydopa treatment on rat brain noradrenaline. Brain Res 60:199–207

Zieher LM, Jaim-Etcheverry G (1975) 6-Hydroxydopa during development of central adrenergic neurons produces different long-term changes in rat brain noradrenaline. Brain Res 86:271–281

Zigmond MJ, Stricker EM (1975) Compensatory changes after intraventricular administration of 6-hydroxydopamine; A neurochemical model for recovery of function. In: Jonsson G, Malmfors T, Sachs Ch (eds) Chemical tools in catecholamine research, vol I. North Holland, Amsterdam, pp 319–326

Chapter 6

General Methods for Characterization of Brain Regions

K. H. Andres and Monika von Düring

1 Introduction

The recognition of the components of the central nervous system is directly related to questions concerning the interconnections of neuronal systems within the brain. Therefore, it is necessary to combine a description of structural details with their exact topographical orientation with respect to other structures. Thus, an analysis of neuronal systems requires a profound knowledge of the localization of the smallest areas. It necessitates a specific preparatory method in order to investigate distinct areas by light and electron microscopic means.

The interference reflecting light technique (Andres, von Düring 1974, 1977) offered the first precise macrophotographic and low magnification documentation of specimens. The present technique allows the examination of topographical and structural details of tissue surfaces and profiles of specimen slices before their preparation when used for procedures such as scanning electron microscopy, transmission electron microscopy, or freeze fracturing. A special frame for sectioning whole brains corresponds to stereotactic coordinates. This frame aids in the three-dimensional reconstruction of areas of the brain and thus can be used for morphometric analyses.

Supported by German Research Council
SFB 114 grants

2 Technical Equipment

a) A frame for tissue adjustment, consisting of a Perspex container with coordinates in all planes matching those of a tissue-sectioning frame. The bottom plate contains a turntable with microscrews. On the top of these screws are very fine needles.

b) Tissue-sectioning frame with indentations for the knife. The indentations differ in size and orientation according to the direction of the plane of section (frontal, horizontal, sagittal).
c) Manual vibratome made from an electric razor (type Braun) with an attached knife holder, whereby either razor blades (type Szabo) or microtome knives (type American Optical) are inserted.
d) Photographic equipment:
Nikon SLR camera F 3 with DW-4, 6 × magnification finder and interchangeable focusing screen type M.
Tele-equipment for macrophotography free of parallaxes: telephoto lenses and several extension rings and polarization filters. Equipment for interference reflecting light photography: repro-copy outfit, turntable, black plane dishes for specimens, macrolenses and wide-angle lenses.
Film material with very fine grain (type Agfa ortho 25, development: Rodinal).
e) Illumination:
2 × 150-W halogene lamps with glass-fiber-light conductors, 8 mm caliber (type Schott), two-lens collectors.
f) Flat embedding dishes made of polypropylene with shiny surfaces.
g) Stereomicroscopy with camera lucida.
h) Substance for sectioning procedures:
Agarose L (Behringwerke Marburg)
Agarose LOT Nr. 1568 (L'industrie biologique française).

3 Procedure

3.1 Preparation and Telemacrophotography

The tissue for this procedure is fixed by aldehyde perfusion (see Chap. 2). The osmolarity and pH of the rinsing and fixation solutions must be adjusted to that of the tissue in order to obtain optimal results. During preparation, the pia-arachnoid and parts of the dura mater should be left on the brain surface to avoid injuries.

To diminish distortion due to parallaxes, the photography of the removed brains as well as that of the tissue in the adjusting and sectioning frames is carried out at a distance of 5–20 m, depending on the size of the specimen, by use of a combination of telephoto lenses and extension rings (5–16 cm).

The brain is adjusted in a special frame to guarantee a reproduceable sectioning angle (Fig. 1). The sides of the frame are transparent and bear a system of coordi-

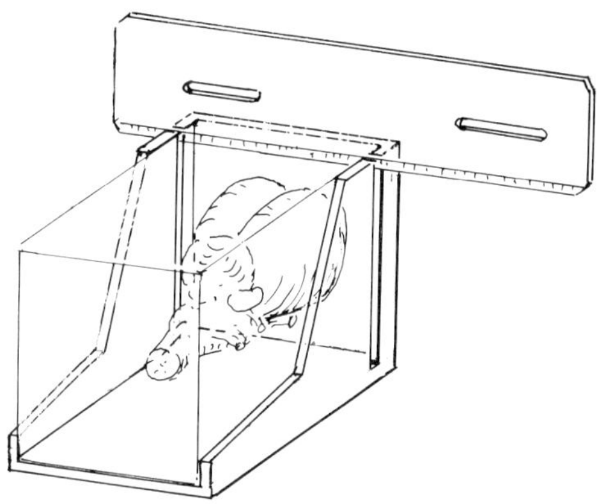

Fig. 1. Apparatus for serial sectioning of brain slices. The brain has been transferred into a block of agarose

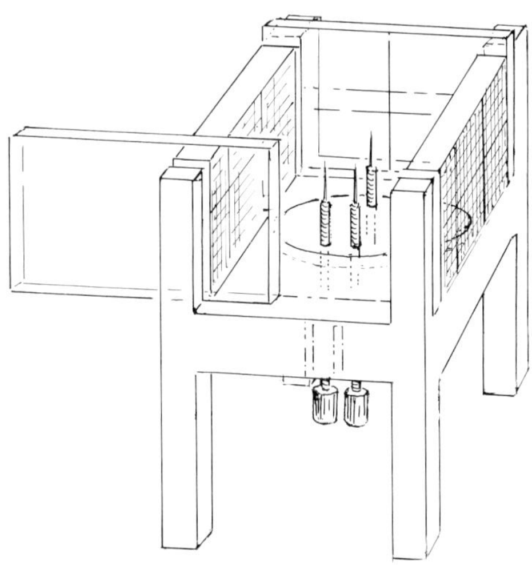

Fig. 2. Adjusting frame with adjusting screws bearing fine needles on top

nates which may correspond to those of a stereotactic apparatus and of the sectioning frame. The bottom plate of the frame contains a turntable with microscrews which have very fine needles on top to impale the brain (Fig. 2, 3). This arrangement allows an adjustment of the coordinates. After documentation of the adjusted brain by telemacrophotography, the space between the brain and the adjusting frame is filled with agarose (3%, +45 °C). The superfluous agarose is pressed out by covering the frame with a warm metal block.

Since the agarose does not shrink during the hardening and cooling phase, the brain remains in its correct position (Fig. 4). This also applies even after removing the adjusting screws from the brain before it is taken out of the frame. Due to the elasticity of neural tissue, the small canals of the needles close almost completely after lifting the brain. The block of agarose is now pushed into a sectioning frame of identical dimensions and adjusted to the cutting indentations for the required slices. The frames differ in their orientation due to the desired plane of sectioning. Before sectioning, the preparation is photographed by telemacrophotography (Fig. 5). Two razor blades placed into the gaps at both sides of the block prevent any movement during the cutting process. All slices should remain together in one block until the sectioning is finished.

3.2 Sectioning

For brain sectioning, a simple apparatus can aid in cutting slices (Fig. 1). To achieve a constant thickness of the slices and to maintain the chosen plane, a more specialized sectioning frame can be constructed (Figs. 2, 3). This frame offers the possibility of cutting the tissue in any of the three spatial planes.

The sectioning is carried out with a manual vibratome which is armed either with a razor blade or a microtome knife (Fig. 6). The manipulation of the vibratome should be controlled through a binocular microscope. The knife is brought through all the cutting gaps. To improve the gliding of the knife, a few drops of glycerine should be dripped onto the frame. After cutting, each gap is marked by a little piece of paper to avoid cutting one slice twice or omitting one. Using a Plexiglass bar of the same size as the block of agarose, the sectioned block is pushed out of the frame and the slices are distributed onto specimen glasses. Usually, the agarose is removed from the slices. In case it is desirable to keep the topography of surface structures such as vessels, the meninges, or nerve roots in their original position, the brain slice should be left under agarose covering. Any blackening of the agarose during the osmification is washed out by buffer.

Fig. 3. Adjusting frame with coordinates on the side planes. A rat brain is mounted on top of the adjusting screws with the aid of needles

Fig. 4. Block of transparent agarose containing the properly positioned rat brain

Fig. 5. a Telemacrophotograph of the rat brain inside the sectioning frame (lateral view). **b** Telemacrophotograph of the rat brain (dorsal view). The asterisks mark at (*a*) the position of the habenula and at (*b*) part of the choroid plexus. Compare Figs. 12, 13, 14b

Fig. 6. Sectioning frame with inserted block of agarose. The vibratome knife is brought through the cutting gaps

Fig. 7a, b. Front and rear aspect of rat brain slice no. 9 shown in interference reflecting light

Fig. 8. Interference reflecting light equipment. The collectors cast the cold light onto the object which, at an angle of 45°, is kept in 70% ethanol. The lens of the Nikon camera is used in a retroposition and in combination with extension rings

Fig. 9. Zoom stereomicroscope with integrated camera lucida (Zeiss). The photograph under the prism is superimposed with the embedded brain slice

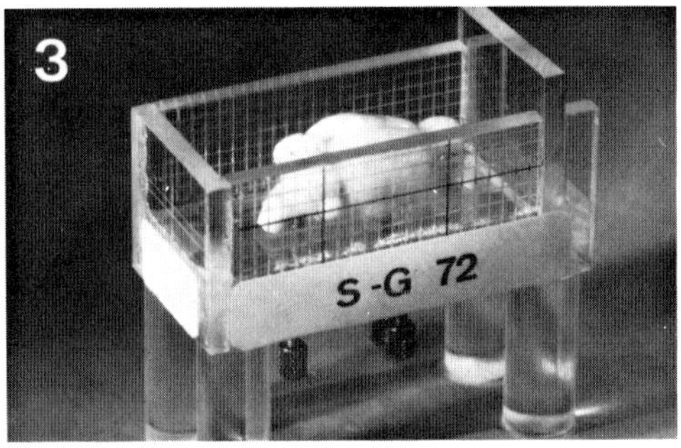
3
S-G 72

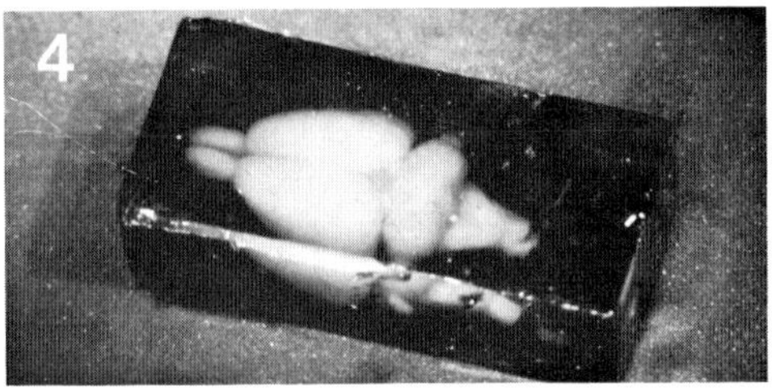
4

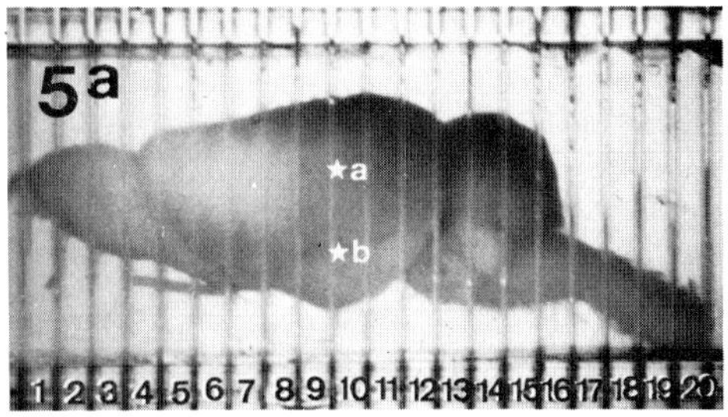
5a
★a
★b
1 2 3 4 5 6 7 8 9 10 11 12 13 14 15 16 17 18 19 20

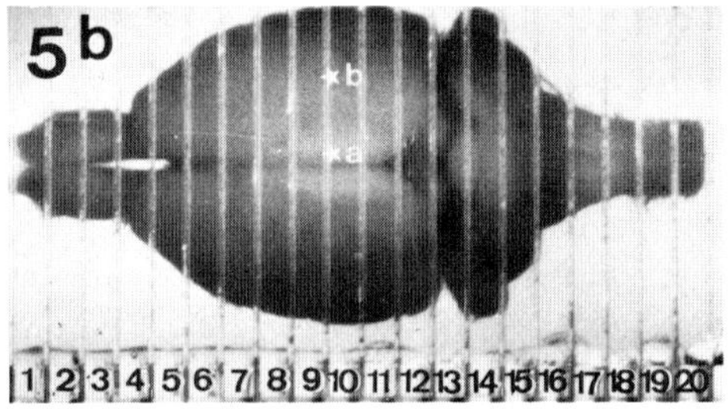
5b
★b
★a
1 2 3 4 5 6 7 8 9 10 11 12 13 14 15 16 17 18 19 20

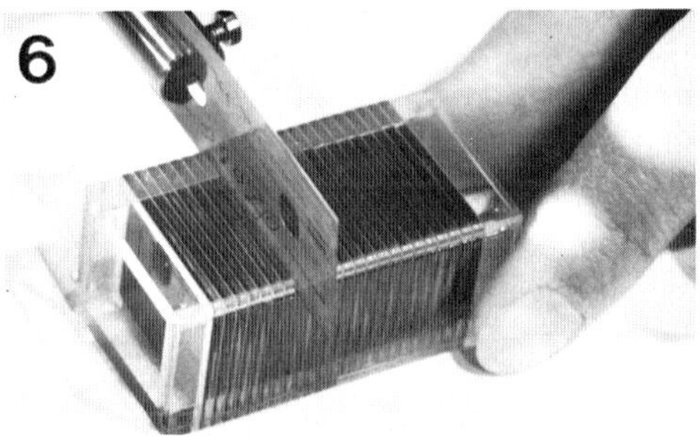
6

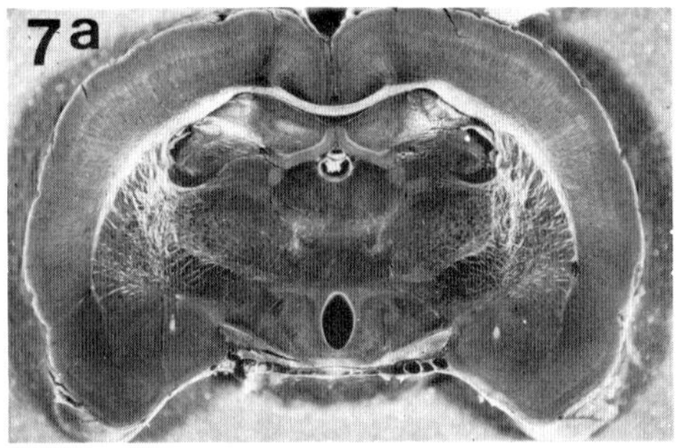
7a

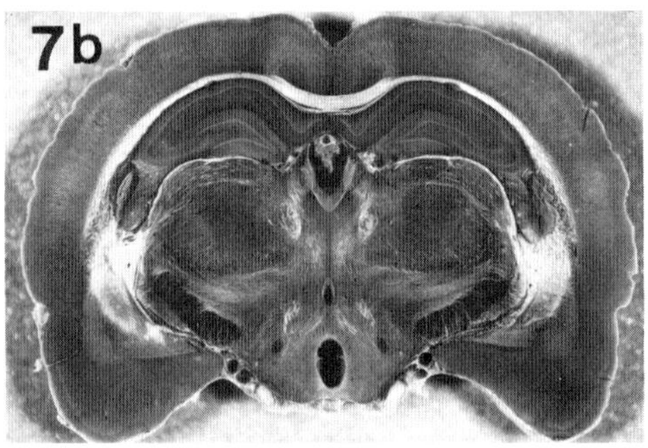
7b

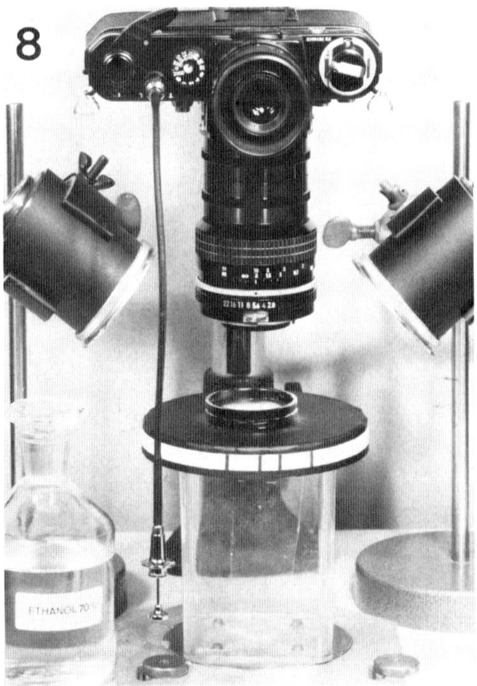
8

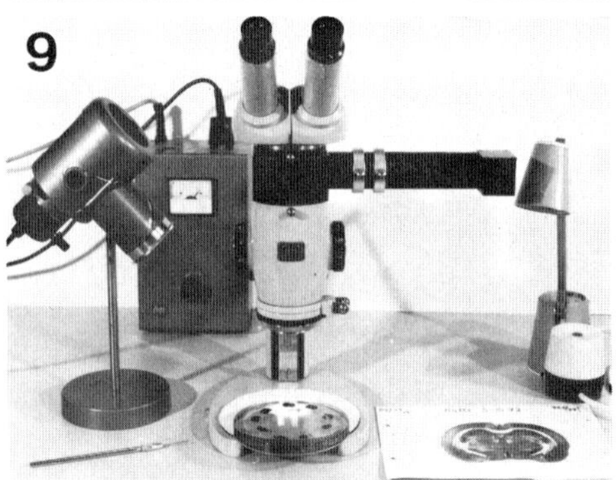
9

3.3 Osmification

After a phosphate buffer wash, the brain slices are postfixed in a solution of osmium tetroxide. It is necessary that the slices are thoroughly rinsed. The glasses must therefore be constantly shaken or turned. Since brain tissuc contains a high percentage of lipids which reduce a high amount of osmium tetroxide, it is important to use the solution in an abundant and highly concentrated amount. The dehydration with ethanol also takes place in the shaker or turning apparatus.

3.4 Interference Reflecting Light Technique

The specimens are processed in 70% or 80% ethanol and then photographed using the interference reflecting light technique. The surfaces of the flat dishes for the specimens must be covered with a dull black foil to minimize scattered radiation during the high intensity illumination.

The reflecting light is partly absorbed by the black specimen surface and partly reflected by interferences with specific surface structures. These structures cast iridescent colors which give a very high contrast to the dark tissue background. In this way, a specific structural pattern of the tissue is illuminated and is the equivalent of a photograph at low magnification of the stained histological specimen. As the clarity of the structure is dependent upon the angle of incidence, it is useful to rotate the specimen dish to find the optimal postion (Figs. 7 b, 10).

Normal and wide-angle lenses in the retroposition in combination with extension rings should be used when photographing. This technique offers a direct magnification of up to tenfold with a working distance of about 4 cm or more, which is needed for the illumination of the surface. The illumination is achieved by use of two 150-W halogene lamps. The cold light is directed from two sides onto the surface of the sample by glass fiber conductors with a caliber of 8 mm. Two-lens collectors are installed in front of the conductors, giving a homogeneous illumination of the specimen (Leitz, Monla-collectors, 4 cm diameter; Fig. 8).

To adjust the section to the size of the film, a turntable is suitable. It also offers the possibility of changing the angle between the illumination and a certain structure. Using only one light directed from one side and rotating the brain slice, the shining and fading fibers on the surface indicate their course through the slice. Utilizing the high resolution of this photographic method, Agfa Ortho 25 film with a Rodinal developer is used (4–500 ml water).

3.5 Embedding

After photographic documentation of the brain slice surfaces, the dehydration and subsequent embedding in Araldite is carried out. The brain slices are placed into narrow and flat dishes made of polypropylene, covered with Araldite and polymerized at +65 °C to +85 °C. After being cooled down the tablets of Araldite can be removed from the dishes.

Fig. 10. Interference reflecting light photograph of the front aspect of brain slice no. 10 of the rat brain

Fig. 11. Left habenula (*h*) and fasciculus retroflexus (*fr*) in detail in interference reflecting light

Fig. 12. Semithin section corresponding to Fig. 11 showing the medial and lateral nucleus habenulae (*hm, hl*) and the stria medullaris (*sm*). Compare the transverse sections of the vessels and nerve fibers

Fig. 13. High magnification of a detail of Fig. 10 showing the lateral ventricle (*lv*) and the choroid plexus

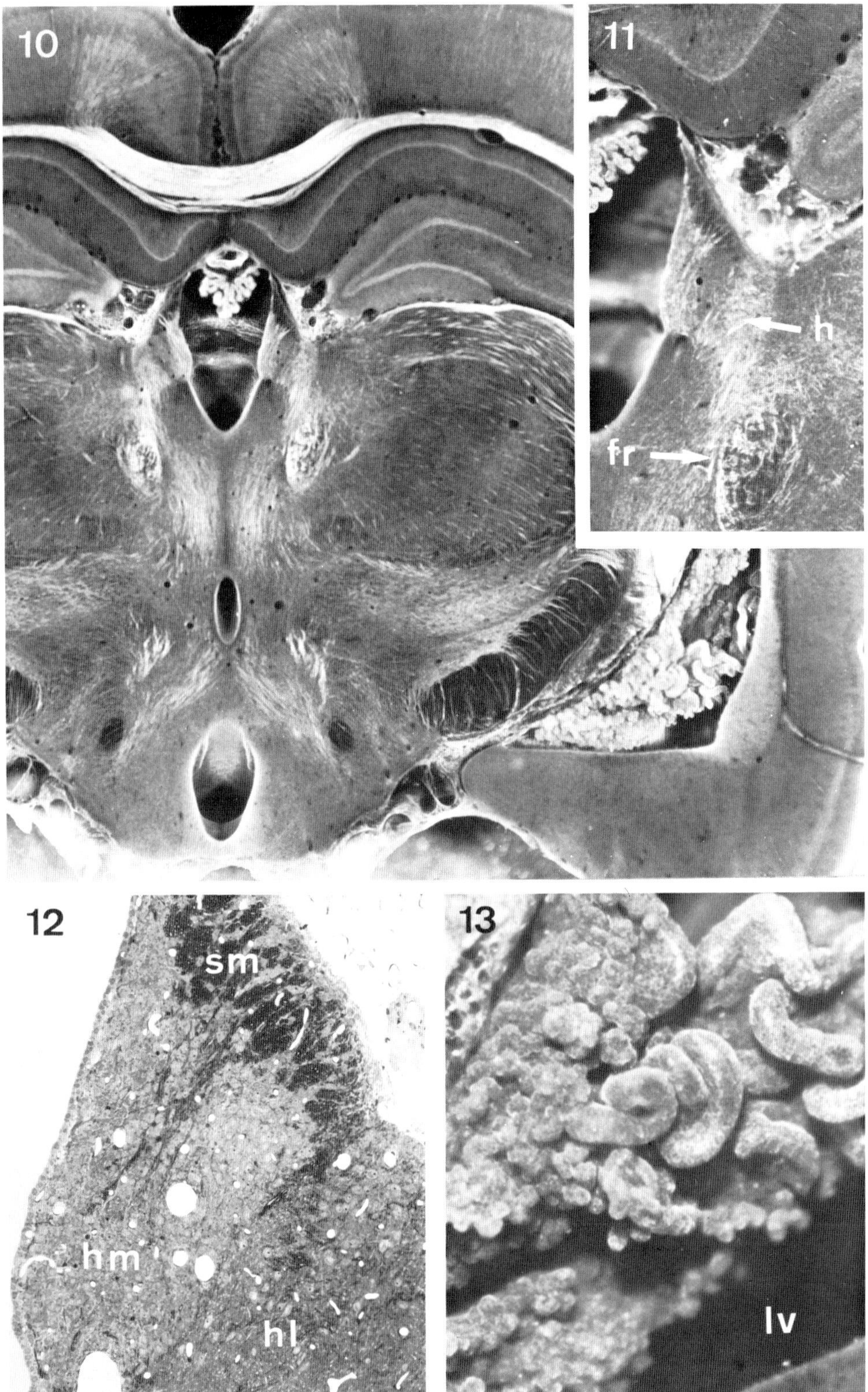
10
11
h
fr
12
sm
hm
hl
13
lv

3.6 Directed Choice of Samples

The complete brain atlas which is achieved by use of the photographs of both sides of all slices provides an orientation for the choice of the slice samples. The chosen area is noted in the brain atlas. The labeled picture is then projected onto the now totally darkly stained brain slice. With the help of a camera lucida which is integrated into a stereomicroscope, both surfaces are then superimposed (Fig. 9). The structures of interest can be marked on the tablet of Araldite by scratching it with a fine needle. The area is now sawn out and heated up to +85 °C. At this temperature the resin becomes soft, enabling one to trim it with a razor blade or any other sharp knife. Thus, the required specimen is taken out for semithin and ultrathin sectioning, whereby the orientation of this sawn out part is still possible with respect to the whole topography of the brain (Figs. 10–13). Remaining sawn out pieces of the brain slice are glued onto a foil in their original places. This makes possible further investigation without loosing the general arrangement of the brain slice.

The mounting of the sample onto a methacrylate cylinder which can be built by cutting bars of plexiglass of the required caliber is carried out with Technovit glue (Kulzer).

3.7 Reconstruction

A more precise localization of interesting areas of the brain slice and their three-dimensional extension can be achieved by producing a graphic reconstruction (Staubesand, Andres, 1953). The overall orientation and the sectioning frame with its coordinates give a reference system. The examined parts of the brain tissue, now photographed, are projected in parallel to the cutting plane of each slice onto the spaces of a grid system of the same dimensions as that of the specimen. The connection of all points of the projected brain results in a projections diagram in accordance with the plane. The shorter the distance between the cutting gaps, the more exact the reconstruction (Fig. 14a).

When demonstrating segments of a neuronal system in their extension inside a single brain slice, it is important to interpolate the space between the front and rear surface of a slice using the photographs gained by the conventional histological serial sectioning of the brain tissue.

The brain used for embedding in paraplast and sectioning is adjusted to a system of coordinates in the same manner as the former one in agarose. This guarantees the concordance of the sectioning planes. Due to the high rate of shrinkage of the embedded brain in Paraplast (Lancer, St. Louis), the total aspect of the brain as well as that of single slices must be brought to conformity by means of photography.

Pictures of those paraplast sections matching the front and rear sides of the investigated brain slice are selected. The depicted method offers a reconstruction of the paraplast sections showing the three-dimensional aspect of the neuronal system inside the brain slice. With the coordinates of one side plane and the top plane, vertical to each other, it is possible to define the spatial extension of a neuronal system in relation to the brain surface (Fig. 14b).

4 Critical Considerations, Possibilities, and Limitations

The photography of the brain slices resembles that of the picture of the tissue under low magnification. The Araldite-embedded samples can then be cut out very precisely for scanning electron microscopy and for freeze fracture studies as well as for semithin sectioning and transmission electron microscopy. Since the spatial orientation of the block is already defined, extensive cut-

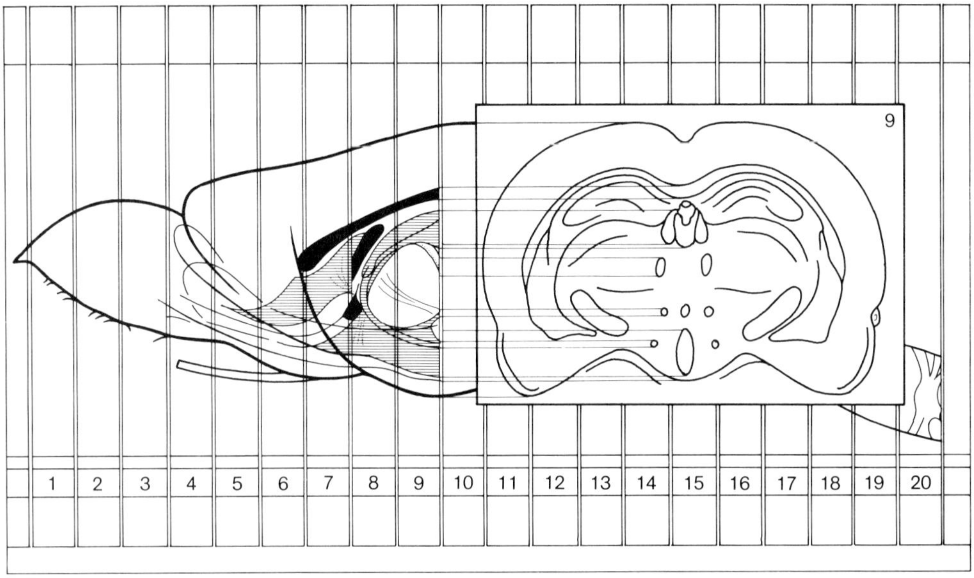

a

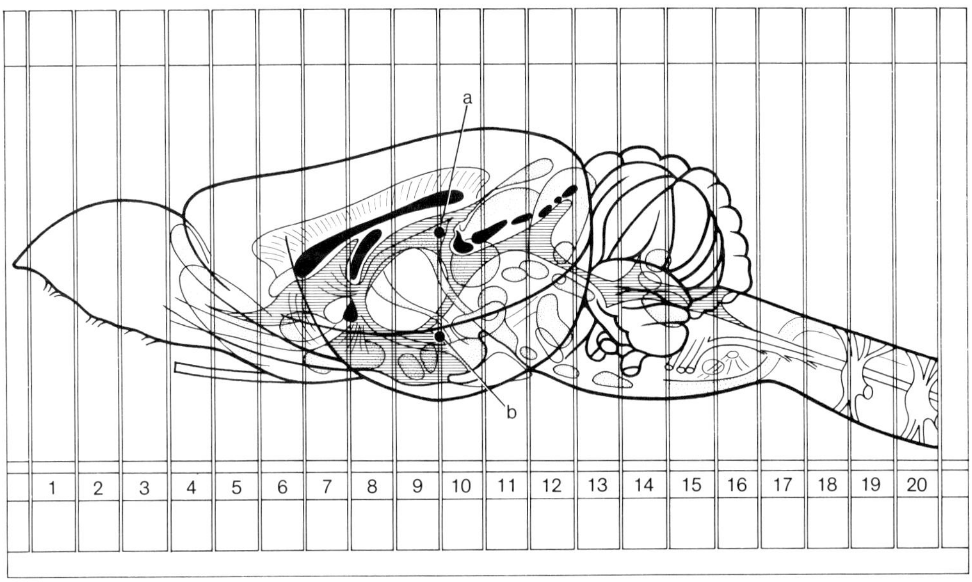

b

Fig. 14. a Graphic reconstruction of brain slices in a parallel projection. The structures of interest in the brain slices are drawn into the gaps of the sectioning frame. **b** Complete reconstruction after interpolation of a light microscopically serially sectioned brain. The positions of the habenula (*a*) and of the chorioid plexus (*b*) are exactly defined. They are marked in the telemacrophotographs in Fig. 5 with the same symbols

Table 1. Some iridescent colours of surface and tissue structures produced by the interference reflecting light method

Surface structures	Iridescent colours normal	Iridescent colours autolytic
Ciliated epithelium Ciliated ependyma	blue – green	grey
Keratinized epithelium	gold – brown	–
Olfactory epithelium:		
Fishes	blue – green	grey
Amphibia	yellow	grey
Reptiles	orange	grey
Birds	copper	grey – yellow
Mammals	silver	–
Collagenous fibres	bright silver	–
Nerve cells	invisible or dark grey	light grey or white
Nerve fibre bundles (CNS) (longitudinally sectioned)		
myelinated	bright copper to silver	light silver
unmyelinated	orange – silver	–
Nerve fibre bundles (cross sectioned)	black	brown

ting becomes unnecessary. Neighbouring regions are kept in their original relationship to each other.

Another important advantage of the method is the possibility of estimating the quality of the fixation and recognizing unexpected pathological alterations (Table 1). Nonsuitable samples can be eliminated before further stages of preparation or even electron microscopy have been carried out. The photographs of the brain slices constitute a complete atlas which can be used for further morphological investigations. Since sections of the vertebrate brain may vary greatly, reference to only one brain is unsatisfactory.

For comparative neuroanatomical studies, which also include rare species, this brain atlas is a valuable asset.

The choice of thickness of the brain slices depends on the task and on the size of a brain. For brains of small animals a thickness of 1 mm is advisable, while for larger ones 1.5–2 mm is recommended. The penetration capacity of osmium tetroxide limits the thickness to 2.5 mm.

An additional advantage of the method becomes obvious for morphometrical studies. The telemacrophotography of the brain in the orientation frame offers a fixed correlation of the brain surface to the side and top plane of the frame. It therefore defines the position in a spatial system of coordinates.

5 References

Andres KH, von Düring M (1977) Interferenzphänomene am osmierten Präparat für die systematische elektronenmikroskopische Untersuchung. Mikroskopie 30: 139–149

Andres KH, von Düring M (1977) Interference phenomenon on osmium tetroxide-fixed specimens for systematic electron microscopy. In: Hayat MA (ed) Principles and Techniques of Electron Microscopy. Biol Appl Vol 8. Van Norstrand Reinhold, pp 246–261

Staubesand J, Andres KH (1953) Graphische Rekonstruktion zur räumlichen Darstellung präterminaler Gefäße und intravasaler Besonderheiten. Mikroskopie 8: 111–120

Part II

Light Microscopical Research Methods in Neuroanatomy

Chapter 7

Enzyme Histochemistry of Nervous Tissue

E. Thomas

1 Introduction

Examination of nervous tissue by light microscopy is rewarding. Many of the methods are easily performed, cheap, and often quick in giving results. These methods are reliable, and comparison with results from biochemistry is satisfactory.

This contribution is a very personal account based on my own experience [1] and is by no means complete as to the methods available. It is written especially for the beginner in the field of neurohistochemistry. Therefore, the reader should also try later additional methods and other procedures which are not discussed here [vid. Gomori 1952; Pearse 1960, 1968, 1972; Deane et al. 1960; Burstone 1962; Barka and Anderson 1963; Kiszeli and Pósalaky 1964; Spannhof 1964; Arnold 1968; Chayen et al. 1973, 1975; Lojda et al. 1976, 1979; Ciba Foundation Symposium 73 (new series) 1980]. Comprehensive texts about enzyme histochemistry of the nervous system (Gerebtzoff 1959; Colmant 1961; Friede 1961, 1966; Koelle 1963; Adams 1965; Arvy 1966; Giacomo 1966; Novikoff 1967 a, b; Manocha and Shanta 1969, 1970;

[1] The former technical collaboration of Miss Ch. Beyer and Miss H. Schucht is acknowledged.

Thomas 1969, 1977; Eränkö 1971; Silver 1974; Davidoff and Galabov 1974; Hallpike 1976) should be consulted for further information.

For enzyme studies, cutting the tissue in a cryostat is essential. As a frozen block is treated, only the included bone, if strong enough, will harm the section. Besides, nearly all histological methods can be performed on cryostat sections (see Sect. 5).

2 Tissue

Nervous tissue is soft, thus careful preparation is of great importance: pressure must be avoided. Enzymes of nervous tissue give reaction products hours and even days after death; therefore undue haste is unnecessary. To kill small laboratory animals, decapitation after ether narcosis or intoxication by gas should be used if a guillotine is not at hand. Be careful to avoid commercially available cholinesterase inhibitors for killing the animal when you intend to study carboxyl ester hydrolases.

Preparation of brains from small laboratory animals is accomplished by breaking away the skull with a slightly rounded nail cutter. Then, letting the brain hang down, the cranial nerves are severed (see also Witte and Matthaei 1980). Preparation of brains of very small animals is not necessary. For example, we cut whole heads of smaller fishes in the cryostat.

Dorsal root ganglia can also be prepared with a nail cutter. For stronger bones surgical instruments are necessary. With man, support (elevate) the shoulder region, take off the clavicula, with forceps take a nerve of the plexus brachialis and cut it out together with the spinal ganglion in the intervertebral foramen, using not too sharply-pointed scissors. Dorsal root ganglia and the spinal cord of adult mice, frogs, small fishes, and of immature rats can be cut, usually transversally, together with the vertebral column and its muscles. Pressure upon the spinal cord must be avoided when cutting the column into pieces before freezing (Thomas and Exss 1967; Maślińska and Thomas 1975).

It is also possible to cut a whole hand or foot of a smaller laboratory animal without any dissection, mounting it on the dorsal side. Then you may have together, for example, sensory end organs in the finger tips, motor endplates, spindles in the Mm. lumbricales, and smaller nerves. For the localization of motor endplates in the various muscles an atlas gives topographical advice (Cöers and Woolf 1959). Peripheral nerves should be freed from adipose tissue because it smears.

Tissue cultures may be incubated without further preliminaries after being air-dried (Tischner and Thomas 1973; see Sect. 3.3).

2.1 Biopsies

Biopsies (e. g., for clinical diagnosis) may be transported dry in a glass container across a small town without any harm (not in a warm pocket). Small specimens, for example, a rectal biopsy of mucosa and submucosa (to see cells of the plexus submucosus, see Thomas 1977: Figs. 17, 25) must not dry out, otherwise sections can no longer be mounted onto glass slides.

For light microscopy nerves are usually orientated longitudinally (stretched slightly with two pairs of forceps during freezing), but muscle biopsies as a rule are cut exactly transversally (fiber diameters). For unknown reasons we have never been able to cut fresh frozen muscle longitudinally without more or less damaging the muscle fibers by cutting.

Brain biopsies for diagnostic purposes (Schröder et al. 1971: Fig. 1c, d) should be prepared immediately in the operation room, but brain tumours can be brought to your laboratory where you can select the tissue wanted for use. Skin biopsies (Krücke et al. 1971: Fig. 7), as all the other biopsies, may be frozen and sent by air freight in a box with dry ice.

For almost all enzymes it is possible to send dry cryostat sections from one town to another by mail (Thomas and Sourander 1977; see also Sect. 3.3).

2.2 Post-Mortem Material

This can be studied after 12–24 h without deterioration of tissue if the corpse is stored in a cooled room. Loss of dehydrogenase activity is insignificant or not seen at all (Chason 1970; Tyrer et al. 1971).

Carboxylic ester hydrolases (Bergner and Durlacher 1951; Moore and Petty 1958; Petty and Moore 1958; Thomas 1968: Figs. 1, 4, 5) and other hydrolytic enzymes will also remain active. Proteases can survive for thousands of years (Steppuhn and Utkina-Ljubowzowa 1930). Moreover, the very high amounts of acid phosphatases, for instance, in spinal ganglia, do not lead to postmortem autolysis.

2.3 Test Tissues

Test tissues with high activities and simple morphology should be taken to try a method when it is used for the first time. Such tissue is, for instance, a spinal ganglion or the ganglion trigeminale Gasseri. The latter is easily found, prepared, and cut. Cerebellar cortex and medulla oblongata are a little more complicated in morphology, but also have high activities in certain cells.

2.4 Experimental Neurobiology

Changes are most instructively demonstrated when altered tissue is cut together with the control tissue in a "sandwich" block (Thomas 1977; Fig. 52). The bilateral organization of the nervous system allows good comparison when only one side is affected, for example, when one studies "retrograde" nerve cell reaction in the spinal cord (Thomas and Exss 1967).

3 Preparation of Material

Brain or muscle (like any other tissue) is cut with two double-edged razor blades touching each other, side by side which are moved in parallel against each other in the line of section. Avoid water, but sometimes a tiny drop is useful to prevent sticking of brain to the blades. It is good to work on a paraffin wax-plate which can be cleaned easily and which does no harm to your knives.

3.1 Freezing

It is not possible simply to put the tissue into a deep freeze because ice crystallization tears the tissue and makes histologic examination impossible.

Once frozen the tissue must be kept in this state. But it is possible to thaw a block at room temperature and fix it afterwards (e. g., muscle in absolute ethanol to stain for glycogen). In contrast to muscle, which always has to be frozen in liquid nitrogen, nervous tissue and especially brain does not need such a very rapid freezing procedure. [If you do freeze in liquid nitrogen the block may break into pieces (if it is mounted on a cork disk you have only the cracking lines, but anatomical orientation is still preserved). In addition, you may get curious malformations in the tissue: for instance, a "fascicle" of spinal cord may appear above the surface level during the freezing process (shrinkage compression?)].

Freezing of brain and other nervous tissues is done on a microtome chuck with carbon dioxide or by dry ice pressed against the metal holder. CO_2 seems better because it envelops the whole tissue, if you cover the chuck with a plastic hood. Freezing the block should be done as quickly as possible, but open the valve slowly at first.

The tissue should afterwards be as hard as a block of ice.

Muscle has to be frozen in liquid nitrogen. Put the muscle in its natural state (fibers transversally cut with razor blades) on a disk of cork; then powder the surface slightly (in order to avoid Leydenfrost's phenomenon; talcum or other kinds of powder will work) and with long forceps hold it in the liquid nitrogen as long as it bubbles heavily (30–60 s). Later mount the block together with the cork on the microtome chuck or store it. If liquid nitrogen is available, peripheral nerves may be pinned onto a cork disk at their ends by spines of a hedgehog (not commercially available), or they may adhere by themselves stretched upon cardboard. Whole hands with the fingers of small laboratory animals can also be fixed onto cork with hedgehog spines (which can be cut in a cryostat).

Whole frontal slices of a human hemisphere can be frozen on a special microtome chuck with CO_2 if you have a microtome for cutting such specimens (e.g., Tetrander model K; Firma Jung, Heidelberg) in a big cryostat (Firma Dittes, Heidelberg) or an "open-top" type refrigerator with such a microtome.

3.2 Storage

Storage of tissues is simplest in plastic tubes which are sealed by heat with a special instrument available commercially. Unsealed material will dry out within a few days and becomes useless. We have kept sealed tissue for years at –70 °C (but at times lost it when the refrigerator did not work). If a deep freeze is not available, material can be stored at –20 °C for long periods without harm.

3.3 Fixation-Drying

Fixation with aldehydes should be avoided because any kind of fixation reduces or destroys enzyme activity. Therefore, cutting unfixed material in a cryostat is a must in enzyme histochemistry. The other essential, in my experience, is to *let the section dry in air at room temperature for at least 1 or 2 days* when you want to examine hydrolytic enzymes. This drying is a kind of fixation. Moisture in the air will spoil your sections (bacterial growth, diffusion of enzyme activity). Air-drying in a country with a wet climate, therefore, may be not possible.

Dried sections can be stored for days or weeks. Even then strong enzyme reactions are achievable. Muscle ATPase activity decreases in dried sections after some days, but in the perineurium ATPase is active, as are some dehydrogenases, even after weeks (Thomas and Sourander 1977). Control reactions with sections stored for a shorter time are advised.

3.4 Freeze Drying

Freeze drying, which according to the textbooks gives good results in various tissues, was tried without success by us on nervous tissues. Structural preservation was bad. We feel freeze drying is not necessary for light microscope enzyme studies of the nervous system.

4 Cutting

Everybody who has experience in histology is happy to find how quickly one can get good fresh frozen sections in a cryostat. The more stable the microtome the better it is. Cutting a nerve exactly longitudinally is not possible with a rotary microtome.

Many useful hints are given in textbooks (Pearse 1968; Lojda et al. 1979). I only mention that a clean knife and a clean anti-roll plate (also with a perfectly smooth upper edge) are of great importance. So, after each section, removal of ice crystals with a stiff paint brush of medium size hog bristle may be necessary. And with "fatty" nerve tissue frequent cleaning with acetone of the knife (including the back side) and the upper edge of the anti-roll plate may be necessary.

Generally we cut 8–10 μm thick sections at –20 °C with an even, not too quick movement of the knife (motor driven microtomes are ideal, a further advantage being that the block can be trimmed down automatically to the desired level). The temperature may be varied; the fattier the tissue, the lower it should be. An ugly artifact often arises when blocks of brain are cut: parallel cracks occur in the section and sometimes demand a very even-tempered technician who has to try everything imaginable to change the cutting conditions (sometimes in vain). Those cracks appear especially when big blocks are cut on a Tetrander K microtome in huge cryostats and the histologic context may then be ruined. The longer duration of the freezing process of those big blocks may lead to freezing artifacts (ice crystallization).

We take the section (or two sections or a triplet) from the knife onto one end of the slide (in order to save incubation medium). The slide is at room temperature. We touch only one part of the section and move the slide away. The rest comes along and sticks immediately to the glass. This can be repeated with the same slide several times, if the object is small. We incubate in a Coplin jar and do not need any more medium than we would if we mounted on cover slips.

5 Staining

Thionin is a useful stain for orientation and thionin staining is performed quickly. Take the cryostat section (a few minutes after it was cut; the surface must be opaque), put it into 1% aqueous thionin for 1–3 min, rinse briefly in water to remove the excess stain, and differentiate according to desired intensity of coloration in a graded ethanol series (1×75%, 2×96%, 2×100%, Xylol).

Other stains. Fresh frozen sections of nervous tissue mounted on glass slides and dried thoroughly can be stained according to nearly all methods used in histology. We use the Heidenhain-Woelcke stain for myelin; Bodian's silver impregnation (prefix in 4% formalin; the results are excellent; unfortunately sections of muscle may float off during impregnation); Haematoxylin-eosin; Fettrot 7B for neutral fats (also applicable, for example, after Gomori's metal salt method for acid phosphatase); the plasmal reaction (especially for peripheral myelin sheaths; even most discrete myelin breakdown products can be visualized in such sections by birefringence of cholesterol esters; also useful as a counterstain after dehydrogenase reactions, e.g., with MTT); the OTAN method; the Gallocyanin-chromalum method; the Periodic-acid-Schiff method; the Congo red stain for amyloid; the Hirsch-Peiffer method for metachromatic substances; etc. Muscle fibers are stained best with 1% aqueous methylene blue. Autofluorescence and birefringence can also be examined in unstained, uncovered sections.

5.1 Counterstains

Counterstains of nuclei after an enzyme reaction depend upon the color wanted. These stains include 2% aqueous methyl green (extracted in chloroform), Mayer's hemalum, and Mayer's carmalum.

6 Enzyme Reactions – A Selection of Methods

The methods given here were applied to nervous tissues by Thomas (1977). In the introduction to each chapter remarks about these enzyme reactions, a guide to relevant literature, and illustrations are to be found.

A modern textbook on methodology is Lojda et al. (1976, 1979). We followed mostly the textbooks of Pearse (1960, 1968, 1972), but others may also be consulted (see Sect. 1). Pearse includes a list of sources for compounds; therefore, only exceptional sources we used are mentioned here.

6.1 Oxidoreductases

The theory of dehydrogenase enzyme histochemistry was discussed by Wohlrab et al. (1979). In nervous tissues with the methods available topological differences of activity in single cell elements and even parts of the cells can be demonstrated.

The tetrazolium salt which should be used, according to our own experience, is not always the commonly used Nitro-BT. With muscle biopsies we feel that MTT (George T. Gurr Ltd.; Coronation Road, Cresswick Industrial Estate, High Wycombe, Bucks, England) gives better results than Nitro-BT, but sections can deteriorate within days or weeks. With nervous tissues generally one uses Nitro-BT as an electron acceptor. But there are hitherto unexplainable situations when Nitro-BT is unsuitable and MTT should be used for the reaction (Thomas 1977). For instance the so-called solitary active cells with a very high activity of NADPH diaphorase are stained more selectively with MTT than with Nitro-BT (Thomas and Pearse 1964).

After cutting the sections should dry for a few minutes until they are opaque. Incubate for 30–45 min at 37 °C. As incubation media are expensive, cover the sections lying in a Petri dish with a few drops of fluid, but be careful that they do not dry out. Stop the reaction by putting the sections in 4% formaldehyde for at least 1 h, wash in tap water, and mount in glycerine jelly (this also applies to sections incubated with Nitro-BT; we don't dehydrate).

For the most part, counterstaining is unnecessary (if desired, use Mayer's carmalum), but an additional enzyme reaction for hydrolases can be performed in a further incubation step (see Sect. 7.2).

In every case adjust pH of the final solution (stock incubating solution plus substrate and coenzyme where used) to 7.1–7.2 with small amounts of 0.2 M Tris or 0.2 M HCl (a tiny drop on the tip of a spatula will often be enough). Test the medium with paper (put a small drop onto it) or better with a pH meter (you need small test tubes; the electrode should just fit in).

All stock solutions for oxidoreductases should be stored at –20 °C (best in small portions).

6.1.1 NADH Diaphorase; NADPH Diaphorase

The incubation medium is prepared with the reduced coenzyme and the stock incubation solution A. Dissolve 2–3 mg $NADH_2$ or $NADPH_2$ (reduced form!; once you are able to estimate the quantity you need not weigh it) in 1 ml of the following stock incubation solution A with Nitro-BT:

Nitro-BT (1 mg/ml demineralized water)	2.5 ml
Tris buffer [1] (0.2 M, pH 7.2)	2.5 ml
Demineralized water	5.0 ml

Alternatively (for muscle; e.g., for "solitary active cells") the following stock incubating solution A with MTT is used:

MTT (1 mg/ml demineralized water)	2.5 ml
Tris buffer (0.2 M, pH 7.2)	2.5 ml
Cobalt chloride (0.5 M)	0.5 ml
Demineralized water	4.5 ml

[1] Stock 0.2 M buffer (pH 7.2): To 22.1 ml Tris (hydroxymethyl) aminomethane (24.2 g Tris/liter H_2O) add 77.9 ml of 0.2 N HCl.

6.1.2 The Bound Enzyme Succinate Dehydrogenase

Succinate dehydrogenase does not need coenzymes except menadione (vitamin K_3). The stock incubating solutions B are the same as the stock incubating solutions A used for the diaphorases (see Sect. 6.1.1) except that they are made with 10% less water (use only 4 ml demineralized water in the prescription given above for the stock incubating solution with Nitro-BT and 3.5 ml with MTT).

The stock substrate solution (0.6 M) is 1.26 g disodium succinate in 10 ml H_2O.

For the reaction mix 0.9 ml of stock incubating solution B with Nitro-BT and 0.1 ml of stock substrate solution and add ~ 0.2 mg menadione (if you touch the surface of the substrate in the bottle just slightly with a spatula, sufficient menadione will stick to it and can be put into the incubating medium). In case of a very high enzyme activity for succinate dehydrogenase menadione can be omitted.

6.1.3 The Bound Enzyme α-Glycerophosphate Dehydrogenase

α-Glycerophosphate dehydrogenase does not need coenzymes except menadione; the method is performed like that described in Sect. 6.1.2.

The stock substrate solution (1.0 M) is 3.15 g disodium-glycerol-3-phosphate in 8 ml H_2O, neutralized with ~ 1.8 ml 0.1 N HCl, and made up to 10 ml with H_2O.

Stock incubating solution B with MTT should also be used, particularly for α-glycerophosphate dehydrogenase (see Thomas 1977: Fig. 72).

6.1.4 Lactate Dehydrogenase

The stock substrate solution (1.0 M) is 1.120 g sodium DL-lactate in 10 ml H_2O.

For the reaction mix 0.9 ml of stock incubating solution B (see Sec. 6.1.2) with 0.1 ml of stock substrate solution and add 2–3 mg NAD (unreduced form!).

6.1.5 Glutamate Dehydrogenase

The method is performed like that described in Sect. 6.1.4.

The stock substrate solution (1.0 M) is 1.870 g sodium L-glutamate (monohydrate) in 8.0 ml H_2O neutralized with ~ 0.05 ml 0.1 N HCl, made up to 10 ml with H_2O.

6.2 Hydrolases

For all reactions well-dried cryostat sections should be used. For adenosinetriphosphatase activity see Sect. 3.3. Prefixation before incubation in 4% formalin for 1 min or a little longer can be useful (e.g., with alkaline phosphatase, ATPase), but generally this can be omitted. Incubation is carried out in Coplin jars.

6.2.1 Alkaline Phosphatases

Results from the two methods available are not always identical (Thomas 1977: Fig. 34). The methods are discussed in Sects. 6.2.1.1 and 6.2.1.2.

6.2.1.1 Gomori's Metal Salt Method

Incubate for 30 min–4 h at 37 °C in the following medium:

3% Sodium β-glycerophosphate (stored at 4 °C)	10 ml
2% Sodium diethyl barbiturate (stored at 4 °C)	10 ml
Demineralized water	5 ml
2% Calcium chloride	20 ml
5% Magnesium sulphate	1 ml

Rinse in running tap water for 3 min, treat with 2% cobalt nitrate for 5 min, rinse thoroughly in demineralized water, and treat with a dilute solution of "yellow" ammonium sulfide for 1–2 min. The solution should be very weak: two to three drops of ammonium sulfide solution G. R. taken with a glass rod into ~ 30 ml H_2O are usually sufficient. Immerse until you see coloration with the naked eye, for instance, when testing a dorsal root ganglion. Ammonium sulfide solution deteriorates in the course of time and then does not work sufficiently. We keep it at 4 °C. Wash in running tap water for 5 min and mount in glycerine jelly. The stain is brown to black.

6.2.1.2 Coupling Azo Dye Method

Take the following freshly prepared solution (pH 9.2):

0.1 M Tris buffer, pH 10.0	20 ml
Naphthol-AS-TR-phosphate	20 mg
Variamine blue B	20 mg

Stir well, filter with two layers of filter paper, and then incubate for 10–60 min at 37 °C. Wash in running water for 10 min, and let the sections remain for at least 1 day in 4% formalin (to avoid gas bubbles) before mounting in glycerine jelly. The stain is blue.

6.2.2 Acid Phosphatases

Results with the four methods given are not identical in staining the fine structure of nerve cells (Fig. 1 a–c). This is also evident when a pathological cell reaction is studied with the methods given below (Thomas 1977: Fig. 23).

6.2.2.1 Gomori's Metal Salt Method

Incubate for 30 min to 16 h at 37 °C in a fresh prepared solution of

0.01 M Sodium β-glycerophosphate (stored at 4 °C)	10 ml
0.05 M Acetate buffer (Walpole; pH 5.0; stored at 4 °C)	10 ml
0.002 M Lead nitrate (stored at 4 °C)	10 ml

This solution should be without turbidity (otherwise take fresh prepared stock solutions). False metal impregnation was avoided or reduced by lowering the concentration of lead nitrate to 0.002 M and by shortening the incubation time to 1–2 h. Washing in demineralized water and then quickly rinsing in 1.5% glacial acetic acid G. R. may help to remove "false" (?) impregnation of fibrils (axons), but may also remove true reaction products (?).

After incubation wash thoroughly in demineralized water, treat with dilute "yellow" ammonium sulfide (see Sect. 6.2.1.1), wash well and mount in glycerine jelly. The stain is brown.

6.2.2.2 Azo Dye Method with Naphthol-AS-TR-phosphate and Fast Blue B

Take the following freshly prepared solution:

0.1 M-Acetate buffer (Walpole; pH 5.2)	20 ml
Naphthol-AS-TR-phosphate	10–30 mg
Fast blue B	20 mg

Shake well, filter with two layers of filter paper, and then incubate for 30–60 min at 37 °C. Wash with running water for 10 min and let the sections remain for at least 1 day in 4% formalin before mounting in glycerine jelly. The stain is between red and blue.

6.2.2.3 Azo Dye Method with Naphthol-AS-TR-phosphate and Hexazotized Pararosanilin
(after Barka and Anderson 1962)

Stock solution A: dissolve 2 g pararosanilin hydrochloride (Merck, Darmstadt; free of acridin: Chroma, Stuttgart-Untertürkheim) in 50 ml 2 N HCl, warm, cool, and filter (stored at 4 °C).

Stock solution B: 4% aqueous solution of sodium nitrite (stored at 4 °C; not more than 4 days old, better freshly prepared).

Stock solution C: Veronal acetate buffer (Michaelis; 0.1 M, pH 9.0).

Stock solution D: dissolve 100 mg naphthol-AS-TR-phosphate in 10 ml *N*, *N*-dimethylformamide (stored at 4 °C).

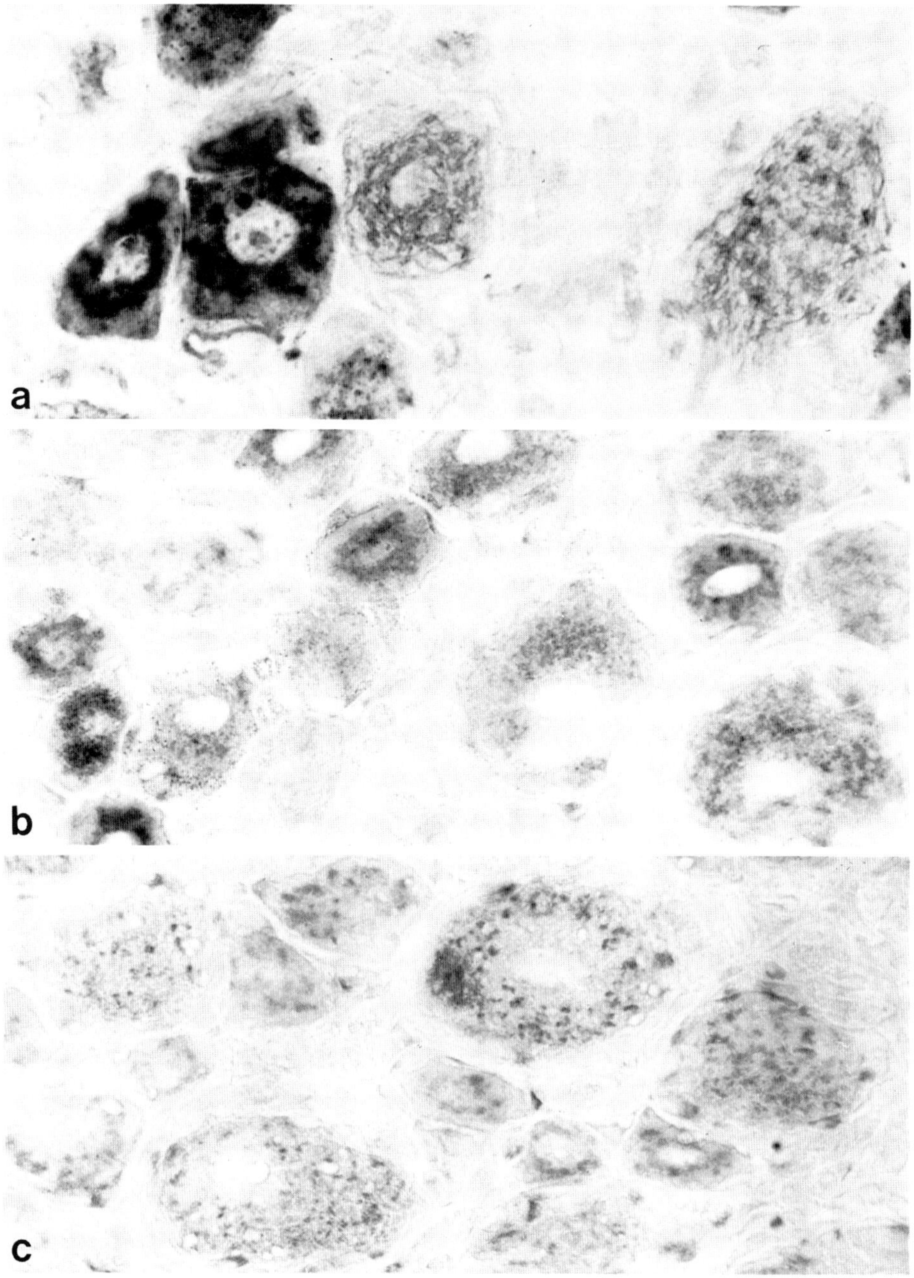

Fig. 1a–c. Acid phosphatases: three different types of intracellular enzyme reaction with three different methods. Dorsal root ganglion cells of rat (Thomas 1977: Figs 22, 23a, c, e). **a** Metal salt method, pH 5.0 (see Sect. 6.2.2.1; incubation 45 min). **b** Coupling azo dye method with naphthol-AS-TR-phosphate and fast blue B, pH 5.2 (see Sect. 6.2.2.2, incubation 60 min). **c** Coupling azo dye method with naphthol-AS-TR-phosphate and hexazotized pararosanilin, pH 5.0 (see Sect. 6.2.2.3, incubation 60 min)

Incubating solution:

Stock solution C	5 ml
Demineralized water	12 ml
Stock solution D	1 ml

Mix 0.8 ml stock solution A and 0.8 ml stock solution B. After about 1 min its color should be amber or pale yellow: add this to the incubating solution. Adjust to pH 5.0 with 1 N NaOH (a few drops; use pH meter). Incubate at room temperature for 30–60 min, wash in running water for 10 min, put into 4% formalin (see Sect. 6.2.1.2), and mount in glycerine jelly. The stain is red. Counterstain if desired with methyl green.

6.2.2.4 Azo Dye Method with α-Naphthyl Phosphate and Hexazotized Pararosanilin
(after Barka and Anderson 1962)

This is performed very similarly to the method in Sect. 6.2.2.3, but instead of stock solution D the following stock solution E (stored at 4 °C) is used: dissolve 400 mg sodium α-naphthyl phosphate in 100 ml Michaelis buffer stock solution C.

Dilute 5 ml stock solution E with 10 ml demineralized water. Pour into this a 1-min-old mixture of 0.8 ml stock solution A and 0.8 ml stock solution B. Adjust to pH 5.4 with 1 N NaOH using a pH meter. Add demineralized water to give a final volume of 20 ml. The stain is reddish-brown.

6.2.3 Adenosine Triphosphatase
(Calcium Method – Padykula and Herman 1955)

Take a freshly prepared solution of

0.1 M Sodium barbiturate (2.062 g/100 ml)	6 ml
0.18 M $CaCl_2$ (1.998 g/100 ml)	3 ml
Demineralized water	9 ml
Adenosine 5'triphosphate (disodium salt)	45 mg

After the ATP is dissolved, adjust the pH to 9.4 with 0.1 N NaOH (~ 2 ml) and make up to 30 ml with demineralized water. Filter with two layers of filter paper and incubate at 37 °C for 5 min to 3 h (various times of incubation are advised). Wash thoroughly in three changes of 1% calcium chloride. Immerse in 2% $CaCl_2$, 3–5 min. Wash in three changes of demineralized water. Immerse in dilute "yellow" ammonium sulfide (see Sect. 6.2.1.1). Wash in demineralized water, mount in glycerine jelly. The stain is dark brown.

6.2.4 Carboxylic Ester Hydrolases

One finds corresponding sites of reaction with the three methods given below. On the other hand a "polar" distribution of acetylcholine esterase on the neuronal side and of "nonspecific" cholinesterases on the extraneuronal side is evident (Thomas 1977). In this case, from the standpoint of a histologist, control reactions with inhibitors seem to be of secondary importance. In addition with respect to inhibitors, studies and text books on carboxylic ester hydrolase histochemistry (Koelle 1963; Härkönen 1964; Kokko 1965; Söderholm 1965; Friede 1967; Silver 1974) should be consulted.

6.2.4.1 Acetylthiocholine Method
(after Gomori 1952)

Stock solution, which keeps infinitely, is:

Copper sulphate ($CuSO_4 \times 5H_2O$)	0.3 g
Glycine	0.375 g
Magnesium chloride ($MgCl_2 \times 6H_2O$)	1.0 g
Maleic acid	1.75 g
1 N Sodium hydroxide solution	30 ml
Hot saturated (about 40%) solution of Na_2SO_4 (68 g/170 ml)	170 ml

The pH is about 6.0. Na_2SO_4 crystallizes out on cooling (leave the crystals in the bottle).

Dissolve about 20 mg acetylthiocholine iodide in a few drops of water (in a clean spoon) and add this to 10 ml of the stock solution. Incubate sections for 20 min to

20 h (peripheral nerves: 3–12 h; dorsal root ganglia: 90 min to 3 h; muscle endplates: 20–30 min). Rinse in three changes of demineralized water, immerse in a dilute solution of "yellow" ammonium sulfide (see Sect. 6.2.1.1), rinse again in water, counterstain if desired with methyl green or Mayer's hemalum, rinse and mount in glycerine jelly. The stain is brown. Sometimes, ugly crystalline precipitates will arise (therefore, avoid the rinse in Na_2SO_4 as stated in the original prescription).

6.2.4.2 Butyrylthiocholine Method

The butyrylthiocholine method is performed like the method described in Sect. 6.2.4.1, but the substrate is butyrylthiocholine iodide instead of acetylthiocholine iodide. Times of incubation may be shorter than those stated above.

6.2.4.3 Indoxyl Acetate Esterase Method
(after Holt and Withers 1952)

Dissolve 4 mg 5-bromo-4-chloroindoxyl acetate (Sigma Chemical Co) in 0.1 ml ethanol (100%, not denatured). One then adds:

0.2 M Tris buffer (Hydroxymethyl amino methane/HCl buffer) pH 6–8 (vid. 6.1.1)	6 ml
0.05 M Potassium ferricyanide (stored at 4 °C)	3 ml
0.05 M Potassium ferrocyanide (stored at 4 °C)	3 ml
0.1 M Calcium chloride	3 ml
Demineralized water	15 ml

Incubate sections at 37 °C for 5 min to 12 h (see Sect. 6.2.4.1). Wash in water, counterstain if desired in Mayer's carmalum, rinse again in water and mount in glycerine jelly. The stain is blue.

7 Combined Methods

The results of combined methods may be more informative than a simple counterstain. The procedures are as stated above, one after the other with a rinse in demineralized water between them. We tried with success the following combined methods:

1. *Acetylthiocholine method + alkaline phosphatase method* (azo dye stain). See Tischner and Thomas (1973: Fig. 4).
2. *Lactate dehydrogenase method* (with MTT) + *indoxyl acetate esterase method.* In this case, both reactions were reduced in intensity (Thomas 1977: Fig. 13).

8 Problems and Facts

The results one gets with the methods given here may vary. This depends upon many factors. Some of these differences have a technical reason. The substrates one uses can vary in quality. For many years we were able to perform the method for arylsulphatase according to Rutenburg et al. (1952) with 6-bromo-2-naphthyl sulphate as substrate (Thomas and Lange 1968; Thomas 1977: Fig. 53). For an unknown reason we no longer get positive results with this compound although we have tried samples from several firms. This is embarrassing. Other failures are mentioned by Gomori (1952), for instance, with his technique for acid phosphatase. They fall into six groups which he discusses in detail. Limitations and pitfalls of the methods when applied to the nervous system are described by Adams (1969).

Moreover, results depend upon many other conditions. I quote here, for example, the following: species differences, changes during morphogenesis, circadian rhythms, and plasticity under physiologic stress. More are discussed by Thomas (1977).

On the other hand the methods given here have been proved for many years to be valuable for anatomical research and to be very sensitive indicators of pathological cell processes which are manifested by increased or decreased enzyme reactivity (Thomas 1981 a, b). They are, therefore, a useful tool in science not only for neurobiology but also for neuropathology.

9 References

Adams CWM (ed) (1965) Neurohistochemistry. Elsevier, Amsterdam London New York

Adams CWM (1969) Enzyme histochemistry: Applications and pitfalls. In: Lajtha A (ed) Handbook of neurochemistry, vol 2. Plenum Press, New York London, pp 525–538

Arnold M (1968) Histochemie. Einfuhrung in Grundlagen und Prinzipien der Methoden. Springer, Berlin Heidelberg New York

Arvy L (1966) Les phosphatases du tissue nerveux. Hermann, Paris

Barka T, Anderson PJ (1962) Histochemical methods for acid phosphatase using hexazonium pararosanilin as coupler. J. Histochem Cytochem 10:741–753

Barka T, Anderson PJ (1963) Histochemistry. Theory, practice, and bibliography. Hoeber Medical Division/Harper & Row, New York Evanston London

Bergner AD, Durlacher S (1951) Histochemical detection of fatal anticholinesterase poisoning. Am J Pathol 27:1011–1022

Burstone MS (1962) Enzyme histochemistry and its application in the study of neoplasms. Academic Press, New York London

Chason JL (1970) Enzyme histochemistry in postmortem nervous system. In: Tedeschi CG (ed) Neuropathology. Methods and diagnosis. Little Brown, Boston, pp 379–384

Chayen J, Bitensky L, Butcher RG (1973) Practical histochemistry. John Wiley a Sons, New York. Deutsche Ausgabe (1975) Histochemie. Grundlagen und Methoden. Verlag Chemie, Weinheim

Ciba Foundation Symposium 73 (new series) (1980) Trends in enzyme histochemistry and cytochemistry. Excerpta Medica, Amsterdam Oxford New York

Coërs C, Woolf AL (1959) The innervation of muscle. A biopsy study. Blackwell, Oxford

Colmant HJ (1961) Ergebnisse der Enzymhistochemie am zentralen und peripheren Nervensystem. Fortschr Neurol Psychiatr 29:61–124

Davidoff M, Galabov G (1974) Lysosomen und lysosomale Enzyme im Zentralnervensystem der Ratte. Progr Histochem Cytochem 6/2: 1–64

Deane HW, Barrnett RJ, Seligman AM (1960) Histochemische Methoden zum Nachweis der Enzymaktivität (Histochemical methods for the demonstration of enzyme activity). In: Graumann W, Neumann K (eds) Handbuch der Histochemie, vol VII/1. Fischer, Stuttgart

Eränkö O (ed) (1971) Histochemistry of nervous transmission. Prog Brain Res 34

Friede RL (1961) Histochemischer Atlas der Gewebsoxydation im Hirnstamm der Katze. Karger, Basel New York

Friede RL (1966) Topographic brain chemistry. Academic Press, New York London

Friede RL (1967) A comparative histochemical mapping of the distribution of butyryl cholinesterase in the brains of four species of mammals, including man. Acta Anat (Basel) 66: 161–177

Gerebtzoff MA (1959) Cholinesterases. A histochemical contribution to the solution of some functional problems. Pergamon Press, London

Giacomo P de (1966) Istochimica enzimatica normale e patologica del sistema nervoso centrale. Quad Acta Neurol XXIV

Gomori G (1952) Microscopic histochemistry. Principles and practice. University of Chicago Press, Chicago

Härkönen M (1964) Carboxylic esterases, oxidative enzymes and catecholamines in the superior cervical ganglion of the rat and the effect of pre- and post-ganglionic nerve division. Acta Physiol Scand [Suppl 237] 63:1–94

Hallpike JF (1976) Histochemistry of peripheral nerves and nerve terminals. In: Landon DN (ed) The peripheral nerve. Chapman & Hall, London, pp 605–665

Holt SJ, Withers RFJ (1952) Cytochemical localization of esterases using indoxyl derivatives. Nature 170:1012–1014

Kiszely G, Pósalaky Z (1964) Mikrotechnische und histochemische Untersuchungsmethoden. Akadémiai Kiadó, Budapest

Koelle GB (1963) Cytological distributions and physiological functions of cholinesterases. In: Eichler O, Farah A (eds) Koelle GB (subed) Handbuch der experimentellen Pharmakologie, vol XV. Springer, Berlin Göttingen Heidelberg, pp 187–298

Kokko Au (1965) Histochemical and cytophotometric observations on esterases in the spinal ganglion of the rat. Acta Physiol Scand [Suppl 261] 66:1–76

Krücke W, von Hartrott HH, Schröder JM, Thomas E, Gibbels E, Scheid W (1971) Licht- und elektronenmikroskopische Untersuchungen zum Spätstadium der Thalidomid-Polyneuropathie. Fortschr Neurol Psychiatr 39: 15–50

Lojda Z, Gossrau R, Schiebler TH (1976) Enzymhistochemische Methoden. Springer, Berlin Heidelberg New York

Lojda Z, Gossrau R, Schiebler TH (1979) Enzyme histochemistry. A laboratory manual. Springer, Berlin Heidelberg New York

Manocha SL, Shantha TR (1969) Enzyme histochemistry of the nervous system. In: Bourne GH (ed) The structure and function of nervous tissue: vol II, Structure II and physiology. Academic Press, New York London, pp 137–240

Manocha SL, Shantha TR (1970) Macaca mulatta. Enzyme histochemistry of the nervous system. Academic Press, New York London

Maślińska D, Thomas E (1975) Enzymehistochemical studies of "retrograde" reaction in motor neurones of immature rats. Acta Neuropathol (Berl) 33:317–323

Moore EJ, Petty CS (1958) A note on cholinesterase activity in post-mortem tissues. J Histochem Cytochem 6:377–379

Novikoff AB (1967a) Enzyme localization and ultrastructure of neurons. In: Hydén H (ed) The neuron. Elsevier, Amsterdam London New York, pp 255–318

Novikoff AB (1967b) Lysosomes in nerve cells. In: Hydén H (ed) The neuron. Elsevier, Amsterdam London New York, pp 319–377

Padykula HA, Herman E (1955) Factors affecting the activity of adenosine triphosphatase and other phosphatases as measured by histochemical techniques. J Histochem Cytochem 3:161–169

Pearse AGE (1960) Histochemistry. Theoretical and applied, 2nd edn. Churchill, London

Pearse AGE (1968) Histochemistry. Theoretical and applied, 3rd edn, vol I. Churchill, London

Pearse AGE (1972) Histochemistry. Theoretical and applied, 3rd edn, vol II. Churchill Livingstone, Edinburgh London

Petty CS, Moore EJ (1958) Histochemical demonstration of cholinesterase. Application to forensic pathology. J Forensic Sci 3:510–520

Rutenburg AM, Cohen RB, Seligman AM (1952) Histochemical demonstration of arylsulfatase. Science 116:539–543

Schröder JM, Thomas E, Kollmann JF (1971) Formvarianten kurvilinearer Zytosomen in Gehirn-, Leber- und Knochenmarksbiopsien bei neuroviszeraler Lipidose. Verh Dtsch Ges Pathol 55:432–437

Silver A (1974) The biology of cholinesterases. Front Biol 36

Söderholm U (1965) Histochemical localization of esterases, phosphatases and tetrazolium reductases in the motor neurones of the spinal cord of the rat and the effect of nerve division. Acta Physiol Scand [Suppl 256] 65:3–60

Spannhof L (1964) Einführung in die Praxis der Histochemie. Fischer, Jena

Steppuhn O, Utkina-Ljubowzowa X (1930) Proteolytische Zellfermente von ägyptischen Mumien (etwa 3000jährig) und Mammut (etwa 30 000 bis 100 000jährig). Biochem Z 226:237–242

Thomas E (1968) Histochemie der Alternsvorgänge des Nervensystems, insbesondere der Alzheimerschen Fibrillenveränderungen. Verh Dtsch Ges Pathol 52:74–92

Thomas E (1969) Histotopochemie und Histopathochemie des peripheren Nervensystems bei Verletzungen und Tumoren. Veröff Morphol Pathol 80

Thomas E (1977) Histochemie der Enzyme im Peripheren Nervensystem. In: Graumann W, Neumann K (eds) Handbuch der Histochemie, vol VII/5. Fischer, Stuttgart New York

Thomas E (1981a) Orthologie und Pathologie der Nervengewebe – Fakten und Probleme. Acta Histochem [Suppl XXIV] (Jena) pp 17–20

Thomas E (1981b) Enzymaktivitäts-Veränderungen in Nerven- und Hüllzellen bei experimentellen Eingriffen. Acta Histochem [Suppl XXIV] (Jena) pp 37–39

Thomas E, Exss R (1967) Histochemische Untersuchungen von Oxydoreduktasen und Esterasen im Perikaryon nach Axondurchtrennung. Acta Neuropathol (Berl) 7:253–260

Thomas E, Lange HP (1968) Histochemische Untersuchungen bei einem Fall von metachromatischer Leukodystrophie. Pathol Eur 3:313–322. Also in: Nunes Vicente A, Dustin P, Lowenthal A (eds) Cerebral lipidoses II. Presses Académiques Européennes, Bruxelles, pp 199–208

Thomas E, Pearse AGE (1964) The solitary active cells. Histochemical demonstration of damage-resistant nerve cells with a TPN-diaphorase reaction. Acta Neuropathol (Berl) 3:238–249

Thomas E, Sourander P (1977) Impaired development of the rat perineurium by undernutrition. An enzyme histochemical study. Acta Neuropathol (Berl) 38:77–80

Tischner K, Thomas E (1973) Development and differentiation of fetal rat sensory ganglia and spinal cord segments in vitro. An enzyme histochemical study. Z Zellforsch 144:339–351

Tyrer JH, Eadie MJ, Kukums JR (1971) The postmortem stability of certain oxidative enzymes in brain and spinal cord. Histochemie 27:21–27

Witte PU, Matthaei H (1980) Mikrochemische Methoden für neurobiologische Untersuchungen. Springer, Berlin Heidelberg New York

Wohlrab F, Seidler E, Kunze KD (1979) Histo- und Zytochemie dehydrierender Enzyme. Grundlagen und Problematik. Barth, Leipzig

Chapter 8

The Golgi Methods

D. Kent Morest

1 Introduction

The Golgi methods continue to be the methods of choice for microscopic study of individual neurons and their processes in the central nervous system. They were introduced over a century ago (Golgi 1873) and went through a period of very productive use for some 30–40 years afterwards. Subsequently, these methods have been relatively neglected for many years. Now again, they are widely employed in the field of neurobiology. They are key techniques, because they provide precisely the most crucial information for organizing, correlating, and interpreting data from a variety of methods and disciplines. And today, virtually all significant research in the neurosciences is interdisciplinary in at least its conception, if not its execution. For example, a study of the neuronal architecture in the medial geniculate body with the Golgi methods provided more insight into the functional organization of this structure than previous years of study with microelectrode recordings (see Morest 1965 a, b). The reason for this is that the Golgi methods provide unsurpassed demonstrations of the processes of neurons, their axons, and dendrites. These are the processes which establish the synaptic organization of the nervous system. Detailed observations of axonal endings, dendritic spines and branches, and geometrical patterns of the axonal plexus and dendritic fields can be made on specific types of neurons. By correlating such observations with silver degeneration methods it is possible to relate the morphology of individual types of neurons to their connections and hence to relate them to specific functional contexts (see Morest 1965 b). In recent years much more elaborate correlations between a variety of techniques have been possible, e.g., between the findings with Golgi, silver degeneration, Nissl, and electron microscopic methods, on the one hand, and electrophysiological data on the other hand (see Morest et al. 1973; Morest 1975 a, b).

More examples could be cited. This situation is being further enriched by the correlations of individual types of neurons and axonal endings recently made possible with new labelling methods, such as horseradish peroxidase histochemistry, immunocytochemistry, and autoradiography. To this list can be added electron microscopic observations of Golgi-impregnated neurons and intracellular dye-marking. None of these techniques will replace the Golgi methods; on the contrary, they can only derive validity when supported by general methods, like those of Golgi. Clearly the Golgi methods provide information indispensable to an understanding of how the brain works.

The Golgi methods comprise several different metallic impregnation techniques. These methods have in common the property of impregnating the cytoplasm with metallic salts which render the entire profile of an individual cell and its processes visible in histological preparations suitable for light or electron microscopy. The methods are simple, and they employ ordinary histological techniques and equipment. They can be applied to well preserved tissue, and the resulting preparations are of permanent value, permitting useful study for decades, if not centuries.

There are two main types of Golgi methods, the silver and the mercurial impregnations. The silver impregnation consists of crystalline deposits of silver mono- or di-chromate, while the mercurial impregnation (Golgi-Cox) contains reduced mercury (Morest and Morest 1966; Fregerslev et al. 1971 a, b). Of the silver-chrome methods there are two main varieties, the rapid Golgi method, employing primary fixation with chrome-osmium mixtures, and the Golgi-aldehyde methods, employing primary fixation with aldehydes. In both of these methods chromation is followed by silvering to produce intracellular crystals.

2 The Rapid Golgi Method

(after Morest and Morest 1966)

This classic method provides the most exquisite impregnations of neurons, their processes and appendages. Some useful discussions have been published previously (e.g., Kallius 1926; Polyak 1941; Morest and Morest 1966).

2.1 Method for Immersion-Fixation

2.1.1 Fixation

Immerse slices of fresh tissue, 3 mm thick, on a layer of cotton gauze in a freshly prepared mixture, containing 3% potassium dichromate and 0.25% osmium tetroxide, "first fixative", at room temperature in a volume of fixative about 50× that of the tissue.

2.1.2 Impregnation

1. Continue fixation in the first fixative for 1–5 days in the dark.

2. Rinse slices briefly with 0.75% silver nitrate, blot briefly by touching them with bibulous paper, and immerse on gauze in a volume of freshly made 0.75% silver nitrate ("first silver solution") about 50× that of the tissue for 2–6 days in the dark.
3. Double or triple impregnations may be prepared by removing the slices from the first silver solution, rinsing briefly with distilled water, gently brushing away surface crystals, and repeating the preceding two steps with freshly made solutions.

2.1.3 Dehydration and Embedding

The impregnated blocks of tissue may be embedded in celloidin before sectioning or cut before embedding in plastic.

2.1.3.1 Celloidin Embedding

1. Gently brush slices free of loose surface crystals and dehydrate in a volume about 50× that of the tissue as follows: 50% ethanol, 1 h; 70% ethanol, 2 h; 95% ethanol, 1 h; 100% ethanol, 1 h; 2:1 diethyl ether:ethanol, overnight, followed by two to three changes of 2–3 h each. During the alcohol treatments gently agitate the solutions (not the specimens!) on a clinical rotator.
2. Immerse the specimens in low viscosity (RS 1/2 sec) nitrocellulose (Hercules, Inc., Wilmington, Delaware) dissolved in 2:1 ether:alcohol in changes of 5%, 10%, 20%, and 30% (wt/vol) for 1 day each. The specimens may be kept for several days in 30% nitrocellulose.
3. Embed the slices individually in "boats" made from a lightweight paper and filled with fresh 30% nitrocellulose.
4. Harden in chloroform vapor in a sealed container, peeling off the paper gradually as the surface hardens.
5. Trim and mount the block on a chuck with 30% nitrocellulose and complete the hardening in chloroform. Do not overharden.
6. Soak the specimens in 70% ethanol overnight at 20 °C to remove any unreacted silver from the tissue.

2.1.3.2 Plastic Embedding

If plastic is the desired embedding medium, the sections are cut before infiltration.

1. Gently brush slices free of loose surface crystals and mount on the stage of a manually controlled tissue chopper (e.g., Smith-Farquhar model) or a Vibratome (Oxford Laboratories, Foster City, California) with cyanoacrylate adhesive and partially included in agar or Carbowax 400 (polyethylene glycol distearate 400).
2. Section at 50–200 μm and infiltrate and embed in a plastic medium suitable for light or electron microscopy (see Chaps. 2, 3).

2.1.4 Cutting and Mounting Celloidin Sections

1. Cut specimens, kept wet with 70% ethanol, at 80–160 μm on a sliding microtome with the hardest available steel knife having a straight inclined bevel. Mount the knife at an angle of 1°–2° to the block face and about 45° to the leading edge of the block.
2. Collect sections serially in 70% ethanol and pass through 95% ethanol, two changes, for 20 min each, and clear in alpha-terpineol for 30 min, then store in fresh alpha-terpineol.
3. Rinse sections in toluene before mounting in a neutral synthetic resin, e.g., Permount (Fisher), under # 1 coverglasses (approx. 150 μm thick or less).

2.2 Commentaries on Immersion-Fixation of the Rapid Golgi Method

2.2.1 Fixation

The quality of the impregnations, as well as the degree of histological preservation, may be improved by fixing the tissue as soon after death as possible. In the case of young kittens and small animals one may induce hypothermia, following general surgical anesthesia, by immersing the shaven body in ice water until the rectal temperature reaches 24°–25 °C. In this condition it is often possible to expose the brain, while minimizing blood loss and preserving respiration and heart beat, until the last cut is made through the caudal medulla and the brain falls into the fixative.

It is important that slices be as close to 3 mm in thickness as possible. If the slice is too thick, the center of the tissue may be devoid of impregnated cells. If the slice is too thin, there is not likely to be any impregnation at all. For samples which are less than 3 mm thick, e.g., the retina, the organ of Corti, early embryos, certain invertebrate organisms, etc., it is advisable to increase the effective thickness of the sample. Sometimes this can be done by leaving intact connective tissue coverings, such as sclera or meninges, or by covering one surface with a protective coating, such as agar. Perhaps the most generally useful maneuver is to wrap the specimen with connective tissue membranes, such as chorioallantois or omentum, and place the tissue between two pieces of porous filter paper at the time of fixation. A pencil drawing may be made of the orientation of the specimen on the paper, and the resulting sandwich processed intact through the remaining steps, including embedding and sectioning.

2.2.2 Impregnation

The optimum times for these steps vary considerably, according to age of the animal, size of the tissue sample, portion of the nervous system, species, and degree of myelination, to mention some of the better known factors. One has to determine the best times empirically. In general, the darkness of the impregnation is proportional to the length of time in silver, but too long a time can darken the background and produce precipitates on the surface of cells and of the tissue block. The extent of the impregnation, i.e., the proportion of cellular structures impregnated per unit volume and the uniformity of the impregnation throughout the sample, generally depends on the length of time in the fixative. However, too long a time in fixative can suppress the Golgi reaction. The most extensive and uniform impregnations are obtained when the fixative is acid, the best preservation, with a pH near neutrality. Multiple impregnations should increase the yield in resistant tissues but also favor the impregnation of the axonal plexus. On the other hand, when successful, single impregnations can provide some of the most demonstrative examples of entire isolated neurons. Some typical impregnation schedules appear in Table 1. For double and triple impregnations it is a good idea to increase the times in the second and third silver solutions, while reducing the concentration of the third silver solution to 0.5%. Because of the use of dilute silver solutions careful attention

Table 1. Some typical impregnation schedules

Days in:	1st Fix.	1st Silver	2nd Fix.	2nd Silver	3rd Fix.	3rd Silver
Single impregnation	3	4				
Double impregnation	3	4	3	4		
Triple impregnation	3	4	3	4	3	5
Single impregnation	2	3				
Double impregnation	2	3	3	5		
Triple impregnation	2	3	3	4	4	6

must be paid to the purity of the water. This should contain less than 0.5 ppm sodium chloride (resistivity greater than 0.5 megohms). In certain cases one may need to resort to extreme variations. For example, successful impregnations of chick embryos at one day of incubation have been achieved after 12–24 hours in each of the solutions. For some fish embryos the specimens were pelleted in a centrifuge and impregnated en masse at 4 °C.

2.2.3 Dehydration and Embedding

Obviously the times for dehydration and infiltration will vary with the size of the specimens. The schedule given is adequate for 3 mm thick slices through the forebrain of an adult cat. If, for some reason, embedding cannot be carried out immediately, the specimens can be stored in 30% nitrocellulose at −10 °C, but this is not recommended as a matter of course. Low viscosity nitrocellulose is preferred to purified collodion preparations, since it permits a rapid, partial infiltration, which is sufficient to hold the sections together during cutting and mounting. The cellular impregnations, consisting, as it were, of delicate crystalline bouquets of microscopic dimensions, are exceedingly fragile. Therefore the specimens are to be treated with the utmost care at all stages of preparation. Never squeeze or jostle the specimens, lest one fracture axons and multilate dendrites. Remember also that the Golgi impregnation is unstable under all of the conditions of the preparatory process.

2.2.4 Cutting and Mounting

In addition to providing an opportunity to produce thin sectioning for electron microscopy, plastic embedments can provide the best light optics as well. However, celloidin embedding remains the most convenient method. The traditional knife bevel for sectioning celloidin does not seem to be necessary for cutting such thick sections. The knife angles recommended are ones likely to minimize crumbling and fractures due to the great friability of the tissue. Because of this property of Golgi preparations successful microtomy demands a very clean and sharp knife edge and avoidance of curling sections. As the sections are cut, while still wet, they are monitored under the microscope and the thickness adjusted, usually to the thickest usable value. During dehydration absolute ethanol should be avoided, since it will dissolve celloidin, leaving the friable sections highly susceptible to the trauma of handling. An alternative dehydration and clearing after 95% ethanol would be two changes of 1-butanol (or chloroform-ethanol), 10 min each, and two changes of oil of cedar wood (white) for clearing, 20 min each. The sections can be stored in alpha-terpineol or cedar wood oil for several months without signs of fading, but this is not recommended. A very brief exposure to clove oil will darken the impregnation, but this is seldom desirable; moreover, this treatment is hard to control and also dissolves celloidin.

Natural or non-neutral resins, such as Canada balsam, should be avoided, as silver chromate crystals are unstable in such media and the Golgi impregnations can decompose or fade, especially when sealed off by a coverglass. However, provided the preparations are carried out as stipulated, Golgi preparations may be kept under coverglasses indefinitely without fading or darkening. At least the author has not seen any sign of deterioration of impregnations for periods up to 25 years. A coverglass is desirable for use with oil-immersion lenses, which are necessary in almost any modern morphological investigation. Because of the limited working distance of such lenses and the relatively great section thickness, a thin coverglass is recommended. In the unlikely event of high magnification photomicrography with a dry lens having no correction collar, the coverglass may have to be replaced with a slightly thicker one.

2.3 Method for Perfusion-Fixation

This procedure results in optimum preservation of fine details, such as dendritic shape, dendritic appendages, and axonal endings.

1. In an anesthetized, fasted animal insert an indwelling catheter into a peripheral vein, such as the superficial saphenous vein of a kitten.
2. 30 min before the perfusion begins slowly inject freshly dissolved sodium acetazolamide intravenously (200 mg/kg, but not more than 100 mg altogether) along with 1000 IU sodium heparin.
3. Install a tracheotomy tube with connection to a tank of a 95% oxygen–5% carbon dioxide mixture, slowly flowing in an open system.
4. Slowly inject 1 ml 1% sodium nitrite (freshly dissolved in the wash-out mixture) intravenously immediately before opening the diaphragm, or inject it into the right ventricle after opening the diaphragm. (Alternatively, hypothermia may be used).
5. Open the diaphragm and start artificial respiration with a 95% oxygen–5% carbon dioxide mixture.
6. After clamping the descending aorta, insert a cannula through the left ventricle into the base of the aorta, open the right atrium, and perfuse enough wash-out rapidly from a height of 1 m, more or less, until the atrial perfusate is nearly, but not quite clear. This usually takes about 15 s in a kitten. At that time a volume of fixative several times that of the head is perfused rapidly. The perfusion mixtures should be administered at 38 °C (25° for hypothermia). The perfusate should be continuously washed away and adequate ventilation provided for protection from the osmic acid fumes. For washing out, one may use 0.1 M dibasic potassium phosphate-sodium acid buffer at pH 7.4 and 0.5% polyvinylpyrrolidone (average molecular weight of 40,000) or McEwen's (1956) saline containing 0.5% polyvinylpyrrolidone. The wash-out should contain 1 ml of 4% lidocaine for each 80 ml of total volume. For fixation one may use a mixture containing 0.25% osmium tetroxide, 0.5% polyvinylpyrrolidone, and 3% potassium dichromate (buffered at pH 5.8 by adding sodium hydroxide).
7. Immediately following the perfusion the tissue should be treated as described under the Method for Immersion-fixation (Sect. 2.1).

2.4 Commentary on Perfusion-Fixation for the Rapid Golgi Method

Extensive experience indicates that each step is essential for a successful perfusion. Overall we have succeeded in about half of our attempts, more often in young kittens and weanling rabbits, less often in adult cats. This leaves room for improvement. The dichromate in the fixative promotes cerebral edema, while osmium tetroxide is a powerful vasoconstrictor and coagulant. These factors combine to thwart perfusions of the cerebral capillaries. Sodium acetazolamide, hypothermia, oxygen, polyvinylpyrrolidone, and a short wash-out help to prevent cerebral edema. Sodium nitrite, carbon dioxide, lidocaine, and warm solutions or hypothermia help to prevent vasoconstriction. For possibly better fixation, but less extensive impregnations, use 0.5% osmium tetroxide and buffer at pH 6.8, particularly for electron microscopy. The first fixative can be buffered at pH 5.8, with the second or third fixatives unbuffered.

3 The Golgi-Aldehyde Methods

These methods offer the advantage of a fixation compatible with a greater variety of other histological methods. The impregnations seldom approach those of the best rapid Golgi preparations in quality or in extent, particularly of fine details, such as dendritic appendages or the axonal plexus. The impregnations do provide useful, if incomplete observations of the cell bodies of neurons and their main dendrites, especially in heavily myelinated regions.

3.1 The Rapid Golgi-Aldehyde Method
(after Kopsch 1896; Colonnier 1964; Blackstad 1965)

3.1.1 Fixation

1. Carry out perfusion-fixation according to one of the standard procedures for light or electron microscopy, using paraformaldehyde and/or glutaraldehyde (see Chaps. 2, 3). A typical formula for the perfusion-fixative would call for a 1% paraformaldehyde and 3% glutaraldehyde mixture in a 0.1 M phosphate buffer. The wash-out might consist of a 0.1 M phosphate buffer containing 1 ml of 4% lidocaine per 80 ml of buffer.
2. Remove the calvarium 4 hours after the perfusion and place the head in cold 10% formol-saline for several days, or longer if convenient, before blocking into 2–4 mm thick slabs. If electron microscopy is contemplated, the head should be immersed in cold perfusion-fixative overnight, the brain removed from the skull the following day, blocked, and placed immediately in the impregnation-fixative without exposure to formol-saline.

3.1.2 Impregnation

1. Fix in a mixture consisting of 3% potassium dichromate and 5% glutaraldehyde for 5–7 days at 20°–25 °C in a volume 25× that of the tissue. (An alternative impregnation-fixative is 3% potassium dichromate and 0.25% osmium tetroxide).
2. Rinse the tissue blocks in 0.75% silver nitrate. Immerse blocks in 0.75% silver nitrate, using a volume 25× that of the tissue for 5–7 days at 20°–25 °C.
3. Double impregnations may be prepared by removing the slices from the silver solution, rinsing briefly with distilled water, gently brushing away loose surface crystals, and repeating the preceding two steps with freshly made solutions.

For dehydration, embedding, cutting, and mounting see Sect. 2.1.

3.2 Golgi-Hortega Method
(after Stensaas 1967)

This method is carried out in much the same way as the rapid Golgi-aldehyde method. It favors the impregnation of somata and dendrites of neurons. Sometimes this method will succeed when the rapid Golgi methods have failed.

3.2.1 Fixation

Fix either by immersion or perfusion with a freshly prepared mixture consisting of 3% potassium dichromate, 3% chloral hydrate, 10% commercial formalin, 1.5% commercial glutaraldehyde, and dimethyl sulphoxide, 5 drops/100 ml. (Dimethyl sulphoxide alters cutaneous permeability and is a potentially dangerous substance, to be handled carefully under a ventilating hood).

3.2.2 Impregnation

1. Immerse tissue in the fixative for one day.
2. Change to freshly made fixative for one more day.

3. Rinse in 0.75% silver nitrate. Immerse in 1.0% silver nitrate for 2 days.

For dehydration, embedding, cutting, and mounting see Sect. 2.1.

3.3 Commentary on Golgi-Aldehyde Methods

Double impregnations may increase the extent of the impregnation, but in general these methods are less flexible than the rapid Golgi method. Many of the same comments about the rapid Golgi method apply to the Golgi-aldehyde techniques as well.

4 Golgi Methods for Electron Microscopy

Material prepared by the rapid Golgi and Golgi-aldehyde methods can be used for electron microscopy, provided adequate fixation is obtained by perfusion and provided the tissue is embedded in a plastic suitable for thin-sectioning. With the method outlined one may study the thick plastic-embedded slices with the light microscope, select structures of interest, and cut these structures out for thin-sectioning. Since there is a tendency for the Golgi reaction product to disintegrate during cutting and when the thin sections are floated on a fluid (Blackstad 1965; Stell 1965), it may be desirable to use a method which removes silver chromate, as in the gold substitution method.

4.1 Gold Substitution Method for Electron Microscopy of Golgi Impregnations

(after Fairen et al. 1977)

1. Dehydrate Golgi-impregnated slices (2 mm thick) in 20%, 40%, 60%, and 80% glycerol, 1 h in each change, and store in absolute glycerol at 4 °C overnight or longer.
2. Cut sections of Golgi impregnations on a tissue chopper or Vibratome (see Sect. 2.1.3.2), collecting sections in absolute glycerol. At this stage sections can be mounted on slides with glycerol under coverglasses and observed with light microscopy to select individual neurons for further study. At this time drawings of the structures of interest and orientating landmarks can be made, and suitable sections selected for gold substitution.
3. The sections are re-hydrated by passing them through changes of 80%, 60%, 40%, 20% glycerol, and distilled water, 20 min each change. Place in 0.05% yellow gold chloride for 20 min in an ice bath in a refrigerator at 4 °C, agitating every 2 min.
4. Following three changes of ice-cold distilled water, 5 min each, the sections are placed in ice-cold 0.5% oxalic acid for 6 min.
5. Rinse in distilled water, three changes, 5 min each, bringing gradually to room temperature.
6. 1% sodium thiosulphate at 20 °C, two to three changes for a total of 60–90 min, agitating periodically.
7. Distilled water, three changes, 5 min each.
8. 0.15 M phosphate buffer at pH 7.3, 20 min.
9. 2% osmium tetroxide in 0.15 M buffer, 30 min.
10. 0.15 M phosphate buffer, three changes
11. 50% methanol, 20 min.
12. 1% uranyl acetate, freshly dissolved in 70% methanol, 2 h in the dark.
13. Dehydrate and embed in plastic for electron microscopy (see Chap. 3). A detailed study of impregnated neurons with the light microscope can be made at this time.

4.2 Commentary on Golgi Methods for Electron Microscopy

By removing silver chromate this method renders Golgi preparations much more suitable for thin-sectioning, while preserving the organelles within the impregnated cells for study with the electron microscope. However, some users do not report uniformly successful results in a variety of materials. Another method, based on a different principle, has been published by Ramón-Moliner and Ferrari (1972).

5 Mercurial Golgi Methods

These are probably the most consistent of the Golgi methods in terms of the extent of the impregnation achieved from sample to sample. For this reason these methods are especially useful in initiating study of an unfamiliar region of the central nervous system. The impregnations seldom attain the delicacy of silver chromate nor do they often demonstrate much of the axonal plexus. The grain of the reaction product is usually much coarser than that of the silver chromate impregnations. Moreover, precipitates all too often encrust the surfaces of cells, especially when the tissue has been fixed too long. Nevertheless, on occasion some of the most exquisite impregnations have been prepared with these methods. The methods have an advantage for study of unfamiliar regions in permitting Nissl-counterstaining of the unimpregnated cells. They are not well suited for electron microscopy.

5.1 Golgi-Cox Method I
(after Ramón-Moliner 1961, personal communications; Morest 1964, unpublished)

5.1.1 Fixation

1. Anesthetize the animal and, if feasible, place in hypothermia at a rectal temperature of 24 °C.
2. Keeping the animal alive as long as possible (see Sect. 2.2.1), remove the brain rapidly and immerse it in the fixative.
3. Cut the brain into slices 4–5 mm thick with sharp scissors and immerse on gauze in a jar containing a volume of fixative 100× that of the tissue at 20°–25 °C for 1 week.
4. Change to fresh fixative for one month.

The fixative is concocted as follows:
Solution A: 5% potassium dichromate. Warm 500 ml of distilled water and dissolve 25 g potassium dichromate.
Solution B: 5% mercuric chloride. Bring 500 ml of distilled water to a boil briefly. Just when the boiling stops add 25 g mercuric chloride to the steaming water.
Solution C: 5% potassium chromate. Dissolve 20 g in 400 ml of distilled water at room temperature.

Cool solutions A and B to room temperature. Mix 5 parts of A with 5 parts of B. Dilute 4 parts of C with 10 parts of distilled water. While stirring continuously, slowly pour the AB mixture into the diluted C solution. Let the mixture sit for at least 5 days, until no more red precipitate forms. Decant and filter the mixture through very retentive filter paper (e.g., Whatman # 42). If the precipitate forms once more, the mixture should be filtered again. The fixative may be stored but should be filtered before use.

For dehydration, embedding, and cutting see Sect. 2.1.

5.1.2 Mounting and Reduction

1. Collect sections in 70% ethanol. Small Gooch crucibles are convenient for carrying the sections in serial order through the subsequent changes.
2. 95% ethanol, 2 min.

3. 3 : 1 ethanol : chloroform, three changes, 5 min each.
4. Toluene, two changes, 5 min each.
5. Soak sections in a mixture consisting of 3 parts chloroform, 1 part methyl benzoate, and 4 parts benzyl alcohol for at least 3 min.
6. Mount sections on slides coated with albumen freshly made from raw eggs as follows: Take the white of an egg and mix it with 500 ml distilled water and 1 ml strong ammonia solution (25%–28%). Mix thoroughly, pour into a staining dish, and store at 60 °C overnight. Remove froth from the surface of the mixture before dipping slides.
7. Dry sections in air for 20 min under a 60-W incandescent lamp, or in a 37 °C oven until the chloroform is completely gone, making sure there are no wrinkles.
8. Soak sections in toluene, three changes, 5 min each, and 95%, 70%, and 40% ethanol changes, 3 min each.
9. Reduce in a mixture of 3 parts strong ammonia water to 2 parts absolute ethanol for 20 min, or, to produce a more delicate impregnation, use the same mixture for 2 min, followed by 3 parts ammonia water to 7 parts ethanol for 60 min.
10. Soak sections in changes of 70% and 40% ethanol, for 2 min each, followed by running tap water, 10 min.
11. 1% sodium thiosulphate until the yellow color of the section is bleached (about 10 min).
12. Running tap water, 10 min.
13. 70% ethanol, 5 min; 80% ethanol, two changes, 5 min each; 95% ethanol, 2 changes, 5 min each; 1-butanol, two changes, 10 min each.
14. Toluene, three changes, 5 min each.
15. Coverslip sections, using a neutral synthetic medium, e.g., Permount (Fisher).

5.2 Golgi-Cox Method II

(after Van der Loos 1959, personal communication)

The same method as above is followed for fixation, dehydration, embedding, and cutting.

5.2.1 Reduction and Mounting

1. Collect sections in 70% ethanol.
2. Immerse in a mixture of 3 parts strong ammonia water to 2 parts ethanol, 20 min.
3. Rinse sections in distilled water, two changes, 5 min each.
4. 5% sodium thiosulphate, 5 min.
5. Distilled water, two changes, 2 min each.
6. Hypo-clearing agent (Kodak), stock solution, 3 min.
7. Distilled water, two changes, 3 min each.
8. 70% ethanol; 80% ethanol, two changes; 5 min each.
9. 95% ethanol, two changes, 5–15 min each, depending on section thickness.
10. 1-butanol, two changes, 10 min each (may be omitted if dehydration in previous step was long enough).
11. Alpha-terpineol, two changes, 20 min each.
12. Rinse in toluene. Mount and coverslip sections with a neutral synthetic medium.

5.3 Nissl-Counterstaining for the Golgi-Cox Method

(after Ramón-Moliner, personal communications; Morest, unpublished)

Sections to be counterstained should be cut at 50 μm thickness, alternating with sections at the thickness used for the regular method. Follow the protocol of "The Golgi-Cox Method I" (Sect. 5.1) through step 12.

Before coverslipping, after 2 min in 25% ethanol, counterstain in the following mixture at pH 3.8 for 90 min at room temperature: 2 g cresylecht violet or neutral red, 185 ml 1 M acetic acid, 15 ml 1 M sodium acetate, 200 ml distilled water; add the preceding mixture to 400 ml 50% ethanol. After staining, coverslip sections with a neutral synthetic medium.

5.4 Commentary on the Mercurial Methods

In the author's experience Nissl counterstaining is not routinely useful, for usually the impregnations are extensive enough to permit adequate orientation with reference to standard Nissl-stained series or atlases. These methods are not recommended for perfusion-fixation. It is traditional to store the tissue in the dark while fixing. It is possible to observe the presence of colloidal mercury bichloride in the cell bodies and dendrites of large neurons in the unreduced sections and to use this observation to monitor the section thickness during microtomy. A common fault with these methods is the appearance of an unimpregnated margin involving a zone of variable thickness around the entire circumference of the tissue block. This phenomenon appears to be a function of the tissue in the fixative and is possibly formed by prolonged fixations. However, a fixation that is too short may result in a faint impregnation or none at all. There is probably an optimum time for any particular sample.

6 How to Use the Golgi Methods

A characteristic property of the Golgi methods is that they typically produce impregnations of only a fraction of the cellular population in a single sample, varying from 0%–20%. Thus, in some preparations it is possible to trace out the three-dimensional configuration of individual neurons and their synaptic processes, unencumbered by the complexities of the surrounding neuropil. Moreover, the Golgi methods are elective, i.e., non-selective, in that the particular cells impregnated in any sample or series seem to have a random distribution with respect to type and location. In other words, in any given sample one may not predict which individual cells will be impregnated. Probably all types of neurons and, indeed, all types of cells in any tissue can be impregnated by one or another of these methods. In fact the author has often observed lovely impregnations of fibroblasts, cartilage cells, osteocytes, capillary endothelium, and hematocytes, to mention a few examples, as well as all types of neurons and glia. However, when sufficient numbers of cells are observable, these methods can be expected to provide a representative sample of any population of cells.

These properties of the Golgi methods endow them with certain limitations and advantages. Some of these have already been mentioned. Two main areas of concern are the special demands made on the microscopic techniques and the sampling errors.

6.1 Microscopic Techniques

6.1.1 Observation

Much useful advice appears in an earlier discussion by Polyak (1941). In the present state of the art the most useful observations of neuronal morphology pertain to those features related to the synaptic organization and electrical properties of neurons. These features nearly always include some of the finest and most delicate parts of cells, such as dendritic appendages and axonal endings. Because of the nature of the impregnations visualization (but not resolution) of structures on the order of 0.1 μm in diameter or less is possible. This has been confirmed by electron microscopic examination of impregnated structures previously observed in the light microscope. However, the optical distortions introduced by the unusually great thickness of the sections and halos from superimposition of precipitates usually make it impossible to approach the limit of resolution of the light microscope and can make it hard to obtain reliable images. In addition to selection of the finest impregnations and quality of embedding medium one must pay sufficient attention to the optical equipment. Generally, oil-immersion objective lenses of the highest numerical apertures (1.25 or greater), fully corrected or at least semi-apochromatic, are required. Unfortunately, most of the commonly available lenses fulfilling these requirements have short working distances, which preclude their use with thick sections mounted under coverglasses. Certain objective lenses with the required features have been manufactured either for optical measurements of cosmic ray tracks or more recently for observation of tissue cultures. Although the former lenses are no longer manufactured, sometimes one can be purchased from a physicist or metallurgist.

The best objectives are ones that were originally designed for measurements of photographic layers. One example is the Leitz KS apochromat 100× oil-immersion objective, which has a numerical aperture of 1.32 and working distance of 370 μm. A similar lens, once made by Koristka (Milan), is a 100× semi-apochromatic oil-immersion lens with a numerical aperture of 1.25 and working distance of 530 μm. With this objective, only a small spot in the center of the field is kept in focus, as one moves the focus spot along the surfaces of the cells. Still available commercially is the Zeiss 63× semi-apochromatic, oil-immersion lens (NA 1.25) with a working distance of about 0.2 mm (formerly 650 μm). Leitz has also made the KS 100× oil-immersion, semi-apochromatic objective, said to focus with an accuracy of 0.2 μm at 4000× magnification in layers up to 650 μm thick. Generally overlooked and still commercially available are the Leitz Ultropak objectives of long working distance for incident light. These lenses are available as apochromatic or semi-apochromatic, oil-immersion objectives with 260–270 μm free-working distance (NA 1.3–1.4). Observations of Golgi impregnations with incident light can provide very colorful images, which can be very useful in rendering visible surface features that would otherwise be lost in the cell's shadow in transmitted light. However, these lenses can also be used for transmitted light or combined dark- and bright-field observation. The Leitz Ultropak objectives were preferred by Polyak (1941) for the Golgi methods. Similar objectives are made by Zeiss (Epiplan HD), including a 100× oil-immersion lens (NA 1.25) with 280 μm working distance.

Other useful lenses, designed primarily for observations of tissue cultures, are those for differential interference microscopy (e.g., the system of Nomarski, manufactured by Zeiss, or that of Smith, manufactured by Leitz). These systems have excellent oil-immersion objectives with ample working distances. Other advantages of these systems for Golgi observations are an effective shallow depth of focus (optical sectioning) and certain special color effects, which can enhance visibility of delicate, lightly impregnated structures. Another advantage is that one can often visualize unimpregnated cell bodies and fiber bundles in the background, thus permitting orientation to the local cytoarchitecture, and sometimes observations of the relations of impregnated axonal endings to unimpregnated cell bodies. This last advantage does not always materialize, but it is more common with the rapid Golgi method than with other variants. However, chrome-osmium staining of unimpregnated cells and myelinated fibers in rapid Golgi preparations usually provides as much, or more orientation to the cytoarchitecture than the usual counterstains, thus providing a distinct advantage over the Golgi-aldehyde methods.

6.1.2 Illustration

The purpose of the microscopic study, of course, is to build up a three-dimensional image of neurons in the mind of the observer. If the microscopist has any ability, he can very quickly do this for a large number of cells, making ample use of the fine focus knob. If accurate measurements in three dimensions are required, he may use photogrammetric or computer-assisted semi-automatic graphic reconstructions (e.g., Mannen 1966; Lindsay 1977). For most purposes a two-dimensional drawing will effectively convey a reliable impression to the reader of the image in the microscopist's mind. This is best accomplished with a microscopic drawing apparatus, e.g., the drawing tubes, manufactured in recent years by Zeiss, Leitz, and Wild, which are the successors to the traditional camera lucida. This equipment will allow any competent microscopist to render a satisfactory drawing rather easily. No particular artistic ability is required, although with a little practice one may learn to enhance certain aspects of the drawing to create the desired impression, often with a suggestion of the third dimension (e.g., Morest 1968; Brawer et al. 1974).

Objectivity is not an issue here. The sole requirement is to convey effectively the observer's perceptions to an audience. Hence to record precisely the silhouette of a complex field of neuronal processes may produce an inaccurate and confused image in the minds of the audience. The microscopist must arrange the drawing so that it corresponds to the information that he wishes to convey. There is no other requirement to be met in the interest of objectivity.

The least objective method of illustration is photomicrography. Many clever tricks have been applied to the problem of focusing on structures in depth while retaining sufficient resolution, including the extensively gerrymandered, but still quite futile montage. Occasionally some limited detail or overall gross impression of the preparations can be represented in photomicrographs (e.g., Morest and Morest 1966). However, photographic methods are generally not worthwhile, for almost never can a photomicrograph depict Golgi impregnations with any accuracy nor convey anything but the most distorted derivative of the microscopist's perceptions.

6.2 Sampling Errors

6.2.1 Age

It is well known that the most extensive impregnations occur in immature animals, especially with the rapid Golgi method. One reason for this is that heavily myelinated axons do not ordinarily impregnate, but the presence of myelin and other differentiated tissue constituents could retard the Golgi reaction throughout the tissue. It is perhaps not so well known that all of the Golgi methods do in fact yield useful, if more fragmentary results in fully mature brains, although one may need considerably more samples than with younger material. Even so, the most informative data will still usually come from young animals. Thus, the question arises as to the extent to which the observations represent the mature state. A good strategy is to prepare material from young or neonatal animals, adolescents, and adults. Then usually enough can be learned from the younger material to elucidate the more limited observations in adults. A good time to look at young mammals is when spontaneous, coordinated motor activity appears, e.g., sometime between the opening of the eyes in kittens and weaning.

6.2.2 Unpredictability of the Impregnations

Because of the variations in results, with many factors often uncontrollable, one should give some thought to general strategy. It is usually necessary to examine a large amount of data before concluding that the findings accurately represent any region or cell type in the nervous system. History shows that the most productive investigators working with these methods directed their attention to those questions which the available material could answer. However, the questions for most investigators will arise in other contexts. Turning to the Golgi methods for answers to specific questions can be a frustrating experience, unless one has access to a large collection of preparations. Indeed the most extensive contributions are likely to come from those investigators fortunate enough to have access to such collections. The alternative is to start a limited collection oneself and hope for the best.

Two strategies predominate. One approach is to determine an optimum protocol, by systematically varying the times and, perhaps to some extent, the temperature and concentrations of the reagents, among other possible variables, for a number of identical samples. It may be possible to settle upon a specific formula for a given region, age, species, etc., but this is not a common outcome in the author's experience. The impatient histologist with tissue to spare may wish to monitor grossly the progress of the diffusion of the reagents into the tissue blocks with razor-thin slices. However, if one follows the instructions for each method, this should be unnecessary. Another strategy is the shotgun approach. One simply processes a large number of samples simultaneously in separate containers, while varying times, double or triple impregnations, etc., for each sample. Usually some good impregnations will result. Then the process is repeated until a large number of specimens is available for study. This is the strategy preferred by the author.

It is wise to process material by more than one method, since rather different kinds of observations can be made this way. When first beginning study of an unfamiliar region, the investigator might well begin with the Golgi-Cox method and Nissl-counterstaining, progress to one of the Golgi-aldehyde methods, and eventually to the rapid Golgi method for the most revealing details. The Golgi-Cox method should provide the quickest orientation to the types of neurons present and their topographical relations to the surrounding nuclei and tracts. The Golgi-aldehyde methods may provide opportunities to focus on clearly isolated examples. In the end the rapid Golgi method will provide the greatest wealth of detail.

The Golgi methods will undoubtedly continue to be useful for the foreseeable future. As in most areas, no doubt the most worthwhile results will accrue to those who devote the most time to their studies. Some investigators will have to make a long-term commitment. "But," to quote Lorente de Nó (1934), "on the other hand, the results of such a study remain." It will not have to be done over and over again by later investigators with newer techniques. Nevertheless, the methods are simple enough that many investigators will want to try them at one time or another. For the unpredictability of the Golgi methods is not always a disappointing feature but sometimes manifests itself in unanticipated discoveries and insights. It was Polyak (1941) who remarked, "as a compensation for frequent failures, preparations of unsurpassed fineness and beauty come along which may, in one stroke, answer the questions that for a long time have baffled even the best scientific minds."

Acknowledgments. The methods reported here are those currently used in the author's laboratory. The author is indebted to many colleagues who have contributed over the years to the development of his understanding both by examples and by personal communications, but most of all to those who have worked with him in the laboratory. Much of the work has been supported by grants from the National Institutes of Health (NINCDS).

7 References

Blackstad TW (1965) Mapping of experimental axon degeneration by electron microscopy of Golgi preparations. Z Zellforsch 67:819–834

Brawer JR, Morest DK, Kane EC (1974) The neuronal architecture of the cochlear nucleus of the cat. J Comp Neurol 155:251–300

Colonnier M (1964) The tangential organization of the visual cortex. J Anat 98:327–344

Fairen A, Peters A, Saldanha J (1977) New procedure for examining Golgi impregnated neurons by light and electron microscopy. J Neurocytol 6:311–337

Fregerslev S, Blackstad TW, Fredens K, Holm MJ (1971 a) Golgi potassium-dichromate silver-nitrate impregnation. Nature of the precipitate studied by X-ray powder diffraction methods. Histochemie 25:63–71

Fregerslev S, Blackstad TW, Fredens K, Holm MJ, Ramón-Moliner E (1971 b) Golgi impregnation with mercuric chloride: studies on the precipitate by X-ray powder diffraction and selected area electron diffraction. Histochemie 26:289–304

Golgi C (1873) Sulla sostanza grigia del cervello. Reprinted in: Golgi C (1903) Opera Omnia, vol I. Hoepli, Milan, pp 91–98

Kallius E (1926) Golgische Methode. In: Krause R (ed) Enzyklopädie der mikroskopischen Technik, 3rd ed, vol II. Urban & Schwarzenberg, Berlin, pp 909–944

Kopsch F (1896) Erfahrungen über die Verwendung des Formaldehyds bei der Chromsilberimprägnation. Anat Anz 11:727–729

Lindsay R (ed) (1977) Computer analysis of neuronal structures. Plenum Press, New York

Lorente de Nó R (1934) Studies on the structure of the cerebral cortex. II. Continuation of the study of the Ammonic system. J Psychol Neurol (Leipz) 46:113–177

Mannen H (1966) Contribution to the quantitative study of the nervous tissue. A new method for measurement of the volume and surface area of neurons. J Comp Neurol 126: 75–90

McEwen LM (1956) The effect on the isolated rabbit heart of vagal stimulation and its modification by cocaine, hexamethonium, and ouabain. J Physiol (Lond) 131:678–689

Morest DK (1964) The neuronal architecture of the medial geniculate body of the cat. J Anat 98:611–630

Morest DK (1965 a) The laminar structure of the medial geniculate body of the cat. J Anat 99:143–160

Morest DK (1965 b) The lateral tegmental system of the midbrain and the medial geniculate body: study with Golgi and Nauta methods in cat. J Anat 99:611–634

Morest DK (1968) The collateral system of the medial nucleus of the trapezoid body of the cat, its neuronal architecture and relation to the olivo-cochlear bundle. Brain Res 9: 288–311

Morest DK (1975 a) Synaptic relationships of Golgi type II cells in the medial geniculate body of the cat. J Comp Neurol 162:157–194

Morest DK (1975 b) Structural organization of the auditory pathways. In: Tower DB (ed) The nervous system: vol I, Human communication and its disorders. Raven Press, New York, pp 19–29

Morest DK, Kiang NYS, Kane EC, Guinan JJ Jr, Godfrey DA (1973) Stimulus coding at caudal levels of the cat's auditory nervous system. II. Patterns of synaptic organization. In: Møller AR (ed) Basic mechanisms in hearing. Academic Press, New York, pp 479–504

Morest DK, Morest RR (1966) Perfusion-fixation of the brain with chrome-osmium solutions for the rapid Golgi method. Am J Anat 118:811–832

Polyak SL (1941) The retina. University of Chicago Press, Chicago, Chap 4

Ramón-Moliner E (1961) The histology of the postcruciate gyrus in the cat. II. A statistical analysis of the dendritic distribution. J Comp Neurol 117:63–76

Ramón-Moliner E, Ferrari J (1972) Electron microscopy of previously identified cells and processes within the central nervous system. J Neurocytol 1:85–100

Stell WK (1965) Correlation of retinal cytoarchitecture and ultrastructure in Golgi preparations. Anat Rec 153:389–398

Stensaas LJ (1967) The development of hippocampal and dorsolateral pallial regions of the cerebral hemisphere in fetal rabbits. I. Fifteen millimeter stage, spongioblast morphology. J Comp Neurol 129:59–70

Van der Loos H (1959) Dendro-dendritic connections in the telencephalic cortex. Stam, Haarlem

Chapter 9

Fluorescence Histochemistry of Biogenic Monoamines

Christine Heym

1 Introduction

Several aldehydes are capable of converting biogenic amines to intensely fluorescent derivates: fluorophores. This reaction, under defined conditions, can be used as a highly sensitive and specific method for the histochemical demonstration of biogenic monoamines at the cellular level.

The localization of monoamine-containing cells by the production of fluorophores with formaldehyde (FA) has first been demonstrated by Eränkö (1951, 1952). It was Falck and co-workers (Falck and Torp 1961; Falck 1962, 1964; Falck et al. 1962; Falck and Owman 1965) who introduced a highly specific and reproducible technique based on the principle of a gas phase histochemical reaction with FA in freeze-dried tissue. Subsequently, this method became widely accepted in the field of neurobiology and initiated a vast number of technical variations and refinements.

The FA reaction is based on a condensation of FA with catecholamines (CA) to yield 6,7-dihydroxy-1,2,3,4-tetrahydroisoquinoline (Pictet-Spengler cyclization reaction), which in a second reaction, promoted by a dry protein layer (Corrodi and Jonsson 1965, 1967), is dehydrogenated to a strongly fluorescent dihydroisoquinoline. This quinoidal compound is in a pH-dependent equilibrium with its tautomeric nonquinoidal form (Corrodi and Hillarp 1963).

Analogous to the reaction with CA the condensation of FA with indolamines, for instance serotonine (5-hydroxytryptamine; 5-HT), yields tetrahydroderivates, which in a second reaction are dehydrogenated to the corresponding dihydrocarbolines (Corrodi and Jonsson 1967).

From a number of reactive carbonyl compounds (Axelsson et al. 1972) glyoxylic acid (GA) was found to be another fluorescence-histochemically applicable reagent (Furness and Costa 1962; Björklund et al. 1972 b; Axelsson et al. 1972, 1973; Lindvall and Björklund 1974). The fluorophores derived from GA and biogenic amines are formed by an initial Pictet-Spengler type cyclization, analogous to that which takes place in the FA reaction.

From the group of aldehydes, o-phthaldialdehyde (OPT) has been found to form a highly fluorescent product when reacting with histamine (H) (Shore et al. 1959).

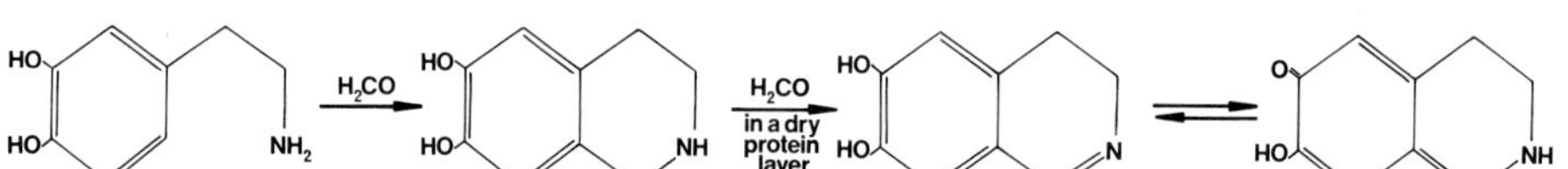

Fig. 1. Dopamine-formaldehyde condensation (Jonsson 1967)

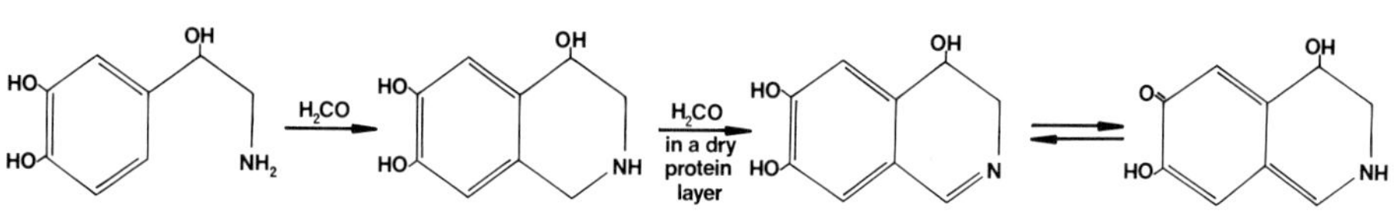

Fig. 2. Noradrenaline-formaldehyde condensation (Jonsson 1967)

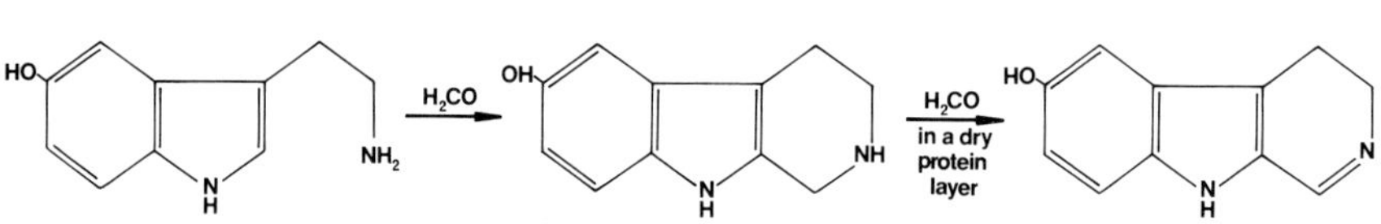

Fig. 3. 5-Hydroxytryptamine-formaldehyde condensation (Corrodi and Jonsson (1965)

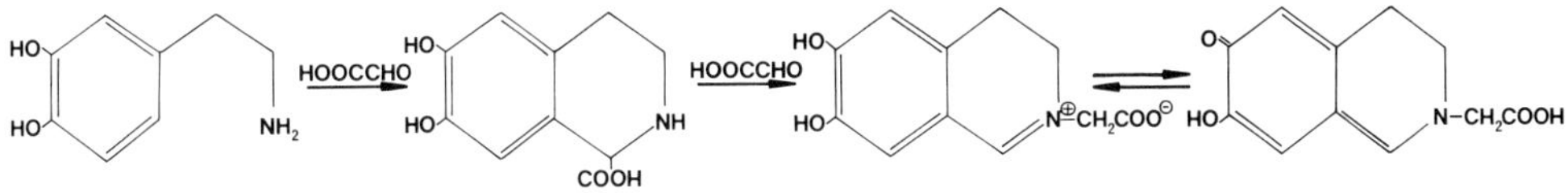

Fig. 4. Dopamine-glyoxylic acid condensation (Lindvall et al. 1974)

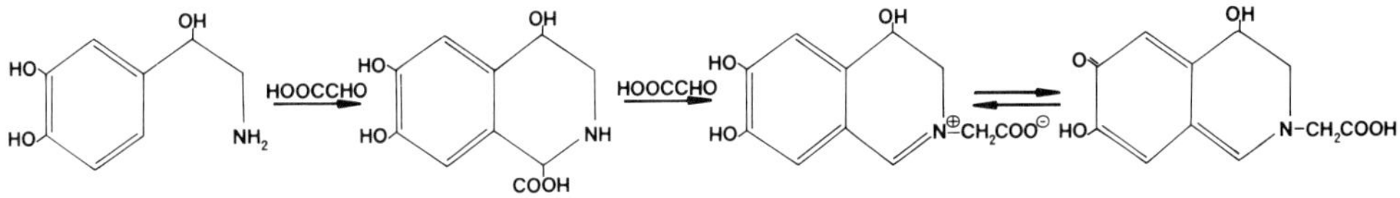

Fig. 5. Noradrenaline-glyoxylic acid condensation (Lindvall et al. 1974)

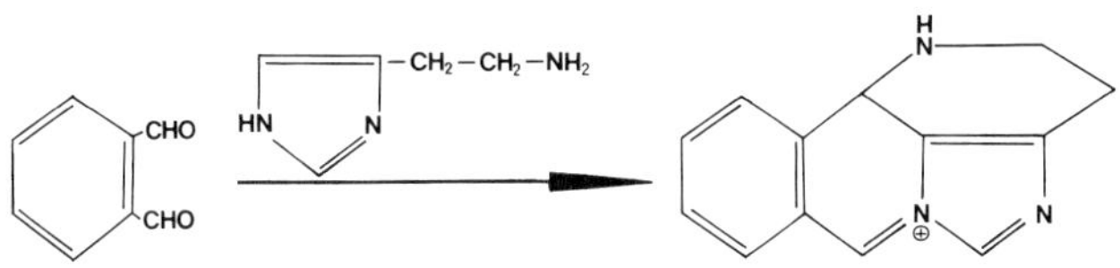

Fig. 6. Histamine-ortho-phthaldialdehyde condensation (Shore et al. 1959)

This reaction has been utilized in methods for the chemical estimation of H in tissues and biological fluids (Juhlin and Shelley 1966; Ehinger and Thunberg 1976). It is probable that the final fluorophore, formed by this reaction, differs from the initial condensation product by rearrangement and oxidation (Shore et al. 1959). At least two fluorophores with different fluorescence characteristics, both of which are dependent on different H-concentrations, can be detected, thus allowing a semiquantitative estimation (Håkanson et al. 1970).

Numerous methodological studies have been carried out in an attempt to improve the sensitivity in the detection of central and peripheral monoamine-containing neuron systems under optimal conditions of tissue preservation at the cellular level. From the enormous variety of methodological descriptions, I will report on a few fluorescence histochemical techniques which are routinely applied in our laboratory for the localization of amine transmitters in the central and peripheral nervous system. With respect to the object of an experiment and in the application to different tissues, each of these methods has its advantages and limitations. For example, a minute, fine, and structural investigation concerns optimal preservation of tissue within small blocks, whereas other studies might involve a brief overall characterization of a large brain region. Therefore, a careful choice should be made in selecting the most convenient technique for each experiment to ensure optimal results.

2 Formaldehyde-Induced Fluorescence (FIF)

The fluorescence characteristics of the CA- and 5-HT-FA products have been established in tissues (Corrodi and Hillarp 1963; Corrodi and Jonsson 1965, 1967; Jonsson 1971; Björklund et al. 1972 a), and the relative fluorescence yield of CA after condensation with FA has been tested in model systems with respect to absorption and emission characteristics, reaction conditions, and influence of water in the specimen (Ritzén 1966).

2.1 Gas Phase Formaldehyde Technique with Tissue Blocks

(Falck-Hillarp technique, after Falck et al. 1962; Falck and Owman 1965)

An extensive review on this method has been provided by Fuxe et al. (1970) and Björklund et al. (1972 a). The formation of fluorophores in this technique is achieved by reaction of FA vapor with monoamines in small blocks of unfixed freeze-dried tissue (see Corrodi and Jonsson 1967; Eränkö 1967). The tissue preparation in this procedure should be carried out under the driest possible conditions. Strict adherence to the following simple precautions should be taken at each step.

2.1.1 Guidelines for the Technical Procedure

2.1.1.1 Preparation of Water-Equilibrated Paraformaldehyde

In general, as is the case in many countries, a mean relative air humidity of 60%–70% is satisfactory for fluorophore formation between monoamines and FA vapor derived from untreated paraformaldehyde powder (PA) in most mammalian tissues. For consistent standardization of the results, however, the water content of the PA used for the fluorophore formation is of critical importance (Falck and Owman 1965; Hamberger 1967); excess humidity causes diffusion of the fluorescent product and too low humidity leads to reduced efficiency of condensation reactions. PA should therefore be water-equilibrated at least 7 days before each experiment.

5 g PA are usually needed for one experiment. The weighed PA is dried in a small Petri dish over P_2O_5 for 1 week. The dried PA is equilibrated for about 10 days at room temperature in a 1000 ml dessicator with a defined relative humidity obtained from an aqueous sulfuric acid solution of defined concentration. Table 1 (modified after Hamberger 1967) is used.

Table 1. Relation between relative humidity, density and weight percentage of aqueous solutions of sulfuric acid

Relative humidity %	Density of sulfuric acid solution	Weight % of H_2SO_4
10	1.58	67.35
20	1.49	59.24
30	1.44	54.49
40	1.39	49.48
50	1.34	44.17
60	1.29	38.53
70	1.25	33.28
80	1.20	27.72
90	1.14	20.08

Example:

For equilibrating PA with a 50% relative humidity, prepare a 44.17 weight% solution of sulfuric acid by diluting a concentrated sulfuric acid (about 98%, density 1.84) in the following manner: $\frac{44.17}{0.98}=45.08$. According to $\frac{45.08}{1.84}=24.5\left(\frac{\text{weight}}{\text{density}}=\text{volume}\right)$, 24.5 ml concentrated H_2SO_4 is pipetted to 70 ml distilled water and filled with distilled water up to 100 ml.

The equilibrated PA can then be used for only one tissue incubation.

2.1.1.2 Condensation of Propane

This step should be performed directly before tissue preparation under a hood to avoid the risk of explosion.

A commercially available propane-propylene mixture is condensed in a metal beaker, which is suspended in a Dewar flask filled with liquid nitrogen. The gas is allowed to flow through a metal tube which is bent around the beaker as seen in Fig. 7.

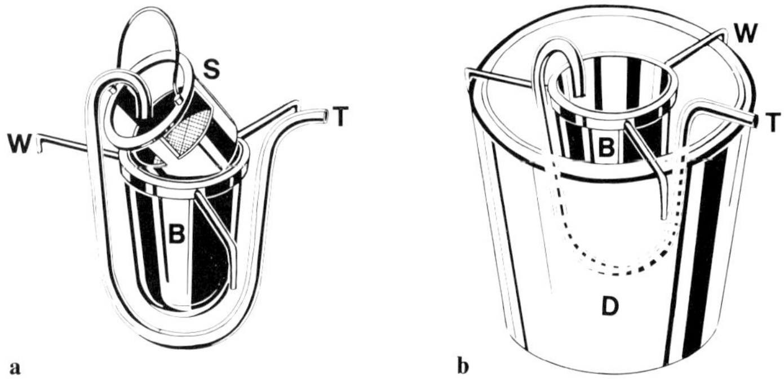

Fig. 7 a, b. Equipment for liquifying propane (modified from Falck and Owman 1965). **a** Metal sieve (*S*) as specimen receptacle fitting in a metal beaker (*B*) for liquid propane. *W*, metal wires for suspending the beaker in a Dewar vessel. **b** The beaker (*B*) is suspended in a Dewar vessel (*D*), filled with liquid nitrogen. A metal tube (*T*) connected by rubber tubing with a propane bottle, is bent around the beaker. The liquid propane drips into it. *W*, suspending rack

2.1.2 Procedure

2.1.2.1 Dissection

The specimen is dissected directly after the animal is decapitated, because narcotic stress can cause depletion of amine stores. When studying tissue with high amine levels the organ can be exposed under general anaesthesia and then the specimen is removed following exsanguination of the animal. Due to the rapid diffusion of monoamines, post mortem amine-containing specimens cannot be used for reliable FM, unless kept in a humid chamber (Penttilä 1968).

Small pieces of tissue are cut with a razor blade. The specimens should not be more than 2 mm thick due to the risk of tissue fracturing. Tissue blocks are placed on aluminium foil, tissue slabs can be placed between two copper sheets.

2.1.2.2 Shock-Freezing

The specimens are shock-frozen (quenched) in the liquid propane (temp. −180 °C). Artifacts by extracellular ice formation are thus avoided, since formation of ice crystals ceases at temperatures below −30° to −50 °C.

After between 30 s and a few minutes the specimens are transferred into the burr holes of a handled special holder of a lead-tin alloy (60/40). The holder is suspended just beneath the surface of the liquid nitrogen (temp. −196 °C) which is kept in another Dewar flask (Fig. 8).

This two-step freezing prevents the formation of a layer of vaporized nitrogen on the warm specimen surface.

All vessels must be covered with a piece of cloth to prevent water condensation on the cold metal. Vaporized nitrogen must be replaced from time to time.

Instead of liquid propane, 2-methylbutane (isopentane) or Freon 12 may be

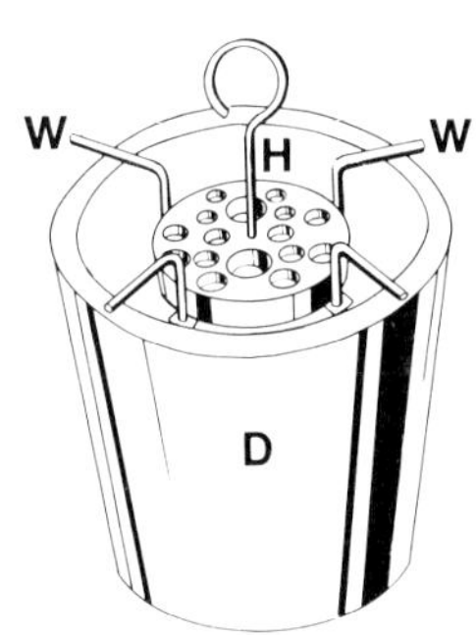

Fig. 8. Specimen holder (*H*) held in a Dewar vessel (*D*) by aid of linked metal wires (*W*); (from Falck and Owman 1965)

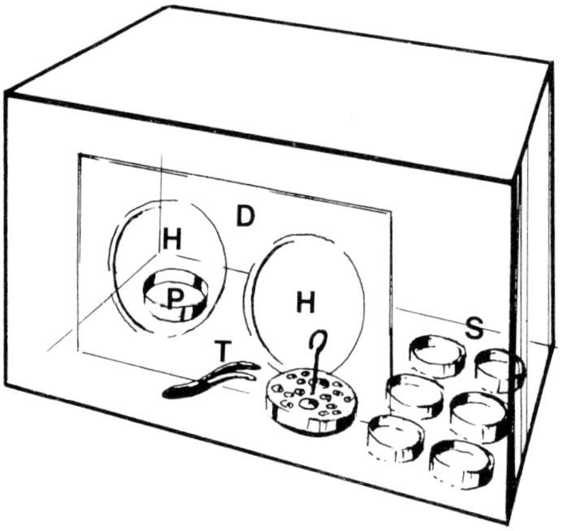

Fig. 9. Plexiglass box with P_2O_5 dishes (*P*) for handling with freeze-dried specimens under driest possible conditions. *D*, sliding door; *H* holes for handling; *S* specimen dishes; *T*, tweezers (modified from Falck and Owman 1965)

applied, diminishing the risk of explosion. However, after shock-freezing in these liquids (at −150 °C in isopentane and at −145 °C in Freon 12) fluorescence yields are not as reliable as in using propane (because the freezing rate of tissue samples is faster in propane).

2.1.2.3 Freeze-Drying

When all samples have been collected in the specimen holder, this holder is transferred to the freeze-drying equipment

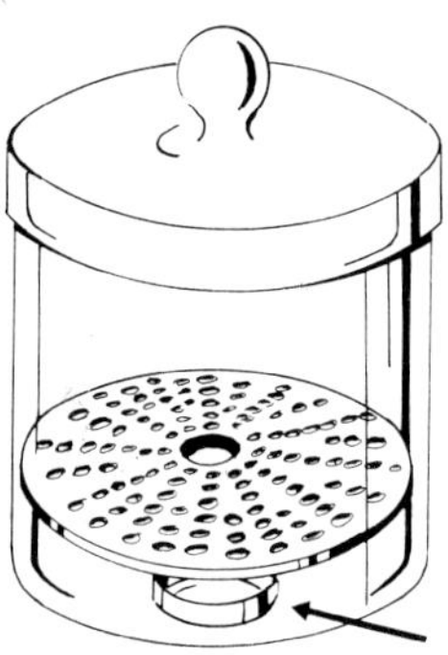

Fig. 10. Airtight glass jar with porcelain shelf for specimens and a Petri dish (*arrow*) containing PA

which has been precooled to −45 °C. We use a WKF, L 05 (Fa. WKF, Darmstadt, Federal Republic of Germany), drying tissue blocks for 4–6 days, tissue sections (see Sect. 2.2) for 2 h. The vacuum should be 10^{-6} mm Hg and the temperature maintained at −45 °C. If the vacuum is greater the drying time is shorter.

After lyophilisation the temperature of the freeze-drying equipment is gradually raised well above room temperature (+45 °C) to avoid water condensation on the preparations. After stopping the vacuum pumps the system is ventilated with air through an evacuation flask filled with silica gel with moisture indicator. For ventilation nitrogen gas can also be used.

The specimen holder is then transported in a dessicator over P_2O_5 to a plexiglass box where the specimens are selected in watchmaker dishes for further treatment (Fig. 9). Some tissue samples should remain without FA treatment for control. All manipulations with dry specimens must be carried out with rubber gloves to avoid remoisturizing the tissue by the "perspiratio insensibilis" of the skin.

2.1.2.4 Formaldehyde Vapor Incubation

Selected watchmaker dishes with tissue blocks are transferred to an airtight glass jar with PA (from normal supply or water-equilibrated; Fig. 10), and exposed to FA vapor in an oven at 70°–80 °C. The FA is derived from PA which releases the gas when heated. We routinely apply PA equilibrated with 50% relative humidity at 70 °C with good results for recording dopamine (DA) and noradrenaline (NA), and at 80 °C for recording adrenaline (A). For optimal fluorescence yield the temperature of exposure and the water content of the PA should be tested for each tissue.

DA and NA fluorescence is yielded after 20 min in tissue sections (see Sect. 2.2) or after 60 min in tissue blocks, whereas optimal A fluorescence is achieved after

1–3 h, respectively. 5-HT fluorescence is improved by treatment with 50% PA for 60 min, followed by vapor exposure of 90% PA for 60 min (Fuxe and Jonsson 1967).

After formation of the fluorophore all further preparatory steps must be performed with artificial light from a 25-W light source. Otherwise (especially in Neon light with its higher UV radiation), fading of the fluorescence intensity may occur (Pearse 1972). The FA-treated tissue should be embedded immediately. If this is not possible, it must be stored in a lightproof dessicator over P_2O_5.

One's aims should be taken into account when choosing an embedding medium. For embedding, sectioning, and mounting see Sects. 6, 7.3, and 7.4.

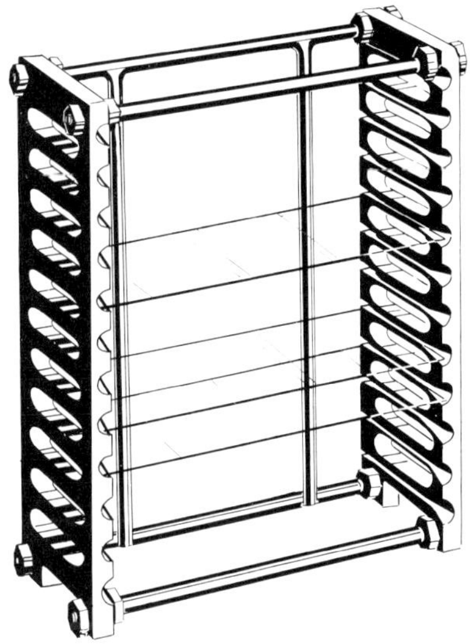

Fig. 11. Holder for coverslips

2.2 Gas Phase Formaldehyde Technique with Tissue Sections

(after Hamberger and Norberg 1964; Heene 1968; Nelson and Wakefield 1968; Fuxe and Jonsson 1973)

The Falck-Hillarp technique can also be performed on fresh-frozen tissue sections.

After dissection (see Sect. 2.1.2.1) the tissue block is placed on a cryostat chuck. The chuck with the specimen is wrapped in aluminium foil and dipped into liquid propane for 30 s. It is then transferred directly to the cryostat.

Sectioning is performed as described in Sect. 7.1. Instead of collecting cryostat sections with a room temperature slide, the sections are picked up with the dry bristles of a fine brush and placed on precooled cover slips in a special holder (Fig. 11) in the sink. The holder is then transferred in a dessicator over P_2O_5 to the freeze-drying equipment and freeze-dried for 2 h. Drying is sufficient when placing the evacuated dessicator into a deep-freezer (–25 °C) overnight. Freeze-drying and FA vapor incubation are explained in Sect. 2.1.2.

2.3 Commentary on the Gas Phase Formaldehyde Technique

This procedure with tissue blocks is rather time-consuming. Results are obtained after approximately 1 week. Nonetheless, the gas phase formaldehyde procedure provides excellent preservation of structural details and a bright specific fluorescence of CA neurons in central and peripheral nervous tissue (Fig. 12). Although the FIF method is considered very sensitive, less than 5×10^{-10} g NA in one nerve varicosity has been calculated (Fuxe et al. 1970; Fuxe and Jonsson 1973), the sensitivity of the technique does not provide complete visualization of all monoamine systems. This applies especially to 5-HT neurons in the central nervous system. Moreover, it is difficult to obtain large-scale histologic surveys on the central nervous system with this technique since fracturing of tissue blocks is a common problem in unfixed shock-frozen and subsequently freeze-dried brain (Winkler 1970 b).

The advantage of applying the gas phase FA procedure to tissue sections is that it saves time. Furthermore, in case no freeze-dryer is available, drying of the frozen sections can be performed in a deep-freezer over P_2O_5 (Csillik and Kalman 1967). Serial sections for parallel histochemical studies are readily produced. On the other hand, the risk of artifacts due to tissue fracturing during shock-freezing is increased by the cryostat manipulations. Thus serial sectioning is extremely difficult. Moreover, the time of tissue storage is limited to a few days.

2.4 Aqueous Formaldehyde Technique

(after Hoyt et al. 1979)

Early histochemical techniques (Eränkö 1951, 1952, 1955) were applied by immersing tissues in formaline solutions favorable to diffusion of tissue amines. This lowered the sensitivity of the method. The technique has gradually been refined (Eränkö and Räisinen 1966; Laties et al. 1967; Sakharova and Sakharov 1971; Hökfelt and Ljungdahl 1972). It is especially recommended for 5-HT neurons and APUD-cells in peripheral tissues (Hoyt et al. 1979).

Tissues are fixed by perfusion with or immersion in an ice-cold 0.1 M phosphate buffer containing 6% FA. For maximum fluorescence it is necessary to prepare the fixative immediately before use. The technique of perfusion has been described in Chaps. 1 and 2.

2.4.1 Solution (6% FA in phosphate buffer)

A 0.2 M sodium-phosphate buffer is made up of stock solution A: 27.6 g $NaH_2PO_4 \cdot H_2O$ in 1 liter distilled water; and stock solution B: 35.6 g $Na_2HPO_4 \cdot 2\,H_2O$ in 1 liter distilled water. 115 ml of stock solution A and 385 ml of stock solution B make up 500 ml of 0.2 M phosphate buffer, which is diluted with 500 ml distilled water to the final volume of 1 liter of 0.1 M phosphate buffer.

Thirty grams PA powder are dissolved in 500 ml preheated (95 °C) 0.1 M phosphate buffer. The solution becomes clear when a few drops of 1 N NaOH are added. The solution is filtered and cooled to room temperature before final adjustment to pH 7.2 with a pH-meter.

2.4.2 Procedure

For perfusion the vascular beds are flushed briefly with 50 ml Ringer-solution at room temperature (see Sect. 4.2.1) containing 0.1 ml of heparin (5000 u/ml aqueous solution) followed by about 10 min perfusion with 500 ml of the fixative at 2°–4 °C. Tissues can stay in the fixative for several days. For embedding and sectioning procedures see Sects. 6 and 7.

2.5 Commentary on the Aqueous Formaldehyde Technique

Because of its simplicity this technique is well-suited to work requiring serial reconstructions of peripheral tissues containing 5-HT neurons or cells of the GEP system. Pre-injection of the animal with an amine precursor (see Sect. 11) is advisable.

Using both the vibratome or the cryostat sectioning on formaline-fixed tissue, it is possible to combine histochemical or immunohistochemical studies with the fluorescence histochemistry on the same section, since a brief formaline fixation usually does not inhibit enzymal activity. We do not advise the use of buffers other than phosphate buffer, because their effect on CA levels has not been fully elucidated. Tris buffer (Tris-[hydroxymethyl]-aminomethan-HCl), for instance, has been shown to degrade granule CA as well as cytoplasmic CA (Gonzalez et al. 1979).

3 Glyoxylic Acid-Induced Fluorescence (GIF)

As in the case of FA fluorophore, optimal development of the GA fluorophore requires an initial excess of moisture in the tissue. This moisture must be driven off during development and the tissue protected from further moisture (Furness and Costa 1975). Since GA is quite inadequate as a fixative, the consistence of tissues after Ga-perfusion is not suited to sectioning with the vibratome. On the other hand, the quality of cryostat sections of perfused tissue does not markedly exceed that of native tissue sections immersed in the fixative. Therefore, we prefer a simple and rapid GA-immersion technique for demonstrating CA-containing neurons as described by De la Torre and Surgeon (1976 a, b). It is also an easily accessible research tool to investigators inexperienced in histofluorescence techniques.

3.1 Glyoxylic Acid Immersion Technique with Tissue Sections or Whole Mounts

[Sucrose-phosphate-glyoxylic acid (SPG) method, after De la Torre and Surgeon 1976 a, b; De la Torre 1980]. This technique can be applied to tissue sections as well as to stretch preparations.

3.1.1 Solution

(1% GA in sucrose-potassium-phosphate)

The reacting solution should be freshly prepared each day. In exceptional cases, it may be used the following day, if kept refrigerated.

For a 75 ml solution fitting into a small beaker, the following reagents are needed: 5.1 g sucrose and 2.4 g KH_2PO_4. These are dissolved in 50 ml distilled water. 0.75 g glyoxylic acid (98% free acid monohydrate) are added and stirred until the solution is clear. The solution is titrated to pH 7.4 with 1 N NaOH and diluted to a final volume of 75 ml with distilled water. This should not change thc pH.

3.1.2 Procedure

The dissected tissue slabs (not thicker than 3 mm) are quickly glued on precooled cryostat chucks with a few drops of water or tissue tec (Tissue tec II, OCT compound, Slee, Mainz FRG). They are immediately placed into the cryostat and the temperature set to –30 °C. A low-temperature thermometer is useful for monitoring the inside temperature (an average freezing rate of 8 °C/min is recommended).

When frozen (after 5–10 min), 10–30 μm sections are picked up with a clean microscope slide and immersed for 30 s in the glyoxylic acid solution.

After immersion, rims of the slide are blotted dry with absorbent paper. The specimens are dried with a cold air stream (hair dryer or pressurized air) for 15–30 min. Several slides can be collected at this step of the procedure. Whole mounts (iris, etc.) are directly immersed in the SPG solution for 2–5 min, blotted dry, then stretched on glass slides and dried as described above.

Dry tissue sections or whole mounts are covered with a few drops of paraffinum perliquidum (light USP mineral oil). The slides are then transferred to the preheated oven, set at 95 °C, and are left there for 2–3 min. Undesirable air bubbles which have been trapped under the sections are eliminated during incubation. Finally, the slides are mounted with one additional drop of paraffinum perliquidum under a coverslip.

3.2 Commentary on the Glyoxylic Acid Immersion Technique

The relative fluorescence yields obtained from DA and 5-HT in dried protein

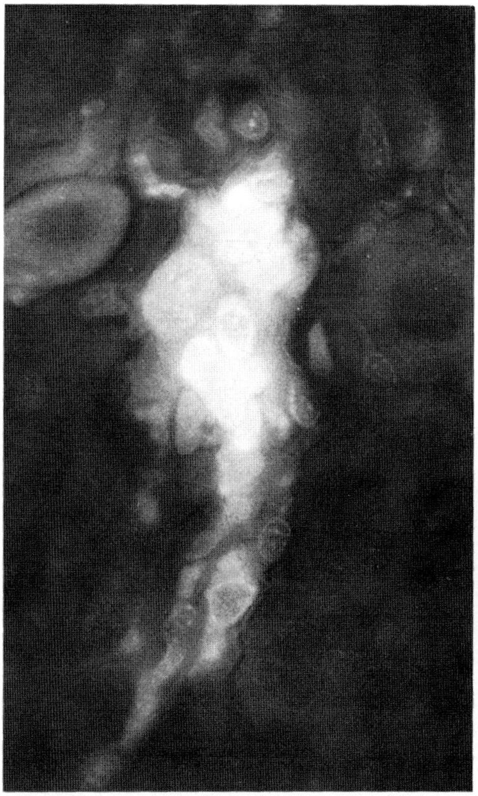

12

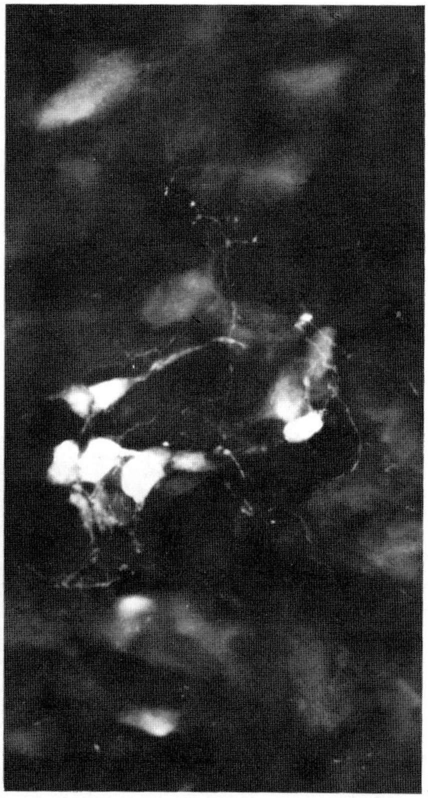

14

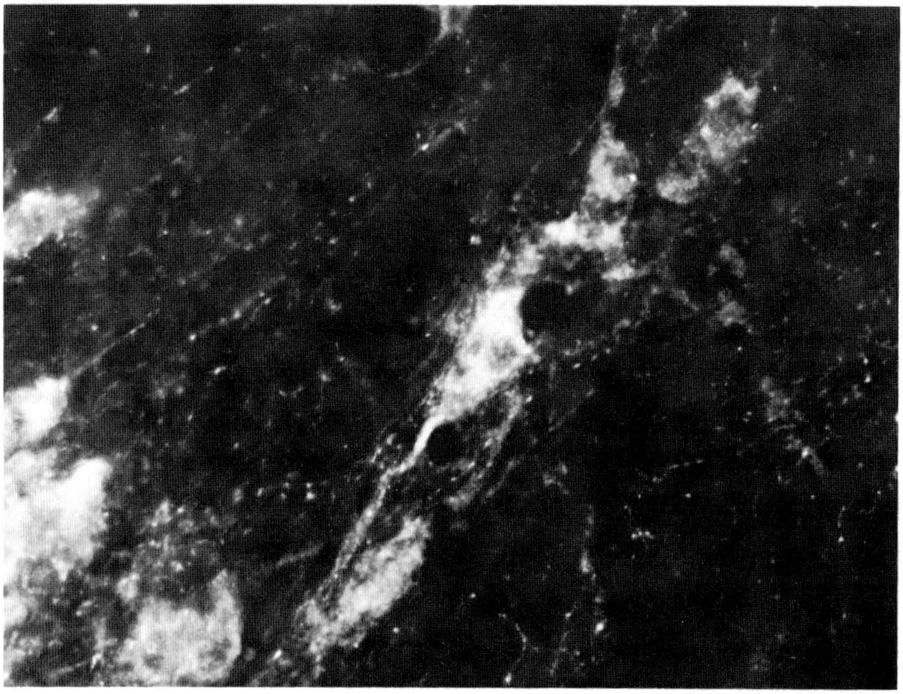

13

droplets after exposure to FA or GA have been shown to be higher after the latter treatment (Axelsson et al. 1972). The high reactivity of GA as compared with FA has been explained by the enhanced catalyzing properties of the GA carboxyl group which leads to fluorophores (Axelsson et al. 1972). In histochemical application to peripheral sympathetic ganglia, however, the counted number of CA-containing, small, intensely fluorescent cells was for unknown reasons much smaller after GIF (Chiba and Williams 1975) than after FIF (Eränkö and Eränkö 1971). Moreover, the morphology of fluorescent pericarya is less distinct after GIF (Fig. 13) than in reactions obtained by FIF. Monoaminergic fibres and terminals can nevertheless be excellently traced with the GA technique. Consistently good results have been obtained especially from the evaluation of terminal and non-terminal portions of CA-containing neurones in central and peripheral tissue (Kyösola 1979), whereas in our experience visualization of 5-HT-fluorophore is not significantly improved by GA. For these reasons GA immersion techniques are especially suited for the rapid evaluation of CA-innervated peripheral tissues. Furthermore, they are ideal for obtaining an overall view of CA neurons in the brain and for neuroanatomical tracing of central CA pathways (Fig. 13). This method can readily be used in combination with immuno-histochemical reactions.

4 Combined Aqueous Aldehyde Techniques

From a number of combined aqueous aldehyde techniques which made the fluorescence histochemical methodology widely accessible (e.g., Grillo et al. 1974; Lorén et al. 1976; Furness et al. 1977 a, b; Lorén et al. 1980) we have chosen four technical procedures as examples (Bloom and Battenberg 1976; Chiba et al. 1976; Ajelis et al. 1979; Furness et al. 1979). With slight modifications they have been applied in our laboratory with consistently good results.

4.1 Guidelines for the Technical Procedure

The following points should be observed for the perfusion procedures given:

All chemicals used are of analytic grade.

Stock solutions for buffers and physiological saline solutions can be stored for only a few days.

Final solutions are made freshly every day and are filtered through membrane filters (Sartorius, Göttingen, Federal Republic of Germany) with 3 μm and 0.6 μm pore size before use.

In variation to the original procedures, a 2.5% solution of polyvinylpyrrolidone (PVP 40, Sigma – MW 40.000) as a poly-

Fig. 12. SIF cells in the rat superior cervical ganglion following gas phase formaldehyde procedure (Sect. 2.1, 50%, 70 °C, 1 h). ×520

Fig. 13. Catecholamine cells in the rat locus coeruleus after immersion in glyoxylic acid (Sect. 3.1). ×410

Fig. 14. Catecholamine neurons in the guinea pig superior cervical ganglion following successive perfusion of glyoxylic acid and formaldehyde/glutaraldehyde (Sect. 4.4). ×410

meric plasma expander is added to the fixatives when studying peripheral tissues (Gorgas, personal communication; see also Chap. 2). Applying PVP, the use of hypermolaric agents as cryoprotectants (e.g., sucrose) can be avoided or clearly reduced.

The amounts of solutions are calculated for small laboratory animals between 200 and 500 g.

After anaesthetizing the animal 0.1 ml heparin (5000 μ/ml aqueous solution) is administered intraperitoneally to minimize blood coagulation.

The perfusion is carried out as described in Chap. 2. The pressure should be approximately 120 mm Hg. The fluids should flow through tubing 8 mm in diameter and kept as short as possible.

For optimal perfusion, the blood is flushed out with 0.9% NaCl containing 0.03% $CaCl_2$, 0.9% gallamine triethiodide (Flaxedil, Boehringer Ingelheim, Federal Republic of Germany, 20 mg/ml), and 0.5% procaine HCl. The solution is prepared as follows: 0.9 g NaCl, 0.03 g $CaCl_2$, and 0.5 g procaine HCl are dissolved in 80 ml distilled water with 1 ml Flaxedil added. The solution is diluted with distilled water to the final volume of 100 ml and kept oxygenated with pressurized air until used. Approximately 10–20 ml of the solution are needed for one experiment.

In most tissues a stable fluorescence has been reported after aldehyde perfusion at room temperature (Furness et al. 1979). We nonetheless prefer, after the initial saline solution perfusion, to carry out all further steps at low temperatures (2°–4 °C) in order to minimize the danger of monoamine diffusion (Jonsson 1971; Hökfelt and Ljungdahl 1972).

With the onset of fixation the animal is covered with crushed ice.

4.2 Simultaneous Perfusion with Glyoxylic Acid and Formaldehyde

(after Bloom and Battenberg 1976)

4.2.1 Solution

(2% GA/0.5% FA in 0.15 M phosphate-buffered Ringer's solution)

A 0.3 M sodium phosphate buffer is prepared as described in paragraph 2.4.1, but with one variation. The agents for the stock solutions are each dissolved in 750 ml instead of 1 Liter. Combining 115 ml of stock solution A and 385 ml of stock solution B 500 ml of 0.3 M phosphate buffer is made up and titrated to pH 7.4 with 1 N NaOH.

500 ml Ringer's solution are made up by separately dissolving 0.1 g $CaCl_2$ (anhydrous), 0.2 g KCl, 0.1 g $MgSO_4 \cdot 7\,H_2O$, 3.4 g NaCl, 1.1 g $NaHCO_3$, 0.07 g $NaH_2PO_4 \cdot H_2O$, and 0.5 g glucose in 60 ml distilled water. The solutions are mixed in the order indicated and diluted with distilled water to the final volume of 500 ml. The pH should be at 7.3.

Then 5 g PA are dissolved in 500 ml 0.3 M phosphate buffer, preheated at 90 °C. The solution becomes clear when a few drops of 1 N NaOH are added. The solution is chilled to 4 °C and titrated to pH 7.4 with 2 N NaOH. (For the study of peripheral tissues the PA is dissolved in 250 ml phosphate buffer and the solution mixed with a PVP solution made by dissolving 25 g PVP in another 250 ml phosphate buffer.)

Directly before use, 20 g GA are dissolved in 500 ml Ringer's solution, the pH adjusted to 7.4 with 8 N NaOH. The precooled FA and GA solutions are combined in equal volumes to derive 500 ml of the final solution.

4.2.2 Procedure

After flushing out the blood with 10 ml of the initial saline mixture at 21 °C (see Sect. 4.1), the animal is perfused with

500 ml of the ice-cold fixative. The brain is then rapidly removed and cut into suitable slabs for vibratome (Sect. 7.2) or cryostat (Sect. 7.1) sectioning. The vibratome stage is filled with an ice-cold mixture of 50 ml 0.3 M phosphate buffer and 2 g GA in 50 ml Ringer's solution, titrated to pH 7.4 with 8 N NaOH. Cryostat sections can be immersed in the same mixture for 3 min before drying with pressurized air. Incubation of the sections in an oven at 95 °C for 3 min improves the specific fluorescence (see also Sect. 3.1.2).

4.3 Simultaneous Perfusion with Formaldehyde and Glutaraldehyde

(Faglu-method, after Furness et al. 1977 a, b; 1979)

4.3.1 Solution

(4% FA/0.5% GLU in 0.1 M phosphate buffer)

500 ml of 0.2 M phosphate buffer are prepared as described in Sect. 2.4. Then 40 g PA are dissolved in 400 ml distilled water at 90 °C with a few drops of 1 N NaOH being added. The FA solution is cooled to 4 °C. (For the study of peripheral tissues PA and PVP are separately dissolved in 200 ml distilled water and the solutions mixed.) Following this, 20 ml GLU (25% aqueous solution) are added. The solution is mixed with 500 ml 0.2 M phosphate buffer, adjusted to pH 7.0 with 1 N NaOH and diluted with distilled water to the final volume of 1 liter.

4.3.2 Procedure

The blood is flushed out by perfusion with an initial 10 ml of the saline mixture at room temperature (see Sect. 4.1). The perfusion is continued with 500 ml of the ice-cold Faglu mixture. This requires 10–15 min. When the perfusion is complete, the tissue is removed and cut into suitably-sized pieces for sectioning on a cryostat (see Sect. 7.1) or vibratome (see Sect. 7.2). Before sectioning, the tissue pieces should be immersed in the fixative for 1–12 h at 4 °C.

4.4 Successive Perfusion with Glyoxylic Acid and Formaldehyde/Glutaraldehyde

(after Chiba et al. 1976)

4.4.1 Solutions

Solution I (2% GA in saline/procaine HCl): In the original directions solution I is made up by 2% GA in Krebs-Ringer bicarbonate solution. In our experience this solution does not constantly remain stable. For this reason we prefer to apply a saline/procaine HCl solution as pre-perfusate for EM.

First 9.0 g NaCl are dissolved in 900 ml distilled water. (For the study of peripheral tissues 9.0 g NaCl and 25 g PVP are separately dissolved in 450 ml distilled water and the solutions mixed.) Directly before use, 20 g GA and 5.0 g procaine HCl are added and the pH adjusted to pH 7.0 by adding 8 N NaOH drop by drop. The resulting solution is diluted with distilled water to a final volume of 1 l. This should not change the pH. The solution is saturated with a 90% O_2 and 10% CO_2 mixture and used immediately.

Solution II (4% FA/0.5% GLU in Sörensen's buffer): For Sörensen's phosphate buffer, two stock solutions are prepared. Stock solution A contains 56.8 g $Na_2HPO_4 \cdot 2\,H_2O$ in 1 liter distilled water; stock solution B contains 27.6 g $NaH_2PO_4 \cdot H_2O$ in 500 ml distilled water. 770 ml of stock solution A and 230 ml of stock solution B make up 1 liter of Sörensen's buffer, which is titrated to pH 7.2 with 2 N NaOH.

Then 40 g PA are dissolved in 950 ml preheated (90 °C) Sörensen's buffer on a magnetic stirrer. The solution is cooled to 4 °C. (In case PVP has been added to solution I, 40 g PA and 25 g PVP are separately dissolved in 480 ml Sörensen's buffer and the solutions mixed.), 20 ml of GLU (25% aqueous solution) is added and, if necessary, the solution filled up with Sörensen's buffer to a final volume of 1 liter. The pH is adjusted to pH 7.4 with 8 N NaOH.

4.4.2 Procedure

After preceding perfusion of 10 ml saline mixture at room temperature (see Sect. 4.1) the perfusion is continued with 500 ml of the ice-cold 2% GA solution I, followed by 500 ml of the ice-cold 4% FA/0.5% GA solution II. Following perfusion, the tissue is dissected and cut into slabs of less than 5 mm thickness which are immersed in solution II at 4 °C for 2–12 h. For cryostat sectioning (see Sect. 7.1) 10%–20% sucrose are added to the immersion solution to minimize formation of ice crystals when freezing brain tissue. Cryostat sections are dried in the hot air stream of a hair dryer and mounted in paraffinum perliquidum (light USP mineral oil) on a hot plate. Vibratome sections (see Sect. 7.2) can be cut into the ice-cold fixative or into 2% GA in 0.1 M phosphate buffer at pH 7.0. They are dried and mounted in the same way as cryostat sections. In case subsequent EM examination is intended, the sections are mounted either in buffer solution or in glycerin/water (1 : 1).

4.5 Successive Perfusion with Glyoxylic Acid and Aluminium/Formaldehyde

(ALFA method, after Ajelis et al. 1979)

4.5.1 Solutions

Double-strength Tyrode buffer is made up by dissolving 16 g NaCl, 0.4 g KCl, 0.4 g $CaCl_2$ (anhydrous), 0.1 g $MgCl_2$, 2.0 g $NaHCO_3$, 0.08 g $NaH_2PO_4 \cdot H_2O$, and 2.0 g glucose in 1 liter of distilled water. When dissolved separately in 100–140 ml of distilled water, combined in the order indicated, and diluted to the final volume of 1 liter, the chemicals do not precipitate.

Dilute 500 ml of this buffer to 1 liter with distilled water. This results in normal-strength Tyrode buffer for solution I. The remaining 500 ml double-strength buffer are needed for solution II.

Solution I (2% GA in Tyrode buffer): Dissolve 10 g GA monohydrate in 500 ml of normal-strength Tyrode buffer. (For the examination of peripheral tissues 7.5 g PVP are dissolved in the Tyrode buffer previous to GA.) The pH is then adjusted to 7.0 by dropwise addition of 1 N NaOH and the solution kept oxygenized until use.

Solution II (4% FA in Tyrode buffer): In the original recipe solution II contains 5–10 g $Al_2(SO_4)_3 \cdot 18\,H_2O$ in 100 ml of a 4% FA solution, the pH adjusted to 3.8 with $Na_2B_2O_7$. At variance with this solution, which to our experience does not remain stable when titrated, we apply the following method:

Dissolve 40 g PA in 500 ml distilled water at 90 °C with a few drops of 1 N NaOH added. (In case PVP has been added to solution I, 40 g PA and 25 g PVP are separately dissolved in 250 ml distilled water and the solutions mixed.) The FA solution is then chilled and mixed with 500 ml of double-strength Tyrode buffer. 5 g $Al_2(SO_4)_3 \cdot 18\,H_2O$ are dissolved in 500 ml of the resulting solution. A final pH of 3.8 is obtained.

4.5.2 Procedure

After flushing out the blood with an initial perfusion of the saline mixture (see Sect. 4.1) the perfusion is continued in two steps: first with 250 ml of the ice-cold 2% GA solution I, and then with 500 ml of the ice-cold aluminium-FA-(PVP) solution II. After perfusion, tissue pieces are dissected and sectioned on the vibratome (see Sect. 7.2), into solution II or on the cryostat (see Sect. 7.1). The tissue sections on microscope slides are dried with the cold air stream of a hair dryer for 10 min or longer and stored at room temperature in a vacuum over P_2O_5 overnight. After warming up the slides to 80 °C, the sections are reacted with PA of 50% relative humidity at 80 °C for 1 h. For analysis the sections are mounted in paraffin oil.

4.6 Commentary on Combined Aqueous Aldehyde Techniques

Aqueous solutions of GA and FA, applied successively (Figs. 14, 17) or simultaneously (Figs. 15, 16) with the perfusion technique potentiate the effect for mapping the distribution of central catecholamine neurons (Battenberg and Bloom 1975; Bloom and Battenberg 1976; Furness et al. 1979). Perfusion with a mixture of aldehydes, for example formaldehyde and glutaraldehyde (GLU), has the advantage of both fixing central nervous tissue and producing fluorescence of catecholamines (Fig. 16, Grillo et al. 1974; Chiba et al. 1976; Furness et al. 1977 a, b, 1979). Being an aldehyde, GLU itself produces amine-fluorophores to some extent (Harrison 1975).

Advantages, field of application, and the easiest sectioning procedure are given in Table 2.

The addition of high concentrations of metallic sulfate (e.g., $AlSO_4$ or $MgSO_4$) to the perfusion solution at low pH (3.8–4.5) enhances the fluorescence intensity in cryostat as well as in vibratome sections (Fig. 17). Moreover, it reduces the unspecific background fluorescence and the diffusion of the CA fluorophore (Lorén et al. 1977; Ajelis et al. 1979). Similar effects are obtained in other perfusion techniques by the introduction of an immersion bath containing metallic sulfate after the sectioning procedure (Lorén et al. 1977). Procedures involving metallic sulfates provide excellent results especially when

Table 2. Duration, proposed sectioning procedure and field of application of combined aqueous aldehyde techniques

Technique (Section)	2.1	2.2	2.4	3.1	4.2	4.3	4.4	4.5
Duration	7 days	3½ h	2 h	20 min	90 min	2 – 14 h	3 – 14 h	24 h
Tissue	CNS, PNS	CNS, PNS	PNS, GEP	CNS, PNS	CNS, PNS	CNS PNS	CNS PNS	CNS PNS
Microtome	+		+					
Cryostat		+	+	+	+	+	+	+
Vibratome			(+)			+	+	+
CA	+ + +	+ + +	+ +	+ + +	+ + +	+ + +	+ + +	+ + +
5-HT	+	+	+ + +	+	+	+	+	+ +
Visual. of fibers	+ +	+ +	+	+ + +	+ +	+ +	+ + +	+ + +
Cell. preservation	+ + +	+ + +	+ +	(+)	+	+ +	+ +	+ +

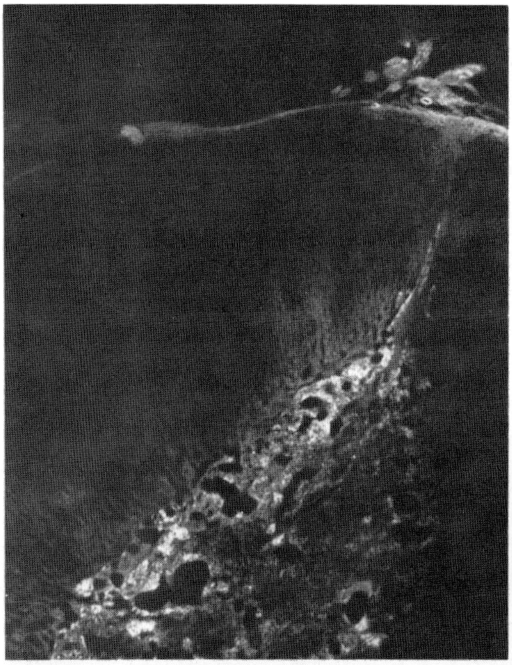

15

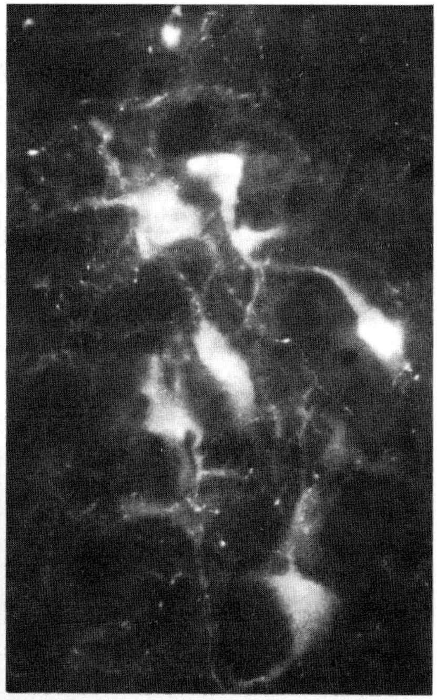

16

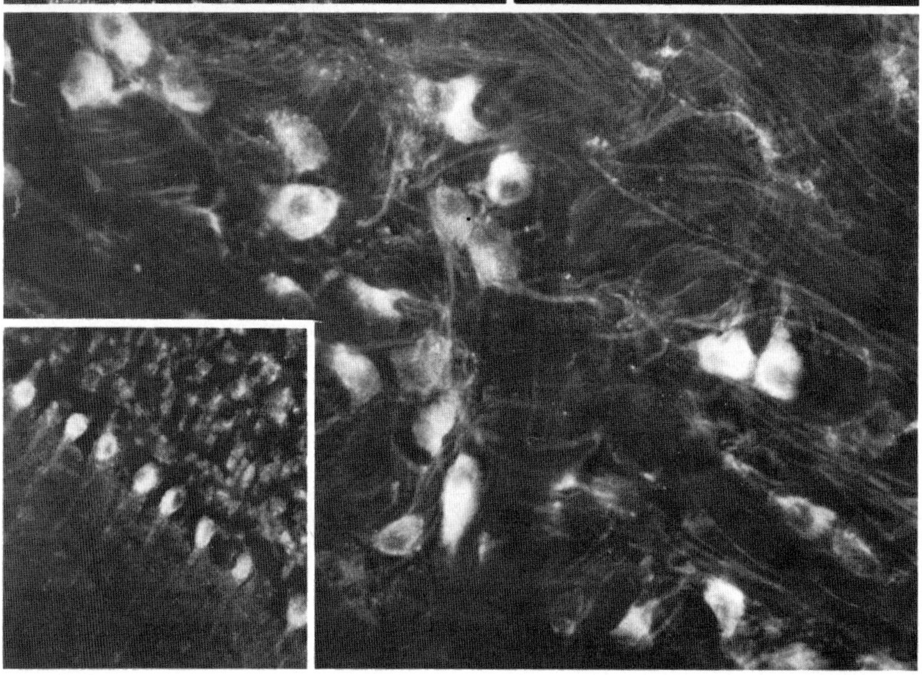

17

Fig. 15. Catecholamine cells in the rat adrenal medulla following simultaneous perfusion of glyoxylic acid and formaldehyde (Sect. 4.2). ×45

Fig. 16. Catecholamine neurons in the rat locus coeruleus following simultaneous perfusion of formaldehyde and glutaraldehyde (Sect. 4.3). ×410

Fig. 17. Catecholamine neurons in the rostral pontine part of the reticular formation following successive perfusion of glyoxylic acid and aluminium/formaldehyde (*inset:* Purkinje-cells in the cerebellar cortex of the same specimen) (Sect. 4.5). ×410; ×200

sectioned with the vibratome or cryostat and when additionally reacted with FA vapor (1 h, 50%, 70 °C) after drying. The beneficial effects of high concentrations of metal ions in the perfusion fixative or in the postfixation immersion fluid have been explained by several factors: Magnesium ions may inhibit release of amines during processing; the hypertonic salt solution may help to dehydrate the tissue and/or metallic ions may act directly on the fluorophore formation in the catalysis of the histochemical reaction (Lorén et al. 1977). The number of fluorescent pericarya and fibers after Al-sulfate treatment (Fig. 17, inset), however, far exceeds that seen with all other histo-fluorescence methods (personal observation). This fact might call into question the specificity of the fluorescence when applying metallic sulfates at acid conditions. For this reason, only regions with identified amine neurons should be registered with this method.

The constituents of the initial rinsing solution are intended for accomplishing proper perfusion of tissues. Procaine HCl serves as a capillary dilatator and $CaCl_2$ is thought to stabilize membranes. Convulsions of the animal induced by the ice-cold fixative are diminished by muscle relaxants (Flaxedil®).

PVP with a molecular weight of 40,000 added to the fixatives serves as an iso-oncotic plasma expander which prevents dilatation of intercellular spaces. This results in good structural preservation of tissue. In addition, PVP in high concentrations (10%–20%) acts as an effective cryoprotectant in binding tissue water molecules and avoiding crystallization. Fixatives with desirably high concentrations of PVP, however, cannot be perfused due to their jelly-like consistency. The cryoprotective effect of 2.5% PVP is, in peripheral tissues, adequate to substitute the effect of hypermolaric substances such as sucrose. Moreover, PVP distinctly improves the elasticity of fixed tissue and thus facilitates shock-freezing.

5 Ortho-phthaldialdehyde-Induced Fluorescence (OPT) of Histamine

Microspectrofluorometric characteristics of the fluorophores from H and OPT were investigated in model systems (Håkanson et al. 1970). A shift of the fluorescence maximum from yellow (excitation max. about 410nm emission max. about 545nm) to blue (excitation max. about 365 nm, emission max. about 425 nm) was found to depend on the H-concentration. Histochemical methods with OPT dissolved in ethylbenzene have been applied to fresh sections (Juhlin and Shelley 1966) and to Carnoy-fixed paraffin sections (Enerbäck 1969). However, methods using OPT in liquid media do not allow the demonstration of H stores in cell systems other than mast cells. The more sensitive vapor phase method (Håkanson and Owman 1967; Ehinger and Thunberg 1976) gives bright yellow fluorescence with highly concentrated H (e.g., in mast cells) and a paler bluish fluorescence with cells containing H in lower concentrations.

5.1 Ortho-phthaldialdehyde Method for Histamine

(after Ehinger et al. 1968; Pearse 1972; Ehinger and Thunberg 1976)

5.1.1 Tissue Preparation

Small tissue blocks are shock-frozen in liquid propane (or 2-methylbutane – see Sect. 1.1) and mounted on cryostat chucks. The cryostat temperature is set at –40 °C (see Sect. 6.1).

Collect 20 μm cryostat sections without thawing with the dry bristles of a fine brush onto prechilled coverslips which have been coated with a thin layer of an albumin-glycerin mixture.

The coverslip holder (Fig. 11) is transferred to a dessicator without allowing temperature to rise above –40 °C, and the dessicator evacuated with a mechanical two-stage pump. The sections are freeze-dried overnight at –40 °C over P_2O_5 in vacuo. The dessicator is warmed to room temperature before being ventilated.

As an alternative, small tissue blocks can be shock-frozen and freeze-dried (Sect. 2.1), embedded in paraplast (Sect. 6.1) and sectioned at 8 μm with a microtome (Sect. 7.3). For the OPT procedure the wax is removed with a few drops of xylene.

Whole mounts of thin tissue may be prepared at room temperature and dried for 1–2 h over P_2O_5.

5.1.2 OPT Procedure

Place 30 mg of crystalline OPT (Fluka AG; freshly purified by recrystallization from hot heptane) in a Petri dish in an airtight glass vessel (Fig. 10, 500 ml capacity), preheated to 100 °C. The OPT is heated to 100 °C for 5–10 min to allow vaporization.

The OPT vessel is removed from the oven and the coverslip holder with dry frozen sections transferred to it for 30–60 s.

The coverslip holder is then placed in a moist chamber (closed glass vessel with blotting paper soaked with water) at 22 °C for 2–10 min.

Deparaffinized sections, instead of being placed in a moist chamber, are exposed to the steam of boiling water for 5 s.

The sections are dried at 80 °C for 5–10 min in order to stabilize the fluorophores. After having cooled to room temperature, the coverslips are mounted with xylene onto microscope slides.

5.2 Commentary on the OPT Method for Histamine

This method has not been practiced in our laboratory. According to the authors, the OPT method has a high degree of sensitivity for cryostat sections as well as for paraffin sections. Paraffin sections are less vulnerable to humidification which gives the paraffin method a higher degree of precision and reproducibility. It has not been fully elucidated whether compounds other than H are also OPT-reactive. In order to secure specificity of the reaction, the histochemical procedure should be combined with parallel quantitative determinations of H in the tissues.

6 Embedding

Precondition for an embedding medium in fluorescence microscopy is the absence of autofluorescence. Paraplast as well as some epoxy resins fulfil this condition. The choice of the embedding medium further depends on the respective goal for the examination. Serial sectioning of large tissue blocks is best performed with paraplast-embedded material. Small specimens are sectioned preferably in epoxy resin. Araldite is found to be superior to other epoxy resins with regard to diffusion artifacts when sections are stretched in water. Specimens fixed with aqueous solutions are usually immediately sectioned on the vibratome or in the cryostat (see Sect. 7) with the advantage of time economy. For serial reconstruction or method combinations embedding of the tissue blocks is however advisible. This mode of processing allows convenient storage of specimens for long periods of time. Wet samples are rinsed in H_2O and dehydrated in graded ethanols before being transferred to the embedding medium. Since tissue dehydration implies the risk of amine diffusion, perfusion-fixed tissues are preferably embedded after shock-freezing and freeze-drying.

6.1 Paraplast

Freeze-dried tissue blocks are transferred into the empty part of a vessel (Fig. 18). The other part is filled with previously degassed paraplast (Melting point 56–57 °C, Fa. Lancer St. Louis, USA) and placed in a

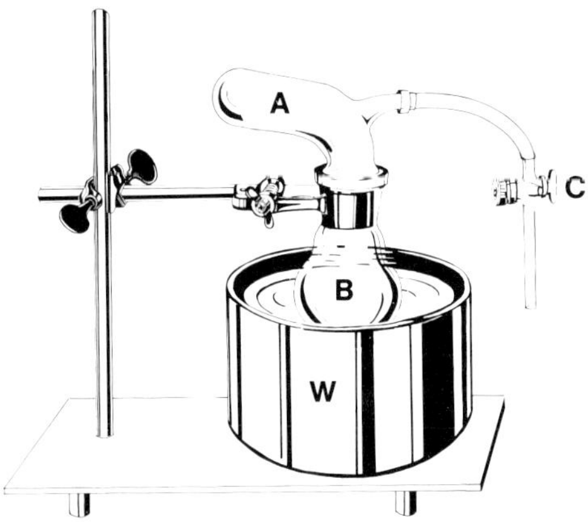

Fig. 18. Equipment for vacuum embedding (from Falck and Owman 1965): Glass vessel consisting of (1) *part A;* which contains paraplast and is immerged in a waterbath at 60–70 °C (*W*), and (2) an empty *part B*, which is connected to a vacuum pump by a 4-way cock (*C*). Parts A and B are airtightly interconnected with silicone grease (medium viscosity)

water bath at 60 °C (Fig. 18). After 15 min of evacuation with a water-jet pump, the specimens are shaken down into the liquid paraplast. They remain there until no more gas bubbles appear (after 20–30 min). Finally, the samples are embedded in embedding molds with paraplast as described in Chap. 1. This last step also applies to ethanol-dehydrated tissue.

6.2 Araldite

To ensure proper infiltration (Hökfelt 1965), freeze-dried tissue blocks are transferred for a short period of time (1–3 min) to vials with propylene oxide until they sink. Dehydrated specimens must remain for 2×20 min in this medium (with one change). Then the samples are placed into a propylene oxide/araldite mixture (1 : 1) in open vials for 6–12 h at room temperature (duration depends on thickness of the samples). The araldite is composed of 65 parts araldite M (CY 212 – Merck, Darmstadt, Federal Republic of Germany), 60 parts DDSA (dodenylsuccinic acid anhydride; Serva, Heidelberg, Federal Republic of Germany), and 3% accelerator 964 (Dy 064; Merck). The mixture should be changed once or twice reducing the accelerator to 2%. When the probes have become transparent, they are put into prewarmed capsules with one drop of araldite. The composition at this step consists of araldite/DDSA mixture (65/60) with 2% accelerator.

The capsules are then filled with epoxy resin. Polymerization is accelerated in an oven at 60 °C. The duration depends on the thickness of the sections to be cut on the ultramicrotome. The best consistency for rather thick sections (3–20 μm) is obtained after 6–12 h, for semithin sectioning (0.5–3 μm) after 12–24 h.

6.3 Glycolmethacrylate

Hoyt et al. (1979) recommend the following procedure: Dehydrated tissues are put into embedding solution A, composed of 80 ml glycolmethacrylate (Electron microscopy sciences Co., Fort Washington, Pa), 16 ml 2-butoxy-ethanol, and 0.405 g benzoylperoxyde. The specimens in solution A are exposed to a mild vacuum for 15 min and steeped overnight. They are then placed in complete medium consisting of 42 parts of embedding solution A and 1 part of embedding solution B (1.5 parts of polyethyleneglycol 400 to 1 part of N,N-dimethylaniline) and are polymerized at room temperature for 4 h.

6.4 Embedding Medium for Light Microscopy (hydroxyethylmethacrylate/butoxyethanol; EFL-67, solution A and B Serva)

This is a variation of the glycolmethacrylate procedure.

Dry tissue samples are transferred to a vessel containing a mixture of EFL-solutions A and B (41 : 0.5) and are degassed several times (8–10×). They are then put into gelatin capsules with the degassed EFL mixture and are sealed with heated paraplast for airtight polymerization. The EFL polymerizes in the refrigerator overnight.

7 Sectioning and Mounting

Tissues in which fluorophores have been formed, must be cut in artificial light. To obtain optimal results all sections should be collected on precleaned glass slides. For cleaning an ether-80%-ethanol mixture (1 : 1) may be sufficient. Clean the slides in chromosulfuric acid overnight, wash in running water for 12 h, rinse in alcohol, dry, and store in an airtight box.

7.1 Frozen Sections

The technique of cryostat sectioning (e.g., in a cryostat HRLM, Slee, Mainz, Federal Republic of Germany) has the advantage of being rapid and offers the possibility of obtaining relatively large sections of good quality (Heene 1968; Winkler 1970 a; see also Sect. 6). Moreover, very small specimens, surrounded by a connective tissue capsule (e.g., spinal or sympathetic ganglia) can be easily sectioned. In peripheral tissues, a polymeric cryoprotectant polyvinylpyrrolidone (PVP 40, SIGMA) dissolved in fixation perfusion solutions is sufficient for light microscopy. When freezing large brain slabs the addition of 10% succrose to the postperfusion fixative is advisable. The tissue samples remain 2–12 h in this solution in the refrigerator.

Attention has to be devoted to the time required to freeze unfixed or perfusion-fixed specimens with respect to the best retention of structural details and maximal fluorescence intensity. Whereas the method of freezing does not significantly influence the fluorescence yield of prefixed tissue, there are differences in the quality of structural preservation. As indicated above, freezing brain slabs (perfused or non-perfused) in liquid propane 2-methylbutane or Freon 12, which maintains optimal structural preservation, frequently results in tissue fracturing. Alternatively, perfused specimens can be frozen within a few seconds on the cryostat chuck in contact with powdered dry ice (e.g., in a CO_2 bench freezer, Slee, Mainz, Federal Republic of Germany) with adequate structural preservation (Bloom and Battenberg 1976). In unfixed specimens not thicker than 2 mm slower freezing within the cryostat (De la Torre and Surgeon 1976 a, b) provides fully acceptable morphologic features.

For cutting frozen sections the specimens are glued onto a cryostat chuck with a few drops of precooled tissue tec (Slee). In order to avoid thawing of the tissue this should be done in the sink of the cryostat which has been set to a temperature of –30 °C. Furthermore, all instruments used (i.e., tweezers and brush) must be prechilled in the cryostat sink.

Sections should be cut at approximately –26 °C. Sectioning brain tissue at –30 °C can be difficult because the sections crumble. Sectioning at higher temperature (–20 °C) is easier but decreases the fluorescence intensity of CA. Fibers appear brighter in thicker sections (20–30 μm), but resolution is improved in thinner sections (5–15 μm). The sections attached to the knife are picked up by pressing a clean, room temperature glass slide against the knife. Structural preservation of perfused tissues is optimized by the use of prechilled slides onto which sections are quickly thawed by finger pressure on the reverse side.

7.2 Vibratome Sections

The vibratome technique (Hökfelt and Ljungdahl 1972) simplifies the mechanical requirements and reduces the overall time of FA-induced fluorescence. The vibratome (Oxford G 501, Oxford, California, USA) procedure was also found to be ideal for the application of GIF (Lindvall et al. 1973). Vibratome sectioning combined with freeze-drying gives very strong fluorescence with low background fluorescence. However, it is difficult to keep sections fracture-free and sections often do not stick to the slide. Better results are obtained by drying the sections with the hair dryer and storing them in vacuo over P_2O_5 overnight. The sectioning procedure of fixed tissue results in large sections of equal thickness when sectioned at 20 µm or thicker. Thin sections of large brain areas of reproducible thickness are difficult to obtain. Their quality largely depends on the consistency of the perfused tissue. For demonstrating fine dopamine fiber networks, e.g., in cortical areas, this technique is superior to the cryostat technique. In thicker sections, processes of cell bodies can often be followed for a considerable distance. Small encapsuled organs cannot be sectioned with the vibratome.

The cold tissue slabs are fixed on the vibratome stage with cyanoacrylic acid methylester (Eastman 910 adhesive). The stage is filled with the solution indicated in the technical procedures or with the ice-cold last perfusate.

Since a cooling device is not available the solution can be kept at 2–4 °C in different ways. Some examples are:

a) By sectioning in a cool chamber
b) By small plastic vials with a mixture of dry ice and alcohol
c) By lead cubes with a handle (as used for coverslipping) which have been chilled in liquid nitrogen.

The temperature must be controlled with a thermometer.

The floating sections are collected on glass slides with the help of a fine brush.

In case the tissue is not sufficiently hardened by the fixation, moistening of the tissue block with a few drops of the ice-cold stage solution (but not completely covering it) facilitates sectioning. The stage is then cooled by crushed ice.

7.3 Paraplast Sections

Sectioning is best done with a rotation microtome at 5–20 µm in a dry atmosphere. Precooling of the block facilitates sectioning. The sections are collected with a dry, fine brush and allowed to stretch in their own melting paraplast on dry and prewarmed slides. For stretching the sections water cannot be employed because the fluorescent compounds then become displaced. Butanol may be used as a convenient medium for stretching wrinkled sections. Cover slips are fixed with paraffin oil or an entellan-xylene mixture (10 : 1).

7.4 Plastic Sections (Araldite, Glycolmethacrylate, EFL)

Semithin sections (0.5–20 μ) cut with a dry glass knife on the ultramicrotome are stretched on glass slides with a drop of water or a mixture of butanol/paraffin oil (3 : 7) on a hot plate. Cover slips are fixed with paraffin oil or butanol/paraffin oil if they are to be removed after examination for further processing (autoradiography, immunohistochemistry, classic staining methods), or with Entellan® when they are to be stored for re-examination.

8 Storage

If not sectioned immediately, all embedded tissue blocks can be stored for months in the dark under the driest conditions possible. For paraplast blocks we use a light-tight dessicator with P_2O_5 placed in the ice-box. Since very low concentrations of PA vapor are sufficient to induce specific fluorescence even at room temperature (Håkanson and Sundler 1974; Sparring and Grube 1977), untreated control specimens must be stored separately.

In sections of plastic-embedded tissue the specific fluorescence of CA and 5-HT can be demonstrated months later. However, paraplast sections of freeze-dried tissue, especially when mounted under coverslips, are rather sensitive to storage with respect to decreasing CA- or 5-HT fluorescence intensity and diffusion artifacts. This occurs after a few hours. Slides with unmounted paraplast sections of CA- or 5-HT-containing tissue may be stored for 24 h without major changes. Tissue sections with H-containing cells should be examined immediately after the OPT-procedure since the pale blue fluorescence of low H concentrations is especially unstable and fades rapidly (Pearse 1972).

9 Specificity of Fluorophores

In the study of monoamine-containing structures it is important to ascertain that the fluorescence observed is due to the presence of one of the reactive monoamines. For this reason, in each experiment control samples of the investigated tissue, which have not been treated for fluorophore formation, should be examined in parallel.

Chemical specificity tests have the advantage of being directly applicable to tissue sections. Specific fluorescent compounds within 1–2 min are readily reduced by a 0.1% sodium borohydride solution in 90% isopropanol at 20 °C to the corresponding non-fluorescent 1,2,3,4-tetrahydro-compounds. Yet, the fluorescence can be regenerated in xylene-dewaxed paraplast sections by renewed FA treatment (Corrodi et al. 1964; Corrodi and Jonsson 1967). The fluorescence is not reestablished in plastic sections when exposed to formaldehyde gas (Hoyt et al. 1979). Non-specific fluorescence (e.g., background fluorescence of tissue proteins; auto-fluorescence of elastic membranes, lipofuscin granules, lysosomes) does not undergo any changes with borohydride treatment.

Differentiation between amine fluorescence and auto-fluorescence can also be achieved by the administration of drugs which reduce amine stores. Specific fluorescence disappears following administration of monoamine-releasing agents, e.g., reserpine (Eränkö and Hopsu 1958). Furthermore, it can be diminished by pretreatment with synthesis inhibitors such as α-methyl-p-tyrosine or p-chlorophenylalanine (Koe and Weissman 1966; Aghajanian et al. 1973).

Specific fluorescence of NA and A is reduced by inhibition of the dopamine-converting enzyme dopamine-β-hydroxylase (e.g., FD-008, Fla 63, or Disulfiram) or by replacement of the physiological transmitter with 6-OH-dopamine (Thoenen and Tranzer 1968) which gives no fluorescent reaction. This false transmitter also causes degeneration of central DA neurons (Ungerstedt 1968). 5-OH-dopamine, forming a fluorophore with aldehydes (Ehinger and Flack 1969) cannot be used for specificity tests. Specific fluorescence of 5-HT can be abolished by administration of the false transmitter 5,7-dihydroxytryptamine (Baumgarten et al. 1974).

10 Discrimination Between Different Monoamines

Many attempts have been made to distinguish between the almost identical spectral characteristics of most fluorogenic amines.

The FIF-induced characteristics of some biogenic amines are given in Table 3 (after Jonsson 1967; Jonsson and Sandler 1969).

Using microspectrofluorometry a safe differentiation between most monoamines can be made. Differentiation between the

Table 3. Excitation and emission maxima of formaldehyde-induced fluorescence of various compounds

Compound giving FIF	Excitation max. (nm)	Emission max. (nm)
Dopamine	410	480
Dopa	410	490
Noradrenaline	410	480
Adrenaline	410	480
Tryptamine	370	490
Tryptophan	375	490
5-Hydroxytryptamine	410	525
6-Hydroxytryptamine	400	505

various CA and between CA and 5-HT requires additional treatment. FA condensation products of NA or DA in tissue sections react differently to HCl treatment. The NA fluorophore is reduced in a two-step reaction to a fully aromatic isoquinoline, whereas the DA fluorophore leads to the conversion of the quinoidal dihydroisoquinoline into its tautomeric non-quinoidal form. The two fluorophores have different excitation spectra as distinguished by microspectrofluorometry (Corrodi and Jonsson 1965; Björklund et al. 1968; Björklund et al. 1971). The resulting spectral changes can also be used for the differentiation between CA and 5-HT. Using microspectrofluorometry, the spectral characteristics of DOPA-thioether fluorophores, e.g., in pigment-forming cells can be distinguished from DOPA and other compounds which are fluorogenic in the Flack-Hillarp method (Agrup et al. 1977).

Fluorescence intensity of 5-HT fluorophores decreases much faster upon continued ultraviolet irradiation than CA fluorophores (Fuxe et al. 1970). This property can be used for microfluorometric differentiation between these two amines (Dahlström and Fuxe 1964; Jonsson 1967). Using a computerized microspectrofluorometer, Geyer et al. (1979) have demonstrated, that a measure of fluorescence fading reliably quantifies 5-HT even in the presence of CA at the cellular level.

While minute fluorescence histochemical differentiation between all closely related amines can be achieved only by very elaborate microspectrofluorometric techniques, a less precise differentiation between some monoamines is readily possible without this expenditure.

In selecting suitable filter systems (Sect. 11.1), distinction between CA fluorescence and 5-HT fluorescence is often possible with the unaided eye. Whereas CA fluorophores are seen as light-yellow to yellow-green, 5-HT fluorophores appear in an orange-yellow color. Different fluorescence intensities, however, can alter the color perceived by the eye (Norberg et al. 1966). Intense fluorescence of primary CA appears yellow, yet moderate fluorescence is green. The best way to provide narrow band irradiation of fluorophores is the use of interference filters with a sharp cut-off at specific wavelengths (Ploem 1969).
5-HT has been found to be readily distinguished from CA following incubation in a glyoxylic acid solution (Sect. 3.1) at acid conditions (Furness and Costa 1975). Whereas 5-HT forms a fluorophore after reaction at pH 3.5, NA does not. Both amines can be visualized after incubation at neutral pH.

Primary amines can be discriminated from secondary amines visually on the basis of kinetic differences in their reactions to FA (Falck et al. 1962; Corrodi and Hillarp 1963; Eränkö 1967): secondary amines are seen to give less fluorescence and require longer exposure to FA vapor. However, this approach remains an estimation; it cannot be considered as a reliable method for amine differentiation (Fixe et al. 1970).

For the differentiation of NA and A cells a fluorescence histochemical technique has been developed by oxidation with gaseous iodine to trihydroxyindole-derivates (THI; Angelakos and King 1965; Angelakos 1967). In this reaction NA and A are oxidized to corresponding adrenochromes and subsequently rearranged to fluorescent lutines with different colors. The reaction gives no visible fluorescent products with DA.

The procedure is described as follows (King and Angelakos 1973):

Place 1–2 g iodine crystals on the bottom of a Coplin jar. A small vial is placed in thc jar with a piece of filter paper on top of it. Freeze-dried cryostat sections are placed on the filter paper and the jar is then covered. The sections are exposed to iodine fumes at room temperature for 2–7 min (to be varied for different tissues).

After iodine oxidation the sections are transferred to the top of a similar vial in another Coplin jar containing 3 ml of concentrated ammonium hydroxyde, and exposed to ammonia fumes for 1 min. The sections are mounted on glass slides with liquid paraffin and examined immediately. A distinct difference in fluorescence colors between NA-blue and A-green cells can be detected visually with the THI method (Sect. 11.1). Control sections are treated in the same manner, except that the order of exposure to iodine and ammonia is reversed.

Dopaminergic cells can be distinguished from NA-containing structures after administration of reserpine (1 mg/kg s.c.) for 3 h followed by i.p. injection of levodopa-methylester (200 mg/kg) in 0.9% saline for 90 min. This treatment results in refluorescence of DA but not NA (Hess 1978).

In tryptophylpeptide-containing cells (e.g., C-cells in thyroid gland), combined formaldehyde-ozon treatment induces a strong greenish fluorescence. Combined formaldehyde-HCl treatment gives only a moderate fluorescence.

When there is the slightest doubt about the fluorescence color and other characteristics, applying one of the procedures described, spectral analysis should be carried out. For differentiation between monoamines by means of immunohistofluorescence of antibodies to CA, 5-HT or to their synthesizing enzymes see Chap. 10.

11 Improvement of Visualization

Fluorescence histochemical detection of monoamines is often difficult in neurons (e.g., nonterminal axons) with low concentrations of monoamines. This problem can be dealt with in several ways:

11.1 Pharmacological Treatment

One possibility of facilitating the localization of monoamines is to increase intraneuronal monoamine levels by pharmacological treatment (Fuxe et al. 1970).

Monoamines or their precursors, when administered by in vivo intracerebral injection, enhance the fluorescence of the corresponding central neurons due to an uptake-concentration mechanism for amines at their cell membrane (Fuxe et al. 1970). Small volumes of saline solutions (5 μl) containing 5–10 μg of DA or NA imply a marked accumulation of these amines in nearby seated CA neurons, whereas, when injected in large volumes (50–100 μl) the CA is taken up by CA nerve terminals in large parts of the brain (Ungerstedt et al. 1969).

Demonstration of nerve cells and of fine nerve plexus in peripheral organs is facilitated by intraperitoneal administration of monoamines or amine precursors (100 mg/kg body wt).

Thus, fluorescence of cells containing 5-HT and of some endocrine GEP cells in peripheral tissues is increased by pre-injection of the animal with 100 mg/kg of the 5-HT precursor 5-hydroxytryptophan (5-HTP, Sigma) or with 5-HT.

Jonsson and Sandler (1969) recommend the administration of 6-HT (100 mg/kg i.p.) which is accumulated in 5-HT nerve terminals, its fluorescence yield being about 4 times higher than that of the physiological transmitter.

Intraperitoneal injection of a *MAO-inhibitor,* e.g., nialamide or iproniazid

(500 mg/kg i.p., Sigma) 4 h before death, decrease the intracellular amine metabolism (Dahlström and Fuxe 1964). For increased 5-HT storage especially pretreatment with pargyline (200 mg/kg, Sigma) 3 h before death is recommended (Azmitia and Henriksen 1976).

Aghajanian and co-workers (1973) administered L-tryptophan in conjunction with MAO-inhibitors in an attempt to increase the intraneuronal 5-HT. However, this combination additionally produces a state of hyperpyrexia, resulting in 5-HT diffusion from its neuronal localization. For this reason the authors recommend pretreatment with an i.p. injection of the sedativum chloral hydrate which effectively blocks the undesired side effect. The drug administration is practiced as follows (Azmitia and Henriksen 1976):

The animals receive an injection with chloral hydrate (400 mg/kg i.p.) 10 min prior to the injection of a MAO-inhibitor (pargyline, 200 mg/kg i.p.). Between 60 and 90 min following MAO-inhibitor treatment L-tryptophan (100 mg/kg i.p.) is administered. The animal is killed 1 h after the last injection.

11.2 Tissue Incubation

Another way to increase the fluorescence intensity in monoamine-containing pathways is the in vitro incubation of the unfixed tissue with monoamines. 5-HT neurons preferentially take up and accumulate 5-HT, whereas DA- and NA-neurons preferentially take up and accumulate NA, DA, or a precursor. After incubation with L-β-3,4-dihydroxyphenylalanine (L-Dopa, Sigma) CA-producing cells become visible. This is due to the primary CA formed intracellularly (Håkanson et al. 1969). The material is incubated for 1 h at 37 °C in continuously oxygenized Tyrode solution containing 50–100 μg/ml L-Dopa.

For improvement of NA visualization small unfixed tissue blocks can also be immersed for few minutes in an oxygenized Ringer solution, containing 12 g/50 ml PVP and 1 mg/50 ml L-NA-bitartrate (Gorgas, personal communication).

For 5-HT neurons I refer to the modification of the Falck-Hillarp technique at the stage of the fluorophore formation (Fuxe and Jonsson 1967; see also Sect. 2.1.2.4): The tissue is initially exposed to relatively dry formaldehyde vapor (65% relative humidity) followed by exposure to a more humid formaldehyde vapor (90% relative humidity). This procedure prevents diffusion of the fluorescent products while improving 5-HT fluorescence.

12 Evaluation

12.1 Microscopy

Fluorescence is an optical phenomenon in which short-waved light is absorbed by a fluorophore and re-emitted as light with a longer wavelength. The spectral characteristics of a fluorophore are composed of two spectra: the excitation spectrum and the emission spectrum. The excitation spectrum is a plot of the total intensity of fluorescence when the specimen is irradiated with light of a specific wavelength. Substantially, the excitation spectrum is identical to the absorption spectrum. Fluorescence is best excited by irradiation with light of a wavelength as close as possible to the peak of the excitation or absorption spectrum. The emission spectrum shows a spectral distribution of the fluorescence emitted by the fluorophore.

Fluorescence microscopy is capable of revealing the presence of very small quantities of fluorophores, because the light emitted from a fluorophore is of a longer wavelength than that used for excitation. For general principles of fluorescence microscopy, refer to Young (1961), Nairn (1969), and Udenfriend (1969).

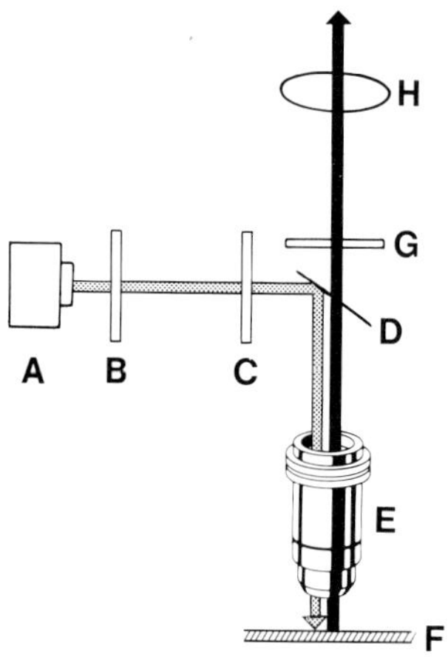

Fig. 19. Optical system of a fluorescence microscope with incident light illumination (epi-illumination). *A*, high pressure mercury lamp; *B*, collector lens and heat absorbing filter; *C*, excitation filter; *D*, dichromatic dividing mirror; *E*, objective; *F*, glass slide with tissue section; *G*, barrier filter; *H*, ocular

Special fluorescence microscopes are offered by all producers of optical instruments. However, any kind of microscope can be used for fluorescence microscopy provided that a suitable source of light, a heat absorbing filter, an excitation (primary or activation) filter, and a barrier (secondary or emission) filter are at hand (Fig. 19). Incident light illumination (e.g., Fluopak-System Leitz; Zeiss epi-illuminator system) guarantees a high fluorescence yield as no loss of light by dispersion or self-absorption in the tissue occurs (Ploem 1969; Pearse 1972). (Fluorescence excitation with transmitted light is achieved by the additional use of dark-field or bright-field condensors.)

In general, a high pressure mercury lamp (Osram, HBO 200) is most suitable as a light source. For absorbing heat the Schott BG 38 filter is recommended because it also cuts out the red end of the spectrum. Heat absorbing and excitation filters are placed between light source and specimen.

The excitation filter provides light from the light source over a narrow band of wavelengths corresponding to the excitation peak of the fluorophore being investigated. Only lightbeams will pass the ultraviolet (UV) or blue excitation filter which are needed by the object for the transformation of the invisible, short-waved UV-radiation into the long-waved, visible radiation. In this manner, unwanted excitation light and disturbing background fluorescence are minimized.

The exciting radiation is focused by a dichromatic dividing mirror through the objective onto the preparation. The intensity of the exciting radiation reaching the section depends on the numeric aperture of the objective; high-aperture objectives such as planapochromates are preferable. Oil immersion objectives are most suitable due to their large aperture (larger than 0.75) and thus their higher fluorescence yield.

The barrier filter is placed between object and ocular. It prevents the light of the excitation wavelength from reaching the observer's eye. Transmission of this filter should range within the spectral region of the emission of the fluorophore, but at the same time it should cut off the light used for excitation as much as possible. The percepted color of the fluorescence depends on the color of the barrier filter. It can be distorted by the yellow or orange tinge of this filter. Thus, the FA-induced fluorescence of NA, apparent as blue-green with a colorless filter, is observed as yellow-green with a yellow barrier filter.

The choice of filters depends on the fluorescence characteristics of a fluorophore. The following filter combinations are recommended for the fluorescence of CA, 5-HT and H (in high concentration):

Excitation filter: Schott BG 3, AL 405. Secondary filter: Zeiss 470 or LP 510
Barrier filter: Schott BG 12. Secondary filter: Leitz K 490 or Zeiss 50

Improved filter systems allow the distinction between blue-green CA fluorescence and yellow fluorescence of 5-HT:

Excitation filter: Toshiba VV-40 + Nikon band pass interference filter
Barrier filter: Schott GG 455

Fluorescence of H (in low concentration) is best visualized with:

Excitation filter: Schott UG 1
Barrier filter: Zeiss 41 or Leitz K 430

Irradiation of fluorophores with UV or blue light will cause a decrease in fluorescence intensity. This fading effect is attributable to photodecompensation. Fading gives rise to difficulties with photography and quantitation. Since fluorescent preparations are particularly subject to this problem general tissue structures should be centered and focused in a phase contrast system with transmitted light from beneath in order to avoid premature fluorescence fading of amines in UV light. (It should be noted, however, that phase contrast lenses reduce the fluorescence yield.) Some recovery may occur if, after examination, the sections are kept in the dark.

12.2 Microphotography

For documentation any kind of microscope camera can be used. In routine assays with automatic exposure times, the photographs are exposed with integrating measurements. For quantitative assays the use of definite exposure times is preferable. In both cases the proportion of the brightness of fluorescent structures to that of the photograph's background is a relative measure for the intensity of the fluorescence.

Fluorescent structures must be photographed before the aldehyde-induced fluorescence has faded under the influence of the irradiation. In order to register even weak fluorescence a sensitive film material should be employed. Satisfactory color photos are achieved with KODAK High Speed Ektachrome artificial light film DIN 22 exposed like DIN 27 (with subsequent special development). A good quality black-and-white photo is guaranteed by KODAK tri-X-Pan, DIN 27 exposed like DIN 30, developed with a fine-grain developer (e.g., KODAK MICRODOL X).

Acknowledgements. The DFG grant He 919/4 supported the methodological research conducted by the author and reported in this chapter. I am grateful to Dr. D. Pfaff for suggestions to the chemical part of the review. I thank Mrs. Christa Wedel and Mrs. Christa Melcher for their technical assistance, as well as Mrs. Hannelore Ehlers for the preparation of the manuscript.

13 References

Aghajanian GK, Kuhar MJ, Roth RH (1973) Serotonin-containing neuronal perikarya and terminals: differential effects of *p*-chlorophenylalanine. Brain Res 54:85–101

Agrup G, Björklund A, Falck B, Jakobsson S, Lindvall O, Rorsman H, Rosengren E (1977) Fluorescence histochemical demonstration of DOPA thioethers by condensation with gaseous formaldehyde. Histochemistry 52: 179–186

Ajelis V, Björklund A, Falck B, Lindvall O, Loren I, Walles B (1979) Application of the aluminum-formaldehyde (ALFA) histofluorescence method for demonstration of peripheral stores of catecholamines and indolamines in freeze-dried paraffin-embedded tissue, cryostat sections, and wholemounts. Histochemistry 65:1–15

Angelakos ET (1967) Demonstration of nerve terminals containing adrenalin by a new histochemical method. Nature 213:391–392

Angelakos ET, King MP (1965) A new histochemical method for the specific demonstration of catecholamine (CA)-containing structures. Fed Proc 24:389

Axelsson S, Björklund A, Falck A, Lindvall B, Svensson LA (1973) Glyoxylic acid condensation: A new fluorescence method for the histochemical demonstration of biogenic monoamines. Acta Physiol Scand 87:57–62

Axelsson S, Björklund A, Lindvall O (1972) Fluorescence histochemistry of biogenic monoamines. A study of the capacity of various carbonyl compounds to form fluorophores with biogenic monoamines in gas phase reactions. J Histochem Cytochem 20: 435–444

Azmitia EC, Henriksen SJ (1976) A modification of the Falck-Hillarp technique for 5-HT fluorescence employing hypertonic formaldehyde perfusion. J Histochem Cytochem 24: 1286–1288

Battenberg ELF, Bloom FE (1975) A rapid, simple, and more sensitive method for the demonstration of central catecholamine neurons and axons by glyoxylic acid-induced fluorescence. I. Specificity. Psychopharmacol Commun 1:3–13

Baumgarten HG, Björklund A, Lachenmayer L, Rensch A, Rosengren E (1974) De- and regeneration of the bulbospinal serotonin neurons in the rat following 5,6- or 5,7-dihydroxytryptamine treatment. Cell Tissue Res 152:271–281

Björklund A, Ehinger B, Falck B (1968) A method for differentiating dopamin from noradrenaline in tissue sections by microspectrofluorometry. J Histochem Cytochem 16: 263–270

Björklund A, Ehinger B, Falck B (1971) Analysis of fluorescence excitation peak ratios for the cellular identification of noradrenaline, dopamin, or their mixtures. J Histochem Cytochem 20:56–64

Björklund A, Falck B, Owman Ch (1972 a) Fluorescence microscopic and microspectrofluorometric techniques for the cellular localization and characterization of biogenic amines. In: Rall JE, Kopin IJ (eds) Methods in investigative and diagnostic endocrinology: vol 1, The thyroid and catecholamines. Elsevier, Amsterdam, pp 318–363

Björklund A, Lindvall O, Svensson LA (1972 b) Mechanisms of fluorophore formation in the histochemical glyoxylic acid method for monoamines. Histochemie 32:13–131

Bloom FE, Battenberg ELF (1976) A rapid, simple, and more sensitive method for the demonstration of central catecholamine-containing neurons and axons by glyoxylic acid induced fluorescence. II. A detailed description of methodology. J Histochem Cytochem 24:561–571

Chiba T, Hwang BH, Williams TH (1976) A method for studying glyoxylic acid-induced fluorescence and ultrastructure of monoamine neurons. Histochemistry 49:95–106

Chiba T, Williams TH (1975) Histofluorescence characteristics and quantification of small intensely fluorescent (SIF) cells in sympathetic ganglia of several species. Cell Tissue Res 162:331–341

Corrodi H, Hillarp NA (1963) Fluoreszenzmethoden zur histochemischen Sichtbarmachung von Monoaminen: I. Identifizierung der fluoreszierenden Produkte aus Modellversuchen mit 6,7-Dimethoxyisochinolinderivaten und Formaldehyd. Helv Chim Acta 46: 2425–2430

Corrodi H, Hillarp NA, Jonsson G (1964) Fluorescence methods for the histochemical demonstration of monoamines: 3. Sodium borohydride reduction of the fluorescent compounds as a specificity test. J Histochem Cytochem 12:582–586

Corrodi H, Jonsson G (1965) Fluoreszenzmethoden zur histochemischen Sichtbarmachung von Monoaminen. 5. Identifizierung des fluoreszierenden Produktes aus Modellversuchen mit 5-Methoxy-tryptamin und Formaldehyd. Acta Histochem (Jena) 22:247–258

Corrodi H, Jonsson G (1967) The formaldehyde fluorescence method for the histochemical demonstration of biogenic monoamines. A review on the methodology. J Histochem Cytochem 15:67–78

Csillik B, Kalman G (1967) Vacuumless freezing-drying: its application in catecholamine histochemistry. Histochemie 2:275–280

Dahlström A, Fuxe K (1964) Evidence for the existence of monoamine-containing neurons in the central nervous system. Acta Physiol Scand [Suppl] 62:232

Ehinger B, Håkanson R, Owman Ch, Sporrong B (1968) Histochemical demonstration of histamine in paraffin sections by a fluorescence method. Biochem Pharmacol 17:1997–1998

Ehinger B, Thunberg R (1976) Induction of fluorescence in histamine-containing cells. Exp Cell Res 47:116–122

Ehinger B, Falck B (1969) Fluorescence microscopical demonstration of 5-hydroxy-dopamine in adrenergic nerves. Histochemie 18: 1–7

Enerbäck L (1969) Detection of histamine in mast cells by o-phthalaldehyde reaction after liquid fixation. J Histochem Cytochem 17: 757–759

Eränkö O (1951) On the histochemistry of the rat adrenal medulla. Acta Physiol Scand [Suppl] 25:89

Eränkö O (1952) On the histochemistry of the adrenal medulla of the rat, with special reference to acid phosphatase. Acta Physiol Scand [Suppl] 16:17

Eränkö O (1955) Histochemistry of noradrenaline in the adrenal medulla of rats and mice. Endocrinology 57:363–368

Eränkö O (1967) The practical histochemical demonstration of catecholamines by formaldehyde-induced fluorescence. J R Microsc Soc 87:259–276

Eränkö O, Eränko L (1971) Small intensely fluorescent granule-containing cells in the sympathetic ganglion of the rat. Prog Brain Res 34:34–51

Eränkö O, Hopsu V (1958) Effect of reserpine on the histochemistry and content of adrenaline and noradrenaline in the adrenal medulla of the rat and the mouse. Endocrinology 62: 15–22

Eränkö O, Räisinen L (1966) Demonstration of catecholamines in adrenergic nerve fibers by fixation in aqueous formaldehyde solution and fluorescence microscopy. J Histochem Cytochem 14:690–691

Falck B (1962) Observations on the possibilities of the cellular localization of monoamines by a fluorescence method. Acta Physiol Scand [Suppl] 56:197

Falck B (1964) Cellular localization of monoamines. Prog Brain Res 8:28–44

Falck B, Hillarp NA, Thieme G, Torp A (1962) Fluorescence of catecholamines and related compounds condensed with formaldehyde. J Histochem Cytochem 10:348–354

Falck B, Torp A (1961) A fluorescence method for histochemical demonstration of noradrenaline in the adrenal medulla. Med Exp 5: 429–432

Falck B, Owman Ch (1965) A detailed methodological description of the fluorescence method for the cellular demonstration of biogenic monoamines. Acta Univ Lund Sect 2, 7:6–23

Furness JB, Costa M (1962) The use of glyoxylic acid for the fluorescence of catecholamines and related compounds condensed with formaldehyde. J Histochem Cytochem 10: 348–354

Furness JB, Costa M (1975) The use of glyoxylic acid for the fluorescence histochemical demonstration of peripheral stores of noradrenaline and 5-hydroxytryptamine in whole mounts. Histochemistry 41:335–352

Furness JB, Costa M, Blessing WW (1977 a) Simultaneous fixation and production of catecholamine fluorescence in central nervous tissue by perfusion with aldehydes. Histochem J 9:745–750

Furness JB, Costa M, Wilson AJ (1977 b) Water-stable fluorophores, produced by reaction with aldehyde solutions, for the histochemical localization of catechol- and indolethylamines. Histochemistry 52:159–170

Furness JB, Heath JW, Costa M (1979) Aqueous aldehyde (FAGLU) methods for the fluorescence histochemical localization of catecholamines and for ultrastructural studies of central nervous tissue. Histochemistry 57: 285–295

Fuxe K, Hökfelt T, Jonsson G, Ungerstedt U (1970) Fluorescence microscopy in neuroanatomy. In: Nauta WJ, Ebbesson SO (eds) Contemporary research methods in neuroanatomy. Springer, Berlin Heidelberg New York, pp 275–314

Fuxe K, Jonsson G (1967) A modification of the histochemical fluorescence method for the improved localization of 5-HT. Histochemie 11: 161–166

Fuxe K, Jonsson G (1973) The histochemical fluorescence method for the demonstration of catecholamines. J Histochem Cytochem 21: 293–311

Geyer M, Dawsey W, Mandell J (1979) Fading: a new cytofluorimetric measure quantifying serotonin in the presence of catecholamines in the cellular level in brain. J Pharmacol Exp Ther 207:650–667

Gonzalez C, Fidone S, Obeso A (1979) Tris buffer: effects on catecholamine synthesis. J Neurochemistry 32:1143–1145

Grillo MA, Comroe TH Jr, Jacobs L (1974) A combined fluorescence histochemical and electron microscopic method for studying special monoamine-containing cells (SIF cells). J Comp Neurol 153:1–14

Håkanson R, Juhlin L, Owman C, Sporrong B (1970) Histochemistry of histamine: microspectrofluorometric characterization of the fluorophores induced by o-phthaldialdehyde. J Histochem Cytochem 18:93–99

Håkanson R, Lilja B, Owman C (1969) Cellular localization of histamine and monoamines in the gastric mucosa of man. Histochemie 18: 74–86

Håkanson R, Owman C (1967) Concomittant histochemical demonstration of histamine and catecholamines in enterochromaffin-like cells of the gastric mucosa. Life Sci 6:759–766

Håkanson R, Sundler F (1974) Formaldehyde condensation at reduced temperature. Increased sensitivity and specificity of the fluorescence microscopic method for demonstrating primary catecholamines. J Histochem Cytochem 22:887–894

Hamberger B (1967) Reserpine-resistant uptake of catecholamines in isolated tissues of the rat. Acta Physiol Scand [Suppl] 71:295

Hamberger B, Norberg K (1964) Histochemical demonstration of catecholamines in fresh frozen sections. J Histochem Cytochem 12: 48–49

Harrison F (1975) A simple method for the intracytoplasmic localization of biogenic monoamines in the anterior lobe of the pituitary gland. Histochemistry 44:119–121

Heene R (1968) Histochemischer Nachweis von Katecholaminen und 5-Hydroxytryptamin am Kryostatschnitt. Histochemie 14:324–327

Hess A (1978) A simple procedure for distinguishing dopamine from noradrenaline in peripheral nervous structures in the fluorescence microscope. J Histochem Cytochem 26: 141–144

Hökfelt T (1965) A modification of the histochemical fluorescence method for the demonstration of catecholamines and 5-hydroxytryptamine using araldite as embedding medium. J Histochem Cytochem 13:518–520

Hökfelt T, Ljungdahl A (1972) Modification of the Falck-Hillarp fluorescence method using the vibratome. Simple, rapid, and sensitive localization of catecholamines in sections of unfixed or formalin-fixed brain tissue. Histochemie 29:315–339

Hoyt RF, Bartlett RA, Sorokin SP (1979) A simple fluorescence method for serotonin-containing endocrine cells in plastic-embedded lung, gut, and thyroid gland. J Histochem Cytochem 27:721–727

Jonsson G (1967) Fluorescence methods for the histochemical demonstration of monoamines. 7. Fluorescence studies on biogenic monoamines and related compounds condensed with formaldehyde. Histochemie 8:288–296

Jonsson G (1971) Quantitation of fluorescence of biogenic monoamines. Prog Histochem Cytochem 2:299–334

Jonsson G, Sandler M (1969) Fluorescence of indolylethylamines condensed with formaldehyde. Histochemie 17:207–212

Juhlin L, Shelley WB (1966) Detection of histamine by a new fluorescent o-phthalaldehyde stain. J Histochem Cytochem 14:525–528

King MP, Angelakos ET (1973) Differentiation of noradrenaline and adrenaline-containing cells in the adrenal medulla by the trihydroxyindole histochemical reaction. Acta Histochem 45:61–70

Koe BK, Weissman A (1966) P-chlorophenylalanine: a specific depletor of brain serotonin. J Pharmacol Exp Ther 154:499–516

Kyösola K (1979) Comparative formaldehyde-induced and glyoxylic acid-induced fluorescence histochemical studies on the intrinsic innervation of the intestines and the liver of normal and vagotomized cats. Acta Histochem 62:188–199

Laties AM, Jakobowitz D, Lund R (1967) A simplified method for the histochemical localization of cardial catecholamine-containing nerve fibers. J Histochem Cytochem 15:535–541

Lindvall O, Björklund A (1974) The glyoxylic acid fluorescence histochemical method: A detailed account of the methodology for the visualization of central catecholamine neurons. Histochemistry 39:97–127

Lindvall O, Björklund A, Hökfelt T, Ljungdahl A (1973) Application of the glyoxylic acid method to vibratome sections for improved visualization of central catecholamine neurons. Histochemie 35:31–38

Lindvall O, Björklund A, Svensson LA (1974) fluorophore formation from catecholamines and related compounds in the glyoxylic acid fluorescence histochemical method. Histochemie 39:197–225

Lorén J, Björklund A, Falck B, Lindvall O (1976) An improved histofluorescence procedure for freeze-dried paraffin-embedded tissue based on combined formaldehyde-glyoxylic acid perfusion with high magnesium content and acid pH. Histochemistry 49: 177–192

Lorén J, Björklund A, Lindvall O (1977) Magnesium ions in catecholamine fluorescence histochemistry. Application to the cryostat and vibratome techniques. Histochemistry 52:223–239

Lorén J, Björklund A, Falck B, Lindvall O (1980) The aluminum-formaldehyde (ALFA) histofluorescence method for improved visualization of catecholamines and indolamines. Application on the central nervous system. J Neurosci Methods 2:277–300

Nairn RC (1969) Fluorescence microscopy and photomicrography. In: Nairn RC (ed) Fluorescent protein tracing. Livingstone, Edinburgh London, pp 68–108

Nelson JS, Wakefield PL (1968) The cellular localization of catecholamines in frozen-dried, cryostat sections of the brain and autonomic nervous system. J Neuropathol Exp Neurol 27:221–233

Norberg KA, Ritzen M, Ungerstedt U (1966) Histochemical studies on a special catecholamine-containing cell type in sympathetic ganglia. Acta Physiol Scand 67:260–270

Pearse AGE (1972) Biogenic amines. In: Pearse AGE (ed) Histochemistry. Theoretical and applied, vol 2. Churchill Livingstone, Edinburgh London, pp 1101–1127

Penttilä A (1968) Effect of incubation in Krebs-Ringer solution or humid air on the amine content, fluorescence, and staining characteristics of the duodenal enterochromaffin and dopamine cells. Virchows Arch B 1:269–282

Ploem JS (1969) Ein neuer Illuminator-Typ für die Auflicht-Fluoreszenzmikroskopie. Leitz Mitt Wiss Tech IV:225–238

Ritzén M (1969) Quantitative fluorescence microspectrophotometry of catecholamine-formaldehyde products. Model experiments. Exp Cell Res 44:505–520

Sakharova AV, Sakharov DA (1971) Visualization of intraneuronal monoamines by treatment with formaline solutions. Prog Brain Res 34:11–25

Shore PA, Burkhalter A, Cohn VH Jr (1959) A method for the fluorometric assay of histamine in tissues. J Pharmacol Exp Ther 127: 182–186

Sparring H, Grube D (1977) Die aldehydinduzierte Fluoreszenz-Methode und Anwendungsbereiche. Leitz Mitt Wiss Tech VII: 6–11

Thoenen H, Tranzer JP (1968) Chemical sympathectomy by selective destruction of adrenergic nerve endings with 6-hydroxydopamine. Naunyn Schmiedebergs Arch Pharmacol 261: 271–288

Torre De la JC (1980) Standardization of the SPG histofluorescence method for tissue monoamines. J Neurosci Meth 3: 1–5

Torre De la JC, Surgeon JW (1976 a) A methodological approach to rapid and sensitive monoamine histofluorescence using a modified glyoxylic acid technique: the SPG method. Histochemistry 49: 81–93

Torre De la JC, Surgeon JW (1976 b) Histochemical fluorescence of tissue and brain monoamines: results in 18 min using the sucrose-phosphate-glyoxylic acid (SPG) method. Neuroscience 1: 451–454

Udenfriend S (1969) Principles of fluorescence. In: Fluorescence assay in biology and medicine, vol II. Academic Press, New York, pp 1–41

Ungerstedt U (1968) 6-hydroxydopamine-induced degeneration of central monoamine neurons. Eur J Pharmacol 5: 107–110

Ungerstedt U, Butcher LL, Butcher SG, Anden NE, Fuxe K (1969) Direct chemical stimulation of dopaminergic mechanisms in the neostriatum of rats. Brain Res 14: 461–471

Winkler J (1970 a) Kontrollierte Gefriertrocknung von Kryostatschnitten. Histochemie 22: 234–240

Winkler J (1970 b) Zum Einfrieren von Gewebe in Stickstoff-gekühltem Propan. Histochemie 23: 44–50

Young MR (1961) Principles and techniques of fluorescence microscopy. Q J Microsc Sci 102: 419–449

Bibliography for Microspectrofluorometry, Cytofluorometry, Microfluorometric Quantitation, and Fluorescence Cytophotometry

Agnati LF, Benfenati F, Cortelli P, D'Allesandro R (1978) A new method to quantify catecholamine stores visualized by means of the Falck-Hillarp technique. Neurosci Lett 10: 11–17

Agrup G, Björklund A, Falck B, Jacobsson S, Lindvall O, Rorsman H, Rosengren E (1977) Fluorescence histochemical demonstration of DOPA thioethers by condensation with gaseous formaldehyde. Histochemistry 52: 179–186

Björklund A, Ehinger B, Falck B (1968) A method for differentiating dopamine from noradrenaline in tissue sections by microspectrofluorometry. J Histochem Cytochem 16: 263–270

Björklund A, Ehinger B, Falck B (1972 a) Analysis of fluorescence excitation peak ratios for the cellular identification of noradrenaline, dopamine, or their mixtures. J Histochem Cytochem 20: 56–64

Björklund A, Falck B (1973) Cytofluorometry of biogenic monoamines in the Falck-Hillarp method. Structural identification by spectral analysis. In: Thaer AA, Sernetz M (eds) Fluorescence techniques in cell biology. Springer, Berlin Heidelberg New York, pp 171–181

Björklund A, Falck B, Owman Ch (1972 b) Fluorescence microscopic and microspectrofluorometric techniques for the cellular localization and characterization of biogenic amines. In: Rall JG, Kopin IJ (eds) The thyroid and biogenic amines. North-Holland, Amsterdam, pp 318–368

Björklund A, Lindvall O, Svensson LA (1972 c) Mechanisms of fluorophore formation in the histochemical glyoxylic acid method for monoamines. Histochemie 32: 113–131

Chang CC (1964) A sensitive method for spectrophotofluorometric assay of catecholamines. Int J Neuropharmacol 3: 643–649

Corrodi H, Hillarp NA (1964) Fluoreszenzmethoden zur histochemischen Sichtbarmachung von Monoaminen. 2. Identifizierung des fluoreszierenden Produktes aus Dopamin und Formaldehyd. Helv Chim Acta 47: 911–918

Enerbäck L, Gustafsson B, Mellblom L (1977) Cytofluorometric quantitation of 5-hydroxytryptamine in mast cells: an improved technique for the formaldehyde condensation reaction. J Histochem Cytochem 25: 32–41

Fukuda M, Böhm N, Fujita S (1978) Cytophotometry and its biological application. Prog Histochem Cytochem 11: 1–119

Håkanson R, Owman Ch, Sjölund K (1974) Cytospectrofluorometric characterization of OPT-induced fluorescence in rat pinealocytes. Histochemistry 42: 323–331

Håkanson R, Owman Ch, Sundler F (1971) Fluorescence histochemical and microspectrofluorometric evidence of tryptophyl peptides in thyroid C cells of cat and pig. J Histochem Cytochem 20: 205–210

Jonsson G (1973) Quantitation of biogenic monoamines demonstrated with the formaldehyde fluorescence method. In: Thaer AA,

Sernetz M (eds) Fluorescence techniques in cell biology. Springer, Berlin Heidelberg New York, pp 191–197

Jonsson G, Sachs Ch (1970) Microspectrofluorometric identification of m-hydroxyphenylethylamines (m-tyramines) in central and peripheral monoamine neurons. Histochemie 25:208–216

Knyazev GG, Spiridonov VK (1979) Quantitative estimation of the fluorescence of catecholamines, detected by Falck's method. Neurosci Behav Physiol 9:244–247

Lindvall O, Björklund A, Falck B, Svensson LA (1975 a) New principles for microspectrofluorometric differentiation between DOPA, dopamine, and noradrenaline. J Histochem Cytochem 23:697–701

Lindvall O, Björklund A, Falck B, Svensson LA (1975b) Combined formaldehyde and glyoxylic acid reactions. I. New possibilities for microspectrofluorometric differentiation between phenylethylamines, indolylethylamines, and their precursor amino acids. Histochemistry 46:27–52

Lindvall O, Björklund A, Svensson LA (1974) Fluorophore formation from catecholamines and related compounds in the glyoxylic acid fluorescence histochemical method. Histochemie 39:197–225

Loefström A, Fuxe K, Jonsson G (1976 a) Microfluorimetric quantitation of catecholamine fluorescence in rat median eminence. I. Aspects on the distribution of dopamine and noradrenaline nerve terminals. J Histochem Cytochem 24:415–429

Loefström A, Fuxe K, Jonsson G, Wiesel FA (1976 b) Microfluorimetric quantitation of catecholamine fluorescence in rat median eminence. II. Turnover changes in hormonal states. J Histochem Cytochem 24:430–442

Paul E, Hartwig HG, Illig L, Möller W (1976) Fluorescenzhistochemische Untersuchungen und mikrofluorometrische Analysen an Pigmentbildenden Tumoren der Haut. Arch Dermatol Res 253–125–144

Ritzén M (1966) Quantitative fluorescence microspectrophotometry of catecholamine-formaldehyde products. Exp Cell Res 44: 505–520

Ritzén M (1973) Microfluorimetric quantitation of biogenic monoamines. In: Thaer AA, Sernetz M (eds) Fluorescence techniques in cell biology. Springer, Berlin Heidelberg New York, pp 184–189

Schipper J (1979) A scanning microfluorimetric study on noradrenergic neurotransmission. PhD Dissertation, University of Amsterdam

Schipper J, Ploem JS, Tilders FJH (1978) Microfluorimetric scanning of sympathetic nerve fibers. An improved method to quantitate formaldehyde-induced fluorescence of biogenic amines. J Histochem Cytochem 26:1057–1066

Sprenger E, Böhm N (1971) Qualitative and quantitative Fluoreszenzmikrospektrographie mit dem Leitz-Mikrospektrographen. Histochemie 25:163–176

Thiessen G, Thiessen H (1977) Microspectrophotometric cell analysis. Prog Histochem Cytochem 9:1–158

Vern B, Schuette WH, Whitehouse WC (1975) Sodium fluorescein: a new reference for NADH fluorometry. Brain Res 98:405–409

Chapter 10

Immunohistochemistry and Immunocytochemistry of Nervous Tissue

W. G. Forssmann, V. Pickel, M. Reinecke, D. Hock, and J. Metz

1 Introduction

During the last decade immunocytochemistry has become one of the most powerful tools for localizing specific substances in the nervous system. The method is based on investigations of Coons et al. (1955), Coons (1978) and of Sternberger (1969). Labeled antibodies directed against purified tissue components or substances are used on tissue sections for localization of their binding sites. This technique may be applied for multiple purposes: at the light and electron microscopical level functional systems of the central or peripheral nervous system can be explored, specific metabolic pathways may be analyzed, and pathologic states of nervous tissue may be recognized. Metabolites, enzymes, neurotransmitters, or receptor systems can be localized in the nervous tissue. Thus specific neuronal pathways, functional systems, and metabolic features of the nervous system are revealed at the macro-, micro-, and molecular-morphological level. Considering morphology as an important tool of understanding living processes and pathologic alterations, the basic importance of immunocytochemistry becomes evident, particularly for neuroanatomy. Almost no technique of comparable importance has been developed in the past decade for neuroanatomic studies.

The following chapter will be devoted to immunocytochemical methods in general and to immunocytochemical identification of substances at the light and electron microscopical level. The systems which are considered are (1) neuropeptide hormones (NPH), (2) neuronal enzymes and proteins, and (3) receptor systems.

2 Immunocytochemical Basis

2.1 Basic Principles of the Technique

The immune system of vertebrates protects the individual from foreign invaders, toxic substances, or many molecules which do not exist in the normal individual. The protection system is complex since both cellular and humoral mechanisms are involved. One mechanism of protection is the response by antibodies, i.e., the production of specific proteins (immunoglobulins) by plasma cells which are capable of binding the foreign substances, the antigens. This humoral antibody-antigen reaction includes several steps: (1) penetration of the antigen into the individual, (2) stimulation of antibody production, (3) circulation of antibodies, (4) interaction with the antigen, and (5) elimination of the antigen.

The antibody formation is known to be one of the most specific biologic interaction systems. Specific antibodies can, therefore, be used as a tool for the recognition of molecules of different characteristics. Histochemists have, since the early work of Coons et al. (1955), used antibodies produced and directed against purified substances for the detection of these substances in tissue sections. The major impact of this idea has been that even substances which normally occur in a species can stimulate antibody production if they are modified by coupling to larger carrier molecules, thus forming an antigen. After formation of an antibody against a neuronal substance, various labeling methods can be applied to detect its distribution or localization. The procedure of immunohistology for neuronal tissue is the following: (1) purification of a neuronal substance, (2) use of the neuronal substance as antigen (immunization), (3) isolation of antibodies against the neuronal substance, and (4) staining of tissue sections by incubation with the labeled antibody system.

2.2 Antigens and Antibodies

2.2.1 Antigens

The immune system is capable of recognizing surface structures of macromolecules with molecular weights over 5000. However, the portion against which the antibody is directed, the antigenic determinant, comprises only a minor part of the molecule. Macromolecules stimulating antibody formation are described as being *immunogenic*. Nonimmunogenic, small molecules (haptens) may become immunogenic if they are attached to a large molecule forming a hapten-carrier system. Then the carrier should not alter the specificity of the hapten and the carrier should not become part of the antigenic determinant. In neurobiology antibodies raised for immunohistochemical or radioimmunoassay techniques are mainly directed against small molecules and this requires coupling of the hapten to a carrier; this principle is illustrated schematically in Fig. 1.

The antigens used are (1) purified enzymes, (2) neuropeptides, (3) membrane constituents, or even (4) steroids and (5) biogenic amines. In addition, during immunization nonspecific stimulants (e.g., Freund's adjuvants) are used to increase the immune reaction.

2.2.2 Antibodies

The antibody which recognizes a specific antigenic determinant is a member of a family of large serum proteins called immunoglobulins. These are of a complex of four polypeptides forming a symmetric Y-like structure and contain two identical low molecular (light chain) and two identical high molecular (heavy chain) parts. The chains are joined by disulfide bridges. At the N-terminus, each chain exhibits a variable portion where the surface recognition for the antigen is located and the antigen-antibody reaction takes place (Fig. 2).

Antibodies may be degraded by papain or pepsin, forming proteolytic fragments. Thus smaller molecular fragments containing the complete univalent (Fab fragment) or divalent [F(ab')$_2$ fragment] binding sites of the antibodies are obtained. This is of importance because the nonbinding site, the Fc fragment which may produce nonspecific interactions in immunohistochemical reactions can be eliminated. In certain systems an immunohistochemical reaction may be carried out using Fab fragments. The schematic drawing indicates the features of this digestion reaction (Fig. 3).

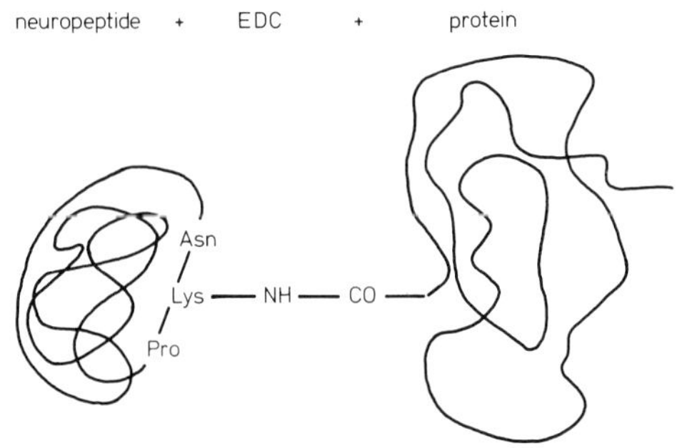

Fig. 1. Schematic drawing of a possible coupling reaction using 1-ethyl 3-(3-dimethylamino-propyl)-carbodiimide-HCl (EDC). The carrier (protein) increases the size and antigenicity of the neuropeptide which becomes a sort of a hapten

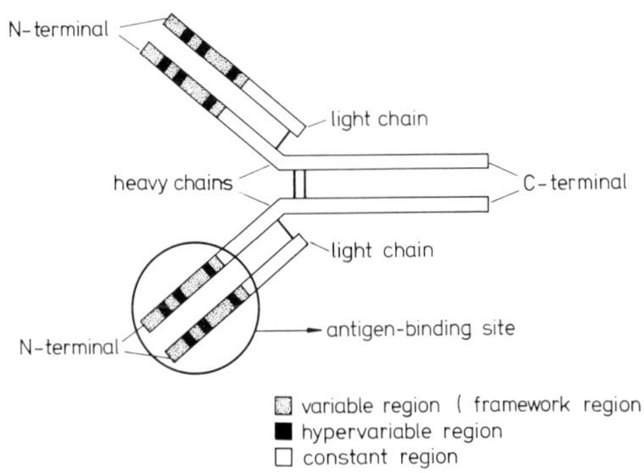

Fig. 2. Schematic drawing of the antibody structure (IgG): Four amino acid chains (two heavy and two light chains) are symmetrically linked by disulfide bridges forming a Y-like molecule. At the variable ends the specific binding sites are expressed according to the antigen used for immunization

2.3 Production of Antisera and Antibodies

2.3.1 Choice and Purification of Antigens

The molecules used as antigens have to be isolated biochemically in highly purified form before immunization since crude mixtures may give heterologous antisera against various tissue components. On the other hand, crude tissue extracts may also be applied for immunization and as a hazard specific antibodies against certain unknown substances of nervous tissue may be obtained which can then be analyzed by immunohistochemical methods. Although, at present, this technique is rarely applied it may be useful for detecting so far unknown substances of specific areas in the central and peripheral nervous system. On the other hand, well-known molecules may be used for immunization not only from

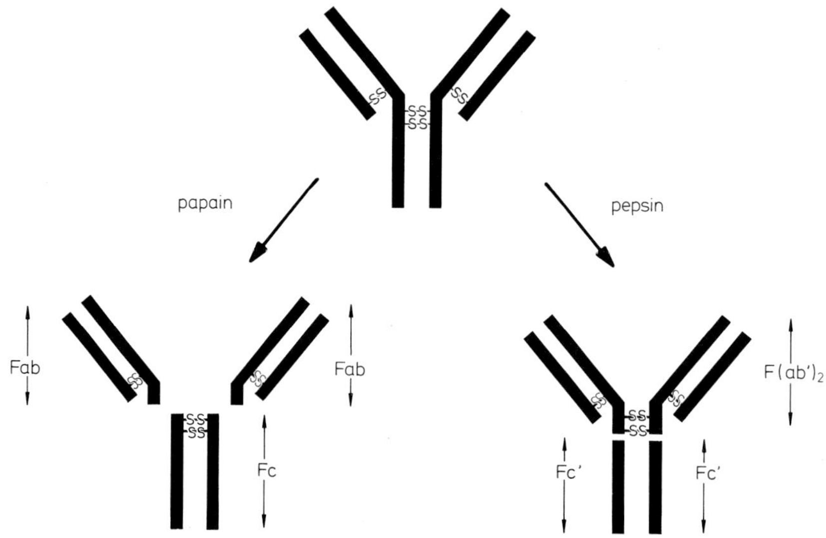

Fig. 3. Digestions of the antibody by papain and pepsin. These reactions provide a possibility to obtain more specific subfractions of the antigen binding site. Radioimmuno-control of the antibody titer after immunization against a neuropeptide

purified tissue extracts but also as synthetic entire molecules or fragments to obtain antibodies which are region specific. Summarized: (1) impure tissue extracts, (2) pure natural molecules, (3) synthetic molecules, or (4) fragments of synthetic molecules may be applied for one or another reason. For detailed description of the purification of neuronal substances biochemical method editions have to be consulted. However, many of the neuronal substances (i.e., neuropeptides) are now commercially available in natural or synthetic form and thus need not be produced by the neuroanatomist.

2.3.2 Techniques of Immunization

Immunization may be carried out with the rabbit, guinea pig, sheep, or goat. As the immune reaction in rabbits is generally easy to stimulate, this species is most commonly used. Various schedules of immunization have been successfully used, including different techniques of coupling smaller molecules with carriers. All these techniques include the application of adjuvants which unspecifically stimulate the immune system:

Adjuvant. A wide variety of substances are known which potentiate the humoral antibody response to injected immunogens. The mixtures mostly used in the preparation of reagent antibodies are "complete" and "incomplete" Freund's adjuvants. In the case of very weak antigens, an additional prestimulation of the immune system with pertussis or diphtheria toxin may be necessary.

Polyvinylpyrrolidone Adsorption. This method is applied for larger peptides and other large molecules. Neuropeptides with less than about 20 amino acid residues give such a limited reaction that these may only be used with a carrier coupling method. One hundred to two hundred milligrams peptide and 1 g polyvinylpyrrolidone are first emulsified with about 1 ml of complete Freund's adjuvants. Various injections are made intracutaneously as described below. The development of the reaction may be controlled by radioimmunoassay or immunohistochemistry. All accessory techniques are as mentioned with the carrier techniques.

Carrier Technique. Larger proteins such as albumin, thyroglobulin, or hemocyanin are coupled with either carbodiimide or glutaraldehyde to the antigen. Also antibodies, for example against somatostatin, conjugated with β-globulin have been used successfully (Arimura et al. 1975). The following methods are recommended:

1. Carbodiimide Coupling. A mixture of neuropeptide, bovine serum albumin (BSA-Serva 11920), and carbodiimide in phosphate buffer is thoroughly stirred for 60 min and dialysed against a 0.05 M sodium phosphate buffer at pH 7.4 for 24 h. The mixture contains 2 mg neuropeptide in 0.5 ml sodium phosphate buffer 0.05 M, 8 mg BSA in 1.0 ml sodium phosphate buffer 0.05 M, and 50 mg 1-ethyl-3 (3 dimethylaminopropyl) carbodiimide HCl (Biomol 04148) in 0.5 ml sodium phosphate buffer 0.05 M.

2. Glutaraldehyde Coupling. A mixture of neuropeptide, bovine serum albumin, and glutaraldehyde (Biomol 11245) prepared as described above is used (1 mg neuropeptide in 1 ml sodium phosphate buffer 0.05 M, 5 mg BSA in 1 ml sodium phosphate buffer 0.05 M and 2.0 ml glutaraldehyde 0.02 M.

To obtain more reliable results, rabbit serum albumin is used and the antigen coupled with glutaraldehyde is purified by column chromatography.

First, in order to remove polymers, the glutaraldehyde (Taab Laboratory Equipment, Reading, Berkshire, England) is purified prior to use by absorption with activated charcoal Norit A (Sigma) until the purity index (Anderson 1967) is smaller than 0.5. Twenty five milliliters of 25% glutaraldehyde are mixed with 10 ml Norit A and filtered through millipore (0.45 μ pore size). The purity index of the filtrate is calculated according to Anderson (1967) from the ratio of the optical densities at 235 nm : 280 nm.

Further rabbit serum albumin is obtained on a Blue Sepharose CL-6B (Pharmacia) column equilibrated with 0.05 M Tris/HCl buffer (pH 7.0) containing 0.1 M KCl. One hundred milliliters of rabbit serum are applied to the column and then rinsed with the same buffer until the optical density at 280 nm is smaller than 0.01. Albumin is eluated with 0.05 M Tris/HCl pH 7.0 containing 1.5 M KCl. The product is dialyzed with an Amicon pressure chamber, and lyophilized.

The coupling reaction is made in 1 ml 0.1 M sodium bicarbonate buffer at pH 9.5 to which 10–40 mg rabbit serum albumin has been added. This solution is added dropwise to 5 ml glutaraldehyde which is thoroughly stirred. The albumin-glutaraldehyde is run through a Sephadex G 25 column (3.6 × 20 cm) equilibrated with 0.9 g sodium chloride. At extinction 280 µm 30% of the shoulder is disused from the curve. The product is concentrated to about 1–2 ml in an Amicon chamber. Ten to one hundred times the molar ratio of the neuropeptide is reacted for 12 h with the albumin-glutaraldehyde and purified with the same amount of 50 mM glycine and 50 mM ethanolamine (Merck 844) in sodi-

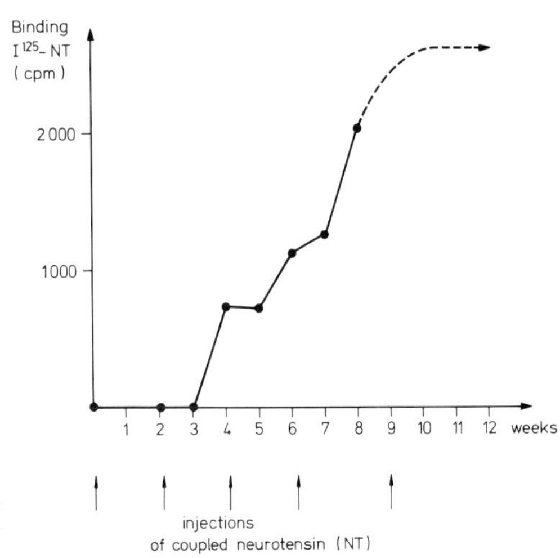

Fig. 4. Example of an immunization against neurotensin (NT) using neurotensin-albumin coupled with glutardialdehyde

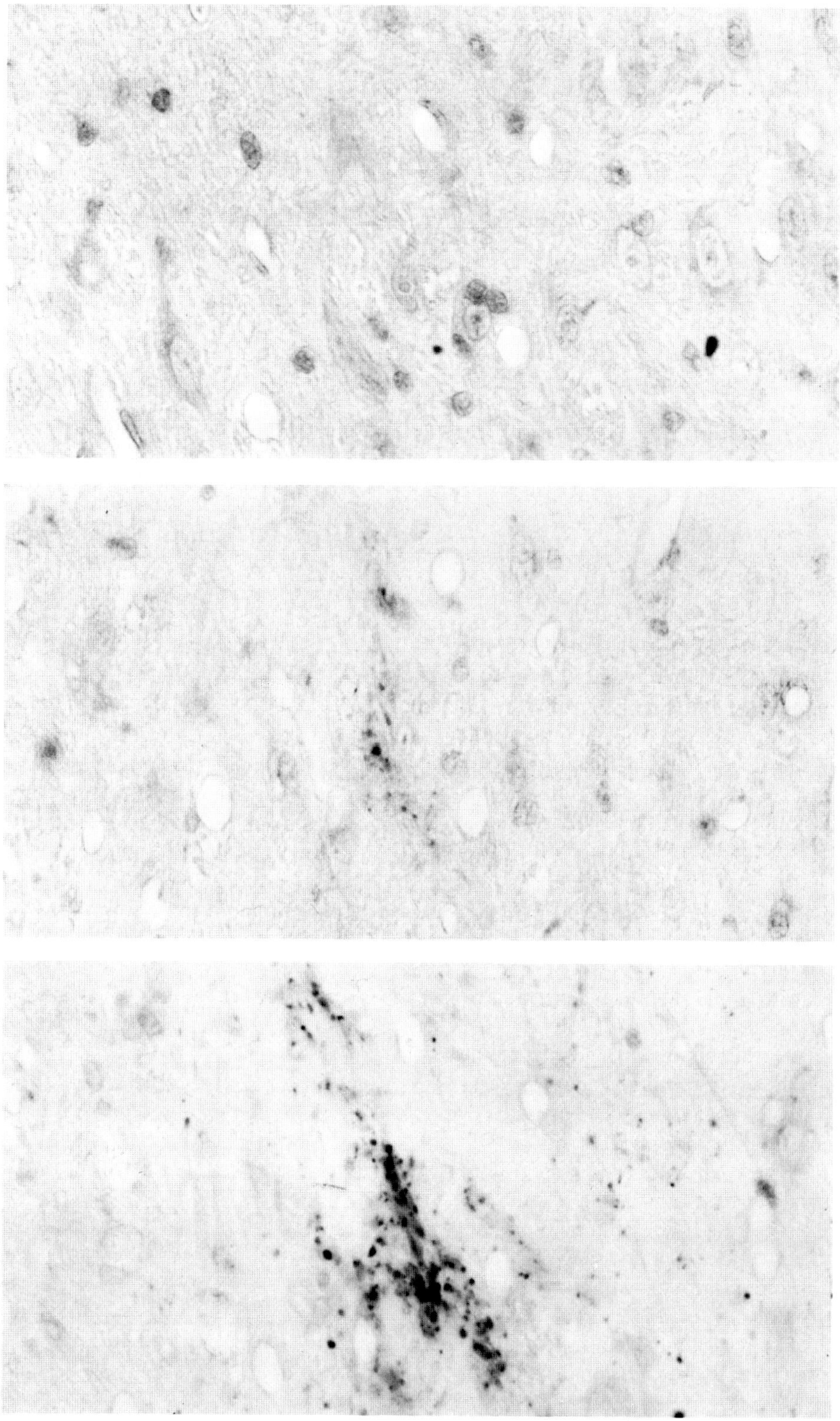

a

b

c

um acetate buffer at pH 4.5 to block the unreacted aldehyde groups on a Sephadex G 25 fine column.

Immunization. For immunization of large animals such as the rabbit, sheep, or goat, small to moderate amounts of antigen should be used (0.01–1.0 mg/kg body wt. for the whole procedure). Among the different routes of administration of the antigen which are used to evoke a humoral response – e.g., intramuscularly, subcutaneously, intradermally, intraperitoneally, or intravenously – the procedure for subcutaneous application will be described in more detail:

The animals are carefully kept in clean cages and small plaques on the paws, and different abdominal and thoracic regions are shaved before the injection. A first series of intracutaneous injections are made with about 50 mg coupled antigen in 50 μl distilled water emulsified in equal volume with complete Freund's adjuvants. The injection is repeated after 14 days and then in time intervals of 14–21 days up to 20 weeks using a five times higher dose of coupled antigen emulsified in incomplete Freund's adjuvants. During the entire period regular controls with serum are carried out to test the titer of antibody formation both by radioimmunoassay (Fig. 4) or by immunocytochemistry (Fig. 5).

2.3.3 Use of Crude Antisera and Purified Antibodies

The precision of the immunohistochemical reaction (Fig. 6) depends on whether crude antisera or purified antibodies are used for the primary antibody incubation (Fig. 7). Without going into further details the steps of precision may be mentioned here:

Crude Antiserum. This contains an undefined number of co-reacting substances, particularly other antibodies which do not result from the specific immunization against a neuropeptide or a neuronal substance.

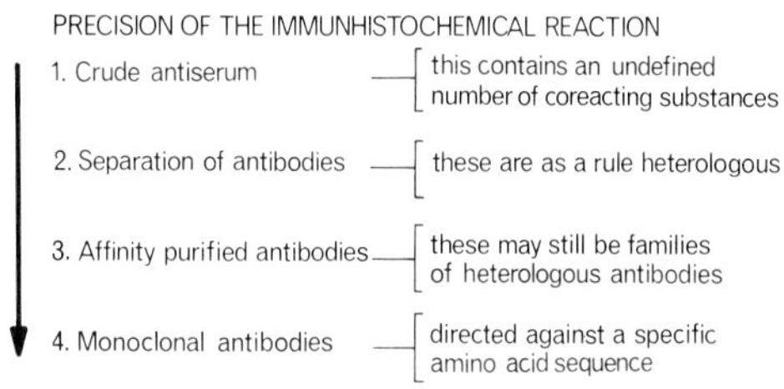

Fig. 6. Possibilities to increase the purity of the antiserum. See also Fig. 7

Purification of Antiserum. The immunoglobulins within the blood serum can be purified using (1) protein A, (2) affinity chromatography, or (3) monoclonal antibody methods:

1. Protein A Method. IgGs of blood serum which consist of a population of heterologous antibodies are separated on a protein A column (Pharmacia). This method offers the advantage that not only antibodies might be separated which are related to several regions of the antigen molecule, but also unspecific antibodies (IgGs fractions) can be removed.

2. Affinity Chromatography. Immunospecific antibodies can be prepared by passing antiserum against a certain neuropeptide through an immunoadsorbent column containing the neuropeptide "as antigen" chemically coupled to an inert solid carrier (glass beads, CNB sepharose). Specific antibody combines with the immobilized neuropeptide and is eluted subsequently with "chaotropic" ions or low pH buffers.

Fig. 5. Immunohistochemical control of immunization against substance P: **a** preimmune serum without any reaction; **b** adjacent section stained with the serum after 6 weeks: Note a few stained varicosities of the zona intermedia of guinea pig spinal cord; **c** strong staining of the same area as in the previous sections by serum taken after the 10th week. ×670

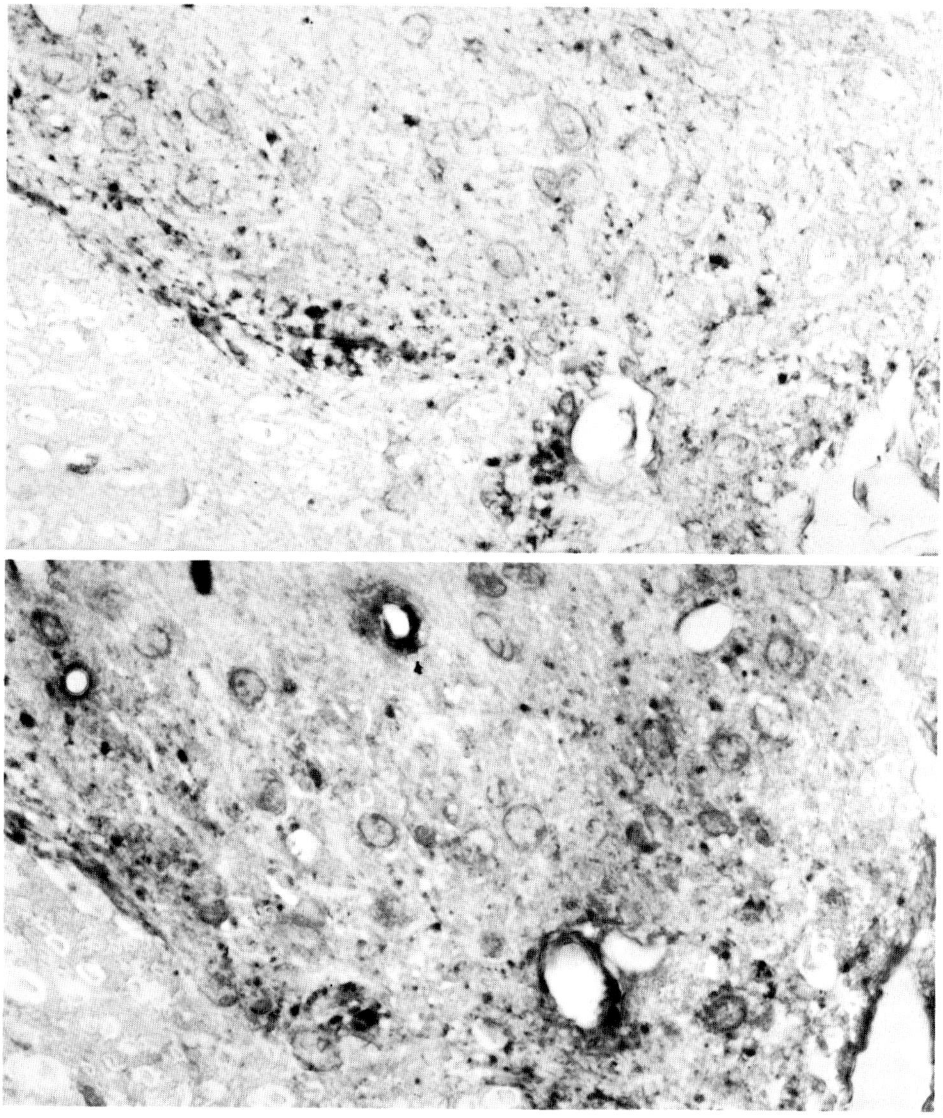

Fig. 7. Immunohistochemical reaction of a crude antiserum and a purified antibody (step 3, Fig. 6) against neurotensin in guinea pig spinal cord (substantia gelatinosa). **a** Crude antiserum. Note false reactions with endothelium and the considerable background. **b** Purified antibody. Only the varicosities are stained; no visible background. ×690

3. Monoclonal Antibodies. This method is the optimal method for the production of region-specific antibodies against neuropeptides (see below).

2.3.4 Monoclonal Antibodies

An extremely valid tool for immunocytochemistry is the production of monoclonal antibodies (Fig. 8). This technique has been developed during recent years for many purposes in immunobiology (Köhler and Milstein 1975; Shulman et al. 1978; Milstein et al. 1979; Galfré et al. 1977; Zarling and Kuns 1980) and has most recently also been applied for the visualization of a neuropeptide (Cuello et al.

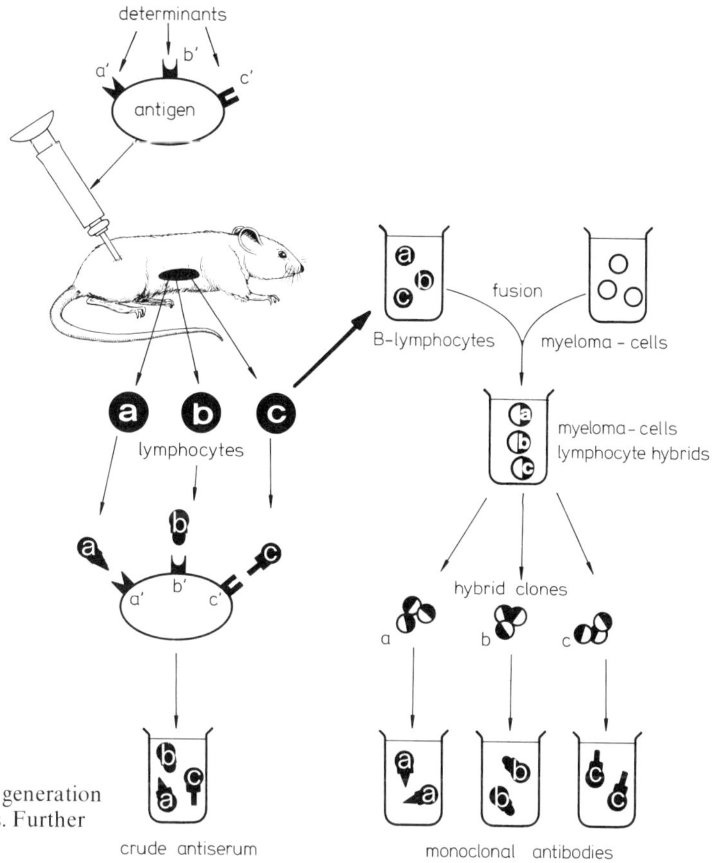

Fig. 8. Principle of the generation of monoclonal antibodies. Further description see text

1979). The basis of this method is seen in Fig. 1. A antigen generally produces heterologous antibodies against several determinants (e.g., segments of amino acid chains in peptides). Thus a reaction with a crude antiserum or purified antibodies may be directed against various parts of the demonstrated molecule. The homologous antibodies of one specific type stem from one clone of B-lymphocytes. If the B-lymphocytes are fused with myeloma cells, the machinery of homologous antibody production can be transferred into a reproducible and long-living cell line. The hybrid cells can be cultured and isolated as clones each of which produces one homologous antibody. The technique although being complicated and expensive will certainly be of the utmost importance in neuroimmunohistochemistry since (1) sequence specific antibodies can be raised, (2) the specificity of antibodies is optimal, and (3) the in vitro synthesis of monoclonal antibodies results in high yields.

For details of this recently developed method publications of Milstein, Köhler, and particularly of Cuello are recommended (Cuello et al. 1979, Cuello and McQueen 1980).

2.4 Immunocytochemical Reactions

The purpose of the immunocytochemical reactions is to localize the specific antibody-antigen complex on the tissue section. As the antibody-antigen complex is not visible directly with microscopic

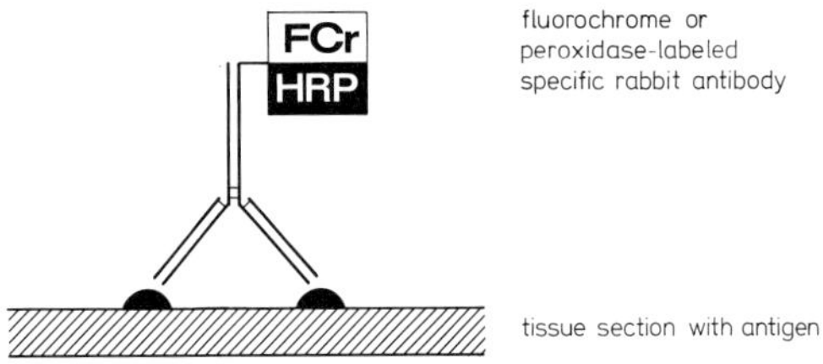

Fig. 9. Schematic drawing of immunohistochemical reactions using the direct antibody labeling

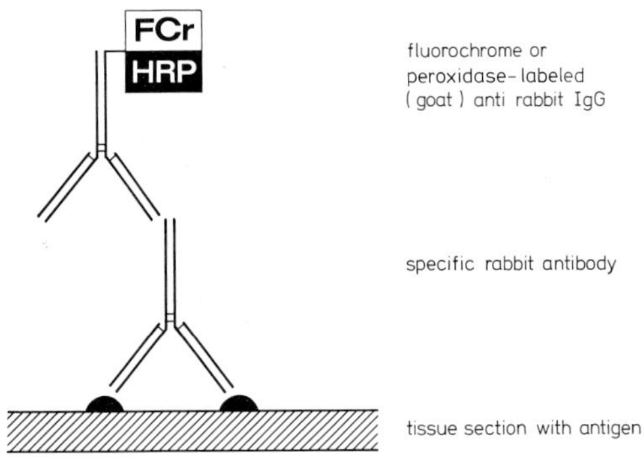

Fig. 10. Schematic drawing of immunohistochemical reactions using the indirect antibody labeling

means, a labeling system has to be combined with the antibody. Various direct and indirect labeling systems have been developed.

Whereas in the direct labeling methods the label is coupled with the specific antibody (Fig. 9), in the indirect methods the antibody-antigen complex is detected with a labeled secondary antibody directed against the specific primary antibody (Fig. 10). The methods have been extensively reviewed by Sternberger (1979) and will only briefly be mentioned here.

2.4.1 Immunofluorescence

The principle of the immunofluorescence methods is that fluorochromes such as fluorescein isothiocyanate (FITC) (Behringwerke 0105 F), giving a green fluorescence or rhodamine B isothiocyanate (RITC) (Sigma, R 5751) giving a red fluorescence are used for the detection of specific antibody after its binding to the antigen. The antiserum applied is either directly labeled with the fluorochrome (direct immunofluorescence) or unlabeled and the fluorochrome is applied in a second step by use of a fluorochrome-labeled antibody directed against the IgG of the species in which the specific antiserum was raised (indirect immunofluorescence).

The sensitivity of the indirect method is tenfold higher than that of the direct method which is the least sensitive of all immunocytochemical methods (Coons 1956). The major disadvantages of both techniques are (1) the high amount of antiserum which has to be applied and (2) the fading of the fluorescence stain.

2.4.2 Enzyme-Labeled Antibodies

The enzyme-labeled antibody methods correspond to the direct and the indirect fluorescence methods, but the fluorochrome is replaced by an enzyme. Mainly horseradish peroxidase is used as an enzyme, 3,3′-diaminobenzidine (DAB) tetrahydrochloride (Fluka 32750) as an electron donor, and hydrogen peroxidase as a substrate (Graham and Karnovsky 1966). The insoluble reaction product is brown. The major advantages of these methods are that they (1) result in permanent preparations and (2) can be applied both for light and electron microscopic studies. However, the sensitivity of enzyme-labeled antibody techniques is not higher than that of immunofluorescence.

2.4.3 Unlabeled Antibody Peroxidase-Antiperoxidase (PAP) Technique

The sensitivity of the unlabeled antibody peroxidase-antiperoxidase (PAP) technique (Sternberger 1969) is 20–125 times higher than that of the other immunocytochemical methods. It consists of the following four steps (Fig. 11):

1. Incubation of the section with a high dilution of the specific primary antiserum raised in species A. This antiserum is directed against the molecule to be detected.
2. Incubation with an excess of an antiserum raised in species B and directed against the IgG of species A.
3. Incubation with peroxidase-antiperoxidase (PAP complex). The antiperoxidase is raised in species A.
4. Incubation with 3,3′-diaminobenzidine tetrahydrochloride (DAB) as electron donor and hydrogen peroxide as substrate for the peroxidase.

For light microscopic investigations the PAP technique can be used also to localize two antigens in tissue sections (Sternberger and Joseph 1979) by carrying out the reaction in two sequences. The first sequence is as described above and thus result in a brown reaction product. However, in the second sequence the antiserum to a second antigen is followed by an anti-IgG, PAP, and then by hydrogen peroxide and 4-chloro-1-naphthol (Merck 1195) yielding a blue reaction product.

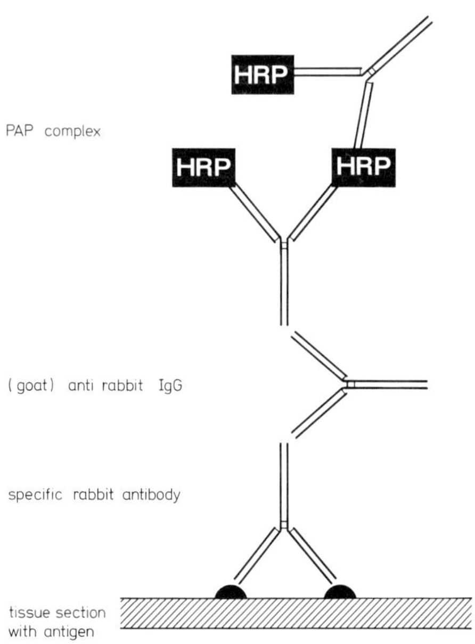

Fig. 11. Schematic drawing of unlabeled antibody peroxidase-antiperoxidase (PAP) technique

2.4.4 Immunocolloidal Reactions

Protein A (pA), a protein of the cell wall of *Staphylococcus aureus,* has a characteristic ability to interact with the Fc fragment of IgG molecules from several species (e.g. Biberfeld et al. 1974; Wright et al. 1977). It has been introduced for the localization of different antigens at the light and electron microscopic levels. The pA technique has been used in combination with ferritin (Bächi et al. 1977; Templeton et al. 1978), peroxidase (Dubois-DalcQ et al. 1977), and especially with colloidal gold (Romano and Romano 1977; Roth et al. 1978) as optic markers.

Colloidal gold is prepared in monodisperse (diameter about 150 Å; Frens 1973) or polydisperse (diameter about 30–120 Å; Zsigmondy and Thiessen 1925) solutions (Faulk and Taylor 1971; Romano et al. 1974). Protein A is added to the colloidal gold suspension forming a noncovalent binding complex by interaction of the positively charged groups of pA with the negatively charged surface groups of the gold particles (Roth et al. 1978).

The staining procedure is performed on thin sections of aldehyde-fixed and Epon-embedded tissue (Roth et al. 1978, 1980). In order to preserve more antigenic sites within the tissue which might be damaged by routinely applied dehydration and Epon embedding, a low denaturation embedding for electron microscopy of thin sections might by useful (Kellenberger et al. 1980).

3 Postembedding Staining Methods in Immunocytochemistry

3.1 General

Most of the immunocytochemical detection is carried out by staining directly on tissue sections. Various fixation methods combined with frozen sections, paraffin sections, vacuum-embedded tissue, and plastic embedding for semithin and thin sections have been developed. These methods are reviewed here. We emphasize methods which have successfully or routinely been used in our laboratory.

3.2 Frozen Sections and Fluorescein-isothiocyanate (FITC) Labeling

Frozen sections of fixed tissue have been widely used for mapping neuropeptides in the central and peripheral nervous system (Hökfelt et al. 1975; 1976; 1978 a–c; Schultzberg et al. 1980). The method is combined with immunofluorescence. This includes three major disadvantages: (1) the sections are difficult to cut and cannot be stored over long periods, (2) rather low dilutions of antisera have to be applied, (3) the fluorescent staining fades after a short time and the label can no longer be seen.

The preparation of frozen sections for FITC staining is carried out as follows (Hökfelt et al. 1975):

The animals are fixed by perfusion (e.g., through the left ventricle or the ascending aorta) with a 4% formaldehyde solution (Pease 1962) at 0 °C–4 °C for 20 min and the specimens are kept in the same fixative after dissection for another 90 min. The dissected tissue is rinsed for 20 h in a phosphate buffer saline (0.1 M, pH 7.2–7.4 containing 5% sucrose) and 10-μm frozen sections are cut. The sections are incubated for 30 min at 37 °C in the humid chamber with the primary antiserum at dilutions of 1:20 to 1:80. After rinsing in phosphate buffer saline for 60 min, the sections are incubated for another 60 min with FITC-conjugated antibodies directed against the antibodies of the species in which the primary antiserum was raised. Subsequently the sections are rinsed again with phosphate-buffered saline, then mounted in a mixture of glycerine and phosphate buffered saline (3:1) on glass slides and observed in a fluorescence microscope (Schott B G 12 activation filter and Zeiss 50 secondary filter). All incubations are carried out in porcelain wells and the solutions contain 0.3% Triton-X-100 (Hartmann et al. 1972). If the sections are not observed directly they should be kept in the cold and protected from light to reduce fading.

3.3 Paraffin Sections and PAP Staining

This method has been routinely used in our laboratory and seems to be the actual method of choice for brain mapping for several reasons: (1) the method is rather sensitive so that low antisera dilutions can be used; (2) reliable serial sections of entire brains can be obtained; (3) the brain structure is adequately preserved; and (4) the staining of the sections does not fade during storing or observation for several years. The application of this method for the study of both central and peripheral nervous system is illustrated in Fig. 12.

3.3.1 Fixation

Animals are perfused under Nembutal or ether anesthesia (see Sect. 4.1) through an abdominal aorta cannula (see Chap. 3). A preceding rinse for 10–15 s with heparin-saline solution (9 g NaCl, 0.1 g heparin, 1000 ml H_2O) may be used to prevent blood clotting. The fixative may also be directly perfused, then the abdominal aorta cannula is opened for a few seconds and the fixative introduced in a quick flush. The fixative, a modified Bouin's fluid, (250 ml acid free, 37% formaldehyde, and 750 ml saturated aqueous picric acid) is perfused for 10–15 min at room temperature using the hydrostatic pressure slightly above the systolic arterial blood pressure (ca. 10% higher) of the experimental animal. After 10–15 min the fixative is rinsed

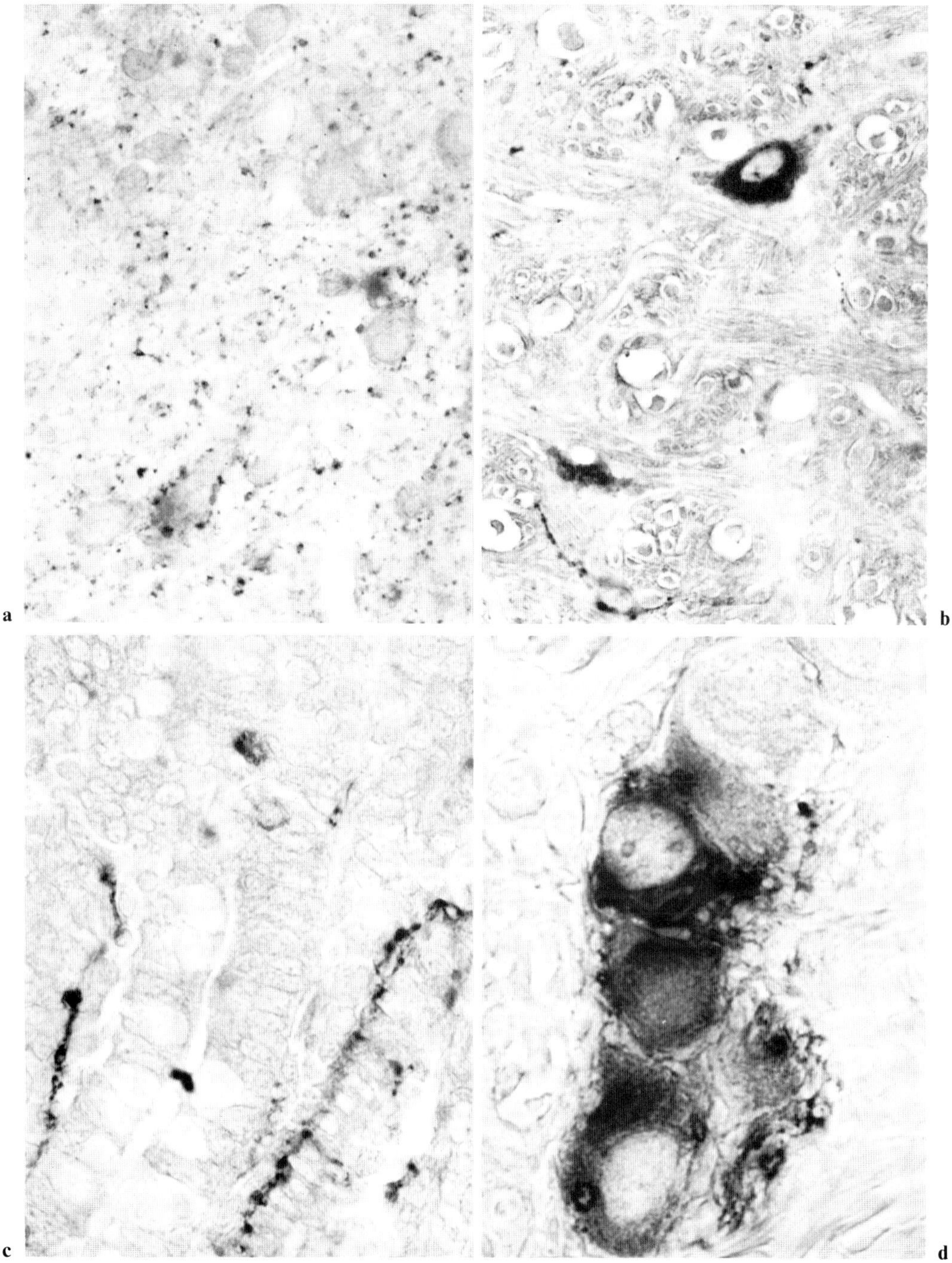

Fig. 12. Various examples of immunohistochemically stained neurons and varicosities in the central or peripheral nervous system using the PAP technique on Bouin-fixed, paraffin-embedded tissue. **a** Somatostatin-immunoreactive nerve fibers and varicosities in Nucleus dorsalis nervi vagi of Tupaia belangeri. Note the high number of stained varicosities at the perikaryon of one neuron. ×600. **b** A somatostatin-immunoreactive perikaryon and several somatostatin-immunoreactive nerve fibers in Nucleus reticularis magnocellularis of Tupaia belangeri. ×530. **c** VIP-immunoreactive nerve fibers in the mucosa of the dog colon. ×640. **d** VIP-immunoreactive perikarya and nerve fibers in a plexus submucosus of the dog caecum. ×1400

out by a saline solution (9.0 g NaCl; 1000 ml H_2O) for about 5 min. The specimens are carefully dissected and placed in 70% ethanol overnight.

3.3.2 Dehydration and Embedding

Dehydration for paraffin embedding is carried out according to the following time schedule: Three changes of 70%, 80%, 90%, and 96% of ethanol for at least 30 min each, then two changes of 100% ethanol for 1 h. According to block size, these times may be prolonged up to 24 h. The time schedule given here corresponds to embedding of entire rat and guinea pig brains.

Thereafter, the tissue is immersed in methylbenzoate (Merck No. 6065) for three changes during 12 h. Then three changes in benzene for 10 min each (Merck, No. 1782) is followed by 2 h paraplast-benzene fluid. Two changes of pure paraplast (Lancer St. Louis, USA) of 60 °C for at least 2 h are made, before the tissue blocks are placed in warm embedding molds which are filled with liquid paraplast. Any bubbles are eliminated with a hot spatula.

The tissue blocks in liquid paraplast are transferred to a cold water bath for 2 h to guarantee a homogeneous hardening of the paraplast block. The blocks are then ready for sectioning.

3.3.3 Serial Sectioning

The oriented block of entire brain may be photographed before final embedding as it is dehydrated or immersed in liquid paraffin. The frontal or sagittal sections are obtained using a routine microtome and mounted on cleaned (ethanol-ether) glass slides covered with a thin glycerin-egg-albumin layer. Two sections of 10 μm are transferred onto each slide and are oriented so that the dorsoventral axis of the brain is perpendicular to the slide and the left brain side is left on the slide, with the label of the slide on the right side (see Fig. 13).

The sections are put on a clean drop of water and the slides kept on a 40 °C hot plate to spread the sections. The sections are dried at 40 °C in an oven for 12 h (overnight). The sections are ready for storing (up to several years) or staining.

In some cases fixation of immunohistochemical procedure may not be adequate due to errors in handling the technique, thus it is recommended that some test slides be stained before the serial sectioning is started.

3.3.4 Staining Procedure

The following solutions have to be prepared for the peroxidase-antiperoxidase (PAP) reaction:

1. Phosphate buffer (PBS):
   Stock solution A (0.2 *M*): Dissolve 27.6 g $NaH_2PO_4 \times 1\ H_2O$ in 1 liter distilled water.
   Stock solution B (0.2 *M*): Dissolve 71.2 g $Na_2HPO_4 \times 2\ H_2O$ in 2 liters distilled water.

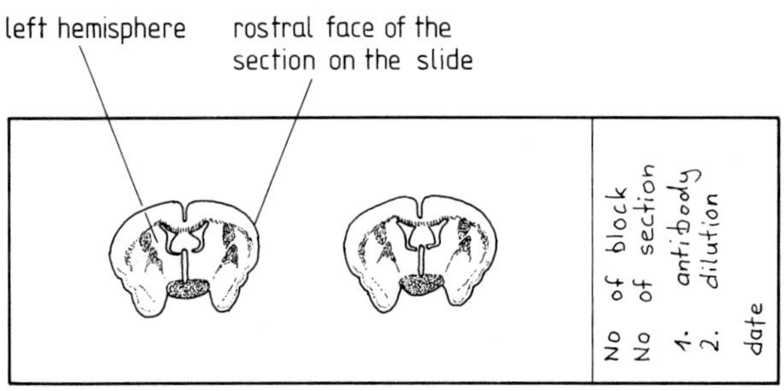

Fig. 13. Schematic drawing of a slide with serial sections used for brain mapping

Prepare the PBS solution as follows:
28.75 ml solution A
96.20 ml solution B
22.40 g NaCl
in 5 liters distilled watcr.
The pH of the final PBS solution is 7.4–7.6.

2. Phosphate buffer (PBS)/normal swine serum (NSS): Dissolve 1 ml NSS in 100 ml PBS.
3. Tris-HCl buffer (0.05 *M*):
Stock solution A: Dissolve 121.14 g tris-(hydroximethyl-)aminomethane in 1 liter distilled water
Stock solution B: 1 *N* HCl
Prepare the final Tris-HCl buffer as follows:
50 ml solution A
40 ml solution B
in 1 liter distilled water.
The pH of the final solution is 7.4–7.6.
4. IgG (Code 21030) is supplied by Boehringer Ingelheim Diagnostika.
5. DAB solution:
Dissolve 37.5 g 3,3′-diaminobenzidine tetrahydrochloride (DAB) (Fluka 32750) in 300 ml Tris-HCl buffer (0.05 *M*) and add 21 μl 30% H_2O_2.
Prepare solution immediately before use.
6. Peroxidase-antiperoxidase (PAP) (Code Z 113) complex is supplied by Boehringer Ingelheim Diagnostika.

3.3.4.1 Schedule for the PAP Technique

1. Deparaffinize sections by transferring the slides in metal racks through two xylol baths, 100%, 96%, 80%, and 70% ethanol, and rehydrate with distilled water (5 min each). Carefully avoid drying of the sections throughout the whole procedure.
2. Rinse sections in PBS/NSS for 10 min.
3. Remove the PBS/NSS carefully all around the sections.
4. Drop a small amount of the diluted (1:2000 to 1:50 000) primary (specific) antiserum (about 10 μl) onto the sections. Incubate the sections in moist Petri dishes for 72–96 h at 4 °C.
5. Rinse twice in PBS/NSS for 5 min and proceed as under 3.
6. Drop anti-rabbit IgG (only if the primary antiserum was derived from rabbits, otherwise an antibody against the IgG of the species in which the primary antibody was raised) diluted 1:10 in PBS/NSS on the sections. Incubate sections for 10 min.
7. Rinse twice in PBS/NSS for 5 min and proceed as under 3.
8. Drop the peroxidase-antiperoxidase (PAP) complex diluted 1:50 in PBS/-NSS on the sections. Incubate for 20 min. The PAP complex must correspond to the species in which the primary antibody was raised.
9. Rinse in TRIS-HCl buffer for 5 min.
10. Incubate in the DAB solution for 10–20 min in the dark while stirring gently with an electric stirrer.
11. Rinse in TRIS-HCl buffer for 2 min.
12. Rinse in PBS for 2 min.
13. Dehydrate sections in ascending concentrations of ethanol and in xylol.
14. Cover sections with "Eukitt".

3.3.5 Evaluation of the Sections (Brain Mapping of Neuropeptides)

Mapping of histochemically demonstrated pathways has become of great importance in understanding brain function, as shown earlier (Dahlström and Fuxe 1964, 1965; Fuxe 1965) for catecholamine neurons and nerves with the Falck-Hillarp method (see also Lackner 1980). Immunohistochemical localization of catecholamine-synthesizing enzymes such as tyrosin hydroxylase, aromatic L-amino acid decarboxylase, dopamine-β-hydroxylase, and phenylethanol-N-methyltransferase has been widely used for mapping (König and Heym 1978). Also, numerous research groups have published immunohistochemical investigations on neuropeptide

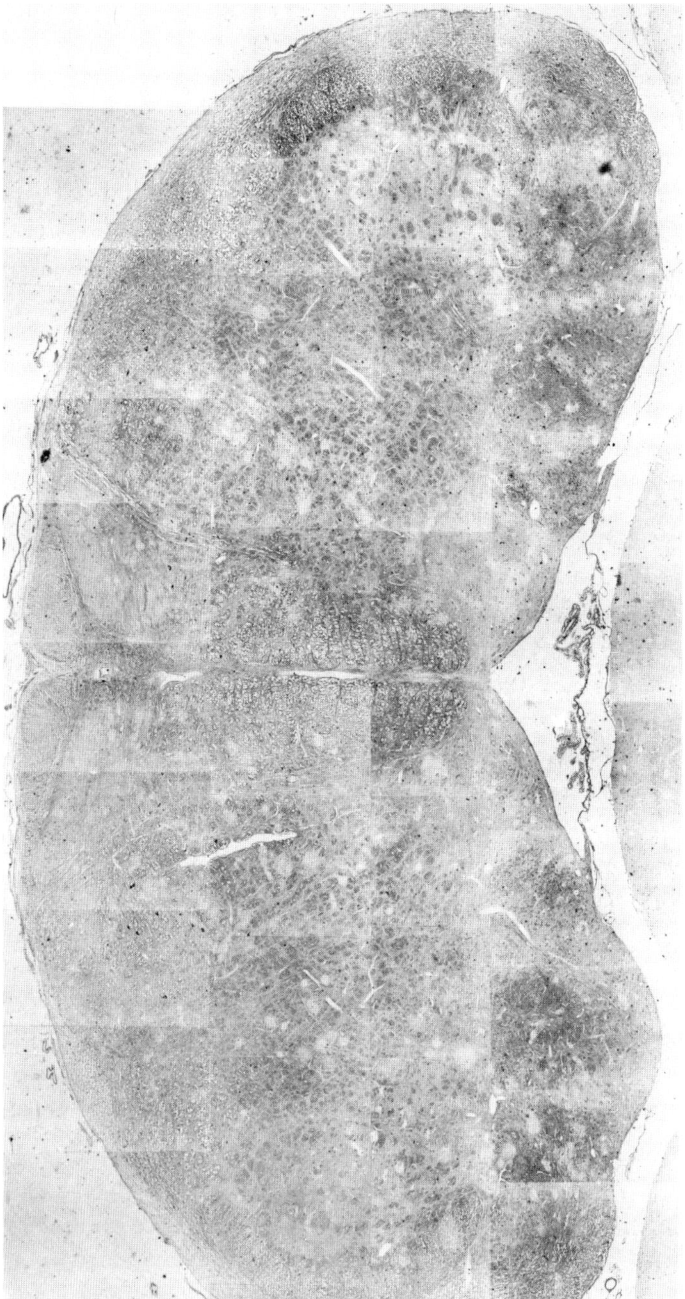

Fig. 14. Montage of a horizontal section of medulla oblongata of Tupaia belangeri. This is a reduced reproduction of a 30×50 cm plate which is used for mapping

Fig. 15. Example of a reproduction of the same horizontal section as in Fig. 14, but from one photograph. This plate can also be used for mapping, but the identification of the tissue structures is inferior compared to that obtained with the montage

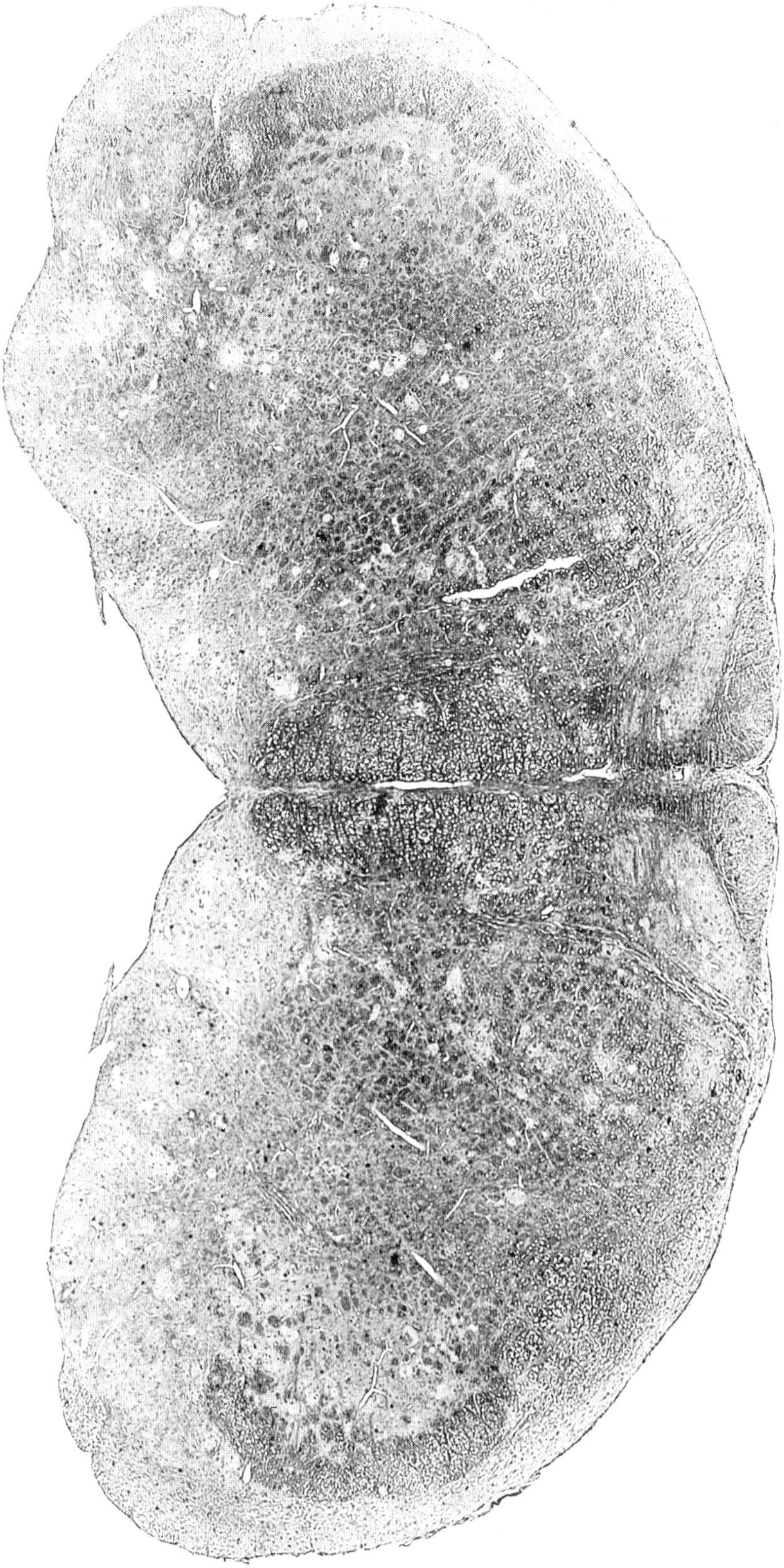

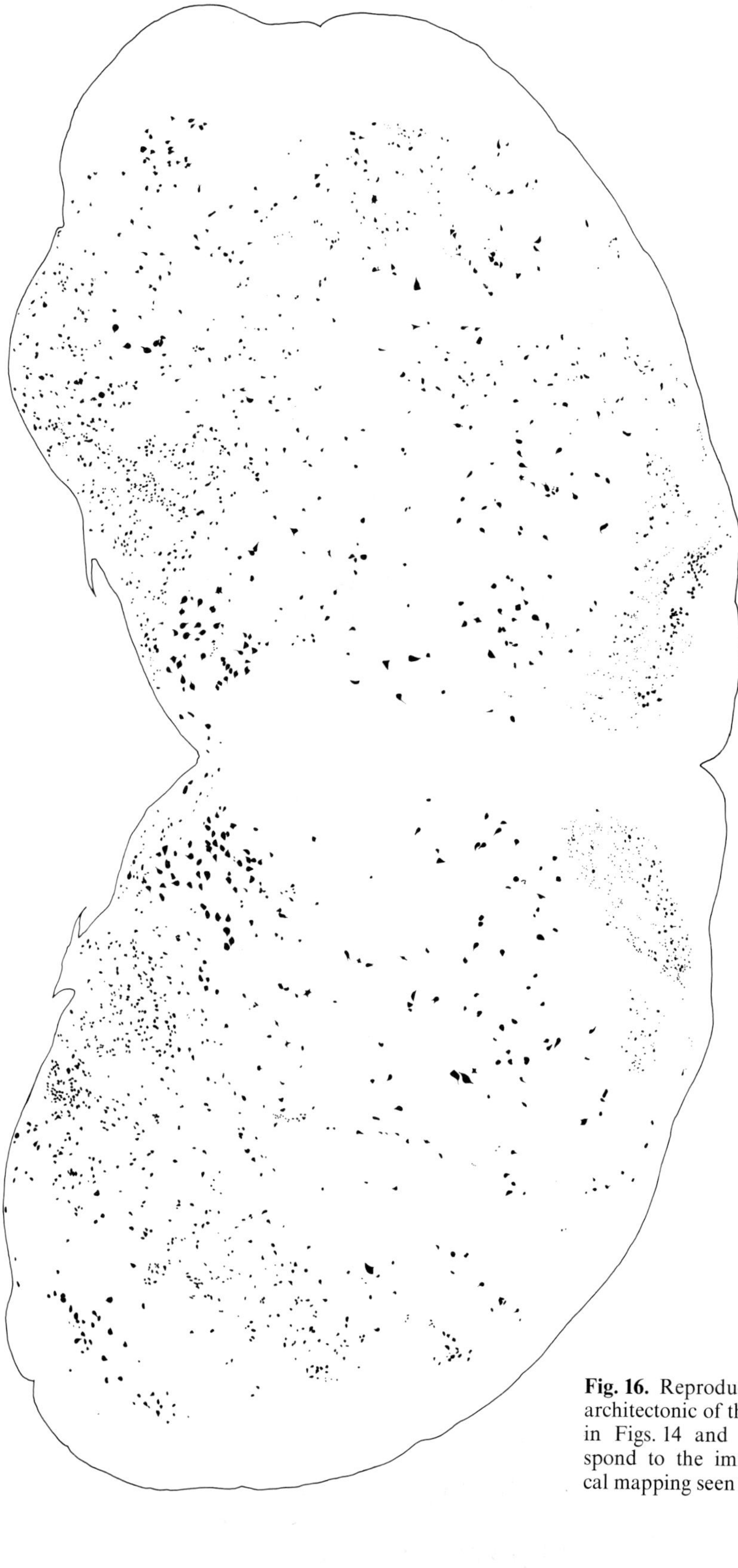

Fig. 16. Reproduction of the cytoarchitectonic of the sections shown in Figs. 14 and 15 which correspond to the immunohistochemical mapping seen in Fig. 17

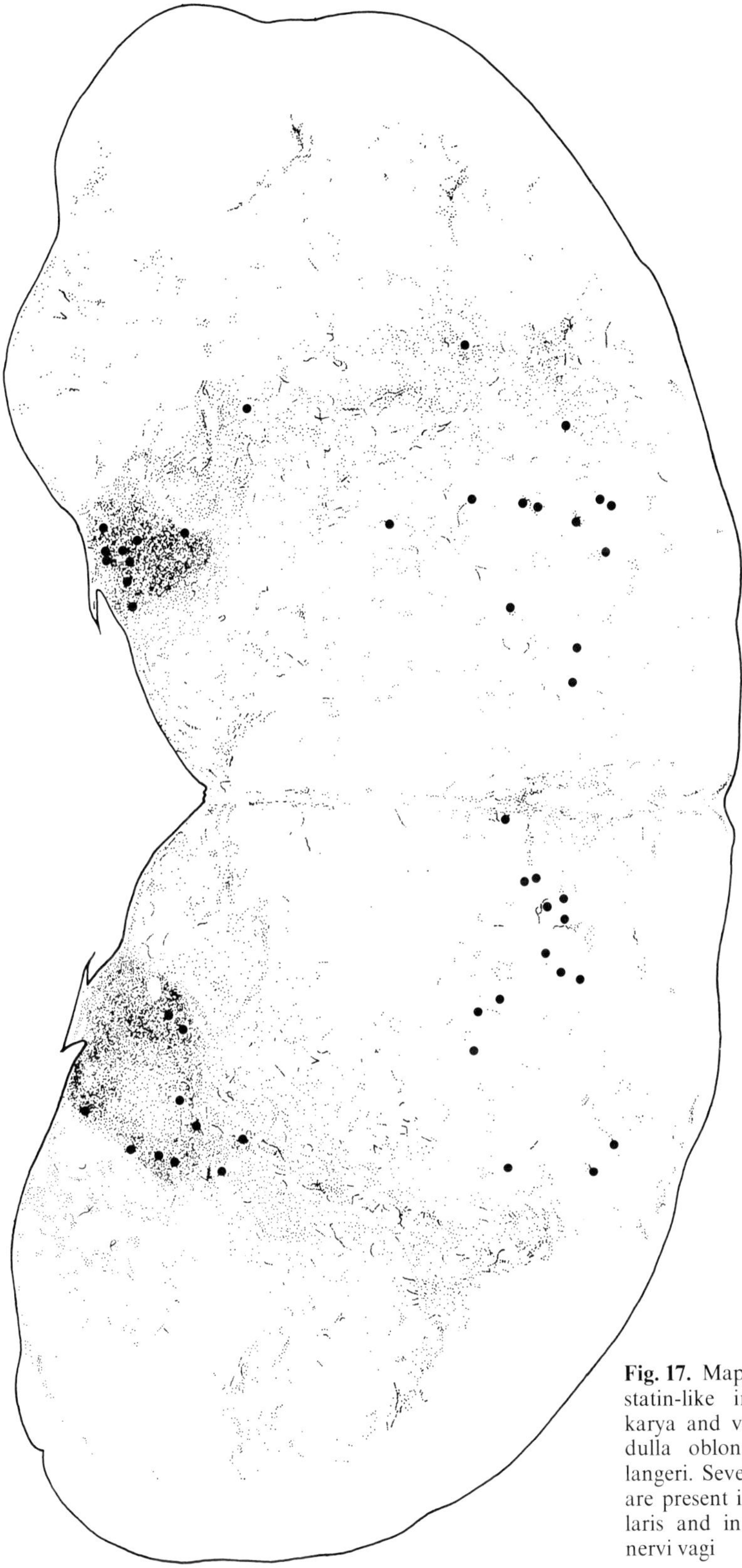

Fig. 17. Mapping of the somatostatin-like immunoreactive perikarya and varicosities in the medulla oblongata of Tupaia belangeri. Several positive perikarya are present in the formatio reticularis and in the nucleus dorsalis nervi vagi

mapping (Hökfelt et al. 1975, 1976, 1977, 1978 a–c, 1979; Pickel et al. 1975 a, b; Cuello and Kanazawa 1978; Ljungdahl et al. 1978; Sar et al. 1978; Burnweit and Forssmann 1979; Costa et al. 1980 a, b; Furness and Costa 1980; Roberts et al. 1980; Sims et al. 1980). However, the mapping methods are quite variable, and mostly semiquantitative. Although many of these studies are carefully carried out, we have tried to improve the mapping technique.

We have therefore used the following method: Sections chosen from the series as mentioned above (see Sect. 3.3.3) are entirely photographed on a Zeiss Axiomat at a determined magnification (objective lens 1:50; optovar 1:3.2) and a montage of the photographed section is made (Fig. 14). Smaller brain sections may be photographed entirely using 9×12 cm glass slide negatives (Fig. 15). Then every positive varicosity and every positive perikaryon is noted on the montage. From this montage a schematic drawing is made containing all information concerning the mapping, including cytoarchitectonic (Fig. 16) and neuropeptide distribution (Fig. 17). Only the size of the positive structures relative to the entire area has changed. The number of positive neuropeptide structures has so far not been so high that the mapping would become inaccurate. At present, the method seems to be optimal until computerized methods become available.

All attempts in our laboratory to use an automatic computerized scanning system for the detection of immunohistochemically stained neurons and varicosities have failed so far because the recognition and discrimination from contrasted but not positive structures (i.e., dirt, precipitations, varying gray tones) was not possible.

3.4 Semithin Sections of Plastic-Embedded Tissue and PAP Staining

The advantage of this technique is that serial sections of cells can be obtained with 0.3–0.5 μm thickness. The method allows the investigation of the same areas of tissue for various antigens and a concomitant localization of several neuropeptides, as well as the performance of adequate control reactions. Although this method has been used mainly for gastrointestinal peptides of endocrine cells (Grube 1980), it is of importance in neuroimmunocytochemistry.

3.4.1 Fixation

The semithin section method can be used with tissue fixed with various techniques depending on the antigen which has to be detected. Therefore, in an initial experiment the appropriate fixation fluid has to be checked. Fixatives such as paraformaldehyde-glutaraldehyde, glutaraldehyde, paraformaldehyde, and picric acid (Bouin's fluid or Zamboni's fixative; Zamboni and DeMartino 1967) may be appropriate.

3.4.2 Removal of the Plastic Embedding Medium (Epon)

For removal of the embedding medium Epon, the sections are exposed to freshly prepared 5% sodium methylate (sodium methoxide) according to Mayor et al. (1961), diluted in methanol and benzol for 1–5 min depending on the section thickness.

The solution is prepared as follows:

5 g of sodium methylate (Merck 806538) are dissolved in 50 ml 100% methanol. Attention! The reaction is exothermic; therefore, a glass of at least 1 liter volume should be used and the procedure should be carried out in a fume cupboard. It is recommended that the methanol level be marked on the glass in order to add

evaporated methanol. Methanol is filled up every 10 min. After dilution of the sodium methylate, 50 ml benzol are added. The solution is gently stirred and another 10–20 ml methanol are added to obtain a transparent mixture. The solution may be filtered before use.

After removal of the Epon the sections are incubated in a freshly prepared methanol-benzol mixture (1 : 1) for 30 s, followed by two changes of acetone (30 s each) and two changes of distilled water (30 s each). Finally the sections are rinsed in phosphate buffer (PBS) for 1–2 min.

After this procedure the sections, together with a small drop of PBS, are transferred by the use of a blunt glass needle onto a glass slide which has been carefully cleaned with ethanol-ether. The glass slide with the sections is dried on a hot plate (90 °C) for about 30 min. Thereafter the sections are fixed on the glass slide and ready for staining.

3.4.3 Staining Procedure

The staining procedure for the PAP reaction with semithin sections of plastic embedded tissue is almost the same as that described for paraffin-embedded tissue. Only three steps in the schedule (see Sect. 3.3.4) have to be changed in the following way:

Step 2: Rinse section in 2% NSS in PBS for 30 min.
Step 6: Incubate sections in anti IgG (dilution 1 : 10 to 1 : 200) for 30 min.
Step 8: Incubate in the PAP complex for 30 min.

4 Preembedding Methods in Immunocytochemistry

4.1 Fixation of Preembedding Staining

For preembedding staining a phosphate-buffered 4% paraformaldehyde-0.2% glutaraldehyde fixative is used. Animals are perfused under Nembutal anesthesia (50 mg/ml Nembutal solution, 0.5 ml per 150–200 g rat, i.p. injection) through the left ventricle for 6 min with the fixative at body temperature. Fixation is continued for another 6 min in situ. The specimens are dissected and left in fixative for another 30–60 min at room temperature before vibratome sections are prepared. If possible the sections should be processed immediately for immunocytochemistry.

Fixation solution:

(A) Prepare a 0.2 *M* sodium phosphate buffer (PBS): Dissolve 17.8 $Na_2HPO_4 \times 2\,H_2O$ (Merck 6580) and 13.8 g $NaH_2PO_4 \times 1\,H_2O$ (Merck 6346) in 500 ml distilled water.

(B) Prepare a 8% paraformaldehyde solution by dissolving 40 g paraformaldehyde in 496 ml H_2O, warm the mixture up to 90°, and add 4% NaOH dropwise until the solution becomes transparent.

(C) Mix (A) and (B) 1:1 to obtain a final solution of 4% paraformaldehyde in 0.1 *M* sodium phosphate, add 30 mg $CaCl_2$, and adjust the pH to 7.4.
For electron microscopy, 4 ml 25% glutaraldehyde are added to 500 ml fixative, giving a final glutaraldehyde concentration of 0.2%.

4.2 Sectioning for Preembedding Staining

Although various methods for sectioning may be used (frozen sections, tissue chopper), for CNS preembedding staining vibratome sectioning seems to be the method of choice. Tissue blocks fixed as indicated are briefly rinsed in 0.1 *M* sodium phosphatase buffer, then glued to a specimen holder using quick setting cement (Loctite 404, Loctite Corp., Newington CT, 06 111). The specimen holder is attached to a vibratome (Oxford, vibratome). The vibratome bath is filled with 0.1 *M* sodium phosphate buffer cooled to 4 °C. Vibratome sections are cut under appropriate conditions (mostly at low speed: 0.5–1, and high amplitude 6–8; knife angle 30°). At room temperature, the sections are then transferred into wells containing 0.1 *M* sodium phosphate buffer.

4.3 Staining Procedure

Antibody staining is carried out in black porcelain spot test plates (A. H. Thomas Co., St. Louis MO). The vibratome sections are transferred during the washes, changes, and incubations by a small wood stick or a brush into new wells containing the appropriate solution. Through all steps the test plates are carefully agitated on a Thomas rotator. The following steps are made:

4.3.1 Tris-Saline Rinse

Two washes with Tris-saline buffer are carried out at room temperature for 5 min. The solution is made from 0.5 M Trizema Base (Sigma Chemical Co., St. Louis, MO), conc. HCl (36%–38%) being added to obtain a pH of 7.6. Then 9.0 g NaCl and 10 ml of goat serum (Grand Island, Biological Company, N.Y., USA) are added per liter of this solution to obtain the final Tris-saline buffer rinse solution.

4.3.2 Triton-Tris-Saline Rinse for Light Microscopy

A 15-min rinse is carried out with Tris-saline solution containing 0.2% Triton X-100 (Grand Island Biological Company) (see Chap. 2). This step provides a deeper penetration of antibodies, but alters tremendously the ultrastructure of the tissue. Thus, it is generally omitted, although in some cases it has been used for electron microscopic studies.

4.3.3 Incubation with Normal Goat Serum

Incubation is carried out for 30 min with normal goat serum (Grand Island Biological Company, N.Y. USA) diluted 1 : 30 to 1 : 50 with Tris-saline. This reaction is carried out to prevent nonspecific binding of the serum with the specific antiserum in step 4.3.4 (see below).

4.3.4 Specific Antiserum Incubation

The specific antiserum is commonly produced in rabbits. If guinea pig, sheep, etc. are used for specific antibody production, the following steps have to be carried out with the corresponding anti-IgG and PAP complex (see below). The antiserum is diluted in Tris-saline containing 1% normal goat serum. The reaction is usually carried out with antiserum dilutions increasing from 1 : 10 to 1 : 10,000 in an initial experiment to check the appropriate dilution for routine studies. Usually dilutions of crude anti-sera between 1 : 500 to 1 : 2000 are finally applied.

The incubation with the specific antibody reaction is carried out at 4 °C for 24 h while continuously rotating the specimens. The antisera in the spot test plates must be kept in a closed moist chamber to prevent evaporation.

4.3.5 Anti-IgG Incubation

This reaction is carried out to produce the link between the bound specific antibody and the PAP complex (see below). Following incubation with primary antiserum the sections are transferred through two washes with Tris-saline containing 1% normal goat serum for 5–8 min at room temperature. Then the sections are incubated for 30 min at room temperature in a 1 : 10 to 1 : 50 dilution of goat-anti-rabbit IgG (Miles Lab. Kankee, Ill.) in Tris-saline. The choice of the dilution depends on the

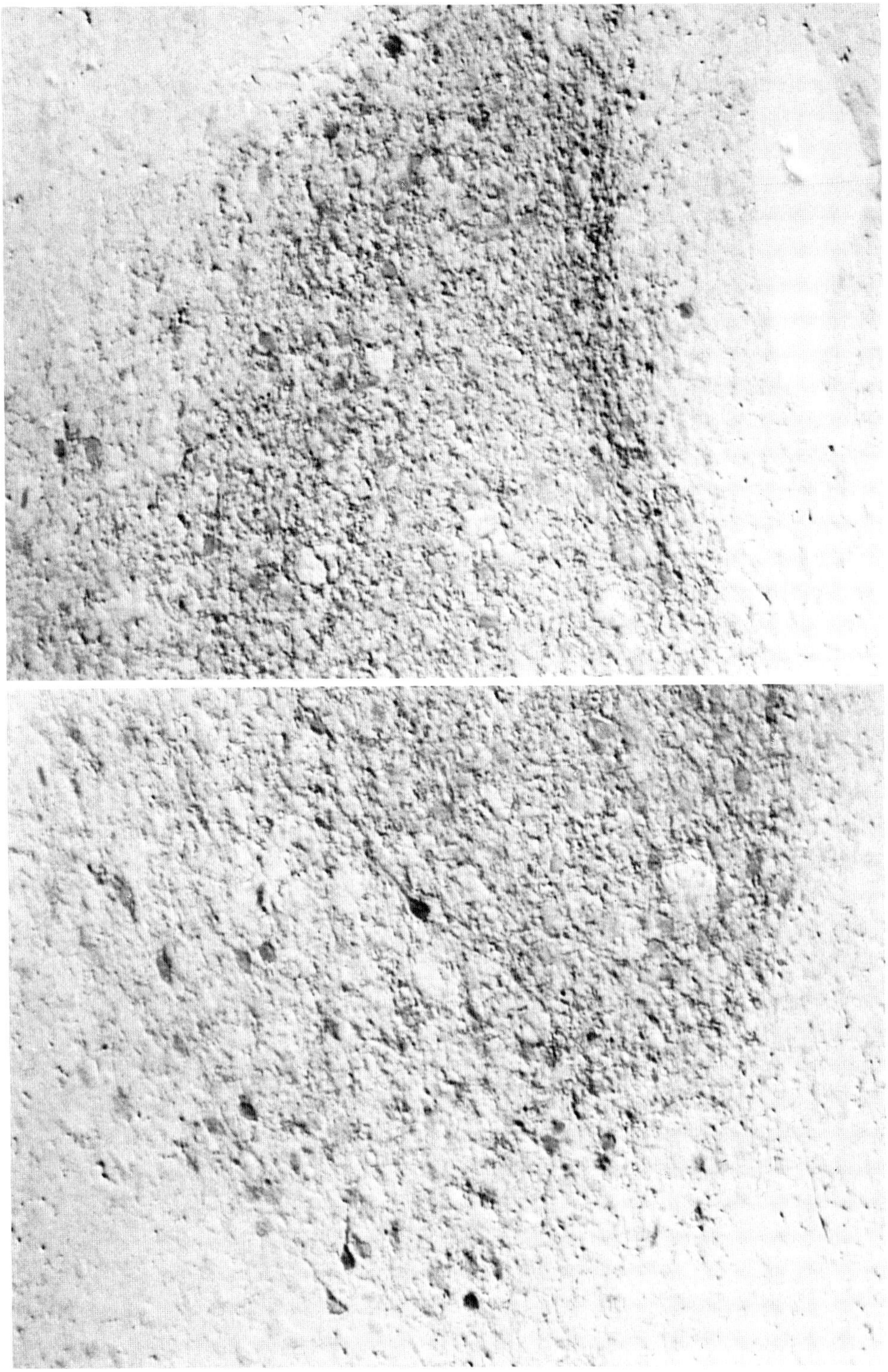

Fig. 18. Light microscopical immunocytochemical localization of substance P in human fetal brain, 17th week of gestation, dorsal tegmental nucleus (Gudden). A dense terminal plexus of substance P is seen throughout the nucleus. Scattered neurons showing immunoreactivity are also seen along the dorsolateral regions of the nucleus. ×400

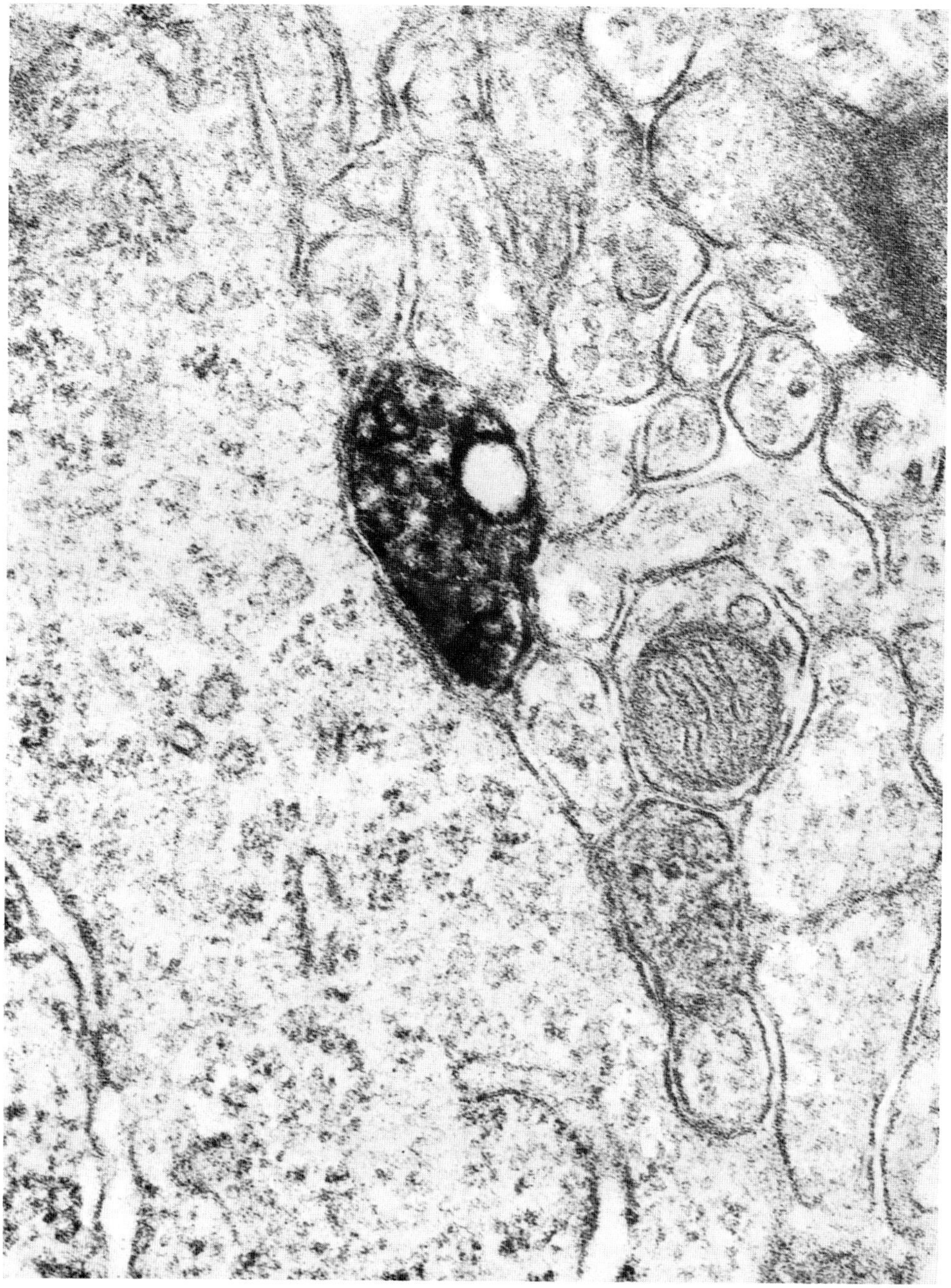

Fig. 19. Neurocytochemical localization of tyrosin-hydroxylase in the caudate nucleus of rat brain. Peroxidase reaction product fills the cytoplasm around the synaptic vesicles. The labeled axon terminal shows a thin postjunctional plaque with the perikaryon of an unlabeled neuron. ×100 000

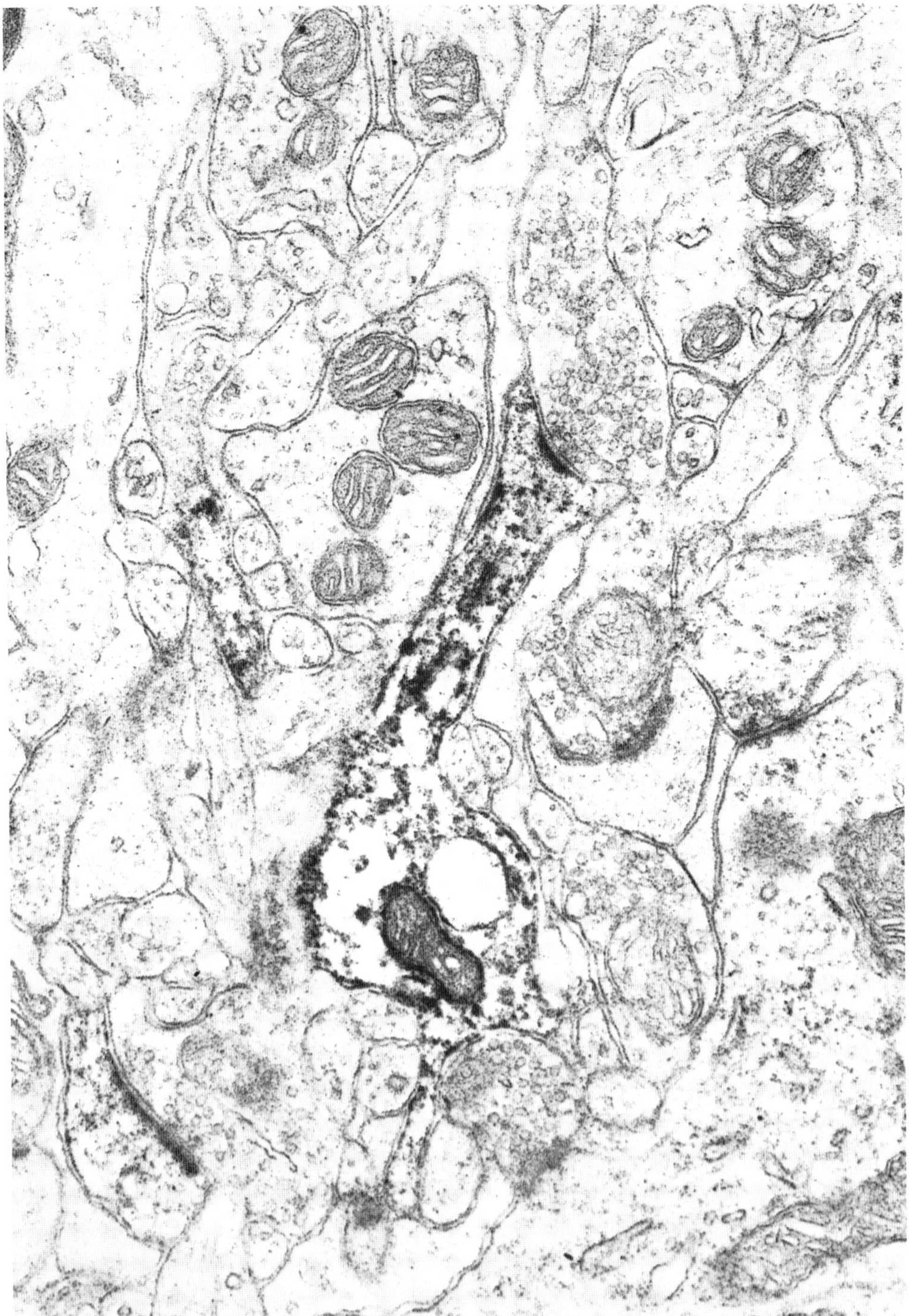

Fig. 20. Neurocytochemical localization of Met-5-enkephalin in a dendrite of a neuron from the rat caudate nucleus. The peroxidase reaction product is located in the entire axoplasm (A). ×50 000

antibody titer and on the final background which increases with the concentration of the IgG solution.

4.3.6 Peroxidase-Antiperoxidase (PAP) Incubation

This reaction is performed to bind the final reacting enzyme peroxidase to the chain of antibodies linked with the detectable antigen. The peroxidase-antiperoxidase complex consists of horseradish peroxidase bound to its antibody obtained from peroxidase-immunized rabbits (or corresponding animals if guinea pig, sheep, etc. specific antisera are used). This method is described extensively by Sternberger (1979). The PAP complex may be produced from Sigma type VI horseradish peroxidase for both immunization and complex formation. The PAP complex is also used from commercial preparations.

The PAP complex is diluted to 1:30 in Tris-saline and the sections are incubated for 30 min at room temperature while being carefully rotated.

4.3.7 Histochemical Peroxidase Reaction

The PAP incubation is preceeded and followed by two washes in Tris-saline for 5–8 min at room temperature. The sections are then incubated in a diaminobenzidine (DAB) solution. The peroxidase enzyme reaction produces a brown reaction product by reducing hydrogen peroxide (Graham and Karnovsky 1966). The reaction is easy to observe on white porcelain test plates. The DAB solution should be freshly prepared and kept from light as long as possible. To 100 ml 0.5 M Tris-HCl at pH 7.6, 12.6 mg 3,3′-diaminobenzidine (Hach Chemical Company, Ames) and 0.12 ml 30% hydrogen peroxidase (Fisher Company) are added. The incubation with this DAB solution is carried out for 5–6 min.

Then the sections are transferred through three 5-min washes with distilled water.

The sections are then processed directly for light or electron microscopic investigation.

4.4 Embedding for Electron Microscopy

For electron microscopy the sections are postfixed for 1–2 h in 2% osmium tetroxide in 0.1 *M* phosphate buffer at pH 7.4 and room temperature (see Chap. 2).

4.5 Evaluation of Preembedding Staining

Results using this technique have been published in numerous papers particularly by Pickel et al. (1975 a, b, 1977, 1979). Light and electron micrographs of preembedding stained nervous tissue are seen in Figs. 18, 19, and 20.

5 Control Reactions in Immunohistochemistry

5.1 The Specificity of the Immunocytochemical Reactions

One of the major problems in the evaluation of immunocytochemistry is the specificity of the localization technique (see Petrusz et al. 1976; Swaab et al. 1977). The ultimate achievement of immunocytochemical localization would be that the localization is restricted to a completely purified antigen of separate identity between the substance used for immunization and that detected in an area of the tissue. For many reasons this can almost never be recommended because antisera or antibodies used in the reaction may detect substances with related antigenicity, the antibodies produced may be related to carrier antigenicity, or nonimmunologic reactions may lead to misinterpretation of the localization technique. There is a wide spectrum of reactions which do not represent the accurate localization mentioned above. In a critical review on immunocytochemistry, Vandesande (1979) divides the reactions into (1) serum nonspecific reactions and (2) method nonspecific reactions. At the actual situation these criteria of evaluation of the specificity can be

BIOCHEMICAL VERIFICATION OF THE IMMUNOHISTOCHEMICAL REACTION

1. Radioimmunoassay (RIA)
2. Combined gel chromatography and RIA
3. Affinity chromatography
4. High pressure liquid chromatography (HPLC)
5. Complete molecular analysis (AA-sequence)

Fig. 21. Biochemical methods which are used as a positive control of immunohistochemical staining

defined more precisely: even if the immunohistochemical reaction may be "correct" and "specific" the representation of a substance may be incorrect. We therefore have to ascertain whether there are (1) cross reactions and (2) false reactions. Also the immunocytochemical reaction should be evaluated by (1) negative and (2) positive controls. The ultimate is that the immunocytochemical localization is shown to be "specific" for a structure which definitively contains the substance biochemically identical to that revealed by the reaction (Fig. 21).

5.2 Cross Reactions

"Cross reaction" is still a term which is variably defined by different authors (Swaab et al. 1977; Sternberger, 1979; Vandesande 1979; Grube 1980). Sternberger (personal communication) includes under cross reactivity the reaction of specific antibodies with tissue constituents which have the same or similar antigenic properties but which are different from the original antigen used for immunization. Vandesande (1979) uses a similar definition. However, in many discussions and publications the term "cross reactivity" is used for any "nonspecific" immunologic reaction in contrast to method nonspecific reactions. In this report we use the terms as follows:

Cross Reactivity: Reactions which are of an immunologic nature related to a stereological configuration of detected antigens which is identical or similar to the stereological configuration in the molecule used as an antigen for immunization. This includes high and low affinity reactions depending on the extent of the molecular similarity:

1. An example for a high affinity cross reaction is that of the detection of neuropeptide families. If gastrin is used as an antigen and an antibody directed against the C-terminal tetrapeptide is obtained, there would also be a high affinity cross reaction with other molecules such as cholecystokinin, caerulein, etc.

2. An example for a low affinity cross reaction is that of the detection of neuropeptides in phylogenesis. Slight variations of the amino acid sequence of peptides do not prevent the immunohistochemical reaction (Reinecke et al. 1980 a, b; van Noorden and Falkmer 1980; Falkmer et al. 1981).

5.3 False Reactions

False reactions are defined similarly to "nonspecific" reactions; however, as the latter includes both immunologic and non-immunologic errors, we prefer this term. A false immunologic reaction is rather frequent and as important as non-immunologic errors.

5.3.1 False Immunologic Reactions

They are due to two reasons: (1) The antigen used for immunization is not highly purified (synthetic or non-synthetic). The antiserum contains antibodies which are not related to the protocolled antigen. (2) The antiserum raised reacts with antigenic determinants directed against the carrier resulting in the detection of carrier-related molecules. Also false immunologic reactions may be caused by antibodies present in a preimmune serum which are not related to the desired immunohistochemical reaction.

5.3.2 False Nonimmunologic Reactions

These reactions are caused (1) by "nonspecific" binding reactions of the primary antibody or (2) interactions of the tissue with the dye. The term "background", which is not precise enough, is frequently used.

Grube and Weber (1980) use the distinctions specific = immunologic = covalent and nonspecific = nonimmunologic = noncovalent binding which can be tested by *quantity* and *avidity* of the binding. If these tests show the nonimmunologic reaction this means either that the antibody is not bound at the variable region of the Fab-fragment or that the antibody is not involved at all in the "false reaction."

5.4 Negative Control Reactions

For both immunologic and nonimmunologic reactions several controls have been offered to suppress the reaction. These are "negative controls", i.e., from the negative reaction it can be concluded whether the initial reaction is specific or non-specific.

5.4.1 Dilution Test with the Primary and Secondary Antisera

The principle of the dilution test is to abolish "co-reactions" with the primary antiserum. At low dilutions the specific antiserum may be even suppressed. Thus, in a dilution series from 1:10 up to 1:10 000 if the reaction appears stronger above 1:2000 then the real dilution effect of a slowly decreasing reaction may become evident. The dilution factor of the primary antisera depends on the method used. In our routine PAP stain (see Sect. 3.3) a specific staining is obtained at 1:2000 or higher. The reactions with lower dilutions of the primary antisera mostly stem from nonimmunologic, nonspecific binding (Buffa et al. 1979; Grube and Weber 1980). Dilution tests of secondary antibodies are of less importance.

5.4.2 Replacement of Steps in the Immunohistochemical Reaction

This control method is also of importance in checking the appropriate immunocytochemical reaction, particularly when testing endogenous enzyme (peroxidase) reaction or nonspecific binding of dye. In the case of replacement of single steps of the PAP procedure this part of the reaction is either completely omitted or carried out using PBS. All the reactivity still appearing afterwards is not related to the specific immunohistochemical reaction.

5.4.3 Absorption Control

The most common way to test an immunohistochemical reaction is the absorption control. This method is based on the principle that the primary antibody is removed or bound by a reaction with the antigen initially used for immunization. Although the removal or blocking of the binding sites suppresses the specific immunologic reaction, an absorption may also suppress other nonspecific reactions, e.g., the complement-mediated reaction etc.; it is doubtful whether it can be concluded that an absorption control discriminates between a specific or nonspecific reaction (Grube 1980).

Absorption control for neuropeptides is carried out as follows: A small amount of the antigen used for immunization is added to the diluted antiserum. The amount of substance to be added depends on the dilution of the primary antiserum. Commonly, 10–50 μg of the antigen are sufficient for absorption, i.e., to abolish the reaction. In a second step the same procedure is carried out with neuropeptides related to the respective antigen. In addition, it may be necessary to preabsorb with other nonrelated peptides. This is indispensable, if the antigen used for immunization is derived from tissue extraction, e.g., immunoreaction against natural glucagon has to be tested by absorption with the other pancreatic polypeptides (insulin, pancreatic polypeptide, somatostatin, etc.).

5.4.4 pH, Ionic Strength, and Suppression of Complement-Mediated Reaction

Recently, the influence of buffer composition (pH, ionic strength) on the specificity of immunoreactions has been investigated using intestinal G cells as a model (Grube 1980). To prevent or, at least, reduce ionic interactions between IgG molecules and the tissue resulting in unspecific staining, the following alterations of the routine PAP procedure (Sect. 3.3.4) are recommended: The PBS used for the dilution of the primary antiserum contains 0.5 M NaCl and the pH of the PBS is elevated to pH 8.6, which is in the region of the isoelectric point of IgG. The rinse of the sections following primary incubation is carried out in PBS also containing 0.5 M NaCl.

Apart from the ionic binding of IgG to tissue components, a binding of IgG molecules mediated by complement may also occur (Buffa et al. 1979). These nonspecific reactions can be avoided in the following ways: The primary antiserum should be used in dilutions higher than 1:500. The antiserum used can be heated at 60 °C for 30 min or treated with complement-fixing antigen-antibody complexes. These are obtained by incubating equal amounts of latex-coated human chorionic gonadotropin and anti-human chorionic gonadotropin antibodies (Immunologic HCG test, Roche, Basel, Switzerland).

5.5 Positive Control Reactions

Positive control reactions are mainly used to confirm the specificity of the immunohistochemical results. The ultimate achievement of the positive control reaction is the proof that the molecule localized by immunocytochemistry is present in the precise region found (Fig. 21). Complete biochemical analyses related to a microarea, are mostly not possible for various regions, such as the separation (microdissection) of the tissue and the small amount (sensitivity of the analysis) of neuronal substances in the tissues. However, positive control reactions should be used as often as possible to substantiate the immunocytochemical reactions.

5.5.1 Parallel Reference Incubation

The specific immunohistochemical reaction may be abolished by numerous factors. If the reaction is carried out with tissue in which the presence of a neuropeptide is not known, parallel reference incubations are of importance to know whether the corresponding incubation can be expected to result in a positive immunohistochemical reaction. Two types of reference incubations are done:

1. Incubation in the same run (on slide) with tissue where the localization of a neuropeptide is established. We use, for example, spinal cord, substantia gelatinosa for somatostatin, neurotensin, or substance P reference incubation. Also gastrointestinal endocrine cells, such as ileal neurotensin cells, pancreatic somatostatin, and

glucagon cells, etc., are used as reference incubation.

2. Incubation in the run with serial sections using various neuropeptides. As a rule this test results in the demonstration of various distribution patterns of the examined substances and gives a hint as to whether the reaction is specific or not.

5.5.2 Control of Immunocytochemical Methods by Radioimmunoassay (RIA)

Immunocytochemical procedures may be controlled by radioimmunoassay. The principle of this method comprises the competitive binding of antigens, e.g., labeled and unlabeled neuropeptides, to specific receptors, in this case the antibodies which have been produced in response to neuropeptides. The amount of the neuropeptide in question is measured after separation of free and antibody-bound antigen by different techniques: electrophoresis, gel filtration, adsorption, fractional precipitation, Seconal antibody precipitation, solid phase antibody (Chard 1978).

Among several possibilities inherent to radioimmunoassay, the activity (titer) of the antibodies which are applied for immunohistochemical reactions can be controlled. However, there exist severe drawbacks in the comparability of radioimmunoassay and immunohistochemical method, since antibodies which are very useful as receptors in RIA do not show any reaction when applied in immunohistochemical methods and vice versa. Probably more importantly RIA is used for confirmation and quantitative measurement of neuropeptides (antigen) in the tissue which have already been or will be characterized and localized by immunocytologic reactions. This procedure provides further information not only about the content of "bound" neuropeptides in the tissue, but also about the level of "secreted" substances in different compartments like the blood.

Additional information to RIA is obtained by radioreceptor assays where a tissue preparation containing receptors for a neuropeptide is used instead of an antibody. This type of assay, when used in correlation with radioimmunoassay, greatly reduces the uncertainty of the identity of the assayed neuropeptide.

5.5.3 Chromatographic Methods Combined with RIA

Analogs of neuropeptides which are suspected when region-specific antibodies of the same neuropeptide give different immunohistochemical results may be identified by separation and isolation procedures in which radioimmunoassays are used as a specific detector system. Tissue homogenates are extracted and then investigated by chromatographic methods to achieve a separation of the analogs according to their differences in molecular weight and size (gel filtration) or isoelectric points (ion exchange chromatography, Fig. 22) or charged groups (high pressure liquid chromatography). The elution profiles which are unspecifically obtained for optical density or protein concentration are specified by identification of the peptides in the picogram range using the RIA (Carraway and Leeman 1976; Rossier et al. 1977).

5.5.4 Control of the Immunocytochemical Reaction by High Pressure Liquid Chromatography (HPLC)

Based upon immunologic criteria a large number of different neuropeptides are thought to be present in nervous tissue. Substances which react with antibodies raised against neuropeptides isolated from tissue extracts, or prepared by chemical synthesis, are presumed to be similar to or often even identical with the neuropeptide used as the antigen. However, before such materials are actually isolated and completely characterized, some doubt about the material present in brain exists.

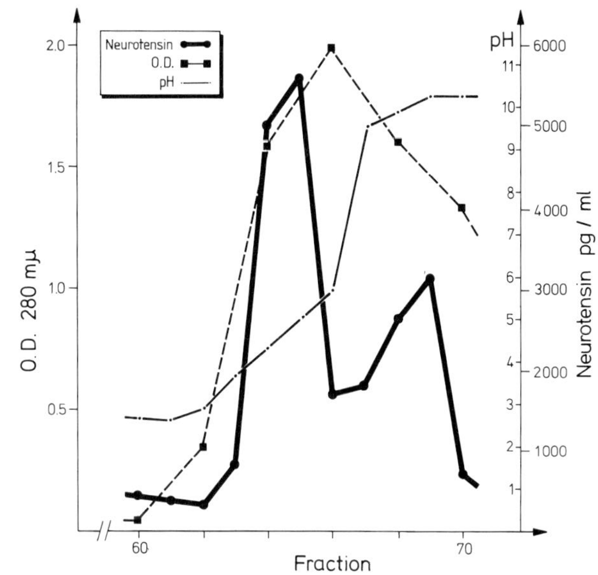

Fig. 22. Gel filtration of a crude preparation of bovin spinal medulla on Sephadex G-25 fine. Column 8–60 cm fluent 0.2 M acetic acid

In order to get more detailed information about the content and structure of neuropeptides which are detected by immunologic methods, high pressure liquid chromatography is the method of choice.

The most powerful tool in chromatographic techniques currently available for separation of small peptides is high pressure liquid chromatography (HPLC). This recently developed technique has already been used in many studies on nervous tissue (Burgus and Rivier 1976; Hancock and Bishop 1976; Monch and Dehnen 1977), including the initial characterization of α- and β-endorphin (Ling et al. 1976), and the confirmation of radioimmunoassay measurements of met-enkephalin concentration in the brain (Bohan and Meek 1978).

Neuropeptides resulting from tissue extractions are chromatographed and/or isolated using reverse phase columns and either isocratic or gradient elution systems. This separation technique depends upon lipophilic (hydrophobic) interactions between the peptides to be separated and the column, a hydrocarbon-covered silica gel (C-18, RP-18). The more hydrophobic the peptide, the stronger its retention by the column. The detection system with a variable wavelength detector is very efficient and more sensitive in combination with a fluorescence detector.

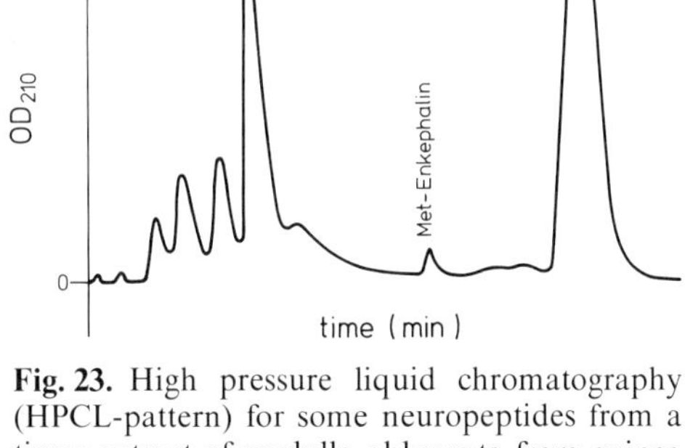

Fig. 23. High pressure liquid chromatography (HPCL-pattern) for some neuropeptides from a tissue extract of medulla oblongata from guinea pig. The separation was made on a 30 cm × 4 mm u-Bondapak C-18 column at room temperature. The elution solvents were methanol and H_2O (60:40). The solvent was pumped at 1 ml/min. The pressure required was 1000 psi. The peptides in the column effluent were detected by absorbens at 210 nm with a variable wavelength detector with a 8 μl flow cell

High pressure liquid chromatography fulfills the requirements by giving precise and reproducible retention time values and quantitative measurements of neuropeptides (Fig. 23). The chromatographic conditions can be adjusted to solve particularly separation problems, e.g., by changing the solvent composition and the gradient.

In conclusion, the versatility of the reverse phase HPLC is a powerful tool for the purification and characterization of both known and unknown peptides from crude extracts of tissue. HPLC is also a very useful method for the rapid analysis and isolation in a preparative scale, of unidentified neuropeptide substances of widely differing polarity on nonpolar stationary phases, by comparison with an authentic sample. Further characterization of the isolated peptides can be obtained by the determination of the amino acid composition and amino acid sequence analysis by the method of Edman and Begg (1967).

6 References

Anderson PJ (1967) Purification and quantitation of glutaraldehyde and its effect on several enzyme activities in sceletal muscle. J Histochem Cytochem 15:652

Arimura A, Sato H, Dupont A, Nishi N, Schally AV (1975) Somatostatin: abundance of immunoreactive hormone in rat stomach and pancreas. Science 189:1007–1009

Bächi T, Dorval G, Wigzell H, Binz H (1977) Staphylococcal protein A in immunoferritin techniques. Scand J Immunol 6:241–246

Biberfeld B, Ghetie V, Sjöquist J (1974) Demonstration and assaying of IgG antibodies in tissues and on cells by labeled staphylococcal protein A. J Immunol Methods 6:249–259

Bohan TP, Meek JL (1978) Met-enkephalin: Rapid separation from brain extracts using high-pressure liquid chromatography and quantitation by binding assay. Neurochem Res 3:367–372

Buffa R, Crivelli O, Fiocca R, Fontana P, Solcia E (1979) Complement-mediated unspecific binding of immunoglobulins to some endocrine cells. Histochemistry 65:15–21

Burgus R, Rivier J (1976) Use of high pressure liquid chromatography in the purification of peptides. Proc Eur Pept Symp 14:85–94

Burnweit C, Forssmann WG (1979) Somatostatinergic nerves in the cervical spinal cord of the monkey. Cell Tissue Res 200:83–90

Carraway R, Leeman SE (1976) Characterization of radioimmunoassayable neurotensin in the rat. J Biol Chem 251:7045–7052

Chard T (1978) An introduction to radioimmunoassay and related techniques. North Holland, Amsterdam

Coons AH (1956) Histochemistry with labeled antibody. Int Rev Cytol 5:1–23

Coons AH (1978) Fluorescent antibody methods. In: Danielli JF (ed) General cytochemical methods. Academic Press, New York, pp 399–422

Coons AH, Leduc EH, Connolly JM (1955) Studies on antibody production. I. A method for the histochemical demonstration of specific antibody and its application to a study of the hyperimmune rabbit. J Exp Med 102: 49–63

Costa M, Cuello AC, Furness JB, Franco R (1980a) Distribution of enteric neurons showing immunoreactivity for substance P in the guinea-pig ileum. Neuroscience 5:323–331

Costa M, Furness JB, Buffa R, Said SI (1980b) Distribution of enteric nerve cell bodies and axons showing immunoreactivity for vasoactive intestinal polypeptide in the guinea-pig intestine. Neuroscience 5:587–596

Cuello AC, Galfré G, Milstein C (1979) Detection of substance P in the central nervous system by a monoclonal antibody. Proc Natl Acad Sci USA 76:3532–3536

Cuello AC, Kanazawa I (1978) The distribution of substance P immunoreactive fibers in the rat central nervous system. J Comp Neurol 178:129–156

Cuello AC, McQueen DS (1980) Substance P: A carotid body peptide. Neurosci Lett 17: 215–219

Dahlström A, Fuxe K (1964) Evidence for the existence of monoamine containing neurons in the CNS. I. Demonstration of monoamines in the cell bodies of brainstem neurons. Acta Physiol Scand [Suppl. 232] 62:1–55

Dahlström A, Fuxe K (1965) Evidence for the existence of monoamine containing neurons in the CNS. II. Experimentally induced changes in the intraneuronal amine levels of bulbospinal neuron systems. Acta Physiol Scand [Suppl. 247] 62:1–36

Dubois-Dalcq M, McFarland H, McFarlin DM (1977) Protein A-peroxidase: A valuable tool for the localization of antigens. J Histochem Cytochem 25:1201–1206

Edman P, Begg G (1967) A protein sequenator. Eur J Biochem 1:80–91

Falkmer S, Carraway RE, El-Salhy M, Emdin SO, Grimelius L, Rehfeld JF, Reinecke M, Schwartz TFW (1981) Phylogeny of the gastroenteropancreatic (GEP) neuroendocrine system. A review with special reference to the occurrence of CCK-like and neurotensin-like polypeptides in lower vertebrates and invertebrates. UCLA Forum Med Sci 23:21–42

Faulk WP, Taylor GM (1971) An immunocolloidal method for the electron microscope. Immunochemistry 8:1081–1083

Frens G (1973) Controlled nucleation for the regulation of the particle size in monodisperse gold solutions. Nature (Phys Sci) 241:20

Furness JB, Costa M (1980) Types of nerves in the enteric nervous system. Neuroscience 5: 1–20

Fuxe K (1965) Evidence for the existence of monoamine neurons in the central nervous system. IV. The distribution of monoamine nerve terminals in the central nervous system. Acta Physiol Scand 64:39–85

Galfré G, Howe SC, Milstein C, Butcher GW, Howard JC (1977) Antibodies to major histocompatibility antigens produced by hybrid cell lines. Nature 266:550–552

Graham RC, Jr, Karnovsky MJ (1966) The early stages of absorption of injected horseradish peroxidase in the proximal tubules of mouse kidney: ultrastructural cytochemistry by a new technique. J Histochem Cytochem 14: 291–302

Grube D (1980) Immunoreactivities of gastrin (G-)cells. II. Non-specific binding of immunoglobulins to G-cells by ionic interactions. Histochemistry 66:149–167

Grube D, Weber E (1980) Immunoreactivities of gastrin (G)cells. I. Dilution-dependent staining of G-cells by antisera and non-immune sera. Histochemistry 65:223–237

Hancock WS, Bishop CA (1976) High-pressure liquid chromatography in the analysis of underivatized peptides using a sensitive and rapid procedure. FEBS Lett 72/1:139–142

Hartman BK (1972) Immunofluorescence of dopamine-β-hydroxylase, application of improved methodology to the localization of the peripheral and central noradrenergic nervous system. J Histochem Cytochem 21:312–331

Hökfelt T, Efendic S, Hellerström C, Johansson O, Luft R, Arimura A (1975) Cellular localization of somatostatin in endocrine-like cells and neurons of the rat with special references to the A1-cell of the pancreatic islets and to the hypothalamus. Acta Endocrinol [Suppl] (Copenh) 200:5–41

Hökfelt T, Johansson O, Fuxe K, Löfström A, Goldstein M, Park D, Ebstein R, Fraser H, Jeffcoate S, Efendic S, Luft R, Arimura A (1976) Mapping and relationship of hypothalamic neurotransmitters and hypothalamic hormones. In: Tvomisto J, Paasonen MK (eds) Proc. Sixth International Congress of Pharmacology, vol 3. Forssan Kirjapaino oy, Forssa, pp 93–110

Hökfelt T, Elde R, Johansson O, Terenius L, Stein L (1977) The distribution of enkephalin-immunoreactive cell bodies in the rat central nervous system. Neurosci Lett 5:25–31

Hökfelt T, Schultzberg M, Elde R, Nilsson G, Terenius L, Said S, Goldstein M (1978a) Peptide neurons in peripheral tissues including the urinary tract: Immunohistochemical studies. Acta Pharmacol Toxicol (Copenh) 43: 79–89

Hökfelt T, Elde R, Johansson O, Ljungdahl A, Schultzberg M, Fuxe K, Goldstein M, Nilsson G, Pernow B, Terenius L, Ganten D, Jeffcoate SL, Rehfeld J, Said S (1978b) Distribution of peptide-containing neurons. In: Lipton MA, Di Mascio A, Killam KF (eds) Psychopharmacology: A generation of progress. Raven Press, New York, pp 39–66

Hökfelt T, Elde R, Fuxe K, Johansson O, Ljungdahl A, Goldstein M, Luft R, Efendic S, Nilsson G, Terenius L, Ganten D, Jeffcoate SL, Rehfeld J, Said S, Perez de la Mora M, Possani L, Tapia T, Teran L, Palacios R (1978c) Aminergic and peptidergic pathways in the nervous system with special reference to the hypothalamus. In: Reichlin S, Baldessarini RJ, Martin JB (eds) The hypothalamus. Raven Press, New York pp 69–135

Hökfelt T, Johansson O, Ljungdahl A, Lundberg J, Schultzberg M, Fuxe K, Goldstein M, Steinbusch H, Verhofstad A, Elde R (1979) Neurotransmitters and neuropeptides: distribution patterns and cellular localization as revealed by immunocytochemistry. In: Fuxe K, Hökfelt T, Luft R (eds) Central regulation of the endocrine system. Plenum, New York pp 31–48

Kellenberger E, Carlemalm E, Villiger W, Roth J, Garavito RM (1980) Low dematuration embedding for electron microscopy of thin sections. Chem. Werke Lowi, Waldkraiburg

Köhler G, Milstein C (1975) Continuous cultures of fused cells secreting antibody of predefined specificity. Nature 256:495–497

König R, Heym Ch (1978) Immunofluorescent localization of dopamine-β-hydroxylase in small intensely fluorescent cells of the rat superior cervical ganglion. Neurosci Lett 10: 187–191

Lackner KJ (1980) Mapping of monoamine neurones and fibres in the cat lower brainstem and spinal cord. Anat Embryol 161:169–195

Ling N, Burgus R, Guillemin R (1976) Isolation, primary structure, and synthesis of α-endorphin and β-endorphin. Two peptides of hypophysical origin with morphinomimetic activity. Proc Natl Acad Sci USA 78: 3912–3916

Ljungdahl A, Hökfelt T, Nilsson G (1978) Distribution of substance P-like immunoreactivity in the central nervous system of the rat. I. Cell bodis and nerve terminals. Neuroscience 3: 861–943

Mayor HD, Hampton JC, Rosario B (1961) A simple method for removing the resin from epoxy embedded tissue. J Cell Biol 9:909–910

Milstein C, Galfré G, Secher DS, Springer T (1979) Monoclonal antibodies and cell surface antigens. Cell Biol Int Rep 3:1–16

Monch W, Dehnen W (1977) High pressure liquid chromatography of peptides. J Chromatogr 140:260–262

Pease DC (1962) Buffered formaldehyde as a killing agent and primary fixative for electron microscopy. Anat Rec 142:342

Petrusz P, Sar M, Ordronneau P, DiMeo P (1976) Specificity in immunocytochemical staining. J Histochem Cytochem 24:1110–1115

Pickel VM, Joh TH, Field PM, Becker CG, Reis DJ (1975a) Cellular localization of tyrosine hydroxylase by immunohistochemistry. J Histochem Cytochem 23:1–12

Pickel VM, Joh TH, Reis DJ (1975b) Ultrastructural localization of tyrosine hydroxylase in noradrenergic neurons of brain. Proc Natl Acad Sci USA 72:659–663

Pickel VM, Reis DJ, Leeman SE (1977) Ultrastructural localization of substance P in neurons of rat spinal cord. Brain Res 122:534–540

Pickel VM, Joh TH, Reis DJ, Leeman SE, Miller RJ (1979) Electron microscopic localization of substance P and enkephalin in axon terminals related to dendrites of catecholaminergic neurons. Brain Res 160:387–400

Reinecke M, Almasan K, Carraway R, Helmstaedter V, Forssmann WG (1980a) Distribution patterns of neurotensin-like immunoreactive cells in the gastro-intestinal tract of higher vertebrates. Cell Tissue Res 205:383–395

Reinecke M, Carraway RE, Falkmer S, Feurle GE, Forssmann WG (1980b) Occurrence of neurotensin-immunoreactive cells in the digestive tract of lower vertebrates and deuterostomian invertebrates. Cell Tissue Res 212:173–183

Roberts GW, Woodhams PL, Bryant MG, Crow TJ, Bloom SR, Polak JM (1980) VIP in the rat brain: Evidence for a major pathway linking the amygdala and hypothalamus via the stria terminalis. Histochemistry 65:103–119

Romano EL, Romano M (1977) Staphylococcal protein A bound to colloidal gold: A useful reagent to label antigen-antibody sites in electron microscopy. Immunochemistry 14: 711–715

Romano EL, Stolinski C, Hughes-Jones NC (1974) An antiglobulin reagent labeled with colloidal gold for use in electron microscopy. Immunochemistry 11:521–522

Rossier J, Vargo TM, Minick S, Ling N, Bloomand FE, Guillemin R (1977) Regional dissociation of β-endorphin and enkephalin contents in rat brain and pituitary. Proc Natl Acad Sci 74:5162–5165

Roth J, Bendayan M, Orci L (1978) Ultrastructural localization of intercellular antigens by the use of protein A-gold complex. J Histochem Cytochem 26:1074–1081

Roth J, Bendayan M, Orci L (1980) FITC-protein A-gold complex for light and electronmicroscopic immunohistochemistry. J Histochem Cytochem 28:55–57

Sar M, Stumpf WE, Miller RJ, Chang K-J, Cuatrecasas P (1978) Immunohistochemical localization of enkephalin in rat brain and spinal cord. J Comp Neurol 182:17–38

Schultzberg M, Hökfelt T, Nilsson G, Terenius L, Rehfeld JF, Brown M, Elde R, Goldstein M, Said S (1980) Distribution of peptide- and catecholamine-containing neurons in the gastro-intestinal tract of rat and guinea-pig: Immunohistochemical studies with antisera to substance P, vasoactive intestinal polypeptide, enkephalins, somatostatin, gastrin/cholecystokinin, neurotensin and dopamine β-hydroxylase. Neuroscience 5:689–744

Shulman M, Wilde CD, Köhler G (1978) A better cell line for making hybridomas secreting specific antibodies. Nature 276:269–270

Sims KB, Hoffman DL, Said SI, Zimmerman EA (1980) Vasoactive intestinal polypeptide (VIP) in mouse and rat brain: An immunocytochemical study. Brain Res 186:165–183

Sternberger LA: Some new developments in immunocytochemistry. Mikroscopy 25, 346–361 (1969).

Sternberger LA (1979) Immunocytochemistry. Wiley, New York

Sternberger LA, Joseph SA (1979) The unlabeled antibody method. Contrasting color staining of paired pituitary hormones without antibody removal. J Histochem Cytochem 27:1424–1429

Swaab DF, Pool CW, van Leeuwen FW (1977) Can specificity ever be proved in immunocytochemical staining? J Histochem Cytochem 25:388–391

Templeton CL, Douglas RJ, Vail WJ (1978) Ferritin-conjugated protein A: a new immunocytochemical reagent of electron microscopy. FEBS Lett 85:95

Vandesande F (1979) A critical review of immunocytochemical methods for light microscopy. J Neurosci Methods 1:3–23

Van Norden S, Falkmer S (1980) Gut-islet endocrinology. – Some evolutionary aspects. Invest Cell Pathol 3:21–35

Wright C, William KJ, Sjödahl J, Burton DR, Dwek RA (1977) The interaction of protein A and Fc fragment of rabbit immunoglobulin G as probed by complement-fixation and nuclear-magnetic-resonance studies. Eur J Biochem 167:661

Zamboni L, DeMartino C (1967) Buffered picric acid-formaldehyde, a new, rapid fixative for electron microscopy. J Cell Biol 35:148

Zarling JM, Kung PC (1980) Monoclonal antibodies which distinguish between human NK cells and cytotoxic T lymphocytes. Nature 288:394–396

Zsigmondy R, Thiessen PA (1925) Das Kolloidale Gold. Akad. Verlagsgesellschaft, Leipzig

Chapter 11

Identification of Single Neurons by Intracellular Application of Tracers

Peter Schubert

1 Introduction

Labeling of individual neurons by direct application of tracers has become a widely used technique in recent years. In contrast to the capricious Golgi impregnation, to which we owe our fundamental knowledge about the nerve cell structure, labeling by single-cell injection of tracers is predictable and allows identification of a particular neuron selected by the investigator. It is now possible to visualize in "Golgi-like" manner the architecture of a certain neuron from which, for example, electrophysiological data have been previously collected. This is the main advantage of the single-cell labeling technique which explains its growing importance; it is not a pure anatomical method but a combined approach which helps to bridge other research disciplines with morphology. Indeed, not only have electrophysiologists become familiar with morphologists' techniques (and vice versa), but some were also attracted by specific problems in the neighboring field. Such a multidisciplinary approach with combined technologies might be a promising way to correlate functional aspects with nerve cell structures and wiring, which are more easily accessible to morphological research. I want to discuss this point to some extent in this chapter.

The development of the single-cell labeling technique was the result of a combination of electrophysiological and morphological know-how, i.e., intracellular recording, application of ionized molecules via iontophoresis, and the use of visualizable

Fig. 1. Labeling of cat spinal motor neurons by intracellular iontophoresis of various radioactive precursors. *Upper row*: incorporation of ^{3}H-orotic acid in the nucleus (*left*) and of ^{3}H-fucose in the perikaryon, accumulated presumably in the Golgi complexes (*right*). *Lower rows*: incorporation of ^{3}H-glycine and transport of radioactive proteins in the dendritic tree (*above*), down the axon (*below*), within the spinal cord (*left*), and in the ventral route (*right*). Autoradiographs counterstained with toluidine blue. (Schubert et al. 1971; Kreutzberg and Schubert 1973; Schubert and Kreutzberg 1975)

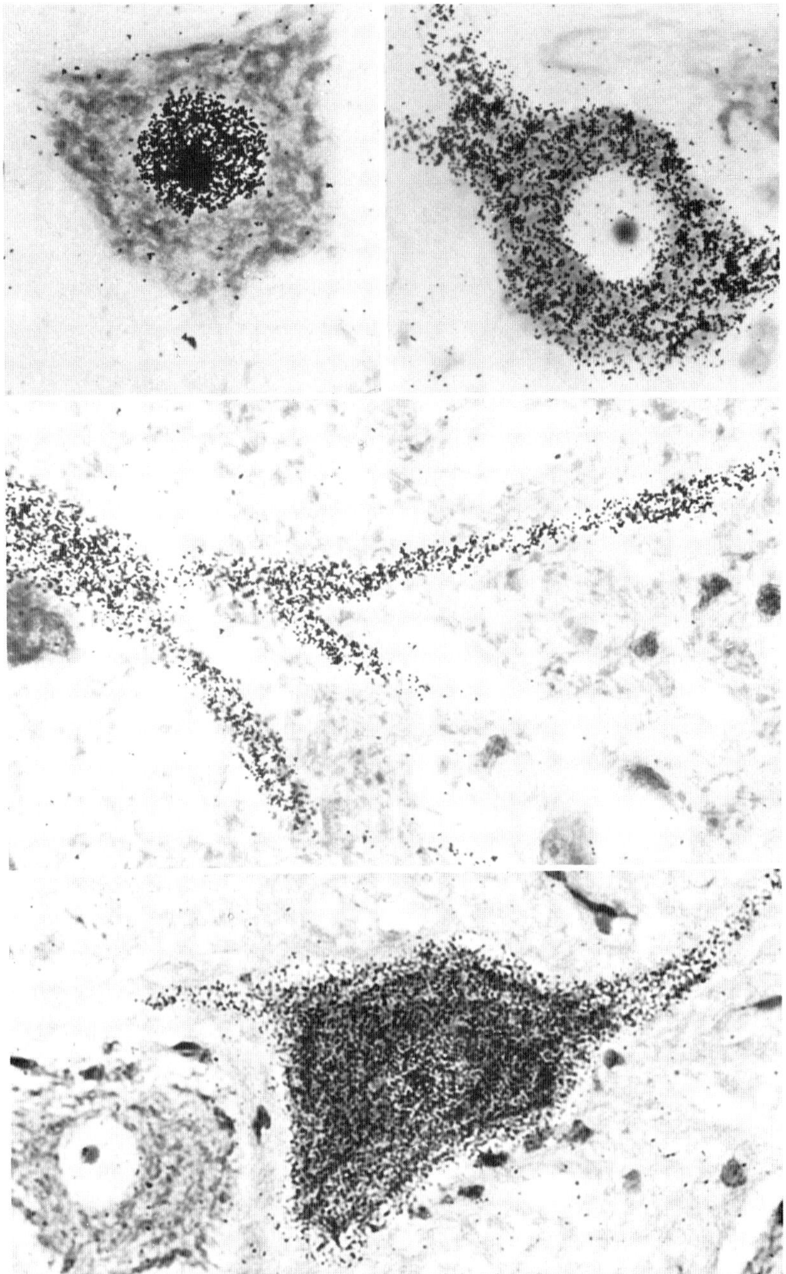

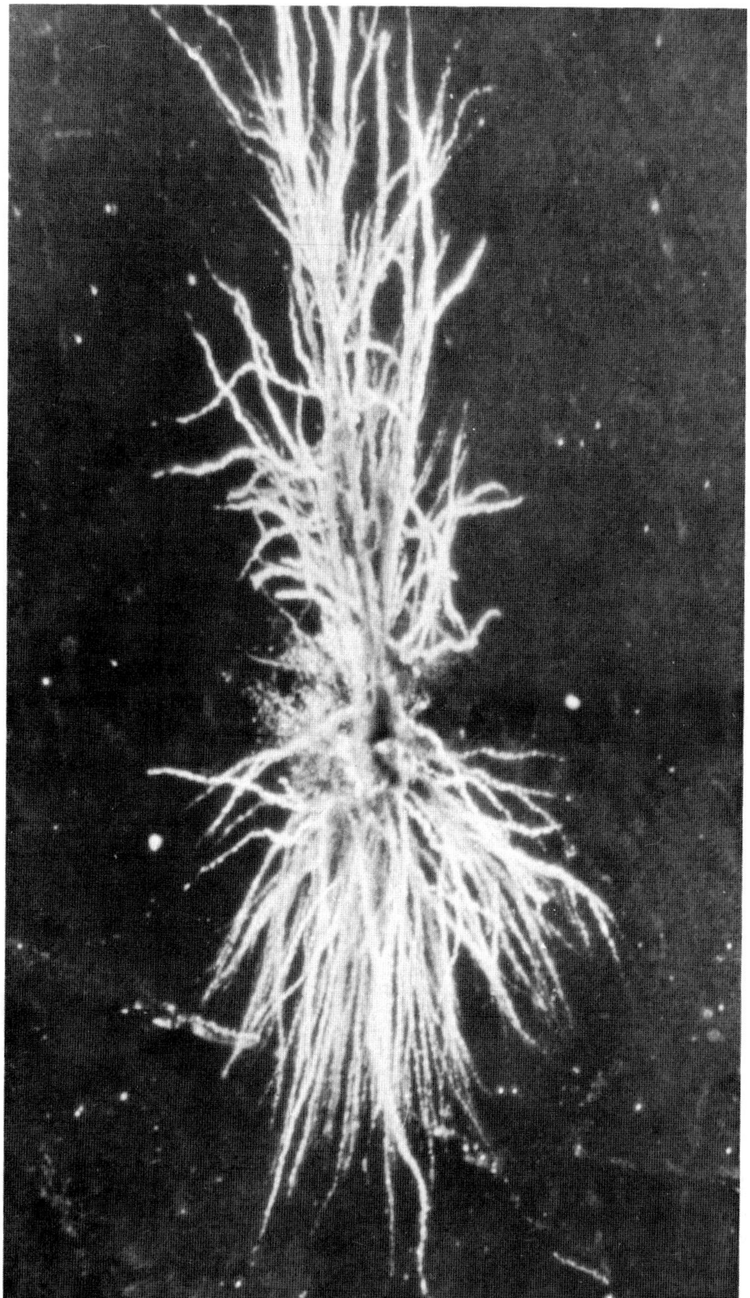

Fig. 2. Labeling of a hippocampal pyramidal neuron by application of horseradish peroxidase, visualized by dark field illumination. I thank Prof. Gary Lynch for permitting the reproduction of this figure. (Lynch et al. 1975)

tracers. In early attempts to localize a neuron from which recordings were made, various metal ions precipitated by a histochemical reaction were tested as intracellular markers, i. e., ferrocyanide (Kerkut and Walker 1962), copper (Lux and Globus 1968), and others. But their intracellular application resulted only in a faint staining of the nerve cell soma with the proximal dendrites and allowed only a rough orientation, as did the application of various dyes such as anilin blue (Behrens and Wulff 1965), Niagara blue (Potter et al. 1966), methyl blue and fast green (Thomas and Wilson 1966).

The first successful morphological identification of an electrophysiologically defined neuron was achieved in 1968 independently by two groups with different approaches. One group, Stretton and Kravitz (1968), used the textile and paper-dye procion yellow, which they localized by fluorescence microscopy; the other group, Globus, Lux, and Schubert (1968), applied a radioactive amino acid, ^{3}H-glycine, followed by an autoradiographic visualization of the newly synthetized proteins. With both techniques, not only a labeling of the nerve cell soma was seen but unexpectedly also of the dendritic tree, traceable up to its peripheral arborization with branches of 1–2 μm. In addition, the axons were labeled up to considerable distances from the cell soma. In a cat spinal motor neuron, for instance, radioactivity could be traced within hours after ^{3}H-glycine iontophoresis for several millimeters down the ventral routes strictly confined to the one axon (see Fig. 1). As investigated in later studies with radioactive amino acids, the convection of the tracer throughout the whole neuron has to be attributed to an effective intraneuronal transport system which not only operates in the axon (Weiss and Hiscoe 1948; Ochs 1972) but also in the arborized dendrites (Schubert et al. 1971).

In 1972 cobalt visualized by precipitation with ammonium sulfide was introduced by Pitman et al. as a third intracellular tracer. This method has been used preferentially for identifying invertebrate neurons, which in cleared whole mount preparations show up nicely as complete entities with all their dendritic and axonal processes.

The most recent approach to labeling nerve cells by iontophoretic application of horseradish peroxidase (HRP) seems to be the most promising and has several advantages. The histochemical visualization of HRP is, in contrast to the autoradiographic method, not time consuming and technically simple. The labeled neuron can be easily localized by conventional light microscopic inspection in relation to the other cells in the section and the accuracy of cell labeling can nearly reach the quality of a Golgi-impregnation. It allows reliable identification of structural details such as dendritic spines. Furthermore, the reaction product of HRP is electron-dense and since, in contrast to cobalt, its application does not seriously affect ultrastructural tissue preservation, the identified neuron can also be examined at the electron microscopic level. Another advantage is that a complete nerve cell labeling is obtained with HRP even if the electrode tip is not properly located inside the neuron but in close proximity to its soma or processes. The reason may be that uptake of HRP is enhanced if a neuron is lesioned by the advancing electrode tip. This allows identification of smaller neurons or even dendrites from which stable intracellular recordings are often difficult to obtain.

A beautiful example of the efficiency of such a quasi-intracellular labeling is given by the hippocampal pyramidal neuron from Lynch et al. (1975) and is shown in Fig. 2. The applicability of HRP as an intracellular marker is based on the work of several laboratories. Graybiel and Devor (1974) worked out parameters for its delivery by microelectrophoresis. Its intracellular application was performed by Snow et al. (1976) and perfected by Kitai et al. (1976).

The technique of intracellular tracer application is basically the same regardless which tracer is used. It will be described in reference to the method developed for radioactive amino acids, since this is covered by personal experimental experience of the author.

2 Technique of Single-Cell Labeling

The technique of iontophoretic tracer application into an electrophysiologically defined neuron is illustrated in the block diagram (Fig. 3). The position of the electrode tip is monitored by recording the nerve cell potentials. Its intracellular location is indicated by an abrupt drop in the membrane potential of up to 80 mV (a large drop means that the neuron is not suffering from injury) and by recording intracellular action potentials. They can occur spontaneously or may have to be evoked by stimulation of the appropriate afferent or efferent fibers. For these measurements basic electrophysiological equipment is needed: an oscilloscope [1], preferably with storage (a band width of 1 M Hz is sufficient), a pre-amplifier [2], and a stimulation unit [2].

2.1 Preparation of Micropipettes

If a recording of high quality and a rather pure application of the tracer is required, double-barreled micropipettes (Theta electrodes) are recommended. They have several advantages:

1) Recording- and tracer-barrels are separated and can be filled with solutions optimal for either purpose. 2) There are no difficulties in rapid and proper filling of the electrode tips. 3) Both barrels may be alternatively filled with tracer, which allows switching the current from one barrel to the other if impedance in one of the barrels is increased during iontophoresis.

These micropipettes are prepared from pyrex glass capillaries subdivided by an inner glass wall (e. g., Fa. Krannich, Göttingen, Federal Republic of Germany). The outer diameter of the capillary is 2.0–2.5 mm, the inner diameter of each barrel is about 0.7 mm. Before pulling the electrodes, the capillaries have to be thoroughly cleaned to optimize their filling properties. The capillaries are washed in chromic and sulphuric acid, in running tap water, distilled water, and then transferred to absolute alcohol, ether, and finally stored in acetone. With the aid of a microelectrode puller (e. g., David Kopf Instruments, USA) with an adjustable heating current appropriate micropipettes are drawn. Shank diameters of about 15 μ at a distance of 200 μ from the tip were found to be convenient for labeling cat spinal motor neurons.

Filling of the pipettes should be performed soon after pulling to avoid contamination. To prevent the formation of fluid bridges between the two barrels and thus a current leakage during iontophoresis, polyvinyl tubes are inserted into the end of each barrel and fixed with melted wax to isolate the barrels from each other. For filling, a syringe without an air space [e. g., Hamilton (Hamilton CO., USA) Type 7105 N] is used. The needle is inserted through the polyvinyl tube into the electrode barrel up to the shoulder and about 2 μl of tracer solution are injected. The immediate filling of the electrode tip should be checked under the microscope. After filling the recording barrel, a 0.15 mm silver wire is inserted into each of the barrels, immersed in the solution, and fixed to the tube with sealing wax. Before use, the tip might be broken to obtain an optimal size by gently

[1] For example, Tektronix, USA (Type 5113) or Phillips, Netherlands

[2] For example, WPI, USA; HiMed, Great Britain; or Neurolog, USA

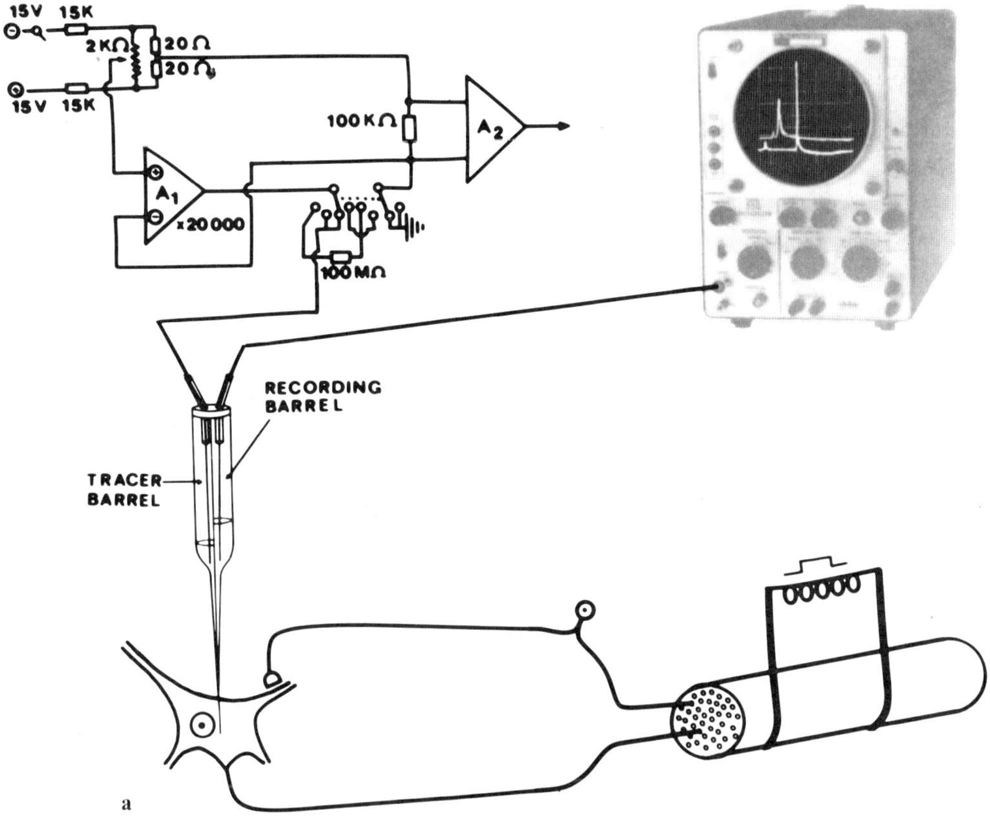

a

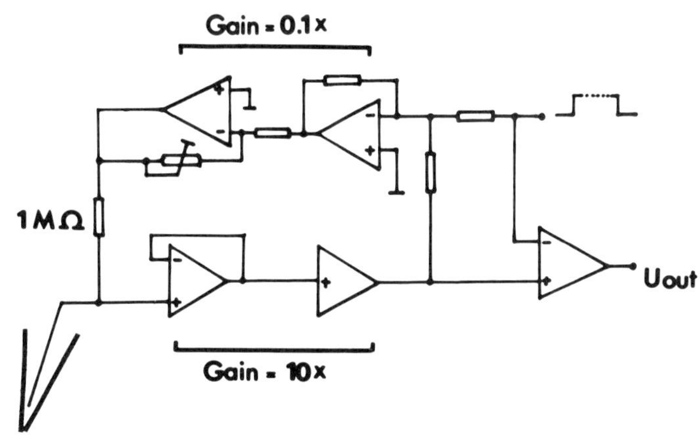

b

Fig. 3 a, b. Block diagram of the iontophoresis devices. **a** as has been used in our laboratory (see also Lux et al. 1970 b); **b** as built by Fa. Meyer und Renz, Munich, Federal Republic of Germany

pushing the electrode tip against a glass rod under microscopic control. These electrodes usually have a resistance of 1–2 MΩ. For labeling neurons the size of cat spinal motor neurons (larger than 30 μ in diameter) a tip size of 1–2 μ allows a stable intracellular recording and provides optimal conditions for passing the iontophoretic current.

For identifying smaller neurons, the use of single-barrel pipettes prepared from capillaries with an inserted glass fiber (e. g., Clark Electromedical Instruments, Pangbourne, G. Britain) are recommended. The glass fiber greatly improves filling properties and also allows the relatively simple filling of the electrodes from the back, as described.

In order to keep the tip size as small as possible, the tip of the pipette might be bevelled instead of broken to allow passage of sufficient iontophoresis current. This procedure is particularly indicated for electrodes filled with HRP as tracer, since they have high impedances of about 100 MΩ. Devices for bevelling electrodes are commercially available (e. g., David Kopf Instruments, USA, K. T. Brown-type Micropipette Beveller) (see Brown and Flaming 1974), but may also be self-made (e. g., by adapting a record player pick-up and turntable for this purpose).

2.2 Preparation of Tracer Solutions

2.2.1 Radioactive Precursors

In order to optimize autoradiographic resolution, tritium-labeled compounds should be used. They are usually supplied by the manufacturer (e. g., Amersham, Great Britain or New England Nuclear (NEN) Corp., USA) in concentrations up to 1 m Ci/ml, dissolved in 0.1 N HCl or in a dilute alcohol solution. Usually 0.5 ml of this solution is dried under a gentle stream of nitrogen and the residue is redissolved in a volume of 20 µl to give a final concentration of about 25 µ Ci/µl. As solvent either 0.01 M acetic acid or 0.01 M KOH is used, depending on whether the tracer is to be applied as an anion or as a cation. Several investigators prefer application as an anion with a negative hyperpolarizing current thus avoiding cell membrane depolarisation. But this does not seem to be essential.

2.2.2 Horseradish Peroxidase

A 4% HRP (Sigma Chemical Company, USA or Boehringer, FR Germany) solution of either Sigma Type VI (Graybiel and Devor 1974; Wong et al. 1979) or a 3 : 1 mixture of Type II and Type VI (Kitai et al. 1976) is recommended, dissolved in 0.05 M HCl buffer (pH 8.6) with KCl (0.2 M).

2.3 Intracellular Iontophoresis

The principle of an iontophoresis apparatus which has been used in our laboratory is demonstrated in the block diagram (Fig. 3). The recording electrode is connected with an oscilloscope via a preamplifier. The iontophoretic current is generated by a battery-operated floating amplifier which serves as a constant current source. The current proportion feed-back signal across a 100 KΩ resistor is amplified by a FET differential amplifier, which provides the necessary power for a panel meter or an oscilloscope display. The device permits direct current measurements with an accuracy of about 5%. The current can be passed between barrels or between either barrel and ground.

Helpful instructions for building such an iontophoresis apparatus are given in the booklet by E. Neher (1974), providing some basic information about electronics to biologists inexperienced in electronics. Several types of iontophoresis apparatuses are commercially available. (e. g., WPI,

USA; HiMed, Great Britain; or Medical Systems Corp., New York, USA). A relatively simple and elegant device for passing current to a single-barrel electrode is schematically shown in Fig. 3. Here, the preamplifier is equipped with a current pump which allows currents of up to 10 nA to be passed through the tracer-containing recording electrode. This current is automatically kept constant up to electrode resistances of 100 MΩ. If iontophoresis currents of higher strength are to be applied, this apparatus can be connected to an external voltage source of up to 100 volts.

During the experiment the microelectrode is fastened in a stereotoxic holder permitting three-dimensional movement. When the pipette is advanced through the tissue, a current of some nano-amperes of a polarity opposite to that of the tracer ion may be applied to the tracer barrel in order to prevent leakage. In our experience with ^{3}H-amino acids leakage was never found to be a problem. For intracellular iontophoresis of amino acids, a current of 5–20 nA was usually applied for 2–4 min, sufficient to obtain an intense autoradiographic labeling of the injected neuron. Application of ^{3}H-glycine as either anion or cation was found to be equally efficient. For applying HRP, 100 ms pulses of 10–20 nA depolarizing constant current at 5 pulses per second for 10–20 min are recommended (Kitai et al. 1976).

During iontophoresis, the correct intracellular site and effect of injection are continuously controlled by recording the nerve cell potentials. Usually tracer application does not interfere with the nerve cell function which in correctly impaled neurons remains undisturbed several hours after injection. (Globus et al. 1968; Schubert et al. 1971; Wong et al. 1979). Survival times should be in the range of 15 min to several hours after ^{3}H-amino acid application and 3–10 h after HRP injection. Fixation and the following tissue processing procedures are the same as described in detail in those chapters dealing with the autoradiographic and histochemical visualization of these tracers after extracellular application.

2.4 Intracellular Pressure Injection

The pressure injection from microelectrodes is recommended as an alternative technique if the substances to be applied cannot be properly ionized to be carried by an iontophoretic current. This is presumably the case if drugs or proteins of higher molecular weight are injected, which might also be relevant for morphological research, as discussed below.

The technique of pressure injection has been applied by Llinás et al. (1972) for determining intracellular calcium levels with the aid of the bioluminescent protein aequorin. Its usefulness fo applying tiny amounts of markers has been demonstrated recently by Hofmeier and Lux (1980). Small amounts of 0.0002 μl can be delivered from micropipettes with a tip size of approximately 1 μ. In the pipette, the solution to be injected is overlayered with a marker solution, e. g., an oil treated with sudan black, which allows estimation of the applied volume by inspecting the shift of the tracer solution-oil miniscus. The open capillary end of the microelectrode is connected to the compressed air supply via polyethylene tubing, tightly fastened in a metal holder. By inserting into this connection an electronically triggered pressure valve operated, e. g., by a stimulator apparatus, controlled pulse injections (with pressures in the range of several kg/cm^2) can be made. Again, such a device as a unit is now commercially available [e. g., Medical Systems Corp. New York, USA, (Type PPM-2)] but can also be self-constructed with relatively little effort.

3 Single-Cell Labeling as an Instrument for Multidisciplinary Research

The single-cell injection technique finds its main application in localizing and morphologically identifying the neuron from which electrophysiological data have been obtained. An extended evaluation of this technique and the use of fluorescent dyes and cobalt as tracers is given by Kater and Nicholson (1973). But as outlined above, the more recently introduced horseradish peroxidase seems to be emerging as the most suitable tracer for this purpose. This tracer even enables the investigator to localize intracellular recordings from dendrites and to identify the neuron to which the dendritic branch recorded from belongs (Wong et al. 1979). In this study it was also shown that the single-cell labeling technique can be successfully applied to a hippocampal slice preparation, thus further extending the applicability of this in vitro technique for multidisciplinary research (see also Lynch and Schubert 1980). The possibility of directly correlating electrophysiological and morphological data allows an approach to more basic electrophysiological problems intimately related to the nerve cell structure. One can, for example measure the cable properties of a given neuron by which the signal propagation in the dendritic tree is determined (Lux et al. 1970a; Lux and Schubert 1975). In this case we used ^{3}H-glycine as a tracer which allowed accurate measurements of the dendritic tree and its detailed reconstruction in serial section autoradiographs.

The technique has been further used to study the parameters of intraneuronal transport in axon and dendrites at the single cell level (Lux et al. 1970b; Schubert et al. 1971). Incorporation site and intraneuronal convection not only of proteins but also of glycoproteins, phospholipids, nucleotides, and RNA can be demonstrated after the application of the respective precursors (Fig. 1, Schubert and Kreutzberg 1975). Among the amino acids, ^{3}H-glycine was the most suitable marker since labeling, in contrast to, for example, basic amino acids, remained strictly confined to the injected neuron.

It is likely that intraneuronal transport is becoming an interesting subject for morphological research since the force-generat-

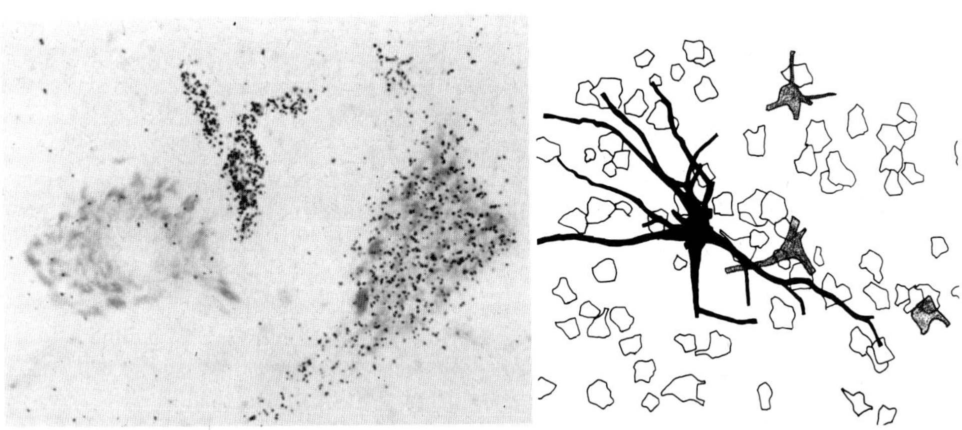

Fig. 4. Lightly labeled neuron in the vicinity of densely labeled dendritic branches belonging to the injected neuron. A partial reconstruction from serial section autoradiographs shows the position of lightly labeled neurons (*dotted*) in relation to the injected neuron (*black*) with many nerve cells interspersed which do not show any radioactivity. This points to a selective interneuronal transfer. (Kreutzberg et al. 1975)

ing mechanism is thought to be provided by the actomyosin system which has recently received considerable study by neuroanatomists. An experimental approach which we have used to test this hypothesis is to apply intracellularly, by means of pressure injection, substances which are known to interfere with the filamentous proteins and to test their effect on the transport of radioactively labeled proteins (see Isenberg et al. 1980).

Another question addressed to morphologists is to what extent are neurons interconnected by gap junctions. The concept of information processing in neuronal "microcircuits" (Schmitt et al. 1975) is

a

b

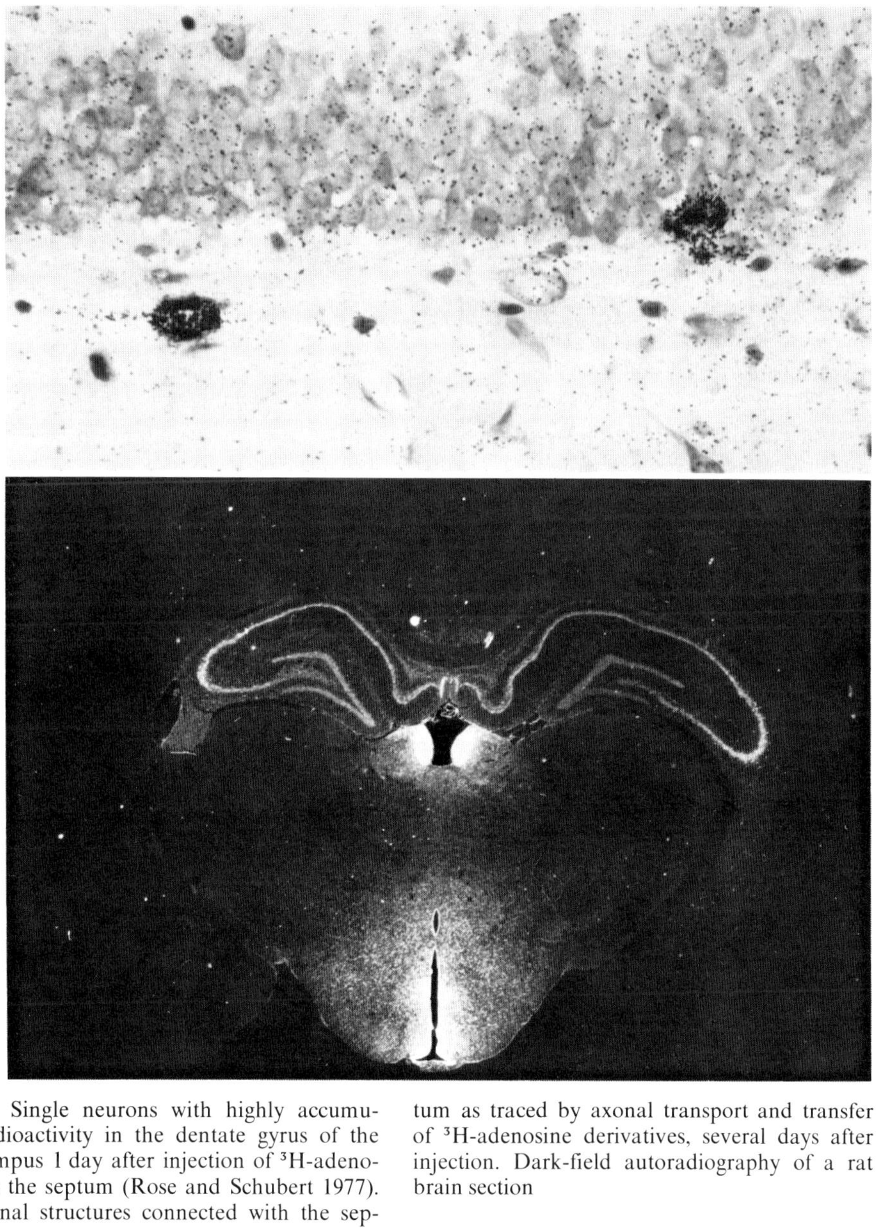

Fig. 5. a Single neurons with highly accumulated radioactivity in the dentate gyrus of the hippocampus 1 day after injection of ^{3}H-adenosine into the septum (Rose and Schubert 1977). **b** Neuronal structures connected with the septum as traced by axonal transport and transfer of ^{3}H-adenosine derivatives, several days after injection. Dark-field autoradiography of a rat brain section

based on the finding of such interneuronal bridges representing not only low resistance connections for signal transmission but also pathways of material transfer (see, e. g., Rieske et al. 1975). The single-cell injection technique might be helpful for tracing such interneuronal cennections. Thus, following the application of ^{3}H-glycine into a single cat spinal motor neuron, 2–3 more lightly labeled neurons are usually seen in the vicinity of the injected neuron (Fig. 4; Globus et al. 1976; Schubert 1974; Kreutzberg et al. 1975). Similar observations were made after iontophoresis of procian yellow (Zieglgänsberger and Reiter 1974). Although the way of transfer, whether via axon collatorals or via the dendrites, has not been identified with certainty, there is some evidence that material passage occurs between the dendritic branches.

A transneuronal transfer of cell constituents relased from axon terminals to target neurons has been described as a general phenomenon in the CNS for ^{3}H-labeled adenosine derivatives (Schubert et al. 1979). Tracing of adenosine derivatives might be included as useful technique to the array of single-cell labeling methods, if an afferent pathway is not diffusely terminating on the whole neuronal population within the target area but selectively on specific neurons. Tracing with ^{3}H-adenosine might be helpful in identifying the target cells. This is suggested by the observation shown in Fig. 5. Here, ^{3}H-adenosine has been injected extracellularly into the septum (25 µCi in 0.25 µl). After allowing one day for transport, a selective labeling of individual neurons is seen in the hippocampal target area; this is most probably reflecting interneurons receiving a dense projection from septal fibers (Rose and Schubert 1977). But the usefulness of ^{3}H-adenosine as a neuroanatomical tracer is restricted, since nerve cell labeling both by anterograde transsynaptic transfer and also by retrograde transport (Hunt and Künzle 1976) has to be considered.

The examples given merely spotlight the possible application of the single-cell labeling technique in biological research. Recently, a fascinating new approach has been presented i. e., combining several morphological tracing techniques: Golgi staining, retrograde transport of horseradish peroxidase, and anterograde degeneration in the same material for an investigation at both the light and electron microscopic levels (see Somogyi et al. 1979). As outlined by Heimer (1980), the single-cell injection technique might be successfully introduced into this chain of techniques, allowing one to determine exactly the input and output relationships of an identified and electrophysiologically characterized neuron at the electron microscopic level.

4 References

Behrens ME, Wulff VJ (1965) Light-initiated responses of retinula and eccentric cells in the *Limulus* lateral eye. J Gen Physiol 48: 1081–1093

Brown KT, Flaming DG (1974) Beveling of fine micropipette electrodes by a rapid precision method. Science 185:693–695

Globus A, Lux HD, Schubert P (1968) Soma dendritic spread of intracellularly-injected tritiated glycine in cat spinal motoneurons. Brain Res 11:440–445

Graybiel AM, Devor M (1974) A microelectrophoretic delivery technique for use with horseradish peroxidase. Brain Res 68:167–173

Heimer L (1980) The continuing evolution of tract-tracing methods. Neurosci Lett 5:S 5

Hofmeier G, Lux HD (1980) Three distinct effects mediated by calcium ions on electrical membrane properties of Helix neurons. Proc XXVIII Intern Congr Physiol Sci, Budapest, Akadémiai Kiadó

Hunt SP, Künzle H (1976) Bidirectional movement of label and transneuronal transport phenomena after injection of (^{3}H) adenosine in the central nervous system. Brain Res 112:127–132

Isenberg G, Schubert P, Kreutzberg GW (1980) Experimental approach to test the role of actin in axonal transport. Brain Res 194:588–593

Kater SB, Nicholson C (1973) Intracellular staining techniques in neurobiology. Springer, Berlin Heidelberg New York

Kerkut GA, Walker RJ (1962) Marking individual nerve cells through electrophoresis of ferrocyanide from a microelectrode. Stain Technol 37:217–219

Kitai ST, Kocsis JD, Preston RJ, Sugimori M (1976) Monosynaptic inputs to caudate neurons identified by intracellular injection of horseradish peroxidase. Brain Res 109:601–606

Kreutzberg GW, Schubert P (1973) Neuronal activity and axonal flow. In: Genazzani E, Herken H (eds), Central nervous system – Studies on metabolic regulation and function. Springer, Berlin Heidelberg New York, pp 84–93

Kreutzberg GW, Schubert P, Lux HD (1975) Neuroplasmic transport in axons and dendrites. In: Santini M (ed), Golgi Centennial Symposium: Perspectives in neurobiology. Raven Press, New York, pp 161–166

Llinás R, Blinks JR, Nicholson C (1972) Calcium transient in presynaptic terminal of squid giant synapse: detection with Aequorin. Science 176:1127–1129

Lux HD, Globus A (1968) Effect of IPSPs of cat spinal motoneurons due to intra- and extracellular iontophoresis of $CuSO_4$. Brain Res 9:377–380

Lux HD, Schubert P (1975) Some aspects of the electroanatomy of dendrites. Adv Neurol 12:29–44

Lux HD, Schubert P, Kreutzberg GW (1970a) Direct matching of morphological and electrophysiological data in cat spinal motoneurons. In: Anderson P, Jansen JKS (eds), Excitatory synaptic mechanisms. Universitetsforlaget, Oslo, pp 189–198

Lux HD, Schubert P, Kreutzberg GW, Globus A (1970b) Excitation and axonal flow. Autoradiographic study on motoneurons intracellularly-injected with ^{3}H-amino acid. Exp Brain Res 10:197–204

Lynch G, Schubert P (1980) The use of in vitro brain slices for multidisciplinary studies of synaptic function. Ann Rev Neurosci 3:1–22

Lynch G, Smith RL, Browning M, Gall Ch (1975) Evidence for bidirectional dendritic transport of horseradish peroxidase in vivo and in vitro. Adv Neurol 12:297–313

Neher E (1974) Elektronische Meßtechnik in der Physiologie. Springer, Berlin Heidelberg New York pp 1–154

Ochs S (1972) Fast transport of material in mammalian nerve fibers. Science 176:252–260

Pitman RM, Tweedle CD, Cohen MJ (1972) Branching of central neurons: intracellular cobalt injection for light and electron microscopy. Science 176:412–414

Potter DD, Furshpan EJ, Lennox ES (1966) Connections between cells of the developing squid as revealed by electrophysiological methods. Proc Natl Acad Sci USA 55: 328–336

Rieske E, Schubert P, Kreutzberg GW (1975) Transneuronal transfer of radioactive material between electrically-coupled neurons of the leech central nervous system. Brain Res 84:365–382

Rose G, Schubert P (1977) Release and transfer of (^{3}H) adenosine derivatives in the cholinergic septal system. Brain Res 121: 353–357

Schmitt FO, Dev P, Smith B (1975) Electronic processing of information by brain cells – Recent research augurs an important role for neuronal local circuits in higher brain function. Science 193:114–120

Schubert P (1974) Transport in Dendriten einzelner Motoneurone. Bull Schweiz Akad Med Wiss 30:56–65

Schubert P, Kreutzberg GW (1975) Parameters of dendritic transport. Adv Neurol 12:255–268

Schubert P, Lux HD, Kreutzberg GW (1971) Single-cell isotope injection technique, a tool for studying axonal and dendritic transport. Acta Neuropathol [Suppl] (Berl), V:179–186

Schubert P, Reddington M, Kreutzberg GW (1979) On the possible role of adenosine as a modulatory messenger in the hippocampus and other regions of the CNS. Prog Brain Res 51:149–165

Snow PJ, Rose PK, Brown AG (1976) Tracing axons and axon collaterals of spinal neurons using intracellular injection of horseradish peroxidase. Science 191:312–313

Somogyi P, Cowey A (1980) The synapses formed by Cajal's "cellules à double bouquet dendritique" in the visual cortex of the cat and monkey. A combined Golgi and electron microscopic study. Neurosci Lett 5:S 118

Somogy P, Hodgson AJ, Smith AD (1979) An approach to tracing neuron networks in the cerebral cortex and basal ganglia: combination of Golgi staining, retrograde transport of horseradish peroxydase and anterograde degeneration of synaptic boutons in the same material. Neurosci. 4:1805–1852

Stretton AOW, Kravitz EA (1968) Neuronal geometry: determination with a technique of intracellular dye injection. Science 162:132–134

Thomas RC, Wilson VJ (1966) Marking single neurons by staining with intracellular recording microelectrodes. Science 151:1538–1539

Weiss P, Hiscoe HB (1948) Experiments on the mechanism of nerve growth. J Exp Zool 107: 315–395

Wong RK, Prince D, Busbaum A (1979) Intradendritic recordings from hippocampal neurons. Proc Natl Acad Sci USA 76:986–990

Zieglgänsberger W, Reiter C (1974) Interneuronal movement of procian yellow in cat spinal neurons. Exp Brain Res 20:527–530

Chapter 12

Light Microscopical Autoradiography of Nervous Tissue

H. Korr

1 Introduction

Autoradiography represents a method for the identification of radioactivity with the aid of photographic film. Due to the close contact between the object to be studied (e.g., a tissue section) and the film layer, not only the occurrence of radioactivity but also its distribution within the histologic specimen can be demonstrated. The advantage of autoradiography lies in the fact that the source of radiation can be exactly localized within a certain area. This area can even be reduced to the subcellular level when autoradiography is combined with electron microscopy.

Apart from providing information on the distribution of radioactivity in cells and tissues, autoradiography can be used to demonstrate metabolic processes, i.e., dynamic processes during the time interval between the application of the labeled substance and the fixation of the tissue. Consequently, autoradiography is used for investigations of metabolic processes, whereas histochemical studies demonstrate amounts of substances present at the moment of fixation.

With respect to the duration of measurement, autoradiography is a slow but basically a very sensitive method. Since the photographic emulsion stays in contact with the tissue for longer periods (e.g., weeks or months), the passage of ionizing particles can be registered during the whole time and it is therefore possible to demonstrate very small rates of decay (up to less than one decay per day per cell).

On the other hand, in studies of metabolic processes autoradiography has the general disadvantage of only demonstrating the occurrence of radioactivity. It provides no information on the chemical binding of this radioactivity. This can often only be elucidated by further investigations. The source of radioactivity may be the substance applied, but it may also be a labeled metabolite of this substance.

Before deciding on the methodological procedure of an autoradiographic study of a certain metabolic process in the tissue, it must be determined whether the whole range of labeled metabolic products of the injected substance or the end-product in the line of synthesis is to be evaluated. In the latter case, it is important to know whether this end-product – in contrast to the metabolites – is firmly incorporated in the examined tissue so that the histologic and autoradiographic process (fixation solution, staining solution, liquid photo emulsion) does not lead to a dislocation of the labeled compounds. The methods described in detail in the following paragraphs are suitable means of investigation only if a dislocation of the labeled compounds can be excluded. If the identification of labeled diffusible substances and their distribution is the objects of the study (e.g., following application of radioactively labeled hormones), other, more special methods have to be used. These methods are described in Chap. 20.

The aim of this chapter is a critical review of the methodological and technical procedures involved in autoradiographic investigations – ranging from animal experiments or in vitro incubations to the evaluation of the complete autoradiograph. The data refer to studies of the DNA, RNA, and protein synthesis in the brain, as well as to studies of neuronal connectivities and the localization of neurons with specific neurotransmitters. For a more intense study of the method of autoradiography and its field of application, see the monographs by Schultze (1969), Fischer and Werner (1971), Amlacher (1974), and Rogers (1979).

2 Labeling of Nervous Tissue

2.1 Choice of the Precursor

A decisive factor for the efficacy of an autoradiographic investigation is the choice of the suitable labeled precursor. For this purpose the following paragraphs will provide information on studies of the DNA, RNA, and protein synthesis. Information on substances for the localization of transmitter-specific neurons in the brain (a field of application of autoradiography in neuroanatomy) can be obtained from Schon and Iversen (1974) and Hertz (1979). These substances are partly demonstrated by labeling the routes of biosynthesis and partly by labeling due to specific high affinity uptake mechanisms.

2.1.1 DNA Synthesis

A cell – whether in the periphery or in the CNS – synthesizes DNA, in contrast to the biosynthesis of other macromolecules, only during a specific time interval of its cell cycle: the DNA synthesis phase or S-phase. A specific precursor of DNA synthesis is thymidine (TdR). An injection of radioactively labeled TdR exclusively leads to labeling of the nuclei of those cells which at the time of injection are in the DNA synthesis phase of their cell cycle. For details referring to an insignificant incorporation of labeled TdR into proteins or mitochondria, and labeling as an indication for cell proliferation, see Korr (1980).

2.1.2 RNA Synthesis

The nucleosides cytidine and uridine are precursor substances commonly used for the labeling of RNA. To a small extent, however, these nucleosides are also incorporated into DNA. Only uridine, which is labeled in the 5-position, can be regarded as a selective precursor of RNA synthesis (for details see, for example, Schultze 1969).

In autoradiographic studies of RNA synthesis in the brain as well as in other organs of the adult mouse, ^{3}H-cytidine reveals the same labeling pattern as ^{3}H-uridine. The grain density after injection of ^{3}H-uridine is, however, about 5 times smaller than after injection of ^{3}H-cytidine under the same experimental conditions (Schultze et al. 1961; Schultze and Maurer 1967).

2.1.3 Protein Synthesis

For studies of the protein synthesis in a cell, radioactively labeled amino acids are applied in the form of a single amino acid or as a mixture of several amino acids. In both cases it must be guaranteed that the amino acid(s) applied is (are) also present in the cells to be studied. It has been demonstrated in various studies (for review see, e.g., Droz 1969, 1975) that the labeled amino acids are peptide bound to protein provided the tissue has been appropriately fixed (see Sect. 3.1).

For labeling the whole brain via the blood stream, suitable substances include tyrosine, lysine, phenylalanine, and arginine in addition to the frequently used leucine. Citoler et al. (1966) found identical labeling patterns for these amino acids in the brain of the adult mouse. This also applies to the oral administration of thioamino acids (Oehlert et al. 1958, 1960; Schultze and Maurer 1967).

Nerve cells show a very high rate of protein synthesis. Moreover, the newly synthesized proteins are continuously transported to the dendrites and particularly to the axon, which results in a somatofugal movement up to the periphery of neuronal processes. Today, the time course of these processes frequently serves to demonstrate fibrous connections between various brain nuclei. Based on empirical studies (see Cuénod and Cowan 1975), leucine or proline are mostly applied in such investigations following a stereotactic intracerebral injection. Furthermore, the precursors of glycoproteins, labeled fucose, or mixtures of leucine, proline, and fucose can be injected. For details, especially on the pros and cons of certain precursors, see the excellent book by Cowan and Cuénod (1975).

2.2 Choice of the Isotope

Particularly suitable for autoradiographic studies are those isotopes which emit low-energy β-particles or, as in the case of ^{125}I, eject a high percentage of electrons with very low energy. A record of isotopes commonly applied in autoradiographic studies and their physical data is given by Rogers (1979).

For studies of nervous tissue the precursors used are mainly tritium labeled. Due to the extremely short range of tritium β-particles (maximum range in tissues about 5 µm; mean range only about one-third of the maximum range, i.e., about 1–2 µm), a very good coordination of the silver grains in the film and the source of radiation is achieved. Light microscopically, the source of radiation can be located directly below the silver grains. A similarly good coordination is achieved with ^{125}I. This isotope, which has been applied only recently in autoradiographic studies on nervous tissue, has a half-life of only 60 days. Thus, there is not as much time for the histologic preparation of the tissue as in the case of tritium (half-life 12.3 years). Examples of recent studies with ^{125}I-labeled substances in the CNS are given by Van Houten et al. (1979, 1980).

Substances labeled with ^{14}C or ^{35}S are also frequently used. Both isotopes show a similar energy-distribution of their β-particles (maximum energy of particles in ^{14}C is 155 keV, in ^{35}S, 167 keV). The mean range of their β-particles is about ten times larger than that of ^{3}H-β-particles. Due to their lower ionization density, less silver grains are produced compared with tritium in the thin emulsion layers which are commonly applied (see also Sects. 3.4.2.1, 3.4.2.2). This disadvantage can, however, be compensated for by the use of a thick emulsion layer (see Sect. 3.4.2.3), since β-tracks can then be observed.

The use of ^{14}C and ^{35}S, however, is advantageous compared with tritium, if sections thicker than 5 µm have to be quantitatively evaluated. Due to the high range of radiation, structures located in the deeper parts of the sections (e.g., split nuclei) are also recognized as being labeled (see also Sects. 3.2, and 5.1).

2.3 Route of Application

Before deciding on the route of application of a substance it should be considered whether this substance can be transported to the brain via the blood stream (systemic application) or whether an injection directly into the brain is necessary (intraventricular or intracerebral application). When using the first mode of application in studies of DNA, RNA, or protein synthesis, the route of application of the substance is of virtually no importance (Schultze 1968, 1969). Except for experiments with very short postinjection survival times, it is thus possible either to inject the substance i.p., i.v., or s.c. or to administer it orally (e.g., for studies of protein synthesis). This is an important factor in experiments with very young animals. Here, an s.c. injection in the skin of the back is much easier to perform than an i.p. injection. It might even be impossible to give the substance intravenously.

If the substance is injected intraventricularly it will not be distributed homogenously throughout the total brain parenchyma (Altman and Chorover 1963). Neither can a selective labeling of the ependyma or slightly deeper regions be achieved nor can the whole brain be equally supplied with the substance injected. Thus, a quantitative comparison of the labeling intensity (grain number per area) of various brain areas is not possible. Furthermore, the labeled substance may enter the blood vessels and get into the blood circulation (see Shaw 1974).

2.4 Amount and Activity of the Labeled Substance Applied

A rule that must be obeyed in all experiments with radioactively labeled substances is that the metabolic processes to be studied should not be impaired by the substance applied. The following factors should be observed:

2.4.1 Amount of Labeled Substance

In general, the amount of labeled substance applied should not exceed the "tracer dose," i.e., it should not influence the physiologic conditions. In most cases this can be achieved by applying only a small percentage of the amount physiologically present in the body as the so-called endogenous precursor pool. Studies by Maurer et al. (1954) have shown, for instance, that the amount of free methionine in the rabbit totals 13.8 mg. In consequence, a dose of 0.3 mg labeled methionine (2% of the methionine pool) injected into a rabbit in studies of protein synthesis can be regarded as the tracer dose.

Data on the concentration of various free amino acids in rat plasma and brain water (wet weight minus dry weight of the brain) are given in a study of Appel et al. (1960), who found values between 10 and 40 μg amino acids per milliliter plasma or brain water. On the basis of these data, it can be estimated that, e.g., by an injection of 10 μCi ^{3}H-leucine of high specific activity per gram body weight only a small percentage of the total amount of free endogenous leucine is administered and the requirement not to exceed the "tracer dose" is thus fulfilled. For information on the significance of the endogenous amino acid pool in intracerebral injections, see also Lajtha (1975).

The tracer dose for TdR has been measured by Lang et al. (1968) and Maurer et al. (to be published): For five different cell types of the mouse the tracer dose was found to be 0.5 μg exogenously applied TdR per gram body weight. The tracer dose for ^{3}H-cytidine used to study the hepatocytes of the adult mouse was estimated to be 0.1 μg cytidine per gram body weight (Schmid and Maurer 1973).

For studies of the RNA, and DNA synthesis in the CNS of adult animals with systemically injected ^{3}H-TdR or ^{3}H-cytidine, the presence of a blood-brain barrier for these nucleosides should also be taken into consideration (Schultze et al. 1972 a). After injection of ^{3}H-TdR the mean grain number per cell nucleus in the brain (neuroglia, cells of the subependymal layer, endothelial cells) is about ten times smaller than that of other cell types in the organism (Mares et al. 1974; Korr 1978 a; Korr et al. to be published). For this reason, higher amounts of labeled TdR must be injected. A blood-brain barrier similar to that for ^{3}H-TdR or ^{3}H-cytidine has also been identified for the amino acids alanine, glycine, and serine (Citoler et al. 1966; Schultze et al. 1972 b).

Examples of the amounts of ^{3}H-labeled neurotransmitter substances that have been applied intracerebrally or intraventricularly are given by, for example, Hökfelt and Ljungdahl 1972 (^{3}H-GABA), Kelly and Dick 1976 (β-^{3}H-alanine, ^{3}H-DABA, ^{3}H-GABA, ^{3}H-glycine), and Calas et al. 1974 (^{3}H-serotonin).

2.4.2 Activity of the Labeled Substance

Since the number of silver grains above a labeled structure in an autoradiograph results from the product of radioactivity and the time of exposure, the general aim of the investigator will be to apply as much radioactivity as possible. A free choice of the amount of radioactivity is, however, only possible if substances with different specific activities are available. If the substance to be administered is only available with one specific activity, the alternatives for the selection of the amount of activity are reduced by the "tracer dose."

For the use of ^{3}H-labeled substances with high specific activities, the following requirements should be met:

a) The labeled substance should be used up as soon as possible after its preparation, because processes of self-decomposition may occur within the substance (even after a few weeks) (for details see Evans 1976).
b) In the case of systemic injection it should be considered whether or not the high specific activity of the substance applied will lead to erroneous results; these can be caused by only slight losses of injection fluid.

When deciding on the activity to be applied, one should also consider possible effects of β-irradiation, i.e., damage to the cells caused by the incorporated radioisotope. This may, however, only occur with longer postinjection survival times. The risk of radiation injuries has often been discussed in studies of DNA synthesis after application of ^{3}H-TdR. In various tissues of the organism radiation effects will occur – with varying intensities depending on the respective organs – when activities considerably beyond the value of 1 μCi per gram body weight are applied (survey: e.g., Schultze 1969). So far, radiation effects on brain cells have only been described by Lewis (1968), this after intraventricular injection of 50 μCi ^{3}H-TdR into adult rats. Yet, with regard to this study it is questionable whether the observed alterations (prolongation of cell cycle phases G_2 + ½ M and S; presence of a large number of abnormal nuclei) may not also be caused by the relatively high local concentration of TdR or by the relatively large amount of liquid injected compared with the ventricle volume (see Sect. 2.4.3). On the other hand, in adult mice no alteration of the proliferative behavior of glial and endothelial cells was observed after an i.p. injection of about 30 μCi ^{3}H-TdR per gram body weight followed by an injection of 0.37 μCi ^{14}C-TdR per gram body weight 4 h later (Korr et al. 1973 b, 1975). This also applies to results gained in Schwann cells in the sciatic nerve of adult mice (Asbury 1970): following daily applications of 10 μCi ^{3}H-TdR per gram body weight during the first 10 days postnatally, faintly labeled and very strongly labeled Schwann cells had similar proliferation capacities 5 months after the transection of the sciatic nerve.

Summarizing the data on the factors "amount of substance" and "radioactivity of the applied substance," the following values may be taken as guidelines for autoradiographic studies in the nervous tissue (Schultze, pers. comm.):

a) ^{3}H-TdR (5–7 Ci/mmol): ca. 10 μCi per gram body weight
b) ^{3}H-cytidine or ^{3}H-uridine (5–30 Ci/mmol): ca. 20 μCi per gram body weight
c) ^{3}H-amino acids (e.g., ^{3}H-leucine, 40–60 Ci/mmol): ca. 10 μCi per gram body weight.

In the case of intracerebral injections of ^{3}H-labeled amino acids or neurotransmitter substances, about 5–50 μCi are applied depending on the aim of the experiment and the species investigated. For the demonstration of fiber connections better results were obtained by the injection of ^{3}H-labeled amino acids with high specific activity than by that of ^{3}H-labeled amino acids with low specific activity (Künzle 1975).

2.4.3 Volume of the Labeled Substance

Concerning the volume of the liquid injected – only this mode of application will be discussed in this chapter – the route of injection is important. Here too, the physiologic conditions must be taken into account. For instance, in the case of injection into the blood stream (e.g., i.v. injection), the animal's total blood volume must be considered. The total blood volume of a rat is about 65 ml/kg body weight (64.1 ml/kg: Altman and Dittmer 1964; 67 ml/kg: Hagemann and Schmidt 1960) and that of a mouse, about 80 ml/kg body weight (77.8 ml/kg: Altman and Dittmer 1964; 89±11 ml/kg: Shaw 1974). According to my own experience, a volume of up to about 10% of the total amount of blood in the animal is justifiable as an *i.v.* injection. If larger volumes have to be injected i.v., a slow injection (over some minutes) is advisable.

In *i.p.* injections, volumes of up to about 0.4 ml (adult mouse) and up to 1.0 ml (adult rat) are tolerated. *Subcutaneous* injections (particularly in the case of young animals, e.g., under the skin of the back) should not exceed volumes of about 0.2 ml.

Intraventricular injections should be carried out cautiously because of the small size of ventricles. The following average values for the adult rat may act as the basis for the interpretation of the "physiologic injection volume" (Levinger 1971): volume of the lateral ventricle, 43 μl; of the IIIrd ventricle, 38 μl; and of the IVth ventricle,

10 μl. In adult rabbits the total volume of the ventricular system amounts to about 1 ml (Schwarzberg et al. 1971).

In *intraocular* or *intracerebral* injections for studies of the neuronal connectivities, the choice of the injection volume depends to a greater extent on the purpose of the study than on physiologic conditions (see Künzle 1975). For intraocular injections, volumes between 20 and 100 μl are usually applied for cats and monkeys, whereas 1–5 μl are injected intraocularly in smaller animals like guinea pigs and rats. Most intracerebral injections have volumes between 0.02 and 0.2 μl. In order to ensure that enough activity is applied despite small injection volumes, commercially available solutions are condensed by evaporation (see Cowan et al., 1972). It should be noted that no volume is injected in the case of iontophoretic applications. For details on intracerebral injections, see Schubert et al. (1972) and Schubert and Holländer (1975).

2.5 Postinjection Survival Time

A general scheme for the time interval to be chosen for the period between application of the labeled substance and killing of the animal cannot be given, since the survival time depends on the purpose of the experiment. But it seems reasonable to give a few data on the time course of the biosyntheses to be studied, particularly with regard to short-term experiments.

2.5.1 DNA Synthesis

In the blood plasma of mice a high concentration of ^{3}H-TdR can be determined as early as 1 min after injection (Skougaard and Stewart 1966). This concentration decreases exponentially with increasing time, i.e., very rapidly, which is indicative of a pulse labeling. Within the cell nucleus, an amount of ^{3}H-labeled DNA sufficient to be demonstrated autoradiographically can be identified a few minutes after the injection of ^{3}H-TdR. This not only applies to various cell types in the organism like epithelial cells of jejunal crypts (Quastler and Sherman 1959; Koburg and Maurer 1962), but also to proliferating glial and endothelial cells in the brain of 14-day-old rats (Korr et al., in preparation). In the nuclei of these brain cells ^{3}H-TdR is available up to 60 min after ^{3}H-TdR injection. Up to this time precipitable ^{3}H-DNA is synthesized from the injected ^{3}H-TdR. However, the majority of labeled DNA is synthesized within 40 min after ^{3}H-TdR injection. This can be demonstrated by the increase of the mean grain number per nucleus as a function of time after injection of ^{3}H-TdR. The maximum grain number is reached after 60 min and is maintained until the cell has passed through the G_2-phase and mitosis. For brain cells this may take a period (T_{G2+M}) of 1.5 –5 h, depending on the cell type and the ontogenetic age of the animals (survey: Korr 1980).

Based on these experimental findings a survival time of no more than 1 h should be chosen for the determination of the relative number of labeled cells in a certain cell type after ^{3}H-TdR injection (= labeling index).

2.5.2 RNA Synthesis

Like TdR, the precursors of RNA synthesis cytidine and uridine are also available to brain cells only a few minutes after injection (Schultze et al. 1972 a). Here too, the injection of labeled cytidine or uridine leads to pulse labeling. Within the cell, labeling is first identified above the nucleolus, where the highest grain density is reached about 10 min after injection. With increasing duration of the experiment the grain number above the nucleolus decreases while it increases above the karyoplasm. Maximum labeling of the karyoplasm is reached between 4 and 8 h. About

16 h after the injection of ^{3}H-cytidine or ^{3}H-uridine the grain density above the cytoplasm reaches its maximum. If investigations on the rat liver can be generalized, the mean life span of the RNA – referring to the entire cell – is about 5 days (Schultze et al. 1961).

In general, it becomes evident that the "duration of the experiment" is of great importance, particularly in studies on RNA synthesis.

2.5.3 Protein Synthesis

Biochemical investigations on the pool of free methionine in the rat with ^{35}S-methionine have shown that free labeled methionine reaches its maximum in the brain about 15–20 min after an i.v. injection. Two hours later the amount of free labeled methionine which is incorporated into protein is already reduced to about one-sixth of the maximum value (Appel et al. 1960). Similar conditions may be supposed for other amino acids, such as leucine, phenylalanine, and tyrosine. An autoradiographic labeling pattern which corresponds to these findings has been found by Droz and Leblond (1963): in the rat brain an increase of the grain number above nerve cell perikarya could be identified up to about 30 min after i.p. injection of ^{3}H-leucine. The maximum labeling was maintained until about 90 min after the injection and then slowly decreased. This decrease may above all be due to the fact that labeled proteins are transferred to the axon (fast axonal transport). These data show that experimental periods of about 1 h should be chosen when protein synthesis in nerve cells is to be studied and if one wants to be sure that the results are not influenced by catabolism and transport of the proteins to the processes of the nerve cell.

For the survival time in studies of neuronal connectivities with ^{3}H-labeled amino acids the intracellular processes must first be considered (for review see, e.g., Heslop 1975): after intracerebral injection the labeled amino acid is absorbed by the neuron and incorporated in the newly synthesized protein. About 2 min after the injection, the labeling is found mainly above the Nissl substance; about 20 min after injection, a labeling peak is observed above the Golgi apparatus. With increasing time, the labeling is found above the axon hillock; here the peak is reached about 90 min after injection. Thereafter, a first wave of labeled protein moves centrifugally in the axon with a speed of roughly 100 mm per day (ca. 4 mm per hour; fast axonal transport). Droz et al. (1973) estimated a life span of about 17 h for these proteins. The fast axonal transport is followed by a period of the so-called slow axonal flow with a speed of 5 mm per day (ca. 210 μm per hour), which is sustained during several days. The proteins involved in this process have a life span of about 22 days. Compared with the amount of proteins involved in the fast axonal transport, that involved in the slow axonal flow is 3–5 times larger.

For studies of terminal projection fields most investigators concentrate on the demonstration of fast axonal transport. According to Cowan et al. (1972) it is recommendable to get a general idea of the postinjection survival times on the basis of the fiber length under study and the speed of transport before starting an autoradiographic study. It may also be useful to set up a time survival series by liquid scintillation counting for about 2–72 h.

For the demonstration of fiber pathways, the slow axonal flow of labeled proteins can be utilized. Survival times of several days are necessary for this type of investigation. For further details on the selection of survival times, see Grafstein (1975).

2.6 Double Labeling Experiments

Due to the introduction of special autoradiographic techniques, for instance, two emulsion-layer autoradiography (see Sect. 3.4.2.3), it is now possible to trace two different isotopes in a single histologic section. Hence, a variety of new approaches for autoradiographic studies have been created (see Van Rooijen 1976).

The autoradiographic identification of different isotopes in one section is based upon the application of isotopes with different energy spectra, i.e., different ranges of their β-particles, or of isotopes with extremely different half-lives. In the first case (and today only experiments of this kind are of any importance), an extremely low-energy isotope (tritium) is combined with an isotope of significantly higher energy (e.g., ^{14}C, ^{35}S, ^{131}I). While the low-energy isotope is traced on the basis of silver grains due to β-particles with a short range, the higher-energetic isotope can be traced according to tracks of grains produced by β-particles with a long range. A summary of the various possibilities for a combination of different isotopes, which have been tested in different tissues, is given by Rogers (1979).

Up to now, double-labeling experiments in the brain with ^{3}H- and ^{14}C-TdR have been carried out in order to evaluate the proliferative behavior of neuroglial and endothelial cells (Korr 1978 a, 1980; Korr et al. 1973 b, 1975) and to elucidate special questions in connection with cell migration of presumptive neurons (Wolff et al. 1978). For a quantitative evaluation of cell kinetic studies, i.e., the exact registration of the relative percentages of purely ^{3}H-labeled, purely ^{14}C-labeled, and double ($^{3}H+{}^{14}C$)-labeled cells in certain brain areas, the application of a two emulsion layer autoradiographic technique (see Sect. 3.4.2.3) and the activity ratio $^{3}H:{}^{14}C$ play an important role. In cell kinetic studies on the brains of adult mice (Korr et al. 1973 b, 1975) and of 14-day-old rats (Korr et al. in preparation), an activity ratio $^{3}H:{}^{14}C$ of 50–80 : 1 has proven advantageous.

A disadvantage of double labeling experiments is that – due to the use of ^{14}C, an isotope the β-particles of which have relatively long ranges – an exact coordination of β-tracks and single labeled cell is no longer possible if the labeled cells are closely situated. Hence, double labeling experiments with ^{3}H- and ^{14}C-TdR are not possible with embryonic tissues or in the subependymal layer of the lateral ventricle of adult mice if the evaluation of the number of differently labeled cells is the aim of the investigation.

For the investigation of tightly packed labeled cells, a modification of the above-mentioned double labeling method seems most appropriate: the application of two ^{3}H-activities of different intensities. According to the results obtained by Pilgrim for various tissues of the adult rat and mouse (Pilgrim 1964; Pilgrim and Maurer 1965), a quantitative distinction can be made in the autoradiograph between weakly ^{3}H-labeled cells and very strongly ^{3}H-labeled cells after an injection of 10 μCi ^{3}H-TdR followed by a second injection of 100 μCi ^{3}H-TdR 1 h later. According to this finding it was possible to measure the duration of the DNA synthetic phase in different cell types.

Presumably this method will also be appropriate for investigations of the brain. In this case, it may be necessary to increase the amount of activity because of the existence of a blood-brain barrier for TdR (see Sect. 2.4.1). It should be noted, however, that this method provides less information, since it only differentiates between two subpopulations (weakly and strongly labeled cells), whereas the application of two different isotopes provides differentiation of three differently labeled subpopulations. Whether this disadvantage can be compensated for depends on the type of investigation.

2.7 Incubation of Nervous Tissue

Autoradiographic studies on nervous tissue in vitro, i.e., after incubation of cultures, pieces of tissue, or fresh sections of several 100 μm thickness with radioactively labeled substances, can be carried out in the same way as in vivo studies. When adding the labeled substance of interest to the incubation medium even greater care has to be taken than in in vivo studies that the dosage is limited to the tracer range. An advantage of in vitro studies, on the other hand, is that it is possible to operate with considerably smaller amounts of substances. This is an important factor in the determination of the highly specific uptake mechanisms of neurotransmitters (see Calas et al. 1974).

The following dosages have been mentioned in the literature: for studies of DNA, RNA, or protein synthesis with ^{3}H-labeled precursors of common specific activities, Amlacher (1974) recommended the addition of 2–5 μCi/ml medium. In the case of ^{14}C-TdR, Jaros et al. (1974) applied 0.1 μCi/ml.

Methodological data on the autoradiographic identification of ^{3}H-labeled neurotransmitters in vitro are given by Matus and Dennison (1972; ^{3}H-glycine), Schon and Kelly (1974; ^{3}H-GABA) and Calas et al. (1974; ^{3}H-serotonin), among others.

3 Autoradiographic Technique

3.1 Fixation of the Tissue

When selecting the fixatives, not only the adequate preservation of the tissue structure should be a decisive factor, but one should also consider whether the fixative could influence the film layer or whether labeled substances could be removed by the fixative.

Fixatives containing sublimate are not suitable for subsequent autoradiography (Kopriwa and Leblond 1962; Kopriwa and Huckins 1972; Korr 1978 b). In these fixatives the presence of mercury salts is likely to provoke a desensitization of the emulsion.

With regard to the loss of labeled substances it should be considered that all substances which are not incorporated into the tissue are washed out. This may even be a desirable phenomenon in studies of DNA or protein synthesis, since it leads to the elimination of all labeled low-molecular metabolites and only the activity incorporated into protein or DNA will be recorded.

According to the results obtained by biochemical experiments concerning the effect of different fixatives on liver tissue (Antoni et al. 1965), activity and mass of DNA and protein are altered only insignificantly when different fixatives are used (neutral formalin; formalin-trichloracetic acid mixtures, Carnoy, methanol). Hence, the choice of the fixative for studies of DNA or protein synthesis is of minor importance. Care should be taken, however, when applying glutaraldehyde mixtures in investigations of protein synthesis. As has been demonstrated in studies on the liver (Peters and Ashley 1967), these fixatives cause unspecific linkages of free labeled amino acids to the tissue.

In investigations of RNA synthesis, however, the choice of the fixative is of vital importance. Comparative autoradiographic studies of various tissues of the mouse 20 min after the injection of ^{3}H-cytidine revealed considerable differences in the grain density depending on the fixative used (Schneider and Maurer 1963). Due to these results, fixation with 6% neutral formalin (pH 7.0) or formalin and 7% trichloracetic acid seems most suitable. The same result has been obtained by Antoni et al. (1965) in biochemical investigations of the rat liver.

For all studies it is recommendable to add a surplus of the nonlabeled precursor substance to the fixative (e.g., 0.1 mg/ml solution) in order to remove by way of an exchange reaction all labeled molecules which are not incorporated into the tissue.

After fixation the fixative should be completely removed by carefully rinsing the histologic specimen in water. Residues of the fixative may increase the background of the autoradiographs by the influence of reducing substances and residues of oxidizing substances in the tissue may cause a fading of the latent image.

For methods to extract certain substances from the section, see Schultze (1969).

3.2 Preparation of Histologic Sections

Autoradiographs can be prepared from frozen sections, paraffin sections, or synthetic resin sections (e.g., methacrylate, Epon, Araldite). When employing frozen sections, it is recommendable to dip the mounted sections briefly into xylene and subsequently into a series of alcohols with decreasing concentrations. This treatment results in a tissue fixation desirable to avoid the danger of chemographic effects (see Sect. 4.1). On the other hand, xylene treatment prevents the development of disturbing cholesterine crystals over myelinated brain structures (Korr et al. 1970, 1973 a).

A defined *section thickness* is important when quantitative evaluations are to be carried out after the application of ^{3}H-labeled substances. Because of the extremely short range of ^{3}H-β-particles, only the most superficial tissue layer (ca. 2–3 μm) contributes to the autoradiographic effect. When using thicker sections, it may happen that a labeled structure (e.g., a split nucleus) is recognized histologically and is thus registered, but that no silver grains are produced, since the β-particles are absorbed in the tissue layer covering this structure. It is therefore recommendable to use thin sections (about 3–5 μm) when applying ^{3}H-labeled substances. When a section is thinner than 1 μm, longer exposure times are necessary, since the grain number then decreases in approximate linearity with the decreasing thickness of the section.

For the *slides* needed for the mounting of the sections, glass containing only small amounts of potassium has proved good. Due to the lowered content of potassium, the amount of naturally occurring ^{40}K in the glass is also reduced, whereby the background of the autoradiographs is diminished. Microscope slides being ground on one side provide the advantage that satisfactory inscriptions can be made with an ordinary pencil – scratching with a diamond pencil creating glass dust is thus avoided – and that an orientation on the upper or lower side of the slide in the dark room is facilitated.

For the mounting of paraffin sections on microscope slides a liquid composed of a mixture of acetone, aqua dest., and albumin-glycerin (20 : 80 : 1) has proved good (Schultze, personal communication).

Paraffin sections must be deparaffinized carefully before they may be brought into contact with the photoemulsion. Paraffin residues cause a blackening of the film. Tissue sections embedded in synthetic resin, however, can be processed without removal of the embedding medium prior to covering with the photographic emulsion.

3.3 Photographic Emulsion

For autoradiographic studies various photoemulsions are available (for review see Rogers 1979). Besides the stripping film AR-10 (Kodak, United Kingdom), the liquid emulsions of Ilford (Essex, United Kingdom) and Eastman-Kodak (Rochester, N.Y., United States) are of special importance. The latter two emulsions differ in the size of the silver bromide crystals and in their sensitivities. The larger the diameter of the crystals the more sensitive is the emulsion. With increasing sensitivity of the emulsion, the background is also raised. In Europe emulsions of Ilford are usually used. This company offers G-emulsions (crystal diameter, 0.27 μm), K-emulsions (0.20 μm), and L-emulsions (0.14 μm). The different categories of emulsion are supplied with different sensitivities, ranging from 0 to 5, the latter being the most sensitive emulsion within each series. The emulsions G-5, K-2, and K-5 are of practical significance for light microscopic autoradiography, and in special cases L-4 is applied, which was originally developed for electron microscopic autoradiography. Its crystal diameter is so small that silver grains can only be registered when the most powerful objectives are used. The emulsions of Ilford, which are provided in the form of gels, are stored in the refrigerator at +4 °C. Freezing of the emulsion must by all means be avoided. After storage for more than 2 months, an increased background cannot be excluded.

Apart from the emulsions in the form of gels, which have been developed for the dipping procedure (see Sect. 3.4.2.2), the stripping film AR-10 (Kodak) is frequently used. In this case, the emulsion layer has been poured onto a glass plate in a constant thickness of 5 μm together with a gelatine underlayer of 10 μm. The crystal diameter in this emulsion is 0.20 μm and is thus equivalent to the K-emulsions of Ilford; its sensitivity is comparable to that of the K-2 emulsion. The AR-10 plates are stored in the refrigerator (+4 °C) and remain applicable for about 6 months.

According to the aim of the study the most suitable emulsion should be chosen. For a preliminary rough orientation on the amount of radioactivity the emulsion Ilford G-5 may be applied. This emulsion is about 3–5 times more sensitive than the emulsion K-2 or the stripping film AR-10. Yet, due to its large silver grains and its high background, the G-5 emulsion is not suitable for grain counting. For a quantitative evaluation including grain counting, the K-2 emulsion is particularly valuable. This emulsion is less sensitive than the K-5 emulsion, but the background remains negligible provided the emulsion layer has been applied and handled properly.

The application of the stripping film AR-10 is advisable when only a few autoradiographs have to be produced. For large numbers of autoradiographs the dipping method is more convenient.

3.4 Preparation of Autoradiographs

3.4.1 Working Conditions in the Darkroom

There are a number of detailed descriptions of the optimal darkroom for autoradiographic studies (Kopriwa 1963; Amlacher 1974; Rogers 1979). Hence, only a few important points will be discussed in the following paragraph.

For reasons of cleanliness, the darkroom needed for the preparation of autoradiographs should not be used for other kinds of photographic work at the same time. In contrast to an ordinary darkroom for photographic work, this room should be absolutely light-tight. Moreover, the darkroom should not be located in the vicinity of machines emitting X-rays, which would produce an increased background on the autoradiographs. The existence of a light trap is absolutely necessary to avoid the need to stay in the darkroom during the long drying period after application of the emulsion. Special requirements have to be fulfilled with respect to temperature and relative humidity of the air. When Ilford emulsions are applied, the room temperature should not exceed +20 °C and the relative humidity should be 45%–50%. When working with the stripping film, +15°–18 °C and 60%–65% relative humidity are recommendable. If fresh air is supplied from the outside, care should be taken that there is no heavy motion of air because whirled up dust tends to collect on drying emulsion layers. The air supplied to the darkroom must not contain traces of H_2S gases (e.g., from dry siphons), since only very small amounts of H_2S cause a high background.

With respect to the illumination of the darkroom, special requirements result from safe-light conditions specified by the producers of photoemulsions. Ilford, for example, recommends the light-brown Ilford "S" safe-light for G-, K-, and L-emulsions. For Kodak AR-10 or Eastman-Kodak NTB emulsions a dark-red Wratten No. 2 filter is recommended. In both cases a 15-W bulb should be used, and the distance between safe-light and photoemulsion should be at least 1 m. If more than just one type of film is applied, it is advisable to use a dark Wratten filter, which can also be applied in preparations with Ilford emulsions. In spite of the recommendations made for special filters, a general rule is that the background becomes less the less light has been used. This especially applies for the use of dry emulsion layers.

As a ceiling light neon light is totally inappropriate. Even several hours after having been switched off, neon tubes emit a dim light which is noticeable to the human eye only after an adequate time of adaptation but which causes an obviously higher background in the photoemulsion. Electric equipment needed in the darkroom consists of refrigerators for the storage of the emulsions and for the exposure of the autoradiographs, and of waterbaths with thermostats for the melting of the emulsion and the development of the autoradiographs. These appliances, as well as switches in the darkroom should be shielded so that no light flashes emitted when turning them on or off can penetrate to the outside. It has proved useful to check the light-tightness of the darkroom from time to time. Small beams of light or a certain translucence will be visible only after an adaptation to the complete darkness of ca. 20–30 min.

3.4.2 Application of the Emulsion

Cleanliness is the major prerequisite for all autoradiographic studies. This applies to the glass equipment, to all chemicals used for the preparation of the developers and fixation baths, as well as to water (aqua bidest. is the safest!). Photoemulsions should never be brought into contact with your fingers! This would cause a chemographic blackening. Moreover, contact of photoemulsions with metals such as copper or iron should be avoided. For the handling of emulsions in the form of gels, forceps made of horn or glass rods should be used.

3.4.2.1 Stripping Film Technique

As a first step the slides with the mounted sections are briefly dipped into a diluted chrome alum-gelatin solution (2.5 g gelatin +0.25 g chrome alum in 500 ml aqua dest.). This chrome alum layer, which has a thickness of about 1–10 nm (in a dry state) serves as a support for the stripping film layer which will be applied in a second step. Without such a chrome alum layer, loosening or slipping of the film layer during development, fixation, and rinsing might occur.

After the chrome alum-gelatin layer has dried (within about 2 h; the time interval between preparation of the chrome alum-gelatin layer and the application of the stripping film should not exceed 24 h), work in the darkroom begins. The film plates are taken out of the refrigerator and sufficiently large pieces of film are separated by careful scratching with a scalpel or razor blade. The subsequent loosening of the film from the glass slide can be critical since electrostatic light flashes may occur and thus may cause an increased background of the autoradiographs. To avoid this source of error, stripping the film off the glass plate in a solution of 20 g sucrose, 0.1 ml KBr 10%, and 1000 ml aqua bidest. is a suitable procedure (Schultze and Maurer, personal communication). The narrow side of the precut piece of film is carefully loosened with the fingertips (by touching the gelatin layer, which is lying directly on the glass). Then the microscope slide with the mounted preparation is transferred close to the loosened end of the film. The film is carefully placed around the edge of the slide, held on the backside, and finally wound around the slide by slowly lifting it with a twisting motion. The film layer is now directly attached to the section with the gelatin layer on the outside. The slides with the attached film are arranged in an upright position for drying. During the drying process they should be protected from direct red light.

At a relative humidity of 60%–65%, the drying process takes about 2 h. If the slides are dried too fast (e.g., at a low relative humidity or when using a fan), artifacts may be produced (for examples see Rogers 1979). After the drying process the slides are stored in light-tight plastic boxes. A drying medium (e.g., Drierite, i.e., anhydrous calcium sulfate with blue indicator) is added in a plastic tube containing small holes, since humidity during exposure causes fading. Finally, the plastic boxes are sealed with black adhesive tape, marked on the cover, and exposed in the refrigerator at +4 °C. The adhesive tape should only be unrolled when all autoradiographs are light-tightly stored, because light flashes may be emitted. Detailed descriptions of the steps taken in the stripping film technique (which do, however, differ in some points) are given by Amlacher (1974) and Rogers (1979) among others.

3.4.2.2 Dipping Technique

When preparing a thin emulsion layer (thickness about 1–2 μm in a dry state before development) for the study of ^{3}H-labeled substances, a certain, previously weighed-out amount of emulsion is first melted in a clean glass vessel in a water bath at +42 °C. This temperature must more or less be maintained since at temperatures higher than +45 °C clumps of silver bromide crystals are formed. The melted emulsion is diluted by the addition of aqua bidest.; a nondiluted emulsion would result in a thicker emulsion layer. For the preparation of a thin film layer as described above with Ilford K-2 emulsion, a dilution of 3 weight parts emulsion with 2 weight parts aqua bidest. has proved to be successful. Emulsion and aqua bidest. should be stirred very carefully (with a glass rod). If they are stirred or agitated too violently, bubbles may be produced which disturb the subsequent dipping process. If the glass vial is touched with the glass rod, the silver bromide crystals may be damaged, which results in a higher background. When emulsion and aqua bidest. have been mixed the mixture is filtered through a double layer of gaze (no bubbles!).

The slides are placed on the plate of a water bath for some time to be prewarmed. Then they are slowly dipped into the emulsion one after the other, removed again at a constant speed, and then dried in an upright position. For the process of dipping, various apparatuses have been constructed (for review see Rogers 1979). Apart from avoiding extremely long or short dipping, it seems to be more important for the production of layers with uniform thickness that the temperature of the emulsion and of the slides to be processed, as well as the conditions in the room (temperature, relative air humidity), are maintained at a constant level.

At a room temperature of +18 °C and a relative air humidity of about 50%, thin emulsion layers are dry after approximately 1 h. The slides with the attached film are stored in the same manner as described above (Sect. 3.4.2.1).

For obtaining regular emulsion layers for preparations with uneven surfaces (e.g., tissue cultures growing on cover slips) or for preparations with very smooth surfaces, one may add a surface-active substance such as Hostapon T (Hoechst, Frankfurt/Main). Approximately 1 drop of a 10% aqueous Hostapon solution is added per 10 ml emulsion.

3.4.2.3 Two Emulsion Layer Autoradiographs

For exact differentiation between ^{3}H- and ^{14}C-labeling in double-labeling experiments, the following double-layer autoradiography has proved to be satisfactory:

a) First Emulsion Layer. A first thin emulsion layer for registration of ^{3}H-β-particles is applied according to the dipping methods with Ilford K-2 emulsion (see Sect. 3.4.2.2).

b) Gelatin Layer. After development, fixation, and drying of the first emulsion layer (see above), the slides are dipped into a +28 °C gelatin solution (10 g gelatin ad 100 ml aqua bidest., diluted at +42 °C) and are dried in an upright position for about 10 h. Thereafter, the slides are put into a formalin solution (1+4) at room temperature for 20 min for hardening of the gelatin layer. Finally, they are carefully washed in tap water for 10 min (danger of washing away the gelatin layer!), rinsed twice with aqua bidest., and dried.

c) Second Emulsion Layer. Ilford K-2 emulsion is melted at +42 °C, then, without further dilution, cooled down in a second water bath to +28 °C. The dry slides are dipped into this emulsion. Subsequently, they are dried in a vertical position in complete darkness for approximately 4 h. With this method, an emulsion layer of about 10 μm thickness (in a dry state before development) is obtained. Details on the preparation of thicker emulsion layers are given by Schultze et al. (1976).

3.4.2.4 Exposure

With regard to the conditions of exposure, it has already been mentioned that the autoradiographs must be stored as dry as possible. This is achieved by the addition of a drying medium. Humidity (moist emulsion layers, high relative air humidity inside the exposure box) leads to the extinction of latent images, the so-called fading. A temperature of +4 °C has proved to be that most favorable for exposure. Special precautions for the exposure of autoradiographs which also emit γ-rays have been discussed in detail by Rogers (1979).

For the determination of the optimal exposure time, no universal recipe can be given. In addition to factors like applied radioactivity and duration of the experiment, the planned method of evaluation also plays an important role. For visual grain counting, about 1 grain per μm² is a desirable grain density. For this purpose shorter exposure times are needed than in cases when a photographic documentation of the autoradiograph is planned.

The photoemulsion becomes sensitive as soon as it is dry. When using liquid emulsions (dipping method), the grain density above a labeled structure increases linearly with increasing exposure time, as long as no saturation has been achieved. A linear increase of the grain density has, for example, been recorded for the emulsion Ilford K-2 over a period of 200 days (perhaps even longer; Schultze, personal communication), and for NTB-2 emulsion (Eastman-Kodak) over 360 days (Kopriwa and Leblond 1962; Leblond et al. 1963). When applying the stripping film, considerable fading may already occur after exposure times of more than 1 week (for survey see, Schultze 1969).

For the practical procedure of the determination of the appropriate exposure time, it has proved useful to expose additional autoradiographs in separate boxes for test developments. Thus, unnecessary warming up (from refrigerator temperature to room temperature) and new packing is avoided for the majority of autoradiographs – all these are factors which contribute to the increase of the background.

3.4.2.5 Development and Fixation

Although the producers of photographic emulsions make special recommendations concerning development, it has been demonstrated that no significant differences exist between the various developers (Leblond et al. 1963). Much more important criteria for reproducible results are the time of development and the temperature of the developer, which both especially affect the background.

For the development of stripping film AR-10 (Kodak) the developer D-19 supplied by Kodak has proved useful. The development can, for example, be performed at +18 °C for 4 min. Instructions for an individual preparation of D-19 and other developers are given by Amlacher (1974).

Ilford recommends the Phen-X developer for the development of emulsion layers produced by the dipping technique. In our institute, the following amidol developer has for years provided good results: amidol (4-hydroxy-m-phenylene-diammonium dichloride) 1.35 g; Na_2SO_3 sicc. 5.4 g; KBr 10% 2.4 ml; aqua bidest. 300 ml. The developer should always be prepared freshly and filtrated before being used. The development is performed at +18 °C for 4 min.

The development of *double-layer autoradiographs* is performed as follows:

a) The *thin* emulsion layer is developed in the same manner as described for the dipping procedure.
b) The *thick* emulsion layer is developed with the following diluted amidol developer for 20 min at +12 °C: 1.125 g amidol; 4.5 g Na_2SO_3 sicc.; 2 ml KBr 10%; 8.75 g H_3BO_3 cryst.; aqua bidest. ad 500 ml.

When compared with the thin emulsion layer the longer time of development of the thick emulsion layer with a diluted developer at low temperatures guarantees a uniform development of the entire thick emulsion layer. In all procedures cited in this chapter, the development is followed without a stopper bath by fixation in 30% sodium thiosulphate solution at room temperature. For stripping film or thin emulsion layers prepared according to the dipping procedure, fixation of 10 min is sufficient, whereas thick layers require 50 min. During development and also during fixation an appropriate movement of the solutions should be guaranteed by slow shaking.

After fixation the slides are washed in running tap water to eliminate all traces of fixation. For thin emulsion layers and stripping film this takes about 20 min, and thick emulsion layers are washed for about 90 min. Rinsing is performed with aqua bidest. and the slides are then dried in a dust-free environment.

3.5 Staining Methods

Not all staining techniques applied in neuroanatomy can also be used in autoradiographic investigations. Staining colors (e.g., toluidine blue or cresyl violet) may, for example, affect the undeveloped photo emulsion, i.e., may cause blackening of the emulsion (positive chemography). Conversely, an impairment of the staining (strong fading of light green) is also possible by photographic processes, i.e., development and fixation. Two principal modes of staining autoradiographs can be differentiated: firstly, prestaining, i.e., staining before the application of the film layer, and secondly, poststaining, i.e., staining through the developed and fixed emulsion layer. Surveys on various stainings that can be applied in autoradiography are given by Boyd (1955), Bélanger (1961), Leblond et al. (1963), and Thurston and Joftes (1963), and special stainings for neuroanatomic studies are described by Sidman (1970) and Hendrickson et al. (1972).

In addition, the following staining methods should be mentioned: Siperstein (1963) gives instructions for the PAS staining of paraffin sections of the hypophysis. This staining is performed before the application of the film layer. An aldehyde-fuchsin-staining especially for autoradiographs of Epon sections is described by Calvert and Pusterla (1974).

Another prestaining method is the Feulgen staining of paraffin and frozen sections. This provides a very clear representation of the nuclear morphology even in brain sections (see Korr 1980), and the subsequent photographic processes do not cause any problems. Therefore, this staining method is also suitable for double-layer autoradiography (Korr et al. 1973 b, 1975).

Feulgen staining is performed as follows:

a) Hydrolysis of the deparaffinized sections in 1 n HCl at exactly +60 °C (water bath) for 6 min.
b) After short rinsing with aqua bidest., storage in Schiff-Reagenz (pararosaniline 0.5 g; $K_2S_2O_5$ 0.5 g; 1 n HCl 10 ml; aqua bidest. 10 ml) at room temperature for about 2 h.
c) Short dipping into tap water and aqua bidest. For the subsequent dipping into the melted emulsion, the sections should remain moist (avoid drops of water, however!).

Feulgen staining leads to a loss of DNA and consequently also to a loss of activity after labeling with ^{3}H- or ^{14}C-TdR (Lang and Maurer 1965). Grain counting on labeled glial cells in the brain of adult mice after injection of ^{3}H-TdR in our laboratory has shown that the loss of grains due to the Feulgen staining mentioned above is only about 10% of that due to hematoxylin staining through the developed film. Autoradiographs of Feulgen-stained sections look even "cleaner" than those stained according to other methods.

Out of the metal impregnations frequently applied in neuroanatomy obviously only those containing no mercury salts can be combined with subsequent autoradiography (see Sect. 3.1). Jaros et al. (1974) combined autoradiography with the silver method of Holmes. Korr (1978 b) described a technique for a combination of metal impregnation of frozen or paraffin sections according to the weak silver carbonate method of del Rio-Hortega (1919) with subsequent autoradiography. No labeling in the autoradiographs was obtained when the sections had previously been stained with the gold chloride sublimate method of Ramon y Cajal (1913; see also Sidman 1970).

Other prestaining methods are the combinations of autoradiography with the horseradish peroxidase histochemistry (Nowakowski et al. 1975) and with the immunoperoxidase technique (Latov et al. 1979). A survey of histochemical stainings for autoradiographic studies is given by Oehmichen and Saebisch (1971).

As a poststaining method which can be performed easily, the methyl-green-pyronine staining technique should be mentioned. Instructions for the staining of cryostat sections for autoradiography are given by Stumpf (1970).

Directions for the poststaining of sections of epoxy resin embedded tissues should also be mentioned. A general survey of staining methods that can be applied to material embedded in various epoxy resins is given by Davie (1970). However, this survey does not indicate which stainings are possible for autoradiographs. In some of these staining techniques the section has to be heated, and damage to the emulsion layer may occur. This can be prevented if the emulsion layer is previously hardened by formalin as described by Richter and King (1972). Thus, the Azur-II-methylene-blue staining of Araldite sections according to Richardson (Richardson et al. 1960) through the emulsion can be performed on the heating plate (+45 °C, 3 min) without problems when the autoradiographs have previously been transferred to a 5% formalin solution at room temperature for 4 min.

3.6 Preparing Autoradiographs for Microscopic Analysis

It has proved reasonable to protect the fixed emulsion layer from scratching by a cover slip. Before being covered the sections and the emulsion layer(s) must be absolutely dry. The drying process takes about 1 day, and for double-layer autoradiographs, about 2 days. Autoradiographs of paraffin and frozen sections can be mounted using conventional media containing no xylene (e.g., Entellan, Merck 7960). When "Entellan-new" (Merck 7961) or Eukitt (Kindler, Freiburg) have been used, after some time a steady decrease in the number of developed silver grains and finally their total disappearance have occasionally been observed. Autoradiographs of epoxy resin sections are preferably mounted with Permount (Fisher, New Jersey) or with the same epoxy resin used for embedding medium.

4 Analysis of Autoradiographs

4.1 Background, Artifacts

Before being evaluated, the autoradiographs should be examined with respect to the background level. This includes the background fog, which is distributed more or less uniformly throughout the emulsion layer. It should be definitely below one silver grain/100 μm², so that even weak labeling of the cells can be registered. The background fog is evaluated by grain counting using a grid in the eyepiece which is divided into 100 or 400 small squares; the background is counted above unlabeled section areas or on an autoradiograph of an unlabeled brain section prepared under identical conditions. For methods determining the background fog by grain counting, see Rogers (1979).

Apart from the background fog, which to a certain extent is unavoidable even with proper handling of the emulsion, additional artificial silver grain clusters can sometimes be found. Such artifacts may be observed at section corners (section ruptures, blood vessels) and possibly result from tensions in the emulsion during the drying process. It is much more difficult to detect artifacts due to chemographic effects: positive chemography, i.e., production of silver grains by reducing substances in the section, and negative chemography, i.e., extinction of latent images by oxydizing substances. Daniels and Gilmore (1975) reported on chemographic effects occurring particularly in brain sections. In order not to be deceived by such "results", it is advisable to prepare autoradiographs of inactive sections of the investigated CNS region parallelly to the sections of labeled tissue for the purposes of comparison.

4.2 Visual Grain Counting

When evaluating an autoradiograph the major question is whether a defined structure is labeled or unlabeled. Another interesting factor is the grain number over a certain structure. To answer this question the grain number above a defined area is counted. Visually, this can be performed with the aid of the above-mentioned grids. Grain densities of up to approximately 1 grain/μm² can be counted without problems. General directions for visual grain counting are given by Rogers (1979).

Furthermore, grain counting plays a role in the differentiation of labeled and unlabeled structures. When a great number of silver grains or tracks (in the case of higher-energy β-particles like ^{14}C in thick emulsion layers) is detected, the decision whether a defined structure (for instance a cell nucleus) is labeled or unlabeled does not cause any problems. It is, however, much more difficult to distinguish a weak labeling from the background. For the definition of the lower counting limit, i.e., the number of grains or tracks which is sufficient to regard a structure as being labeled, two methods can be applied:

a) The first method starts from the background, i.e., the highest grain density or track density that has been obtained above unlabeled areas. The area above which the background was estimated should correspond to that of the investigated structure and should not lie outside the section. If, for instance, in investigations after injection of ^{3}H-TdR, a maximum of two grains per nucleus is only occasionally found in unlabeled areas, cells with three or more grains per nucleus can certainly be regarded as being labeled.

b) The second method is based on the distribution of the grain density or the frequency distribution of the tracks per area of *all* cells, whether labeled or unlabeled. The result of this approach generally is a histogram consisting of two peaks: the first peak (mostly with a maximum of 0 grains per area) is related to the background; the second, larger peak refers to the labeled cells. The lower counting limit is the grain or track density corresponding to the minimum point of the density distribution graph. An example for this mode of determining the counting limit is given by Schultze et al. (1976). Compared to the method described in a), the second method has the advantage of enabling us to determine the error caused by a false classification of the cells due to the chosen counting limit. After extrapolation of both parts of the graph from the counting limit to the abscissa, the planes of the respective parts of the graph indicate how many weakly labeled cells have not been counted and, on the other hand, how many cells have been counted as labeled by mistake on account of the background. These specifications play a role in quantitative cell kinetic studies after the injection of ^{3}H- or ^{14}C-TdR.

A technique for the determination of counting limits in double-labeling experiments with ^{3}H- and ^{14}C-TdR is described by Schultze et al. (1976).

4.3 Photometric Measurements of Grain Density

Instead of visual evaluations, grain counting is often performed with the aid of special photometers. In these techniques either the amount of light reflected by the silver grains or the degree of absorption of transmitted light by the silver grains is measured. With this method, the grain density along any line through a brain section can be measured in order to identify terminal projection fields after intracerebral injection of ^{3}H-labeled leucine. A critical survey on the most frequently used methods for the photometric evaluation of autoradiographs is provided by Rogers (1979).

Due to the possibility of combining a photometer with a microscope-scanning table on the one hand, or with a computer system for the accumulation and preparation of the evaluated data on the other, the photometric analysis of autoradiographs can nowadays be carried out automatically (see, e.g., Mai and Junger 1977). In addition, there are systems which imply the scanning of autoradiographs by a television camera and the subsequent analysis of the pictures by a computer. For details on the more simple computer systems which have proved suitable for the evaluation of brain autoradiographs, see, for example, the review articles of Price and Wann (1975) and Bisconte (1976, 1979).

5 Quantitative Evaluation of the Autoradiographs

5.1 Grain Counting

For the interpretation of grain densities measured, the significance of β-self-absorption in studies with ^3H-labeled substances must be known. Due to the short range of ^3H-β-particles, a great portion of these β-particles is absorbed within the tissue and does not reach the emulsion. The extent of this β-self-absorption strongly depends on the mass density of the labeled cell structure. Although the maximum range of ^3H is about 0.5 mg/cm², its high-energy β-particles scarcely contribute to the autoradiographic effect, as has been demonstrated in studies by Maurer and Primbsch (1964). Of all silver grains, 90% are produced by β-particles emitted from the most superficial layer of the section with a mass density of 0.05 mg/cm². In fixed tissue, after the removal of the embedding medium this superficial layer has a thickness of about 1.8 μm in cytoplasm, about 2.8 μm in karyoplasm, and only about 0.5 μm in the nucleolus. Hence, if on the autoradiograph of a 5-μm section different grain densities are observed above the cytoplasm, the karyoplasm, and the nucleolus, these grain densities can only give evidence of the activity ratio of the investigated structures if the different mass densities are taken into consideration. The following example will elucidate these correlations: After injection of ^3H-uridine, Schultze and Maurer (1963) found an ^3H-activity ratio of nucleolus : karyoplasm : cytoplasm of 25:70:5 for the cells of the esophagus epithelium, if the relative activity was derived simply from grain counts. After consideration of β-self-absorption in the corresponding cell structures this ratio was changed to 60:36:4, i.e., the highest ^3H-activity did not correspond to the highest grain density above the karyoplasm but to the lower grain density above the nucleolus.

A correction of measured data on account of β-self-absorption can only be neglected if the sections investigated are not thicker than 0.1 μm. In these thin sections the grain number above all structures is proportional to the ^3H-activity (Maurer and Primbsch, 1964). β-Self-absorption can also be neglected in thicker sections if isotopes with higher-energy β-radiation, such as ^{14}C or ^{35}S, are applied.

In the following sections the significance of the grain density for DNA, RNA, and protein synthesis will be explained in more detail.

5.1.1 DNA Synthesis

In short-term experiments after application of ^3H-TdR the grain number per cell nucleus is often interpreted as a measure of the DNA synthetic rate, i.e., the amount of DNA newly synthesized during the experiment. Experimental results on various cell types in the organism under physiologic conditions seem to confirm this conclusion (for review see Schultze, 1969). For some cell types in the fetal rat, however, the grain number per nucleus does not seem to be in line with the DNA synthetic rate (Wegener et al. 1964).

Problems arise if the mean grain number per nucleus is taken as a measure of the DNA synthetic rate under altered experimental conditions, i.e., after pretreatment of the animal, e.g., with drugs. It is then presumed that a constant proportion of the injected exogeneous ^3H-TdR is incorporated into newly synthesized DNA of both experimental and control animals. This assumption is important for a comparison (see Lang et al. 1968). Yet, when considering the small amount of exogenously applied ^3H-TdR participating in endogenous DNA synthesis, the great susceptibility of this participation to any changes of the physiologic conditions, i.e., a variation of the precursor pool, becomes evident. As has been demonstrated by Lang et al. (1968), in the normal animal only

0.1%–1% of the ^{3}H-TdR injected is incorporated in the newly synthesized DNA. In summary, this shows that a different grain number per cell nucleus in an experimental animal in comparison with the control animal should not necessarily be regarded as proof for the alteration of the DNA synthetic rate.

5.1.2 RNA Synthesis

When studying RNA synthesis with ^{3}H-uridine or ^{3}H-cytidine, the interpretation of the grain density as a measure for the RNA synthetic rate is even more problematic. The participation of the exogenously applied ^{3}H-cytidine in RNA synthesis has been investigated in the rat liver by Schmid and Maurer (1973). They observed important deviations ranging from 0.002% to 10%, and a linear increase in the participation of ^{3}H-cytidine in the formation of newly synthesized RNA with increasing amounts of exogenously applied ^{3}H-cytidine. Even if the participation of ^{3}H-cytidine in RNA synthesis (when applied in the usual dose) is higher than that of ^{3}H-TdR in DNA synthesis, the proportion is still so small that pool alterations by pretreatment of the animal will still have a great impact.

Far more important is the fact that even macromolecular RNA can be removed from the tissue during fixation. The portion of extracted RNA can vary for different cell structures (see Schneider and Maurer 1963), Thus, the measured grain densities refer only to the remaining part of macromolecular ^{3}H-RNA. It has not yet been investigated whether the remaining portion is always the same, also in pretreated animals, and hence corresponds to that of control animals.

5.1.3 Protein Synthesis

Under certain conditions the grain density measured on an autoradiograph after the application of labeled amino acids can be regarded as a relative measure of the rate of protein synthesis of different cell types. The similarity of the incorporation pattern of different labeled amino acids, i.e., the similarity of the autoradiographs, also suggests that actually the synthesis of protein molecules is measured. According to Maurer (1960, 1972) the radioactivity incorporated into protein is equal to the product of the rate of amino acid incorporation, the mean specific activity of the free amino acid during the experiment, and the duration of the experiment. That means the activity incorporated into protein, i.e., the grain density on the autoradiograph, is not simply proportional to the amino acid turnover rate but also to the specific activity of the free amino acid.

Provided the injected labeled amino acid is rapidly and uniformly distributed in the pool of the free amino acids in the organism, the mean specific activity should be the same in the whole organism. Only in this case is the relative autoradiographic grain density a relative measure of protein synthesis. In the brain, however, some amino acids show a different behavior after systemic injection: as has already been mentioned in Sect. 2.4.1, a blood-brain barrier exists for alanine, glycine, and serine. An injection of these amino acids leads to lower specific activities of the free amino acid in the brain compared with the rest of the body. This also applies to the cerebellum after injection of labeled proline (Garweg 1969). Hence, in these cases a weak labeling of the cells in the brain does not necessarily indicate a reduced protein synthetic rate of these cells.

Apart from the dependency on the specific activity of the free amino acid, the amino acid incorporation rate (grain density) also depends on the amino acid composition of the cellular protein. If a cellular protein contains much more, for example, cystine, the amount of the corresponding labeled amino acid which is incorporated into this protein will be much higher than that of other amino acids (for details see Schultze et al. 1960, 1965; Citoler et al. 1966). Thus, if the protein synthetic rate is derived from the mean grain density on autoradiographs after application of labeled amino acids, the amino acid composition of the protein must also be considered.

5.2 DNA Synthesis and Cell Proliferation

The quantitative evaluation of autoradiographs after injection of labeled TdR not only provides the usual information on whether or not cells of a certain histologic type are labeled and on the grain density of those labeled cells, but also gives additional information: for instance, the labeling index (LI), i.e., the percentage of labeled cells of a certain cell type shortly (about 1 h) after the injection of ^3H- or ^{14}C-TdR, can be determined. This LI can be regarded as a rough estimate of the proliferative activity of the tissue. Moreover, it corresponds to the relationship between the S-phase duration and the cycle time. This relationship is important for the estimation of cell kinetic parameters. In the case of an exponential growth, i.e., when both daughter cells of a mitosis continue to proliferate (e.g., neural epithelial cells in embryonic brains), the following relationship exists:

$$LI_{(\text{exponential growth})} = 2^{T_{G_2+M}/T_C}\,(2^{T_S/T_C} - 1) \quad (1)$$

(where T_{G_2+M} is the duration of the phases G_2 and M, T_S is the duration of the S-phase, and T_C is the cycle time). If T_{G_2+M} and T_S are known the duration of the cycle T_C can be calculated with formula (1). For application to neural epithelial cells in the brain of fetal rats, see Schultze et al. (1974).

In the case of steady state growth, i.e., if only one of the two daughter cells after a mitosis continues to proliferate (like neuroglia in the brains of younger and adult rats and mice) the relationship between the LI and the duration of the cycle phases is the following:

$$LI_{(\text{steady state growth})} = T_S/T_C \cdot GF \quad (2)$$

(where GF = growth fraction, i.e., fraction of proliferating cells related to all cells). The determination of GF is quite difficult (see Korr 1980).

For the experimental determination of the duration of the various cell cycle phases two methods of measuring these cycle phases can be applied: the first method is based on the observation of labeled and unlabeled *mitoses* of the cell type studied, i.e., on the percentage of labeled mitoses as a function of time after a single injection of ^3H- or ^{14}C-TdR. This method is known as the "percent-labeled-mitoses" method (PLM method: Quastler and Sherman 1959). The second method is based on the observation of labeled *interphase cells*. For this purpose, either double-labeling experiments with ^3H- and ^{14}C-TdR are carried out and the ratio of purely ^3H- to double-labeled cells is evaluated on double-layer autoradiographs, or (for a rough estimate of T_C) the mean grain number per nucleus as a function of time is counted after a single injection of ^3H-TdR (see Korr et al. 1973 b, 1975). Another method can be used for studying cell proliferation in embryonic brains, where T_S and T_C can be determined by the method of continuous infusion (or multiple injections) of ^3H-TdR. For the increase of the percentage of labeled cells measured at different times after the beginning of the continuous infusion of ^3H-TdR the pertinent cell cycle parameters can be derived (Fujita 1962). For details on the application of different methods for studies of the proliferative processes in the CNS, see Korr (1980).

Additional conclusions can be drawn from *long-term experiments* after the injection of ^3H- or ^{14}C-TdR. If even after long time intervals after labeling, for instance, after several weeks, labeled cells are found, it must be concluded that these cells, after their labeling, have passed through only a few cell cycles and have then lost their proliferative activity. Since the grain number per nucleus is reduced to about half its initial value after each mitosis, continuous cell divisions would have led to a steady decrease of the labeled DNA up to the complete disappearance of the label. Hence, these experiments provide the possibility to trace the fate of the cells after their labeling.

The proliferative behavior of neurons may serve as an example: it is a well-known fact that the precursor cells of many neurons prenatally pass through their last S-phase and shortly thereafter through their last mitosis. During this prenatal phase the further development of a precursor cell cannot be predicted on the basis of its morphology. With the aid of autoradiography after injection of ^{3}H-TdR, however, a determination of the moment at which the precursor cells of defined neurons will have undergone their last mitosis is possible. This moment of the formation of neuroblasts is described in the literature as the "time of birth" or "cell birthday" (for review see Jacobson, 1978). For the autoradiographic determination of the cell birthday the pregnant animal is injected with ^{3}H-TdR at different times during its pregnancy, and the brains of the offspring are then postnatally (25th day) investigated with respect to labeled cells of specific cell types. Thus, for the Purkinje cells of the rat cerebellum it could be demonstrated that injections of ^{3}H-TdR lead to labeling of the precursor cells of the Purkinje cells up to the 15th day of gestation (E 15). If the ^{3}H-TdR is, however, injected at E 16 or even later, labeled Purkinje cells can no longer be observed. This means that neural epithelial cells which will differentiate into Purkinje cells have terminated their proliferation at E 16 at the latest. If, in addition to this information, the percentage of labeled Purkinje cells up to E 16, the duration of the S-phase of the neural epithelial cells, and the total number of Purkinje cells in the brain of young animals are known, the start of proliferation of the corresponding neural epithelial cells can be determined (see Schultze et al. 1974). This beginning of proliferation has been found to coincide with the development of the neural plate.

When the postinjection survival time after prenatal labeling with ^{3}H-TdR is confined to a few days, the migration processes of neuroblasts in certain brain areas can be demonstrated. Thus, the formation of the cerebral cortex layers from inside to outside could be demonstrated in this way (for review see Berry 1974). Details on the technical procedure of such studies are given by Richter and Kranz (1979, 1980) among others.

Generally, in studies of DNA synthesis, and particularly in the brain, a variety of information can be obtained due to the intervals of proliferation which are different for the different cell types in the course of ontogenesis. The duration of the experiment and the method for the quantitative evaluation after injection of ^{3}H- or ^{14}C-TdR must, however, be carefully selected.

Acknowledgment. I would like to thank Professor Brigitte Maurer-Schultze for her advice and criticism during the preparation of the manuscript.

6 References

Altman J, Chorover SL (1963) Autoradiographic investigation of the distribution and utilization of intraventricularly injected adenine-^{3}H, uracil-^{3}H and thymidine-^{3}H in the brains of cats. J Physiol (Lond) 169:770–778

Altman PL, Dittmer DS (1964) Biological data book. Federation of American Societies for Experimental Biology, Washington, DC

Amlacher E (1974) Autoradiographie in Histologie und Cytologie. Fischer, Stuttgart

Antoni F, Köteles GJ, Hempel K, Maurer W (1965) Über die Eignung verschiedener Fixationen und perchlorsäurehaltiger Lösungen für autoradiographische Untersuchungen des

RNS-, DNS- und Proteinstoffwechsels. Histochemie 5:210–220

Appel KR, Appel E, Maurer W (1960) Konzentration und Austauschrate des freien Methionins im Gehirn der Ratte. Biochem Z 332: 293–306

Asbury AK (1970) The histogenesis of phagocytes during Wallerian degeneration: radioautographic observations. In: Proc VI Intern Congr Neuropath. Masson, Paris, pp 666–682

Bélanger LF (1961) Staining processed radioautographs. Stain Technol 36:313–317

Berry M (1974) Development of the cerebral neocortex of the rat. In: Gottlieb G (ed) Studies of development of behavior and nervous system, vol 2, aspects of neurogenesis. Academic Press, New York, pp 7–67

Bisconte J-C (1976) Quantitative radioautography and kinetics of cellular populations. J Microsc Biol Cell 27:177–184

Bisconte J-C (1979) Kinetic analysis of cellular populations by means of the quantitative radioautography. Int Rev Cytol 57:75–126

Boyd GA (1955) Autoradiography in biology and medicine. Academic Press, New York

Calas A, Alonso G, Arnauld E, Vincent JD (1974) Demonstration of indolaminergic fibres in the median eminence of the duck, rat and monkey. Nature 250:241–243

Calvert R, Pusterla A (1974) Epon-embedded tissue stained with aldehyde-fuchsin for radioautography. Stain Technol 49:323–327

Citoler P, Citoler K, Hempel K, Schultze B, Maurer W (1966) Autoradiographische Untersuchungen mit zwölf ^{3}H- and fünf ^{14}C-markierten Aminosäuren zur Größe des nucleären und cytoplasmatischen Eiweißstoffwechsels bei verschiedenen Zellarten von Maus und Ratte. Z Zellforsch Mikroskop Anat 70: 419–448

Cowan WM, Cuénod, M (1975) The use of axonal transport for studies of neuronal connectivity. Elsevier/North-Holland Biomedical Press, Amsterdam Oxford New York

Cowan WM, Gottlieb DI, Hendrickson AE, Price JL, Woolsey TA (1972) The autoradiographic demonstration of axonal connections in the central nervous system. Brain Res 37: 21–51

Cuénod M, Cowan WM (1975) Some future developments in the use of axonal transport mechanisms for tracing pathways in the central nervous system. In: Cowan WM, Cuénod M (eds) The use of axonal transport for studies of neuronal connectivity. Elsevier/North-Holland Biomedical Press, Amsterdam Oxford New York, pp 337–346

Daniels JS, Gilmore SA (1975) Chemography associated with specific anatomic areas in autoradiographs of brain stems from adult rats. Brain Res 98:343–347

Davie F (1970) Reference list to literature on histological stains applicable to sections of resin-embedded tissue. Science Tools 17: 59–61

Droz B (1969) Protein metabolism in nerve cells. Int Rev Cytol 25:363–390

Droz B (1975) Autoradiography as a tool for visualizing neurons and neuronal processes. In: Cowan WM, Cuénod M (eds) The use of axonal transport for studies of neuronal connectivity. Elsevier/North-Holland Biomedical Press, Amsterdam Oxford New York, pp 127–154

Droz B, Koenig HL, DiGiamberardino L (1973) Axonal migration of protein and glycoprotein to nerve endings. I. Radioautographic analysis of the renewal of protein in nerve endings of chicken ciliary ganglion after intracerebral injection of ^{3}H-lysine. Brain Res 60:93–127

Droz B, Leblond CP (1963) Axonal migration of proteins in the central nervous system and peripheral nerves as shown by radioautography. J Comp Neurol 121:325–346

Evans EA (1976) Self-decomposition of radiochemicals: principles, control, observations and effects. The Radiochemical Centre, Amersham, Review No 16

Fischer HA, Werner G (1971) Autoradiographie. De Gruyter, Berlin New York

Fujita S (1962) Kinetics of cell proliferation. Exp Cell Res 28:52–60

Garweg G (1969) Unterschiedliche Verteilung von L-Histidin und L-Prolin im Autoradiogramm des Mäuse-Kleinhirns. Naturwissenschaften 56:463–464

Grafstein B (1975) Principles of anterograde axonal transport in relation to studies of neuronal connectivity. In: Cowan WM, Cuénod M (eds) The use of axonal transport for studies of neuronal connectivity. Elsevier/North-Holland Biomedical Press, Amsterdam Oxford New York, p 47–67

Hagemann E, Schmidt G (1960) Ratte und Maus. Versuchstier in der Forschung. De Gruyter, Berlin New York

Hendrickson A, Moe L, Noble B (1972) Staining for autoradiography of the central nervous system. Stain Technol 47:283–290

Hertz L (1979) Functional interactions between neurons and astrocytes I. Turnover and metabolism of putative amino acid transmitters. Prog Neurobiol 13:277–323

Heslop JP (1975) Axonal flow and fast transport in nerves. Adv Comp Physiol Biochem 6: 75–163

Hökfelt T, Ljungdahl A (1972) Autoradiographic identification of cerebral and cerebellar cortical neurons accumulating labeled gamma-aminobutyric acid (^{3}H-GABA). Exp Brain Res 14:354–362

Jacobson M (1978) Developmental neurobiology, 2nd edn. Plenum Press, New York London

Jaros GG, Sensenbrenner M, Wittendorp E, Rechenmann RV, Mandel P (1974) Etude trace-autoradiographique de la prolifération des cellules nerveuses en culture. CR Acad Sci [D] (Paris) 279:1101–1104

Kelly JS, Dick F (1976) Differential labeling of glial cells and GABA-inhibitory interneurons and nerve terminals following the microinjection of (β-^{3}H)alanine, ^{3}H-DABA and ^{3}H-GABA into single folia of the cerebellum. Cold Spring Harbor Symp Quant Biol XI:93–106

Koburg E, Maurer W (1962) Autoradiographische Untersuchungen mit ^{3}H-Thymidin über die Dauer der Deoxyribonukleinsäure-Synthese und ihren zeitlichen Verlauf bei den Darmepithelien und anderen Zelltypen der Maus. Biochim Biophys Acta 61:229–242

Kopriwa BM (1963) A model dark room unit for radioautography. J Histochem Cytochem 11: 553–555

Kopriwa BM, Huckins C (1972) A method for the use of Zenker-formol fixation and the periodic acid Schiff staining technique in light microscopic radioautography. Histochemie 32:231–244

Kopriwa BM, Leblond CP (1962) Improvements in the coating technique of radioautography. J Histochem Cytochem 10:269–284

Korr H (1978 a) Autoradiographische Untersuchungen zur Proliferation verschiedener Zellelemente im Gehirn von Nagern während der prä- und postnatalen Ontogenese. Habilitationsschrift, University of Würzburg

Korr H (1978 b) Combination of metallic impregnation and autoradiography of brain sections. A method for differentiation of proliferating glial cells in the brain of adult rats and mice. Histochemistry 59:111–116

Korr H (1980) Proliferation of different cell types in the brain. Adv Anat Embryol Cell Biol 61

Korr H, Fischer HA, Seiler N, Werner G (1970) Cholesterinkristalle in Kryostat-Gefrierschnitten von nervösem Gewebe als Ursache von Artefakten in Autoradiogrammen. Histochemie 23:138–143

Korr H, Fischer HA, Seiler N, Werner G (1973a) Über Auftreten und Unterdrückung der Cholesterinkristallbildung in Kryostat-Gefrierschnitten nervösen Gewebes. Acta Histochem [Suppl] (Jena) XIII:185–188

Korr H, Schilling WD, Dauenhauer M, Schultze B, Maurer W (to be published) Proliferation of glial cells in different areas of the forebrain of the 14-day old rat

Korr H, Schultze B, Maurer W (1973 b) Autoradiographic investigations of glial proliferation in the brain of adult mice. I. The DNA synthesis phase of neuroglia and endothelial cells. J Comp Neurol 150:169–176

Korr H, Schultze B, Maurer W (1975) Autoradiographic investigations of glial proliferation in the brain of adult mice. II. Cycle time and mode of proliferation of neuroglia and endothelial cells. J Comp Neurol 160:477–490

Künzle H (1975) Notes on the application of radioactive amino acids for the tracing of neuronal connections. Brain Res 85:267–271

Lajtha A (1975) Transport and incorporation of amino acids in relation to measurement of axonal flow. In: Cowan WM, Cuénod M (eds) The use of axonal transport for studies of neuronal connectivity. Elsevier/North Holland Biomedical Press, Amsterdam Oxford New York, pp 25–45

Lang W, Maurer W (1965) Zur Verwendbarkeit von Feulgen-gefärbten Schnitten für quantitative Autoradiographie mit markiertem Thymidin. Exp Cell Res 39:1–9

Lang W, Müller D, Maurer W (1968) Prozentuale Beteiligung von exogenem Thymidin an der Synthese von DNS-Thymin in Geweben der Maus und in HeLa-Zellen. Exp Cell Res 49:558–571

Latov N, Nilaver G, Zimmerman EA, Johnson WG, Silverman A-J, Defendini R, Cote L (1979) Fibrillary astrocytes proliferate in response to brain injury. A study combining immunoperoxidase technique for glial fibrillary acidic protein and radioautography of tritiated thymidine. Dev Biol 72:381–384

Leblond CP, Kopriwa B, Messier B (1963) Radioautography as a histochemical tool. In: Wegman R (ed) First Int Congr Histochem Cytochem. Pergamon Press, Oxford London New York Paris, pp 1–31

Levinger IM (1971) The cerebral ventricles of the rat. J Anat 108:447–451

Lewis PD (1968) Radiosensitivity of the subependymal cell layer of the adult rat brain. Exp Neurol 20:208–214

Mai JK, Junger E (1977) Quantitative autoradiographic light- and electron microscopic studies on the retinohypothalamic connections in the rat. Cell Tissue Res 183:221–237

Mares V, Schultze B, Maurer W (1974) Stability of DNA in Purkinje cell nuclei of the mouse. An autoradiographic study. J Cell Biol 63: 665–674

Matus AI, Dennison ME (1972) An autoradiographic study of uptake of exogenous glycine by vertebrate spinal cord splices in vitro. J Neurocytol 1:27–34

Maurer W (1960) Die Größe des Umsatzes von Organ- und Plasmaeiweiß. In: Dynamik des

Eiweißes. 10. Colloq Ges physiol Chem Mosbach. Springer, Berlin Göttingen Heidelberg, pp 1–49

Maurer W (1972) Methodisches zur autoradiographischen Untersuchung des Eiweißstoffwechsels. Acta Histochem [Suppl] (Jena) XII, 65–72

Maurer W, Niklas A, Lehnert G (1954) Messung der Umsatzrate von Serumeiweiß und Körpereiweiß beim normalen Kaninchen mit ^{35}S-Methionin. Biochem Z 326:28–47

Maurer W, Primbsch E (1964) Größe der β-Selbstabsorption bei der ^{3}H-Autoradiographie. Exp Cell Res 33:8–18

Maurer W, Schultze B, Carmona T (to be published) Tracer-Dosis für exogenes markiertes Thymidin und Beteiligung des exogenen Thymidin an der endogenen DNA-Synthese gemessen an den Krypten.

Nowakowski RS, LaVail JH, Rakic P (1975) The correlation of the time of origin of neurons with their axonal projection: the combined use of ^{3}H-thymidine autoradiography and horseradish peroxidase histochemistry. Brain Res 99:343–348

Oehlert W, Schultze B, Maurer W (1958) Autoradiographische Untersuchung der Größe des Eiweißstoffwechsels der verschiedenen Zellen des Zentralnervensystems. Beitr Pathol Anat Allg Pathol 119:343–376

Oehlert W, Schultze B, Maurer W (1960) Autoradiographische Untersuchung zur Frage der Eiweißsynthese innerhalb des Kerns und des Cytoplasmas der Zelle. Beitr Pathol Anat Allg Pathol 122:289–312

Oehmichen M, Saebisch R (1971) Zur Problematik histochemischer Färbungen und autoradiographischer Technik. Acta Histochem (Jena) 41:353–364

Peters T, Ashley CA (1967) An artefact in radioautography due to binding of free amino acids to tissues by fixatives. J Cell Biol 33:53–60

Pilgrim C (1964) Autoradiographische Bestimmung der Dauer der DNS-Verdopplung bei verschiedenen Zellarten von Maus und Ratte nach einer neuen Doppelmarkierungsmethode. Anat Anz 115:128–133

Pilgrim C, Maurer W (1965) Autoradiographische Untersuchung über die Konstanz der DNS-Verdopplungs-Dauer bei Zellarten von Maus und Ratte durch Doppelmarkierung mit ^{3}H- und ^{14}C-Thymidin. Exp Cell Res 37:183–199

Price JL, Wann DF (1975) The use of quantitative autoradiography for axonal tracing experiments and an automated system for grain counting. In: Cowan WM, Cuénod M (eds) The use of axonal transport for studies of neuronal connectivity. Elsevier/North Holland Biomedical Press, Amsterdam Oxford New York, pp 153–172

Quastler H, Sherman FG (1959) Cell population kinetics in the intestinal epithelium of the mouse. Exp Cell Res 17:420–438

Ramon y Cajal S (1913) Contribucion al conocimiento de la neuroglia del cerebro humano. Trab Inst Cajal Invest Biol 11:225–315

Richardson KC, Jarett L, Finke EH (1960) Embedding in epoxy resins for ultrathin sectioning in electron microscopy. Stain Technol 35:313–323

Richter CB, King CS (1972) Formalin as a hardener of photographic emulsions to facilitate staining of epon sections after autoradiography. Stain Technol 47:268–269

Richter W, Kranz D (1979) Autoradiographische Untersuchungen zur Neurogenese und Morphogenese der Regio cingularis der Ratte. IV. Quantitative Untersuchungen zur Ermittlung der Zellursprungszeiten der Cortexschichten. J Hirnforsch 20:581–629

Richter W, Kranz D (1980) Autoradiographische Untersuchungen zur Neurogenese und Morphogenese der Regio cingularis der Ratte. V. Quantitative Untersuchungen des Ablaufs der Migrationsvorgänge. J Hirnforsch 21:11–37

Rio-Hortega P del (1919) El tercer elemento de los entros nervosos. Bol Soc Espan Biol 9:68–83

Rogers AW (1979) Techniques of autoradiography, 3rd edn. Elsevier/North-Holland Biomedical Press, Amsterdam New York Oxford

Schmid G, Maurer W (1973) Prozentuale Beteiligung von exogenem Cytidin an der RNS-Synthese der Leber der Ratte. Exp Cell Res 78:143–151

Schneider G, Maurer W (1963) Autoradiographische Untersuchung über den Einbau von H-3-Cytidin in die Kerne einiger Zellarten der Maus und über den Einfluß des Fixationsmittels auf die H-3-Aktivität. Acta Histochem (Jena) 15:171–181

Schon F, Iversen LL (1974) The use of autoradiographic techniques for the identification and mapping of transmitter-specific neurons in the brain. Life Sci 15:157–175

Schon F, Kelly JS (1974) The characterisation of ^{3}H-GABA uptake into the satellite glial cells of rat sensory ganglia. Brain Res 66:289–300

Schultze B (1968) Die Orthologie und Pathologie des Nucleinsäure- und Eiweißstoffwechsels der Zelle im Autoradiogramm. In: Altmann HW, Büchner F, Cottier H, Holle G, Letterer W, Masshoff W, Meessen H, Roulet F, Seifert G, Siebert G, Studer A (eds) Handbuch der allgemeinen Pathologie, Bd II/5. Springer, Berlin Heidelberg New York, pp 466–670

Schultze B (1969) Autoradiography at the cellular level. In: Pollister AW (ed) Physical techniques in biological research, 2nd edn., vol III b. Academic Press, New York London

Schultze B, Citoler P, Hempel K, Citoler K, Maurer W (1965) Cytoplasmic protein synthesis in cells of various types and its relation to nuclear protein synthesis. In: Leblond CP, Warren KB (eds) The use of radioautography in investigating protein synthesis. Symp Int Soc Cell Biol, vol IV. Academic Press, New York London, pp 107–139

Schultze B, Hörning N, Maurer W (1972 a) Blut-Hirn-Schranke und Placentar-Schranke für ^{3}H-Thymidin und ^{3}H-Cytidin bei der Maus. Z Naturforsch [B] 27:554–558

Schultze B, Maurer W (1963) Größe der RNS-Synthese in Nukleolus und Karyoplasma bei einigen Zellarten der Maus. Z Zellforsch Mikroskop Anat 60:387–391

Schultze B, Maurer W (1967) Nuclear and cytoplasmic protein synthesis in various cell types from rats and mice. In: Goldstein L (ed) The control of nuclear activity. Prentice-Hall, Englewood Cliffs New Jersey, pp 319–349

Schultze B, Maurer W, Hagenbusch H (1976) A two emulsion autoradiographic technique and the discrimination of the three different types of labelling after double labelling with ^{3}H- and ^{14}C-thymidine. Cell Tissue Kinet 9: 245–255

Schultze B, Nowak B, Maurer W (1974) Cycle times of the neural epithelial cells of various types of neuron in the rat. An autoradiographic study. J Comp Neurol 158:207–218

Schultze B, Oehlert W, Maurer W (1960) Vergleichende autoradiographische Untersuchung mit H-3, C-14 und S-35-markierten Aminosäuren zur Größe des Eiweißstoffwechsels einzelner Gewebe und Zellarten bei Maus, Ratte und Kaninchen. Beitr Pathol Anat Allg Pathol 122:406–431

Schultze B, Oehlert W, Maurer W (1961) Über eine allgemeine Beziehung zwischen der Umsatzrate der Ribonukleinsäure und des Eiweißes im Organismus von Maus und Ratte. Biochim Biophys Acta 49:35–46

Schultze B, Rabbani B, Maurer W (1972 b) Blut-Hirn-Schranke und Placentar-Schranke für verschiedene Aminosäuren bei der Maus (Untersuchung mit Ganzkörper-Autoradiographie). Beitr Pathol 147:352–365

Schubert P, Holländer H (1975) Methods for the delivery of tracers to the central nervous system. In: Cowan WM, Cuénod M (eds) The use of axonal transport for studies of neuronal connectivity. Elsevier/North-Holland Biomedical Press, Amsterdam Oxford New York, pp 113–125

Schubert P, Kreutzberg GW, Lux HD (1972) Use of microelectrophoresis in the autoradiographic demonstration of fiber projections. Brain Res 39:274–277

Schwarzberg H, Schulz H, Unger H (1971) Hirnventrikelsystem und Liquorströmung bei Kaninchen. Acta Biol Med Ger 26:341–345

Shaw GG (1974) Some shortcomings of direct intraventricular injection in mice. Br J Pharmacol 50:603–605

Sidman RL (1970) Autoradiographic methods and principles for study of the nervous system with thymidine ^{3}H. In: Nauta WJH, Ebbesson SOE (eds) Contemporary research methods in neuroanatomy. Springer, Berlin Heidelberg New York, pp 252–274

Siperstein ER (1963) Identification of the adrenocorticotrophin-producing cells in the rat hypophysis by autoradiography. J Cell Biol 17:521–546

Skougaard MR, Steward PA (1966) Comparative effectiveness of intraperitoneal and intramuscular ^{3}H-thymidine injection routes in mice. Exp Cell Res 45:158–166

Stumpf WE (1970) Tissue preparation for the autoradiographic localization of hormones. In: Wied GL, Bahr GF (eds) Introduction to quantitative cytochemistry, vol 2. Academic Press, New York, pp 507–526

Thurston JM, Joftes DL (1963) Stains compatible with dipping radioautography. Stain Technol 38:231–235

Van Houten M, Posner BI, Kopriwa BM, Brawer JR (1979) Insulin-binding sites in the rat brain: In vivo localization to the circumventricular organs by quantitative radioautography. Endocrinology 105:666–673

Van Houten M, Posner BI, Walsh RJ (1980) Radioautographic identification of lactogen binding sites in rat median eminence using ^{125}I-human growth hormone: evidence for a prolactin "short-loop" feedback site. Exp Brain Res 38:455–461

Van Rooijen N (1976) The separate detection of two radioactively labeled compounds in tissue sections or cell smears on a lightmicroscopic level: a review on double radionuclide autoradiography. Int J Appl Radiat Isot 27: 547–554

Wegener K, Hollweg S, Maurer W (1964) Autoradiographische Bestimmung der DNS-Verdopplungszeit und anderer Teil-Phasen des Zell-Zyklus bei fetalen Zellarten der Ratte. Z Zellforsch Mikroskop Anat 63:309–326

Wolff JR, Chronwall BM, Rickmann M (1978) Morphogenetic relations between cell migration and synaptogenesis in the neocortex of rat. In: Neuhoff V (ed) Proceedings of the european society for neurochemistry, vol 1, Verlag Chemie, Weinheim New York, pp 158–173

Chapter 13

Brain Localization of Hormones and Drugs by Thaw-mount Autoradiography, Combined Autoradiography-Formaldehyde Induced Fluorescence, and Combined Autoradiography-Immunohistochemistry

Walter E. Stumpf and Madhabananda Sar

1 Introduction

Autoradiography is an important technique for the localization of hormones and drugs. No reliable method was available for the cellular and subcellular localization of non-covalently-bound substances before 1964, when Stumpf and Roth developed the dry-mount autoradiography technique (Stumpf and Roth 1964). Diffusible substances are generally of small molecular weight that include metal ions, amino acids, steroid hormones, and most drugs. Liquid fixatives, dehydration fluids, embedding media, and other fluids commonly used for the preparation of histological sections must be considered a source of translocation and leaching of diffusible substances. Only exceptionally can fixatives be found that interlink such molecules with other tissue constituents at their in vivo sites of deposition, so that translocation during fixation and subsequent treatment can be excluded.

The problems of autoradiography with drugs and hormones have been reviewed repeatedly and standards for the introduction and use of appropriate techniques have been set (Stumpf and Roth 1966; Stumpf 1971). Tests were conducted with two different compounds that are known to be concentrated at certain cellular and subcellular sites (Stumpf and Roth 1966). Subsequently the wet thaw-mount autoradiography has been tested and compared repeatedly with the results obtained with the dry-mount technique that most rigorously excludes fluids, moisture, and melting during tissue preparation until the end of exposure. Results obtained with both of these techniques have stood the test of time. However, since thaw-mount autoradiography is easier to perform than the dry-mount technique, thaw-mount autoradiography has become the technique of choice.

The thaw-mount autoradiographic technique was described first in 1966 as "technique #2" (Stumpf and Roth 1966) and later explained in detail (Stumpf and Sar

---

Supported by PHS Grant NS09914

1975; Stumpf 1976). Its use in neurobiology includes the study of steroid hormone distribution (Stumpf and Grant 1975; Stumpf and Sar 1976), localization of drugs and neurotoxins (Stumpf et al. 1981), 2-deoxyglucose (Pilgrim and Wagner 1981), incorporation of precursor molecules, and tracing of neural pathways (Conrad and Stumpf 1974). The introduction of combination techniques has extended the use of the thaw-mount and dry-mount techniques for the simultaneous demonstration in the same section of a radioactively-labeled compound and an otherwise histochemically or immunohistochemically identifiable substance. These combination techniques include the autoradiography-formaldehyde induced fluorescence applied for the demonstration of steroid hormones and catecholamines (Grant and Stumpf 1973) and the autoradiography-immunohistochemistry applied for the demonstration of steroid hormones and antibodies (Keefer et al. 1975; Sar and Stumpf 1979). A description of these techniques is given and examples of results from these applications are provided.

2 Thaw-mount and Dry-mount Autoradiography

2.1 General

Freezing, storage, and cutting are identical for all of the procedures described here. The radioactively-labeled compound (chemical purity and high specific activity are essential) is administered to the animal by intravenous, intraperitoneal, or subcutaneous injection, depending on the experimental conditions and objectives. The animal is killed by decapitation. The excised brain is placed on a tissue mount in toto or after dissection in a petri dish on ice. Brass tissue mounts are prepared and numbered in advance and minced liver is placed on the mounts in order to serve as adhesive for the tissue. Depending on the size of the tissue block, different size tissue mounts should be used. Before freezing, the tissue is properly oriented for later sectioning. Some liver may cover the sides of the tissue at its base to better anchor it. The mounted tissue is then frozen in propane, freon, isopentane, or a similar hydrocarbon that is cooled by liquid nitrogen. A cooled liquid hydrocarbon rather than liquid nitrogen is used in order to minimize vapor insulation of the specimen during cooling to achieve a more rapid freezing.

Propane and freon need to be liquified with liquid nitrogen in advance of the experiment and then kept in a vessel cooled with liquid nitrogen (see also Chap. 9). Liquified propane and freon, as well as isopentane, have a boiling point much higher than liquid nitrogen. Therefore, heat transfer is facilitated and not delayed by vapors as is the case with liquid nitrogen. Freezing requires experience in order to immerse the tissue into the coolant at a rate fast enough to minimize ice crystal formation and slow enough to prevent cracking of the tissue. Different modes of freezing have been described by Stumpf (1976).

The frozen-mounted tissue is transferred from the coolant to liquid nitrogen for storage until sectioning. Several tissue mounts may be kept in a plastic test tube that may be stored indefinitely within a compartment of a liquid nitrogen tissue storage container.

Frozen-sectioning may be performed in an open-top type cryostat such as the Wide-Range cryostat, which not only houses the microtome but provides space for handling of tissues, storage, or freeze-drying, with easy access from above. A dissecting microscope that is mounted on an arm and pivoted at the side of the cryostat can be swung above the knife. Its use together with fiber optics light facilitates frozen-sectioning. With the dissecting microscope, the cutting procedure can be followed and the quality of the sections judged more effectively.

Frozen sections of 3–5 μm thickness provide a good compromise regarding optimal light microscopic cellular and subcellular resolution and stainability.

2.2 Control Experiments

Controls are required to prevent "false positives" and "false negatives" that may be caused by interaction of tissue constituents, or chemicals used for tissue treatment, with the photographic emulsion. Artifacts due to such sources are called respectively "positive chemography" and "negative chemography." In order to exclude chemography, control autoradiograms need to be prepared from animals or tissues that have received identical treatment, except for the ratioactively-labeled material. Tissues from experiments in which a different radioactively labeled compound is used may serve as controls if conditions and treatment are otherwise identical and the results are different.

It is emphasized that control experiments are essential, since artifacts are reproducible with the same technique and conditions, and, therefore, reproducibility alone cannot be invoked as proof of authenticity.

2.3 Thaw-mount Autoradiography

Sections are picked up from the knife under safelight with a desiccated photographic emulsion (Kodak NTB 3 or 2)-coated slide kept at room temperature. A clamp attached to the knife back may be used as a fulcrum to facilitate the quick down and up section pick-up movement of the slide. Refreezing of the melted section should be avoided, and the knife must be kept free of debris and ice crystals. The section-mounted slide is placed into a light-proof desiccator box at room temperature. After sectioning the box will be sealed and kept in a freezer or refrigerator for exposure. Exposure times are dependent on many factors, such as specific activity and specific concentration of the compound. Since the latter is unknown, the exposure time cannot be calculated but must be determined empirically. Exposure times may vary from a few days to one year or longer. At the end of exposure, the slide box is removed from the freezer. After adjusting to room temperature, the desiccator box is opened and the slide(s) removed for development, with or without prior brief fixation. Since fixation and treatment of the undeveloped slide may cause artifacts, this step, if introduced, needs to be controlled. Photographic processing is done in our laboratory with Kodak NTB3 emulsion under constant temperature conditions (15 °C) of all fluids: 1 min in Kodak D19 developer, a brief rinse in tap water, 5 min in Kodak fixer, a 5 min rinse in tap water, and subsequent staining. As an optimal stain for autoradiography, we had introduced methyl-green pyronin for DNA (blue – the blue color is due to the presence of methyl violet in commercial methyl green) and RNA (red) as a simple 1-step stain that does not obscure silver grains. As an alternate stain for good discrimination of cellular and subcellular structures, another single-step stain with methylene blue-basic (or acid) fuchsin may be used. After staining and brief rinsing in tap water, the slide is allowed to air-dry and the section is mounted with Permount and a coverslip.

For further details on the thaw-mount technique see Stumpf and Sar (1975), Stumpf (1976). Depending on equipment available, experimental conditions, and preferences, modifications can be made of most of the steps outline. However, since any added step may introduce artifacts, proper controls are always required.

2.3.1 Methyl Green-Pyronine (MGP) Staining

Ingredients

0.2 M disodium phosphate, anhydrous, MW 141.98
0.1 M citric acid, monohydrate, MW 210.14
0.5% phenol solution
1.0% resorcinol solution
pyronine GS, CI 45005 (Chroma)
methyl green, CI 42585 (Chroma)

To prepare stock buffer solutions 28.396 g Na_2HPO_4 is dissolved in 1 liter distilled water; and 21.014 g citric acid is dissolved in 1 liter dist. water. Mix 210 ml 0.2 M disodium phosphate and 190 ml 0.1 M citric acid. Add 2 ml 0.5% phenol solution and 10 ml 1% resorcinol solution. To half of this mixture add 1.0 g pyronin; to the other half add 6 g methyl green. Stir until dissolved. Store pyronin and methyl green stock solutions in refrigerator and stir again before combining.

Combine 30 ml of the methyl green solution with 50 ml of the pyronin solution. Allow 2–5 days to age. Filter before each use. The solution remains stable up to 6 months at room temperature.

Procedure

Stain in MGP reagent for 10 s to 1 min.
Wash gently in two changes of tap water.
Air-dry and mount with Permount and a coverslip.

2.4 Dry-mount Autoradiography

With dry-mount autoradiography, thawing of sections is avoided, since thawing is a potential source of translocation and chemographic artifacts. The dry-mount technique excludes or minimizes translocation and may serve as a control.

Instead of thawing, frozen sections are transferred with the bristles of a fine brush from the knife to a vial. Several sections may be dropped into a vial. Vials are transferred within the cryostat to a vacuum flask for subsequent freeze-drying. Freeze-drying is conveniently done with a cryosorption pump (Stumpf 1976). Freeze-drying of frozen sections usually is done overnight at a vacuum of 10^{-4} torr or better. Freeze-drying is a crucial step during which the temperature of the specimen must be kept below −35 °C until the end of drying, since ice crystal artifacts or excessive shrinkage may cause distortion of information. Throughout the procedure the specimen is kept in the cryostat, and only at the end of freeze-drying, the cryosorption pump is transferred to the laboratory bench. The specimen chamber of the pump is allowed to warm up and the molecular sieve compartment of the pump remains immersed in liquid nitrogen. Thus, a vacuum is maintained.

At the end of freeze-drying, when the specimen chamber has assumed room temperature, the vacuum is broken with dry air or nitrogen gas and the freeze-dried sections in their vials are stored in a desiccator until dry-mounting. Since freeze-dried sections and photographic emulsion are hygroscopic, dry-mounting is done under conditions of 20%–40% relative humidity. If this is not observed, autolysis of tissue if too humid, or electrostatic discharge if too dry, may cause artifacts.

Freeze-dried sections are placed on clean Teflon pieces and, under safelight, are pressed against a desiccated photographic emulsion-coated slide. Tissue sections should be without folds, since folds may cause pressure artifacts and detachment of the section during development. When the pressure is released, the Teflon falls off and the sections adhere to the photographic emulsion. The section-mounted slide is placed in a light-proof desiccator box for exposure as described above. At the end of exposure, and immediately prior to photographic development, the section area of the slide is breathed on twice, in order to increase adherence of the sections to the emulsion and to prevent their loss during subsequent photographic processing and staining, which is done as described above for the thaw-mount procedure. For further detail see Stumpf and Sar (1975) and Stumpf (1976).

3 Combination Techniques

Combination techniques enable the simultaneous localization in the same section of a radioisotopically labeled compound and a second substance that can be recognized by another histochemical criterium, such as, fluorescence or staining with immunohistochemical indicators.

3.1 Combined Autoradiography-Formaldehyde Induced Fluorescence

Freeze-dried sections are prepared at 4–6 μm thickness, as previously described, and exposed for 2 h to paaformaldehyde vapor (50% relative humidity) at 80 °C. These vapor-exposed sections may be stored in a desiccator in the dark before dry-mounting as described above. After photographic exposure and development as described, the air-dried and unstained sections are mounted with Entellan and a coverslip.

The slides are then scanned first for visualization of catecholamines, using a dark-field condenser and transmitted ultraviolet light. Once fluorescing catecholamines are located, a combination of ultraviolet and tungsten light is employed in order to observe developed silver grains and fluorescing catecholamines simultaneously. Thus, nuclear aggregates of silver grains that represent ^{3}H estradiol uptake sites are viewed as orange-yellow dots over neuronal nuclei surrounded by cytoplasm with yellow-green fluorescence (BG-12 excitation and Zeiss "50" emission filters). After microscopic observation of the slides and photographic recording, the coverslip is removed and the sections stained with methyl green pyronin for study as conventional autoradiograms. This technique has been described in detail by Heritage et al. (1977).

3.2 Combined Autoradiography-Immunohistochemistry

Either the thaw-mount or the dry-mount approach may be used and the autoradiograms are prepared as described previously until the end of photographic exposure. The following steps are added:

a) Histological Fixation of Exposed Slides Before Photograpmic Development. At the end of exposure, the light-proof boxes containing the autoradiographic slides are removed from the freezer and allowed to equilibrate to room temperature. Histological fixation as well as photographic processing are carried out in the darkroom under safelight. The slides are fixed for 30 s either in cold 2.5%–3% paraformaldehyde or 4% formalin solution buffered in 0.01 M phosphate buffer (PBS), or Bouin's solution, followed by rinsing with PBS, pH 7.5. In case of freeze-dried autoradiograms, the slide is breathed on over the sections before fixation in order to facilitate adherence of sections to the emulsion and to prevent loss of sections from the slide during photographic processing.

b) Photographic Development and Fixation. Immediately after histological fixation, the slides are developed in Kodak D-19 developer, diluted 1 : 1 with PBS, at 18 °C for 60 s, rinsed in PBS and fixed in Kodak fixer for 5 min followed by rinsing in 2 changes of PBS 5 min each and subsequently processed for immunoperoxidase staining.

c) Immunoperoxidase Staining. A modification (Sar and Stumpf 1979) of the unlabeled antibody technique (Mason et al.

1969) is applied using the peroxidase antiperoxides complex (Sternberger 1974).

The autoradiographic slides after photographic development and fixation are passed through hydrogen peroxide-egg albumin (Zehr 1978) in order to reduce nonspecific staining. Accordingly, the autoradiograms are treated for 5 min with freshly prepared 3% hydrogen peroxide in PBS (0.01 M, pH 7.5), and then washed with 3 changes of PBS, 5 min each, followed by immersion in 5%–10% egg albumin for 10 min. After a rinse with PBS the autoradiograms are incubated with primary antiserum: First, the excess PBS from around the tissue section is wiped off. The primary antibodies raised in rabbit are then applied at optimal dilution, one or two drops, depending on the size of the section. Incubation is carried out in a humidified atmosphere at 4 °C for 24 or 48 h. After incubation with the primary antibodies the slides are washed with PBS and 1% normal sheep serum in PBS for 3–5 min each, followed by incubation with one or two drops of second antibodies, sheep anti-rabbit gamma globulin diluted 1 : 100 in PBS/normal sheep serum for 10 min. Following a 3–5 min wash in PBS, the autoradiograms are incubated at room temperature for 20–25 min with rabbit PAP complex (1 : 50 in PBS) and washed with PBS for 3 min.

The antibody-bound peroxidase is then demonstrated by incubating the autoradiograms for 10 min in diaminobenzidine (DAB) solution containing hydrogen peroxide. The DAB solution is prepared as follows: 150 mg 3,3′-diaminobenzidine tetrahydrochloride is dissolved in 200 ml 0.05 M Tris buffer, pH 7.6 (Nakane and Pierce 1966), and 15 μl 30% hydrogen per-

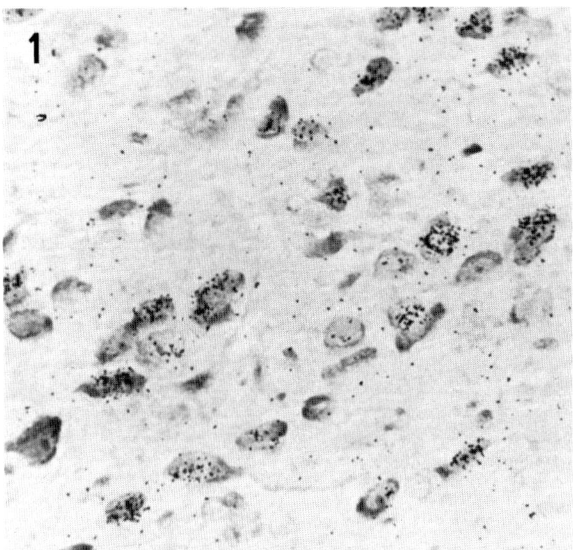

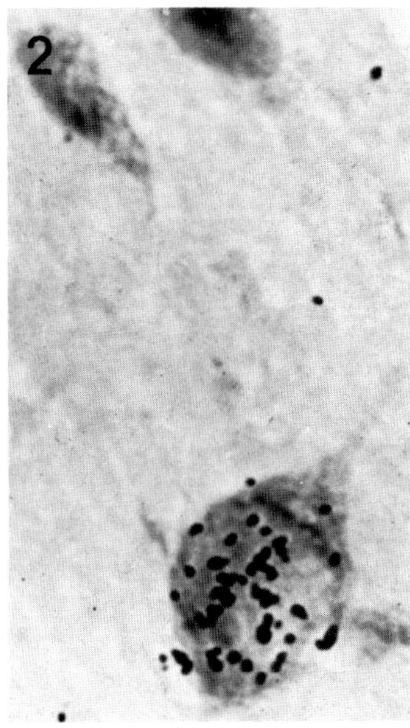

Figs. 1, 2. Dry-mount autoradiography as used for the localization of steroid hormones. Hypothalamic nucleus ventromedialis pars lateralis (Fig. 1, ×200) and the nucleus arcuatus (Fig. 2, ×1500), frontal plane, showing concentration of rdioactivity in nuclei of certain neurons. As is characteristic for steroid hormones, the nucleolus is spared and the cytoplasm contains relatively little radioactivity at 2 h after subcutaneous injection of ^{3}H estradiol-17β into mature ovariectomized female rat. Exposure times: 117 days (Fig. 1), 70 days (Fig. 2). Two μm stained with methyl-green pyronin for DNA and RNA. Reproduced from Stumpf (1968)

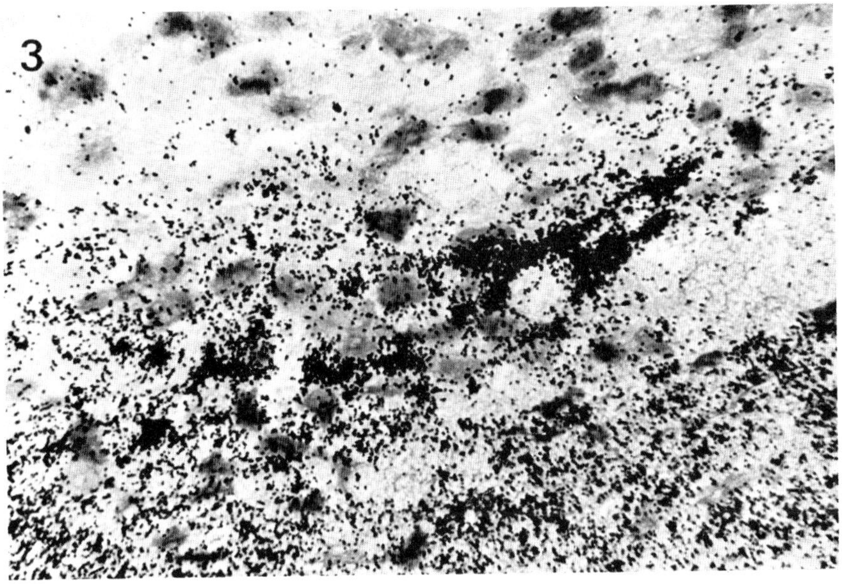

Fig. 3. Thaw-mount autoradiography as used for the tracing of neural pathways. Suprachiasmatic nucleus and optic chiasm of rat. The heavy concentration of silver grains represents nerve endings at neurons (in center) that contrast with weaker labeling of nerve fibers in the optic chiasm (*CO*), obtained after ocular injections of ^{3}H *l*-tyrosine. 4 μm, ×660, stained with methyl-green pyronin. Reproduced from Conrad and Stumpf (1974)

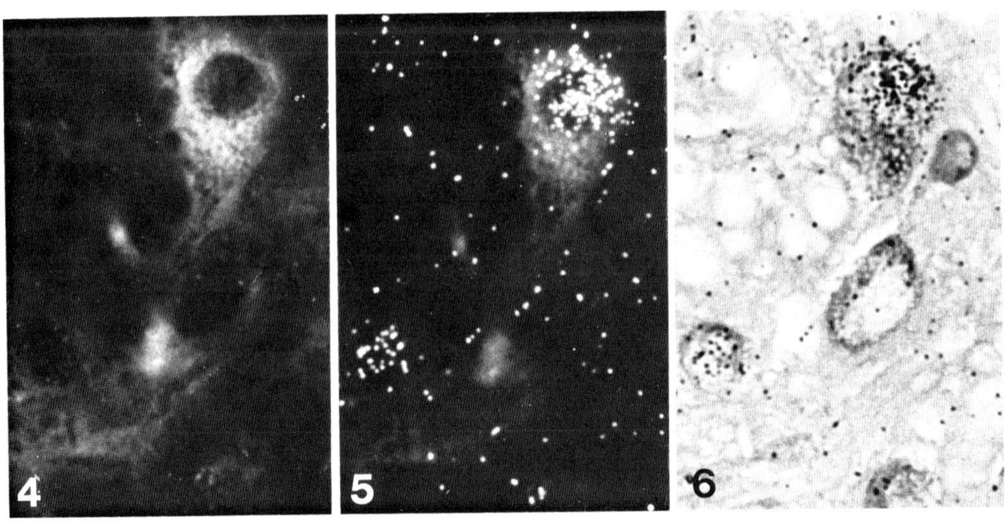

Figs. 4–6. Combined dry-mount autoradiography and formaldehyde-induced fluorescence for the simultaneous demonstration of ^{3}H estradiol and catecholamine in neurons from the region of the nucleus reticularis lateralis of brain stem. Observed under UV-light only (**Fig. 4**), UV-light and tungsten light simultaneously (**Fig. 5**) and after staining with methyl-green pyronin under tungsten light (**Fig. 6**). Reproduced from Heritage et al. (1977). 6 μm, ×470

oxide is added to this solution. After incubation with the DAB solution, the autoradiograms are washed in Tris buffer and PBS for 3 min each and counterstained either with 0.75% methyl green or 0.1% toluidine in PBS, then dehydrated in graded ethanols, cleared in xylene, and mounted with Permount and a coverglass. Specificity of the immunoperoxidase-staining is established by incubating the autoradiograms with preimmune normal rabbit serum or with antiserum which had been preabsorbed with the appropriate antigen. This combination technique has been described in detail (Sar and Stumpf 1980).

4 Examples

The published autoradiogram is the evidence. Therefore, any publication in autoradiography must contain pictorial evidence and the published pictures must be representative. These principles have not always been followed in the literature. Examples are provided in Figs. 1–9 for the different techniques described in this chapter. Figures 1–2 show examples of the dry-mount autoradiographic technique as used for the localization of steroid hormones. Subsequent publications in the literature on steroid hormone distribution as obtained by thaw-mount autoradiography are based on the evidence provided by this approach. Figure 3 shows an example of the thaw-mount technique for the tracing of neurol pathways. Tracing of neural pathways by thaw-mount autoradiography appears superior to the use of embedding techniques regarding sensitivity and completeness, since no radioactive material is lost during tissue processing. Figures 4–6 provide examples for the combined autoradiography and formaldehyde-induced fluorescence. Figures 7–9 show results obtained from the combined use of autoradiography and immunohistochemistry.

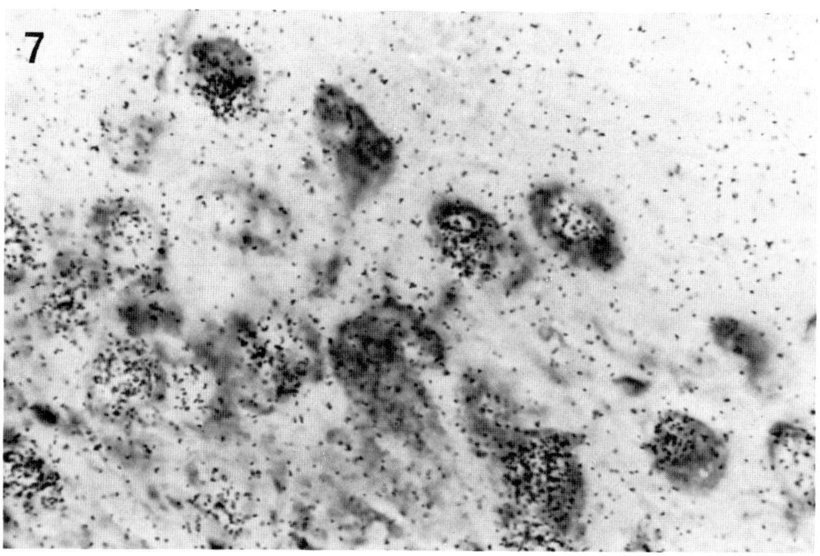

Fig. 7. Combined dry-mount autoradiography and immunohistochemistry of mouse supraoptic nucleus after ^{3}H estradiol-17β injection and staining by the immunoperoxidase method with antiserum to neurophysin 1, 1:2000. 4 μm, ×890. Nuclear concentration of radioactivity in neurophysin-secreting cells. Reproduced from Sar and Stumpf (1980)

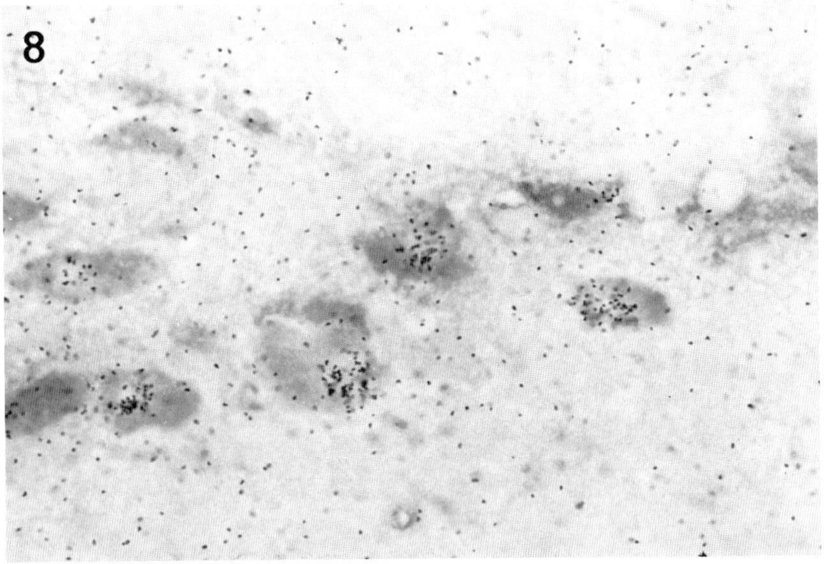

Fig. 8. Combined thaw-mount autoradiography and immunohistochemistry of guinea pig supraoptic nucleus after ^{3}H estradiol-17β injection and staining by the immunoperoxidase method with antiserum to neurophysin I, 1:2000. 4 μm, ×820. Nuclear concentration of radioactivity in neurophysin secreting cells. Reproduced from Sar and Stumpf (1981)

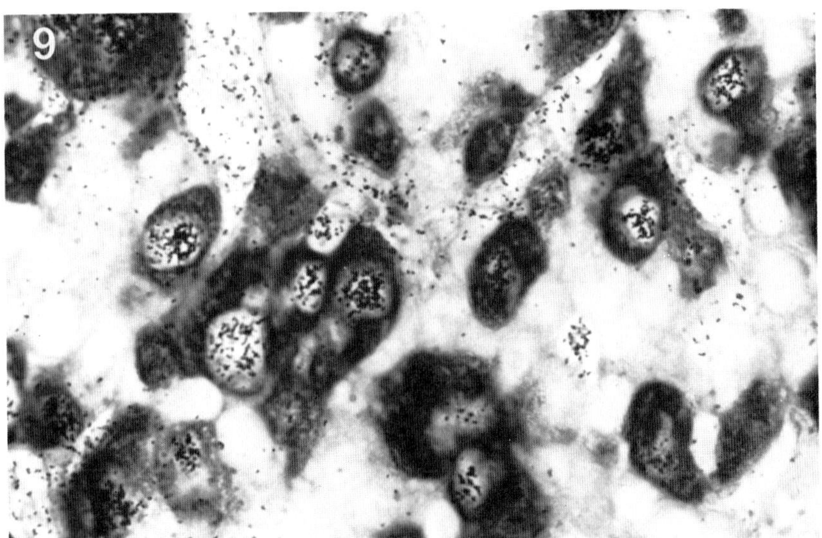

Fig. 9. Combined thaw-mount autoradiography and immunohistochemistry of rat anterior pituitary after ^{3}H dihydrotestosterone injection and staining by the immunoperoxidase method with antiserum to 0-LH, 1:1000. Note the nuclear concentration of radioactivity in LH-secreting cells. Four μm. Reproduced from Sar and Stumpf (1979). ×1020

5 References

Conrad CD, Stumpf WE (1974) Retinal projections traced with thaw-mount autoradiography and multiple injections of tritiated precursor or precursor cocktail. Cell Tissue Res 155:283–290

Grant LD, Stumpf WE (1973) Localization of ^{3}H-estradiol and catecholamines in identical neurons in the hypothalamus (abstr). J Histochem Cytochem 27:404

Heritage AS, Grant LD, Stumpf WE (1977) ^{3}H-estradiol in catecholamine neurons of rat brain stem: combined localization by autoradiography and formaldehyde-induced fluorescence. J Comp Neurol 176:607–630

Keefer DA, Stumpf WE, Petrusz P, Sar M (1975) Simultaneous autoradiographic and immunohistochemical localization of estrogen and gonadotropin in the rat pituitary. Am J Anat 142:129–135

Mason TE, Phifer RF, Spicer SS, Swallow RA, Dreskin RB (1969) An immunoglobulin-enzyme bridge method for localizing tissue antigens. J Histochem Cytochem 17:563–569

Nakane PK, Pierce GB Jr (1966) Enzyme-labeled antibodies: Preparation and application in the localization of antigens. J Histochem Cytochem 14:929–931

Pilgrim C, Wagner H-J (1981) Improving the resolution of the 2-deoxy-D-glucose method. J Histochem Cytochem 29:190–194

Sar M, Stumpf WE (1979) Simultaneous localization of steroid and peptide hormones in rat pituitary by combined thaw-mount autoradiography and immunohistochemistry: localization of dihydrotestosterone in gonadotropes, thyrotropes, and pituicytes. Cell Tissue Res 202:1–7

Sar M, Stumpf WE (1980) Simultaneous localization of ^{3}H-estradiol and neurophysin I or arginine vasopressin in hypothalamic neurons demonstrated by a combined technique of dry-mount autoradiography and immunohistochemistry. Neurosci Lett 17:179–184

Sar M, Stumpf WE (1981) Combined autoradiography and immunohistochemistry for simultaneous localization of radioactively labeled steroid hormones and antibodies in the brain. J Histochem Cytochem 29:161–166

Sternberger LA (1974) Immunocytochemistry. Prentice Hall, Englewood Cliffs

Stumpf WE (1968) Estradiol concentrating neurons: topography in the hypothalamus by dry-mount autoradiography. Science 162: 1001–1003

Stumpf WE (1971) Autoradiographic techniques and localization of estrogen, androgen and glucocorticoid in pituitary and brain. Am Zool 11:725–739

Stumpf WE (1976) Techniques for the autoradiography of diffusible compounds. Methods in Cell Biology 13:171–193

Stumpf WE, Grant LD (1975) Anatomical neuroendocrinology. Karger, Basel

Stumpf WE, Roth LJ (1964) Vacuum freeze-drying of frozen sections for dry-mounting, high-resolution autoradiography. Stain Technol 39:219–223

Stumpf WE, Roth LJ (1966) High resolution autoradiography with dry-mounted, freeze-dried, frozen sections. Comparative study of six methods using two diffusible compounds, ^{3}H-estradiol and ^{3}H-mesobilirubinogen. J Histochem Cytochem 14:274–287

Stumpf WE, Sar M (1975) Autoradiographic techniques for localizing steroid hormones. In: O'Malley BW, Hardman JG (eds) Methods in enzymology: vol XXXVI, hormone action, part A, steroid hormones. Academic Press, New York, pp 135–156

Stumpf WE, Sar M (1976) Autoradiographic localization of estrogen, androgen, progestin, and glucocorticosteroid in "target tissues" and "non-target tissues". In: Pasqualini J (ed) Receptors and mechanism of action of steroid hormones. Marcel Dekker, New York, pp 41–84

Stumpf WE, Sar M, Grant LD (1980) Autoradiographic localization of ^{210}Pb and its decay products in rat forebrain. Neurotoxicology 1:593–606

Zehr DR (1978) Use of hydrogen peroxide-egg albumin to eliminate nonspecific staining in immunoperoxidase techniques. J Histochem Cytochem 26:415–416

Chapter 14

Combined Immunocytochemistry and Autoradiography: In Vivo Injections of Monoclonal Antibodies and Radioactive Amines (Substance P and ^{3}H-Serotonin)

Victoria Chan-Palay

1 Introduction

Recently we have developed a new tool for the investigation of neurons which contain both neuropeptides and biogenic amines. This method includes a simultaneous application of in vivo injections of antibodies against neuropeptides and of radioisotope-labeled biogenic amines. The method will be demonstrated with respect to substance P and ^{3}H-serotonin localized in the medulla oblongata.

Previous investigations (Chan-Palay et al 1978) had demonstrated that some serotonin (5-HT) neurons in the ventral medulla oblongata of rat, particularly those in the reticular formation also contain the peptide substance P (SP). Such neurons have been examined for their 5-HT content exhaustively. They have endogenous amine stores detectable by the Falck-Hillarp technique, verified to be 5-HT by identification of excitation and emission spectra by microspectrofluorimetry on individual cells (Chan-Palay et al. 1978) and have 5-HT immunoreactivity (Hökfelt et al. 1978). The cells have uptake systems for low molarity ^{3}H-5-HT (Chan-Palay et al., 1978), are sensitive to 5-HT uptake inhibitors and monoamine oxidase inhibitors, are unaffected by reserpine, and are destroyed by 5,6-DHT. Their SP content has been identified in fixed material with animal antisera against SP by immunofluorescence (Chan-Palay et al. 1978; Hökfelt et al. 1978) and by PAP immunocytochemistry (Chan-Palay et al. 1978). In addition in vivo application of antibody against SP produced by a monoclonal cell line has been used to identify SP content in these cells based on their antigen-antibody recognition and binding systems in the living unfixed state (Chan-Palay 1979 b).

This chapter represents a novel approach for the demonstration of the coexistence of 5-HT and SP in single cells and terminal plexuses using simultaneous autoradiography and immunocytochemistry on the same preparation. The methods described here are: (1) readily adaptable for use for the detection of numerous other peptides, amines, and other transmitter compounds in locations elsewhere in the nervous system and (2) utilizable for light and electron microscopy so that connections as well as the synaptology of these neurons can be studied.

The present adaptation of in vivo injections of antibody in combination with autoradiography expands the range of this new technique for the exploration of many chemically specific systems in the brain and in peripheral organs.

2 General Comments

SP is detected by immunocytochemistry using in vivo injections of the characterized monoclonal SP antibody (Chan-Palay 1979 b) and the peroxidase-antiperoxidase method (PAP, Sternberger 1979). 5-HT is detected by application of ^{3}H-5-HT for uptake by 5-HT neurons followed by autoradiography (Chan-Palay 1975, 1976, 1977 a, b). The sequence of demonstration of cytochemical labels for SP and 5-HT is limited in practice by several factors: the SP antigen-antibody complexes need to be localized rapidly to prevent loss by lengthy tissue preparation and immunocytochemistry should be done before autoradiography. Once the immuno-reactive material is permanently captured, the lengthy exposures and harsh chemical procedures of developing and fixation in autoradiography can be carried out. Attempts to reverse the process by doing the autoradiography before immunocytochemistry have not been successful. This may be explained by a possible close interaction or coupling of 5-HT and SP receptor binding sites so that preloading of neurons with exogenous ^{3}H-5-HT can mask or inhibit the subsequent revelation of SP. The simultaneous labeling experiments circumvent this problem.

The major steps for ensuring or controlling the cytochemical specificity and sensitivity in terms of preservation of antigen, antigen-antibody complexes, radioactive label through tissue preservation, and subsequent preparation should be taken into consideration. A most important consideration, that of penetration of the label (^{3}H-5-HT) and of the antibody is ensured by their direct application into the region of interest under conditions that would allow for active and specific physiological uptake, recognition, and binding.

3 Description of the Methods

3.1 In Vivo Injections

For these model studies the nucleus raphe pallidus in the midline surface of the ventral medulla oblongata has been used on account of its accessibility to stereotaxic and visual approaches for microinjections, and its demonstrated content of 5-HT, 5-HT-SP, and SP neurons. The nucleus raphe pallidus is approached from the ventral aspect as previously described (Chan-Palay 1977 b; Brown et al. 1977; Chan-Palay 1979 b) in rats anesthetized by chloral hydrate (35%, 0.1 ml/100 g body wt.). The bone of the basiocciput overlying the nucleus raphe pallidus is removed and the basilar artery and ventral medulla visualized after slitting the dura. The mortality rate is less than 1% in acute experiments.

Microinjections are made by pressure (Chan-Palay 1977 b) through glass micropipettes with tip diameters of approximately 10 μm. Two to five separate injections each consisting of a volume of 0.025–0.05 μl are made into the nucleus raphe pallidus. Equivalent results in terms of 5-HT/SP-labeled cells can be obtained regardless of the mode of administration of the two labels: ^{3}H-5-HT and monoclonal antibody to SP from double-barrelled pipettes, together from a single pipette, or antibody applied by pipette and intracisternal infusion of ^{3}H-5-HT. Practically, the single-barrel injections are the simplest to execute. The injection sites are sometimes recognizable by a small region of hemorrhage with

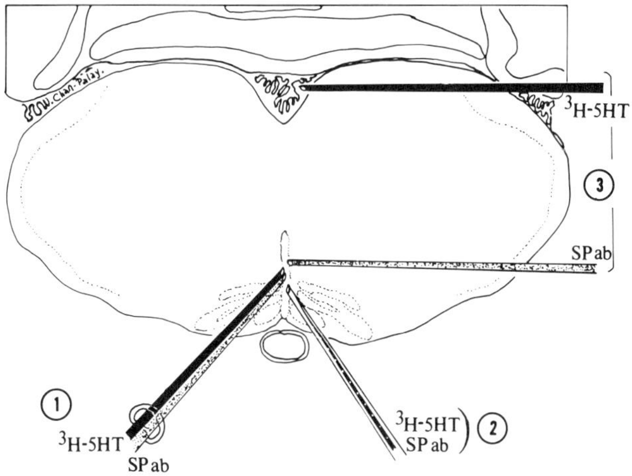

Fig. 1. Diagram to illustrate three experimental paradigms and modes of delivery of the two tracers for combined immunocytochemistry and autoradiography. 1, Double pipette injection with simultaneous delivery from one pipette filled with ^{3}H-5-HT and the other with monoclonal antibody to substance P directly into the nucleus raphe pallidus. 2, Single pipette injection with simultaneous delivery of ^{3}H-5-HT and monoclonal antibody to SP directly into the nucleus raphe pallidus. 3, Injection of monoclonal antibody to SP into the nucleus raphe pallidus with intracisternal injection of ^{3}H-5-HT

red blood cells stained a dark brown by their peroxidatic reaction, unrelated to SP immunoreactivity.

Double-pipette injections. Double-barrelled micropipettes with one barrel filled with ^{3}H-5-HT and the other filled with monoclonal antibody are used. The tip-to-tip separation distances are not greater than 50–80 μm, and the contents of both electrodes are ejected simultaneously by the application of pressure. Each injection site receives equal volumes of 0.025 μl of solution per pipette, a total of 0.05 μl per site.

Simultaneous injection of ^{3}H-5-HT and monoclonal SP antibody from a single pipette. An aliquot of ^{3}H-5-HT is evaporated to dryness and diluted monoclonal SP added. A total of 2–4 μCu of ^{3}H-5-HT with a total of 0.2–0.3 μl of SP antibody is injected in each animal in five separate injections, each containing approximately 0.5 μCu of ^{3}H-5-HT and 0.05 μl of antibody.

Intracisternal infusion of ^{3}H-5-HT (25 μl over 5 min) is administered manually by a Hamilton syringe into animals, which have been pretreated with clorgyline (monoamine oxidase inhibitor) 12 h before. This is followed an hour later by in vivo injections of undiluted monoclonal SP antibody.

3.1.1 Tritiated Serotonin

(^{3}H-5-HT, 10^{-7} m, specific activity 10.8 Cu/mmol, Amersham Searle)

3.1.2 Monoclonal Antibody

Monoclonal antibody against SP is used undiluted in the partially purified form after precipitation with ammonium sulphate and dialysis. The antibody we used is produced and purified by Dr. Cuello and colleagues (Cuello et al. 1979). Radioimmunoassay with ^{125}I-tyrosine-8-substance P is used to assay the titer of the antibody secreted by the hybrid myeloma cell lines. Cuello et al. (1979) demonstrated that 1 : 1000 dilution of the dialysate of ammonium sulphate precipitated antibody does not cross-react with leu- or met-enkephalin, somatostatin, and endorphin. Cross-reactivity experiments indicate that the antibody recognizes a determinant located in the C-terminal portion of substance P. The 5, 6 and 8 amino acid C-terminal fragments of SP and intact SP equally displace labeled SP, indicating complete cross-reactivity. Eledoisin, a *non*-mammalian peptide with the three C-terminal residues in common with SP as well as proline and phenylalanine in the 2 and 7 positions respectively have a cross-reactivity of 5%. Monoclonal antibodies from hybrid myelomas allow the continuous production of highly specific antibodies from permanent cell lines, thus overcoming the significant problem of heterogeneity in antibodies produced in conventional animal preparations.

3.1.3 Control Experiments

All compounds used in these experiments with the exception of the monoclonal antibody which is undiluted are dissolved in 0.9% sterile saline.

3.1.3.1 Control Sera

Undiluted monoclonal antibody absorbed overnight with SP (2.5 ug/10 μl). Three experimental paradigms are tested, and at least six animals are used in each set of experiments. Two animals in each group of the experiments receive injections containing monoclonal SP antibody preabsorbed overnight with SP instead of the actual antibody.

3.1.3.2 5,6-Dihydroxytryptamine

Three rats are treated with 5,6-dihydroxytryptamine-creatinine-sulphate (5,6-DHT, Sigma, 3.0 mg/μl, 10 μl per 100 g body wt.) administered intracisternally 7 days prior to surgery. This neurotoxin is preferentially taken up into serotonin neurons causing their ultimate degeneration as well as a limited amount of tissue damage at the injection site (Baumgarten et al. 1971). The single micropipette injections of combined ^{3}H-5-HT and SP antibody are used.

3.1.3.3 Monoamine Oxidase Inhibitors

Monoamine oxidase inhibitors such as clorgyline used in conjunction with ^{3}H-5-HT autoradiography serve effectively to retard the metabolism of ^{3}H-5-HT into its metabolites, thus ensuring that the label in autoradiograms indicates sites of 5-HT transport and storage rather than that of 5-hydroxyindolacetic acid (5-HIAA) (Chan-Palay and Jonsson, unpublished data from thin layer chromatography experiments). For this reason all animals in the ^{3}H-5-HT intracisternal infusion/SP injection experiments are pretreated with clorgyline (May and Baker; 10 mg/100 g b.w.) 12 h before surgery. Moreover for control experiments at least three animals in each group should receive previously determined effective doses of clorgyline 12 h before surgery.

3.1.3.4 Reserpine

Three rats are treated with reserpine in a single dose (2 g/100 g body wt., i. p.) administered 12 h before surgery. The single micropipette injections of combined ^{3}H-5-HT and SP antibody are used. Reserpine has a documented ability to deplete stored monoamines from neurons in the central and peripheral nervous system (Carlsson 1966).

3.1.3.5 Serotonin Uptake Inhibitors

GE 654 (ASTRA, Sweden; 1 mg/100 g body wt.), Zimelidine (ASTRA; 1 mg/100 g body wt.) and Norzimelidine (ASTRA; 1 mg/100 g b. w.) are used. Each substance is tried separately in groups consisting of three animals and administered 2 h before surgery. The single micropipette injections of combined ^{3}H-5-HT and SP antibody are used.

3.2 Fixation

All rats are maintained for 1–2 h after the last injection and are then perfused with cold Tyrode's buffer (Ca^{2+}-free, 50 ml) followed by 500 ml ice cold 4% formaldehyde with 0.25% glutaraldehyde in 0.2 M phosphate buffer, pH 7.4. Following perfusion the brain is removed and soaked in this fixative for 1–2 h, then rinsed and soaked in Tris buffer (0.05 M, pH 7.6) overnight.

3.3 Immunocytochemistry

Horizontal sections 15–20 μm thick through the entire nucleus raphe pallidus are cut on a vibratome (Oxford Instruments Co.) in cold 0.05 M Tris buffer, pH 7.6, maintained at 10 °C. Serial sections are individually transferred with a fine camel's hair brush into the wells of a disposable culture tray in sequence and their order maintained. The sections are rinsed thoroughly (3×5 min each) with Tris buffer containing 0.05% Triton X-100, pH 7.6, and then treated directly with rabbit anti-rat IgG (1 : 10, in Tris-Triton, at room temperature for 30 min). The sections are rinsed again with Tris-Triton and reacted with rat peroxidase-antiperoxidase (PAP, 1 : 100, in Tris-Triton, pH 7.6, at room temperature for 30 min). After this the sections are washed in Tris buffer, pH 7.6, and soaked in 0.022% diaminobenzidine (DAB) in Tris buffer for 2–3 min. Thereafter H_2O_2 is added with agitation to produce a final concentration of 0.3% and allowed to react for 7 min prior to rinsing in distilled water (3×). Individualized serial sections are examined under a Zeiss stereoscope throughout the procedure to monitor the color of the reaction. Injection sites and groups of labeled cells and terminals can be visualized readily. The sections are then mounted in serial order onto chrome-alum (0.05%) and gelatin (0.5%) treated slides and allowed to air dry in a clean environment.

All sections are examined by phase and Nomarski interference microscopy. Neurons, dentrites, and axons with positive SP immunoreactivity have an unmistakeable orange/brown reaction product.

Attention should be paid to the intensity of the immunoreactivity product. This method of treating the loose sections with the secondary antibody and visualization with DAB-produced cells has far more intense immuno-reactivity than when the vibratome sections were first mounted on slides and then carried through the remaining procedures. An explanation for this may be that loose sections present far greater available surface area for the immunocytochemical reactions.

3.4 Autoradiography

After immunocytochemical evaluation the slides are processed for autoradiography in a light-tight photographic dark room equipped with a sodium lamp having both red and yellow banded filters (Thomas Duplex super safe light, Thomas Instrument Co., New York). A clean dust-free work area covered with absorbent lab mat material is essential.

The nuclear track emulsion (Kodak NTB-2) is diluted as follows: the volume of liquid required to fill the dipping container is determined. This volume height is marked on the side of a plastic beaker, and then the half volume in also marked. The beaker is filled to the half volume mark with distilled water and placed in 45 °C water bath. The temperatures are allowed to equilibrate. Using a glass rod, sufficient emulsion is scraped out of the emulsion packing into the beaker to raise the liquid level to the full volume mark, thus providing a 1 : 1 emulsion to water dilution, and gently stirred.

Once the emulsion mixture is smooth and homogenous, it is slowly poured from the mixing beaker into a dipping container. Sudden agitation should be avoided to

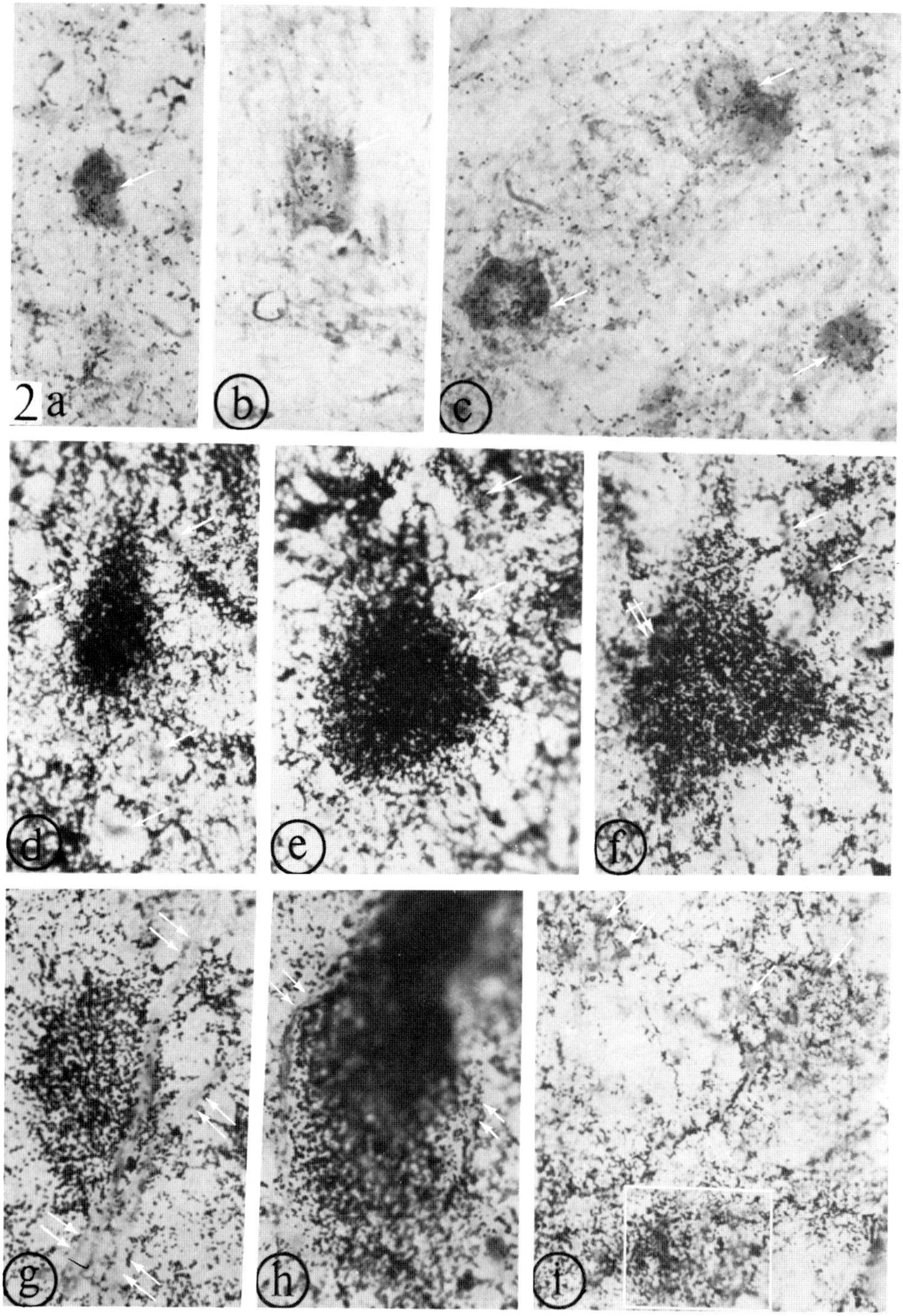
2a
b
c
d
e
f
g
h
i

reduce air bubbles. Several clean empty test slides are dipped sequentially into the emulsion to draw off air bubbles from the surface and to check for even coating of the slides. Between dips gentle stirring is advised.

Slides with sections are individually dipped gently into emulsion and drawn out, using a smooth, even motion for 2–4 s. The slide edges are allowed to make contact with the rim of the container to drain slides of excess emulsion. The slide is then momentarily stood on an absorbent paper towel to absorb excess emulsion. Slides are lined up on a drying rack sequentially, section side forward, labeled and set up right, indicating with labeled tape the various slide groupings. The sections are allowed to dry for 3 h.

Once completely dry the slides are stored in a light-tight slide box that has been provided with small vials filled with phosphorus pentoxide (P_2O_5) stoppered, and covered with Kleenex tissue. The box is placed in a refrigerator during an exposure period of 3–6 weeks. It is advisable to change the dessicant once. In humid areas silica gel is used instead of P_2O_5 to avoid leakage of liquid P_2O_5 onto the slide, as this produces chemical fogging.

After 3–6 weeks several test slides are removed and developed to check the progress of exposure. Remaining slides are left in darkroom if exposure is inadequate.

Properly exposed slides are removed from their box in the darkroom and placed in a stainless steel staining rack. The developing solutions are set out to equilibrate at 18 °C. The slides are developed in full strength D-19 Kodak developer for 4½ min, washed in tap water at room temperature for 30 s, fixed in full strength Kodak rapid fixer at room temperature for 5 min, washed again at 18 °C–20 °C for 30–60 min, and dried.

Completely dry slides are rapidly dehydrated and cleared in xylene prior to coverslipping in Permount, or they are coverslipped directly. No further counterstains are employed. Success of the autoradiograms is judged by examination under dark-field and bright-field microscopy based on the specific accumulation of silver grains on identified neurons and processes at a level over that of the background. The combined study of positive SP immunoreactivity and of autoradiographic label with ^{3}H-5-HT are most convenient in bright-field microscopy.

Neurons with heavy ^{3}H-5-HT accumulation are specifically labeled with autoradiographic silver grains, well above background. Cells and fibers with both ^{3}H-5-HT accumulation and SP immunoreactivity are stained orange/brown and have in addition a superimposed deposit of autoradiographic silver grains.

Fig. 2a–i. Serotonin and SP neurons and their processes in the nucleus raphe pallidus localized by immunocytochemistry and autoradiography after simultaneous injection of ^{3}H-5-HT and monoclonal antibody to SP. **a–c** Small neurons with intense SP immunoreactive-staining and minimal autoradiographic label with ^{3}H-5-HT (*arrows*). **d, e** Larger 5-HT-SP neurons with intense SP immunoreactivity as well as heavy autoradiographic label with ^{3}H-5-HT. *Arrows* indicate boutons or processes in the neuropil with SP immunoreactivity. **f** A large neuron cell body with predominant labeling with ^{3}H-5-HT and minimal SP immunoreactivity. *Crossed arrows* indicate intensely reactive SP boutons upon the somatic surface and *single arrows* indicate similar boutons elsewhere in the neuropil. **g, h** Large neurons of the nucleus raphe pallidus near its boundary with the nucleus reticularis gigantocellularis (pars alpha) labeled in their somata only with ^{3}H-5-HT. They are apposition with processes of other neurons localized by intense SP immunoreactivity (*double arrows*). **i** A cellular neuropil of the nucleus raphe pallidus in which boutons that are intensely SP immunoreactive (*arrows*) lie next to fibers labeled by ^{3}H-5-HT (*crossed arrows*). In the boxed area, the autoradiographic ^{3}H-5-HT label and the SP immunoreactive sites are superimposed indicating possible coexistence of both 5-HT and SP in terminals in this regions. ×320

4 Dynamic Considerations

In vivo injections of antibody provide a rapid and reliable means of marking specific immunoreactive cell groups based upon the antigen-antibody recognition and binding capacities of these cells. They easily allow studies of peptidergic neurons and their connections, whereas the localization of cell bodies has been difficult and has necessitated the use of toxic substances such as colchicine to interfere with fast axonal flow (Hökfelt et al. 1978). This drug is known to inhibit fast axoplasmic transport, thus causing an unphysiological accumulation of many substances including transmitters, enzymes, and precursors in the cell bodies of neurons. It has been used extensively to enhance the detectability of monoamine and peptides for cytochemical localization. The in vivo injection method is invaluable as it reveals peptide-containing neuronal somata reliably without colchicine (Chan-Palay 1979b).

The nucleus raphe pallidus neurons are a mixed population, some cells have a majority of substance P immunoreactivity with little detectable serotonin, others have considerable quantities of both substance P immunoreactivity and serotonin, and still others have only serotonin but are innervated by substance P immunoreactive processes. The subtle differences in neuronal content of the two compounds are made more obvious by avoiding the use of colchicine.

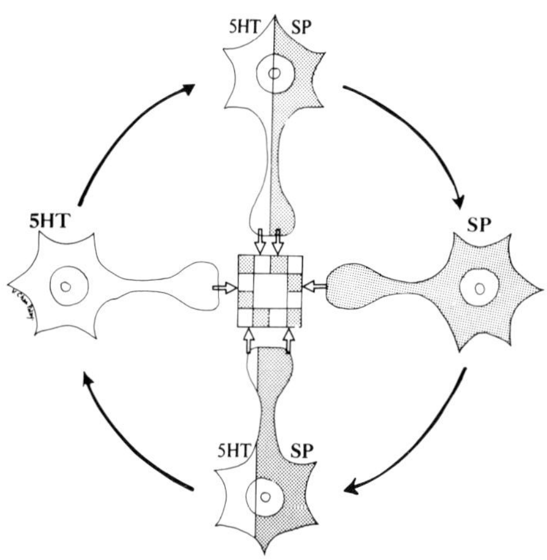

Fig. 3. Schematic diagram to illustrate the concept of dynamic interrelationships between 5-HT and SP in a single neuron. A neuron with both substances in coexistence may have fluctuating levels of one or both substances depending upon parameters of rhythm, time cycle, and physiologic demands for one or another mediator during specific types or phases of activity

The combined immunocytochemistry and autoradiography technique furnishes evidence to suggest that in addition to having two identified putative transmitter substances in coexistence, the amounts of each of these two substances present at any one time may vary. Individual neurons may have more of one, less of another, or have both in large amounts. This heterogeneity in multiple putative transmitter content has been discussed briefly earlier. Our present ideas of the concept of coexistence of putative transmitter substances may have to be expanded to encompass the two critical dimensions of time and the physiological function of the cell. It may be that neurons containing both 5-HT and SP have fluctuating levels of one or both of these substances depending upon parameters of rhythm, demands for one or of the other mediator during specific types of phases of activity (Chan-Palay 1979a).

Detailed studies by electron microscope autoradiography of 5-HT neurons and their axonal projections in the mammalian brain, the insulae of the external nucleus exist in locations as different as the cerebellum, the supraependymal plexus, the caudate nucleus, the locus coeruleus, and the nucleus reticularis paragigantocellularis lateralis. These studies show that there is no consensus on one single constellation of ultrastructural features of the axoplasm that differentiate 5-HT axons from those of other neurons. In fact, identified 5-HT axons are different from one another in one specific region of the brain and they may contain a number of different populations of synaptic vesicles when classified

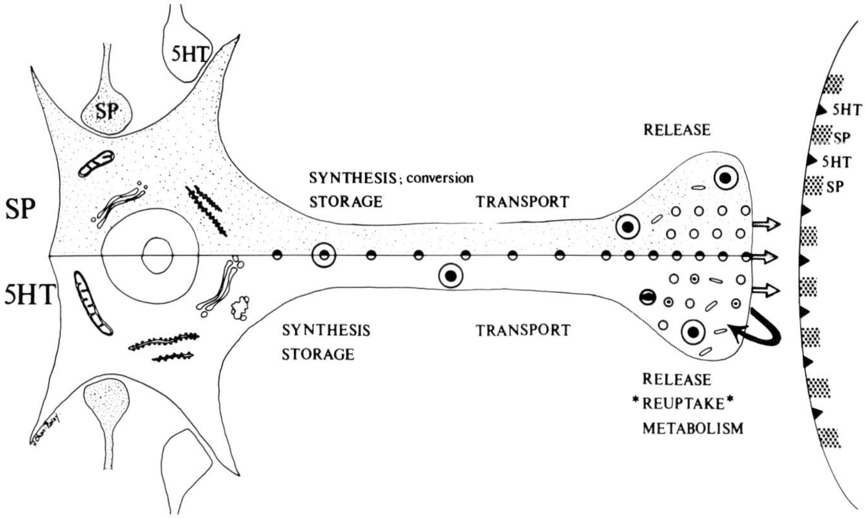

Fig. 4. Schematic diagram of a neuron with 5-HT and SP in coexistence in its soma and processes. The internal cellular machinery to facilitate the synthesis, transport, storage, and release of peptide and amine transmitter, as well as the separate mechanisms required for reuptake and metabolism of the amine alone are depicted. Separate 5-HT and SP receptors are shown on the receptive cell surface to illustrate the need for further recognition/specificity. Dual coupling of 5-HT and SP receptors is also possible, though not illustrated

carefully as to size, shape, and content. Is this heterogeneity in synaptic vesicle morphology an expression of the multiplicity in their neurotransmitter content? A similar situation has emerged from the results of studies of terminals identified with SP immunoreactivity, showing some differences in the synaptic vesicle populations labeled in SP axons. In the light of the present evidence for coexistence of multiple putative transmitters in 5-HT-SP neurons and their terminals, it would be wise to be cautious in discussions as to the vesicular populations primarily identifiable with SP content alone. The question of which chemical mediator for which synaptic vesicle, or if vesicles are involved at all, cannot be definitely decided on the basis of the present insufficient evidence.

The fundamental scheme of simultaneous injection of multiple labels, one radioactive, another a specific characterized monoclonal antibody for the detection of multiple and separate transmitter systems opens vast avenues for future investigation.

5 References

Baumgarten HG, Björklund A, Lachenmeyer L, Nobin A, Stenevi U (1971) Long lasting selective depletion of brain serotonin by 5,6-dihydroxytryptamine. Acta Physiol Scand [Suppl] 373:1–14

Brown JT, Chan-Palay V, Palay SL (1977) A study of afferent input to the inferior olivary complex by retrograde axonal transport of horseradish peroxidase. J Comp Neurol 176:1–22

Calas A, Besson MJ, Gaughy G, Alonso G, Glowinski J, Cheramy A (1976) Radioautographic study of in vivo incorporation of ^{3}H-monoamines in cat caudate nucleus: Identification of serotoninergic fibers. Brain Res 118:1–13

Carlsson A (1966) Drugs which block the storage of 5-hydroxytryptamine and related amines. In: Erspamer V (ed) 5-Hydroxytryptamine and related indolealkylamines. Springer, Berlin Heidelberg New York (Handbook of experimental pharmacology, vol XIX [Suppl], pp 529–592)

Chan-Palay V (1975) Fine structure of labelled axons in the cerebellar cortex and nuclei of rodents and primates after intraventricular infusions with tritiated serotonin. Anat Embryol 148:235–265

Chan-Palay V (1976) Serotonin axons in the supra- and subependymal plexuses and in the leptomeninges; their roles in local alterations of cerebrospinal fluid and vasomotor activity. Brain Res 102:103–130

Chan-Palay V (1977a) Indoleamine neurons and their processes in the normal rat brain and in chronic diet-induced thiamine deficiency demonstrated by uptake of ^{3}H-serotonin. J Comp Neurol 174:467–493

Chan-Palay V (1977b) Cerebellar dentate nucleus organization, cytology, and transmitters. Springer, Berlin Heidelberg New York

Chan-Palay V (1979a) Combined immunocytochemistry and autoradiography after in vivo injections of monoclonal antibody to Substance P and ^{3}H-serotonin. Coexistence of two putative transmitters in single raphe cells and fiber plexuses. Anat Embryol 156:241–254

Chan-Palay V (1979b) Immunocytochemical detection of substance P neurons, their processes and connections by in vivo microinjections of monoclonal antibodies: Light and electron microscopy. Anat Embryol (Berl.) 156:225–240

Chan-Palay V, Jonsson G, Palay SL (1978) Serotonin and substance P coexist in neurons of the rat's central nervous system. Proc Natl Acad Sci USA 76:1582–1586

Cuello AC, Galfre G, Milstein C (1979) Detection of substance P in the central nervous system by a monoclonal antibody. Proc Natl Acad Sci USA 76:3532–3536

Hökfelt T, Ljungdahl A, Steinbusch H, Verhofstad A, Nilsson brodin E, Pernow B, Goldstein M (1978) Immunohistochemical evidence of substance P-like immunoreactivity in some 5-hydroxytryptamine-containing neurons in the rat central nervous system. Neuroscience 3:517–538

Palay SL (1967) Principles of cellular organization in the nervous system. In: Quarton GC, Melnechuk T, Schmitt FO (eds) The neurosciences. Rockefeller University Press, New York, pp 24–31

Sternberger LA (1979) Immunocytochemistry, 2nd edn. In: Cohen S, McCluskey (eds) Basic and clinical immunology. John Wiley, New York

Part III

Electron Microscopical Research Methods in Neuroanatomy

Chapter 15

Quick-Freezing Methods in Neuroanatomy

J. Metz

1 Introduction

Routine procedures employed in tissue preparation for electron microscopic studies, such as chemical fixation, dehydration, and embedding in polymers, have been primary influences in the wide field of ultrastructural investigation in the past. They, however, also limited the potency of electron microscopy and of analytical attachments available, e.g., X-ray microanalysis, autoradiography. Cryofixation deserves special interest as a method of preparation, since unrestricted information on the native state of a specimen can now be obtained.

Although cryofixation of biological tissue as an alternative to chemical fixation was investigated by Altmann as early as 1890, and many studies have been conducted since, the major disadvantages of this method have only been overcome in the last few years. Freeze damage affects not only the ultrastructure by segregation artifacts, but also limits the "resolution" of other analytical methods, since atoms and molecules become dislocated. Treatment of tissue with cryoprotectants prior to freezing largely prevents the damage. Therefore, preparatory methods in electron microscopy such as freeze-fracturing almost exclusively include the use of antifreeze agents, e.g., glycerol. Unfortunately, these antifreeze agents are known to have deleterious effects on native tissue and thus introduce artifacts of their own (Plattner et al. 1972; Echlin et al. 1977; Farrant et al. 1977; Franks 1977). Chemical fixation of tissue applied prior to treatment with cryoprotective agents not only insufficiently stabilizes the ultrastructure (e. g., Van Deurs and Luft 1979), adding considerably to further uncertainties in the interpretation of the results achieved, but also fails the original aim of analyzing the native state. In order to fix the natural distribution pattern of all cellular constituents any chemical pretreatment, such as fixatives and cryoprotectives, has to be avoided. Antifreeze agents, however, are dispensible only if the freezing rates within the specimens are so high that the ice crystals formed are too small to interfere with the image seen in the electron microscope.

Quick or ultrarapid freezing are terms applied to procedures for freezing tissue in its native state and are further differentiated from freezing procedures utilizing pretreatments such as chemical fixation or cryoprotectants.

One of the most important advantages of the quick-freezing method in comparison with conventional ultrastructural approaches is that it enables living specimens to be instantaneously frozen (Van Harreveld et al., 1974). Since in the past, kinetic sequences of rapid events at the ultrastructural level could only be deduced from static electron micrographs of chemically fixed specimens, the ability to undertake direct kinetic studies represents a significant breakthrough in cell biology. Events occurring within the millisecond range may be captured and the accumulation of intermediate stages which might occur during slow death by aldehyde fixation is avoided.

A further advantage of ultrarapid freezing is that, by being able to freeze delicate biological specimens in dilute aqueous solutions in the absence of chemical cryoprotectants one can expose the outer surface of the membrane, extracellular structures, and intracellular cytoskeletal elements by deep etching.

Critical evaluations of the artifacts produced in biological specimens by the alternative biochemical fixation and cryoprotection techniques normally used by electron microscopists should be expected. Further preparatory steps which can be applied after quick freezing such as freeze-fracturing, freeze-substitution, freeze-drying, or autoradiography (Chap. 18) and subsequent analytical methods, e. g., transmission electron microscopy or X-ray microanalysis, open a wide range of possibilities for ultrastructural investigations.

2 Quick-Freezing Methods

2.1 High Pressure Method

Tissue is frozen by a liquid nitrogen jet under a high pressure of about 2000 bar (Moor and Riehle 1968; Riehle and Hoechli 1973). Under these hyperbaric conditions the freezing point of water is lowered to −22 °C. A vitrification of a specimen tissue of 0.5 mm thickness without chemical fixation and cryoprotection is claimed. Since this procedure necessitates an elaborate and costly apparatus and new artifacts might be introduced by the high pressure, the method still remains restricted to experiments with model systems.

2.2 Spray Freezing

This method is applied under the supposition that solidification in a microcrystalline state is achieved if an ideally cold cryogen acts upon a biological sample of the smallest possible size, so that the surface-to-volume ratio is high. Bachmann and Schmidt (1971) devised the spray-freezing method for freeze-fracture replication of solutions. Plattner et al. (1972) and Bachmann and Schmitt-Fumian (1973) adapted this procedure to suspensions of cells and subcellular fractions. Samples contained in their culture or isolation medium are sprayed by a special apparatus (spray freezing apparatus, Balzers, Lichtenstein) as minute droplets into a cooled container filled with an appropriate cooling agent. Liquid propane (–180 °C) is most frequently used. The droplets produced by the sprayer should be not more than about 10–20 μm in diameter so as to achieve a sufficiently rapid freezing rate. The droplets should be immersed in the freezing agent in a liquid state and not, as could happen due to low velocity, freeze within the gaseous phase of the coolant. The following steps in preparing the frozen droplets, especially for freeze-fracturing, are performed in a glove box. The frozen droplets are warmed to –78 °C within a CO_2 cool bath and propane is evaporated. The specimen particles are embedded in an inert organic medium at a temperature just above its melting point. Butylbenzene (–88 °C), isobutyryl-isobutyrate, pentanol, or butanol are employed as embedding media. The frozen specimen droplets are mixed with a droplet of the medium and transferred with a platinum loop to the object holder. After transfer, the medium is solidified by cooling and the preparations are treated as regular freeze-fracture specimens.

Spray freezing involves disadvantages that derive (1) from the size of the specimen which is limited to the size of unicellular microorganisms, and (2) from difficulties in handling the spray gun, frozen droplets, and adhesives. In addition, the surface area of the replicas useful for investigation is limited.

2.3 Freezing by Liquified Gases

Native tissue is either simply dipped into a coolant or superfused in situ with a freezing medium. Varying approaches were employed to improve the freezing process and to adapt this method to the steps of the following analytical procedures.

Fernandes-Morán (1960) used helium II to freeze biological tissue for electron microscopy. Bullivant (1970) plunged unprotected tissue into Freon 12. Invariably, relatively large intracellular and extracellular ice crystals were found which generally varied in size from 50 to 250 μm.

Somlyo et al. (1977) quickly clipped tissue into a silver wire which was fired into supercooled Freon 22 with an air gun operated at a velocity of 60 cm/sec. Supercooled Freon 22 was found to yield results superior to methods employing liquid nitrogen slush.

Steinbrecht (1980) dropped antennae of an insect which have a high surface-to-volume ratio into liquid propane.

Stolinski and Breathnach (1976) transferred small pieces of tissue into thin-walled stainless steel tubes (1.5 mm diameter) to be rapidly frozen in liquid propane at –180 °C. Part of each sample was kept protruding about 0.5 mm above the rim of the tubular holder in order to allow subsequent fracturing.

Schlote et al. (1978) used a C-type specimen holder for shock-freezing of biological tissue in situ which was further studied by X-ray analysis of ultrathin sections. The cylindrical holder was specially designed for the freezing of tissues consisting of longitudinally oriented elements such as muscles, nerves, vessels, or connective tissue. This aluminium holder is formed like a shell with a length of 7 mm, an outer diameter of 3 mm, an inner diameter of 1.5 mm, and has a long slot of 1 mm width. The tissue is shock-frozen either in situ by superfusing the holder with a freezing medium (liquid propane) or in tabula by dipping the specimen holder with a tissue sample into the freezing medium. The undamaged part of the tissue which projects from the holder is selected for cryosectioning.

It should be considered when using the dipping method, that the entry and immersion velocity can affect the transfer of heat under certain conditions (Costello and Corless 1978). The cooling rate at a given entrance velocity appears to be codependent on the viscosity and surface tension of the coolant and the size and shape of the holder. Furthermore, the depth of specimen travel into the coolant clearly affects the freezing rate and can be optimized for each specimen (Costello and Corless 1978). In model experiments these authors found that liquid propane at −180 °C gave the most rapid cooling rates as compared with different Freons (22, 13, 12), isopentane, liquid nitrogen, or solid/liquid nitrogen slush. It should, however, be noted that a number of diverse approaches have been conceived to optimize, infer, or evaluate the cooling rates of biological samples in liquified gases, with equally diverse and often conflicting results and conclusions (Costello and Corless 1978; Rosenkranz 1975; Umrath 1975; Heuser et al. 1976).

2.4 Thin Sandwich Method

In the thin sandwich method, native, suspended material is "sandwiched" between two metal (copper, gold) plates using a 20 µm-thick spacer ring which is then pushed into a coolant e. g., propane (Gulik-Krzywicki and Costello 1977; Müller and Pseid 1979). The thickness of the aqueous layer can be, at least theoretically, increased by a factor of 4 if the specimen is sandwiched between two metal plates and cooled from opposite directions. It has been shown that the freezing rate can be improved when the specimen mass is reduced, the surface area of the specimen in contact with the metal is increased, and the metal plates are very thin and of high heat conductivity (Costello and Corless 1978).

2.5 Cryogen-jet Method

As compared with dipping, the cooling rate can be increased about 30 times by directing a high speed cryogen stream, in this case by shooting liquid propane onto the sandwich surface as described by Moor et al. (1976). These authors developed a device (Cryo-Jet QFD 101, Balzers, Lichtenstein) in which the specimen is placed between two specially shaped copper plates or gold platelets of very low mass. This sandwich is then fixed in a holder and placed between two nozzles through which liquid propane (−180 °C) is blown from opposite directions onto the sample. This method allows "vitrification" of any object which can be prepared as a thin platelet. The frozen sandwich can be cleaved parallel to the specimen plane by use of a double-replica technique.

2.6 Freezing on Cold Metal Surfaces

This method of cryofixation which was already applied to light microscopy was refined by Van Harreveld and Crowell (1964) and Van Harreveld et al. (1965) for electron microscopy, both using freeze-substitution and embedding for thin sectioning. This method of freezing has subsequently been applied to the study of frozen thin sections of pancreas and liver (Christensen 1971) of the extracellular space in the vertebrate central nervous system (Van Harreveld, 1972), and of membrane structure in mouse cerebellar cortex (Landis and Reese 1974). Dempsey and Bullivant (1976a, b) in principle used the original design of a simple copper block freezing apparatus cooled by liquid nitrogen and adapted it to freeze-fracturing. We used this approach to freeze blood platelets and exposed unfractured surface structures by deep etching (Figs. 1, 2).

Heuser et al. (1976, 1979) improved this technique of cryofixation on cold metal surfaces applying the apparent advantages of a colder initial block temperature for the ultrastructural preservation of biological specimens.

When using a liquid helium-cooled block, Heuser et al. (1979) found that the freezing rates were 50%–100% faster than

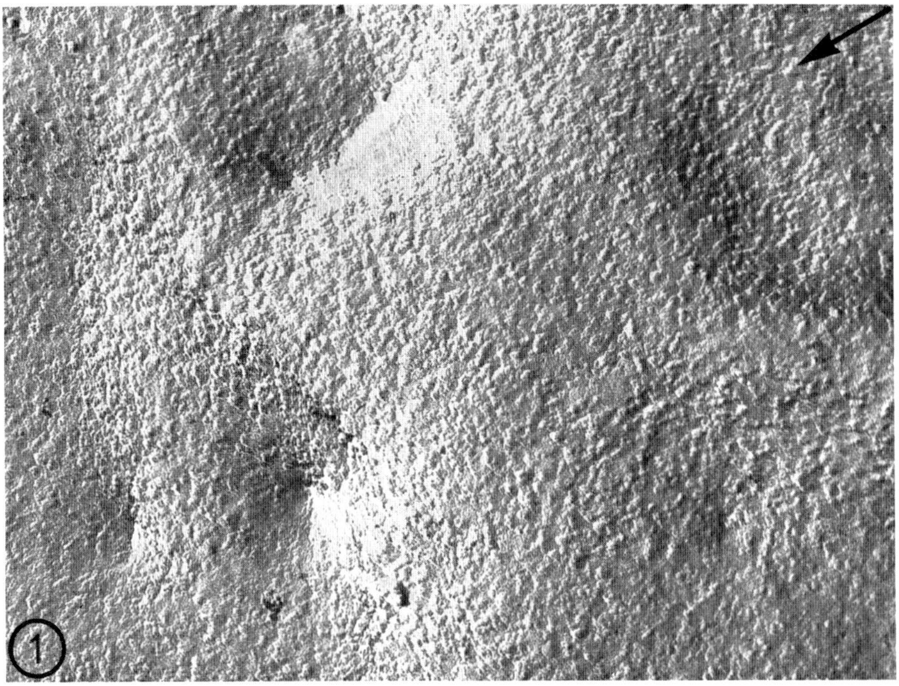

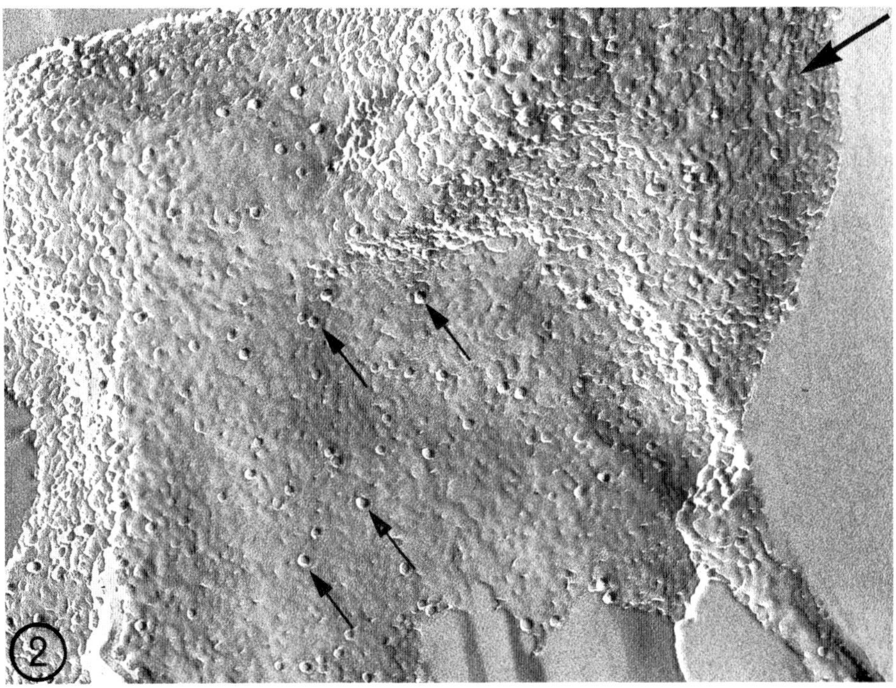

Fig. 1. Deep-etched outer surface of a chemically fixed blood platelet, quick-frozen in distilled water. The specimen was not fractured before deep etching. *Large arrow*, shadowing direction. ×100,000

Fig. 2. Deep-etched blood platelet with ferritin particles (*arrows*) on the outer surface. (Same conditions as in Fig. 1.) ×100,000

in a liquid-nitrogen-cooled block. A copper block was used instead of silver, since silver seems to be slightly less heat-conductive than copper at low temperature.

In principle, the freezing is accomplished by bringing the tissue into contact with a polished metal surface (copper, silver) at the temperature of liquid nitrogen slush or helium (–269 °C). Devices for the controlled and reproducible plunging of samples onto the solidly frozen block were described by several authors (Luyet and Gonzales 1951; Van Harreveld and Crowell 1964; Heuser et al. 1976; Costello and Corless 1978) (Fig. 3), and arc commercially available (The Slammer, Polaron Model Q.F-1, USA; KF 80, Reichert, Austria). A descent of about 30 cm/s produces blocks 0.1–0.2 mm thick from specimens with a thickness of 2–3 mm. The specimen surface which is to come into contact with the cooled metal surface should not have a water layer. To prevent excess drying of this surface the mount is covered by a small, moist styrofoam bucket until just before freezing (Heuser et al. 1979). Contamination of the metal surface

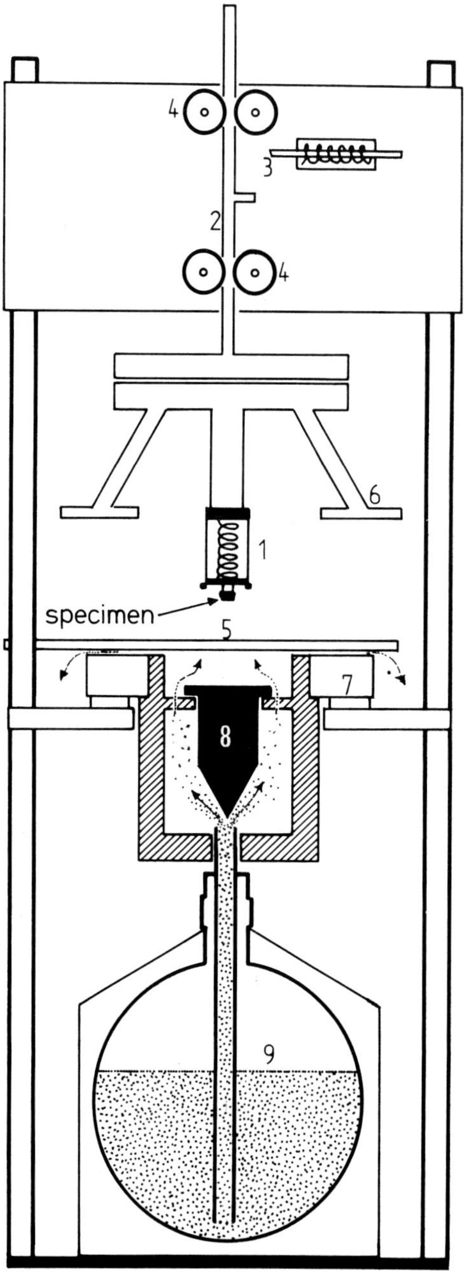

Fig. 3. Quick-freezing machine in which the tissue is smashed against a cold copper block (after Heuser et al. 1979). The specimen is mounted on a metal disc shaped, e. g., to fit on the stage of the freeze fracture apparatus. A filter paper is glued to the disc and absorbs some of the tissue's solution, which when becoming frozen binds the specimen tightly to the metal disc. The disc is mounted to the freezing head (*1*) which is a metal tube, containing a spring inside, which is detachable from the end of a long plunger (*2*). The plunger is suspended above the cooled metal block and after release (*3*) glides down on ball bearings (*4*). A shutter (*5*), which at the latest possible moment is moved away from the entrance to the freezing device during the fall of the plunger and helium gas blowing over the metal surface (utilizing the vapor generated by the spray of liquid helium), keeps the surface of the cooled block free from condensation of atmospheric gases or water vapor. At the time of impact of the tissue on the metal surface, the freezing head telescopes against the spring mounted inside until the iron ring (*6*) hits the electromagnet (*7*) surrounding the copper block. The magnet prevents the freezing head from bouncing away from the copper block after impact. The copper block (*8*) is cooled by liquid helium (*9*) which is produced by pressurizing the liquid helium Dewar underneath the freezing apparatus. The copper block is removable from above and is warmed and dried between runs

by water or air is prevented by passing cooled dry helium gas over it.

One particular advantage of the copper block ultrarapid-freezing method as compared to other methods is that the well frozen layer of the specimen is physically flat and parallel to the specimen support. It is assumed that the freezing starts on a planar freezing front along the area of contact with the copper block and proceeds inwardly.

Dempsey and Bullivant (1976a, b) reported that when using liquid nitrogen as coolant, the first 12 μm of the tissue would be free of visible ice crystals, which then increase in size exponentially with depth. Heuser et al. (1979) claimed that the ice-crystal-free superficial layer is larger when liquid helium is used as coolant. They reported that freezing occurs in 2 ms or less at a depth of about 10 μm, where ice crystal damage is still minimal. Occasionally, an additional sectioning of the tissue was performed immediately before the freezing process (Bernard and Krigman 1974; Van Harreveld and Fifkova 1975; Sitte et al. 1977). The advantage of an automatic freezing machine in combination with electrophysiological stimulation of nerves was described by Heuser et al. (1979). Raviola et al. (1980) used their method to study the configuration of gap junctions in different organs.

3 Preparatory Methods Following Quick Freezing

3.1 Freeze-Cleaving

The freeze-cleaving technique is an effective means of demonstrating the organization of the membrane of neuronal tissues (see Chap. 3). Since in most quick-freezing methods only a very superficial layer (about 10–30 μm) of the tissue is frozen without ice crystals, freeze-cleaving has to be performed with great care. Heuser et al. (1979) maintained their specimen at −105 °C for 30 min to 2 h under vacuum conditions and then just barely grazed it with a specially sharpened razor blade which was replaced for each cleavage.

3.2 Freeze-Fracturing

In freeze-fracturing care must be taken to ensure that the fracture plane passes through the solidified superficial layer. This procedure, therefore, is mainly performed using the thin sandwich method (cryogen-jet method). Preferably, the sandwich plates should be identical with the specimen holder used in the fracture apparatus.

3.3 Freeze-Etching (Deep Etching)

This technique involves sublimation of frozen solute to expose macromolecules or membrane surfaces just below the fracture plane, e.g., freeze-fracturing, freeze-cleaving (Heuser et al. 1979), or of an unfractured specimen surface (Figs. 1, 2; Metz, unpublished work) before replication (see also Chap. 3).
Extracellular details such as the surface of the membrane and intracellular details, e.g., the cytoskeleton of the cell, can be studied by this method. The quick-freezing method is especially advantageous in performing freeze-etching, since no cryoprotectants are used and etching rates are rapidly reached. Rotary shadowing was employed to improve the ultrastructural image (Heuser et al. 1979).

3.4 Freeze-Substitution

In this method tissue water is substituted by an organic medium in the cold and simultaneously fixed for electron microscopy

(Bullivant, 1965). Dempsey and Bullivant (1976a) kept the quick-frozen tissue for 40 days at –70 °C in dry ethanol or dry acetone containing 2% OsO_4. Tissue was then warmed in stages to 0 °C, 4 °C, and room temperature over several hours. Shorter time periods of fixation in OsO_4 were used by Van Harreveld and Crowell (1964), who kept the tissue for three days in 2% OsO_4, in acetone at –85 °C, and increased the temperature in steps, keeping the tissue for 1 h at –25 °C, for 1 h at 0 °C, and then warming it to room temperature. Since only a superficial 10–15 μm layer of the tissue is well preserved, shorter time periods of postfixation in OsO_4 can be used (Raviola, personal communication).

3.5 Frozen Sectioning Techniques (Cryo-ultramicrotomy)

Several methods and devices for cutting frozen thin sections of fresh tissue have been developed and described in detail, e. g., Christensen (1971).

4 Applications and Limitations of the Quick-Freezing Method

The aim of cryofixation is to preserve the native organization of the cellular components by solidification of the specimen by freezing. Freezing damage, such as ice crystals, segregation of macromolecules and small cytoplasmic organelles, which may alter and even completely destroy structures, can only be avoided if the specimen is frozen so rapidly that solidification in the vitreous state takes place. Although true vitrification is not possible within biological samples, the growth of ice crystals should at least be restricted to such a level that they do not interfere with the ultrastructural and analytical methods employed. Since heat can only be extracted through the surface by conduction, the low thermal conductivity of the tissue water reduces the zone in which the critical freezing rate can be achieved to a very thin superficial layer. Beneath this layer, large ice crystals and consequent tissue damage result from the inherently low thermal conductivity of biological tissue, that is, from the limited rate of heat loss.

According to Moor (1971), a specimen can only be solidified in the native state if the temperature interval from 0 °C to –100 °C is passed in less than 0.01 s, which is equivalent to a freezing velocity of about 10 000 °C/s. From model experiments, Van Venrooij et al. (1975) concluded that a reduction in the dimensions of samples will increase the freezing velocities proportional to the square of the reduction. Specimens with a diameter less than 0.1–0.3 mm can probably be frozen without changes in structure and chemical properties. In larger specimens only superficial layers can be expected to be frozen without changes. In biological tissue, however, ice-crystal-free regions have been observed within a superficial 10–30 μm layer only.

Besides these more general conditions, the composition of the investigated tissue may affect the depth to which a rapid frozen tissue is free of ice crystals. The size of cells or cytoplasmic processes has a significant but unexplained effect on the size of intracellular ice crystals (Steinbrecht 1980). Also, the correlation between ice crystal size and distance from the specimen surface is not a strict one. It seems that freezing velocity is higher at the border and in the center of the sample than halfway between these areas (Van Venrooij et al. 1975).

The different approaches to solidification of native tissue by freezing have already permitted various investigations, particularly of ex situ tissue. Small tissue preparations (organ cultures), cell cultures, and subcellular fractions which can be studied by several of the described methods might be prepared under experimentally controlled conditions. Critical restrictions exist, however, when methods of preparation are used in which tissue is removed from an organism and subjected to a freezing procedure. Unfortunately, only the superficial layer of the tissue which may be damaged during the removal is sufficiently preserved by cryofixation. Despite these limitations this method will occupy a firm place in neuroanatomical research in the future.

5 References

Altmann R (1890) Die Elementar-Organismen und ihre Beziehungen zu den Zellen. Viet, Leipzig

Bachmann L, Schmitt WW (1971) Improved cryofixation applicable to freeze-etching. Proc Natl Acad Sci USA 68:2149–2152

Bachmann L, Schmitt-Fumian WW (1973) Spray-freeze-etching of dissolved macromolecules, emulsions, and subcellular components. In: Benedetti EL, Farvard P (eds) Freeze-etching, techniques and applications. Soc Franc Micr Electr, Paris

Bernard SA, Krigman MR (1974) Ultrastructural analysis of the deeper layers of freeze-substituted guinea pig cortex. Brain Res 76:325–329

Bullivant S (1965) Freeze-substitution and supporting techniques. Lab Invest 14:1178–1195

Bullivant S (1970) Present status of freezing techniques. In: Parsons DF (ed) Some biological techniques in electron microscopy. Academic Press, New York London, pp 101–146

Costello MJ, Corless JM (1978) The direct measurements of temperature changes within freeze-fracture specimens during rapid quenching in liquid coolants. J Microsc 112:17–37

Cristensen AK (1971) Frozen thin sections of fresh tissue for electron microscopy, with a description of pancreas and liver. J Cell Biol 51:772–804

Dempsey GP, Bullivant S (1976a) A copper block method for freezing non-cryoprotected tissue to produce ice crystal-free regions for electron microscopy. I. Evaluation using freeze-substitution. J Microsc 106:251–260

Dempsey GP, Bullivant S (1976b) A copper block method for freezing non-cryoprotected tissue to produce ice crystal-free regions for electron microscopy. II. Evaluations using freeze-fracturing with a cryo-ultramicrotome. J Microsc 106:261–272

Deurs Van B, Luft JH (1979) Effects of glutaraldehyde fixation on the structure of tight junctions. J Ultrastruct Res 68:160–172

Echlin P, Skaer MB, Gardiner BO, Franks F, Asquith MH (1977) Polymeric cryoprotectants in the preservation of biological ultrastructure. II. Physiological effects. J Microsc 110:239–255

Farrant J, Walter CA, Lee H, Morris GE, Clarke KJ (1977) Structural and functional aspects of biological freezing techniques. J Microsc 111: 17–34

Fernandes-Morán H (1960) Low-temperature preparation techniques for electron microscopy of biological specimens based on rapid-freezing with liquid Helium II. Ann NY Acad Sci 85:689–713

Franks F (1977) Biological freezing and cryofixation. J Microsc 111:3–16

Gulik-Krzywicki T, Costello MJ (1978) The use of low temperature x-ray diffraction to evaluate freezing methods used in freeze-fracture electron microscopy. J Microsc 112:103–116

Harreveld A Van (1972) The extracellular space in the vertebrate central nervous system. In: Bourne G (ed) Structure and function of the nervous system, vol 4. Academic Press, New York, pp 447–511

Harreveld A Van, Crowell J (1964) Electron microscopy after rapid-freezing on a metal surface and substitution fixation. Anat Rec 149:381–386

Harreveld A Van, Fifkova E (1975) Rapid-freezing of deep cerebral structures for electron microscopy. Anat Rec 182:377–386

Harreveld A Van, Crowell J, Malhorta SK (1965) A study of extracellular space in central nervous tissue by freeze-substitution. J Cell Biol 25:117–137

Harreveld A Van, Trubatch J, Steiner J (1974) Rapid-freezing and electron microscopy for the arrest of physiological processes. J Microsc 100:189–198

Heuser JE, Reese TS, Dennis MJ, Lan Y, Jan L, Evans L (1979) Synaptic vesicle exocytosis captured by quick-freezing and correlated with quantal transmitter release. J Cell Biol 81:275–300

Heuser JE, Reese TS, Landis DMD (1976) Preservation of synaptic structure by rapid-freezing. Cold Spring Harbor Symp Quant Biol 40:17–24

Landis D, Reese TS (1974) Membrane structure in rapidly-frozen, freeze-fractured cerebellar cortex. J Cell Biol 63:184a

Luyet B, Gonzales F (1951) Recording ultra-rapid changes in temperature. Refrig. Engng. 59:1191

Moor H (1971) Recent progress in the freeze-etching technique. Philos Trans R Soc Lond [Biol] 261:121

Moor H, Kistler J, Müller M (1976) Freezing in a propane jet. Experientia 32:805
Moor M, Riehle U (1968) Snap-freezing under high pressure: A new fixation technique for freeze-etching. Proc 4th Eur Reg Conf Electron Microsc 2:33
Müller W, Pseid P (1979) A new inexpensive specimen carrier for freeze-fracturing. J Microsc 115:113–116
Plattner M, Fisher WM, Schmitt WW, Bachmann L (1972) Freeze-etching of cells without cryoprotectants. J Cell Biol 53:116–126
Raviola E, Goodenough DA, Raviola G (1980) Structure of rapidly-frozen gap junctions. J Cell Biol 87:273–279
Riehle U, Hoechli M (1973) In: Benedetti EL, Favard P (eds) Freeze-etching, techniques, and applications. Soc Franc Micr Electr, Paris
Rosenkranz J (1975) The course of temperature variation in an object during the freeze-etching procedure. Arzneim-Forsch 25:454–458
Schlote W, Wolburg H, Wendt-Gallitelli MF (1978) Shock-freezing of biological tissue in situ with C-type specimen holders for x-ray microanalysis of ultrathin cryosections. Drug Res 29:1812
Sitte H, Fell H, Höbl W, Kleber H, Neumann K (1977) Fast-freezing device. J Microsc 111: 35–38
Somlyo AV, Shuman H, Somlyo AP (1977) Elemental distribution in striated muscle and the effects of hypertonicity. J Cell Biol 74: 828–854
Steinbrecht RA (1980) Cryofixation without cryoprotectants. Freeze-substitution and freeze-etching of an insect olfactory receptor. Tissue Cell 12:73–100
Stolinski C, Breathnach AS (1976) Freeze-fracture replication of organized tissue without cryoprotection. J Anat 122:271–281
Umrath W (1975) Rapid freezing in open cooling baths. Arzneim-Forsch 25:450–453

Chapter 16

Ultrastructural Histochemistry of Nervous Tissue

J. G. Richards

1 Introduction

Electron histochemistry is the visualization of chemical substances in ultrathin sections of biological tissues at a subcellular level by the use of electron dense stains, i.e., stains which confer a selective contrast when observed by electron microscopy. In neuroanatomical research perhaps the most exciting field of application of this technique is the localization of neurotransmitter amines (Richards, 1978).

The distribution of biogenic monoamines in peripheral sympathetic neurons and in the brain has been demonstrated at the light microscopical level by the Falck-Hillarp formaldehyde-induced fluorescence histochemical technique. These biologically highly active substances are most concentrated in nerve terminals but are also present in high amounts in dendrites and in lesser quantities in neuronal perikarya and nonterminal axons. Neurotransmitters such as dopamine (DA), noradrenaline (NA), adrenaline (A), and serotonin (5-hydroxytryptamine, 5-HT) are stored in numerous small (50 nm) and occasional large (100 nm) vesicles in nerve terminals. The storage of high concentrations of these substances in an osmotically stable form within vesicles is probably achieved by complex formation with 5′-phosphonucleotides, such as adenosine-5′-triphosphate (ATP), which are also highly concentrated in these vesicles.

The electron histochemical demonstration of endogenous monoamines can be achieved by a modification of the chromaffin reaction (Tranzer and Richards, 1976) and of 5′-phosphonucleotides by the uranaffin reaction (Richards and Da Prada, 1977). More recent findings on the application of these techniques have been reported by Richards and Da Prada (1980). Amine storage sites can also be identified by selectively labelling them with exogenous amines ("false" transmitters) (Thoenen and Tranzer, 1971) such as 5-hydroxydopamine which are highly osmiophilic, i.e., electron dense. After release of the endogenous amine (physiological transmitter) upon arrival of a nerve impulse, its interaction at the transmitter receptor of a target neuron is terminated by either re-uptake at the presynaptic neuronal membrane or by enzymatic degradation. The interspecific nature of the high affinity uptake mechanism results in the accumulation of "false" transmitters in the storage vesicles. Labelling with "false" transmitters is a useful alternative to the chromaffin or uranaffin reactions in tissues in which the endogenous amine or nucleotide is difficult to localize, e.g., in the central nervous system.

2 Fixation and Staining of Neurotransmitter Amines

2.1 Crosslinking Amines and Tissue Proteins

Glutaraldehyde is an excellent fixative for preserving cytological detail and for retaining (fixing) biogenic amines (Hayat, 1970; Hopwood, 1972). This bifunctional aldehyde reacts covalently, predominantly with free amino groups of terminal amino acids

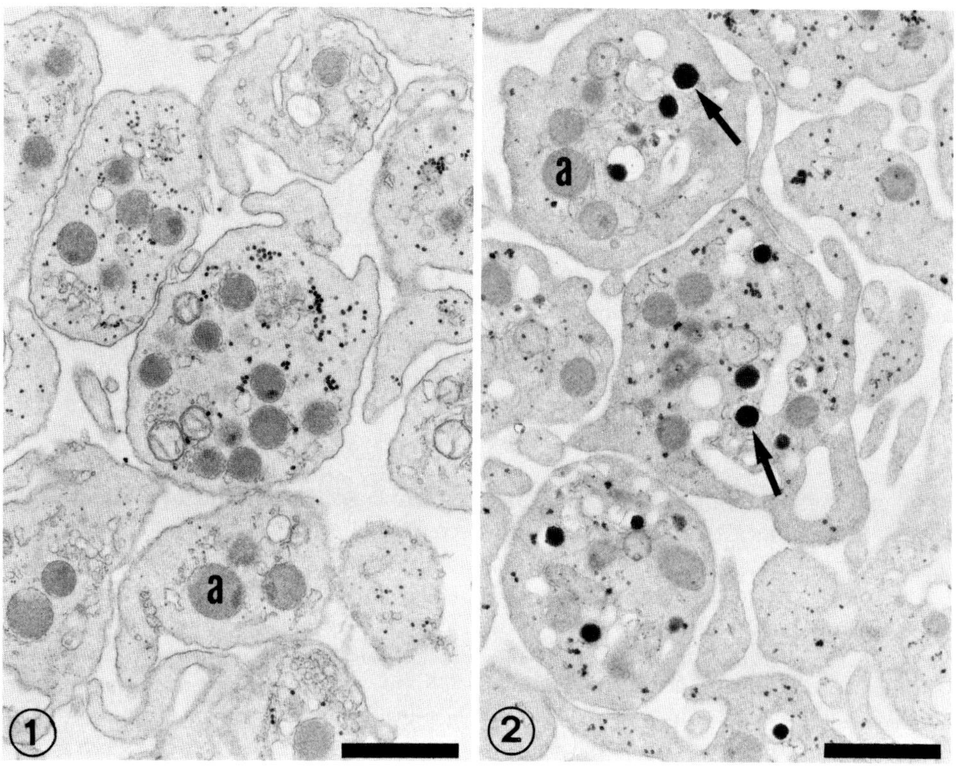

Figs. 1, 2. Rabbit blood platelets. Osmium vs glutaraldehyde and osmium fixation. Note the presence of highly electron dense granules (→) in platelets fixed in glutaraldehyde and osmium (Fig. 2) but their absence in osmium-fixed platelets (Fig. 1) *a*, *α*-granule. bar = 1 μm, × 16,500

of proteins, e.g., lysine and of neurotransmitter amines, e.g., NA, through the formation of Schiff bases. The latter crosslink with either further proteins or amines:

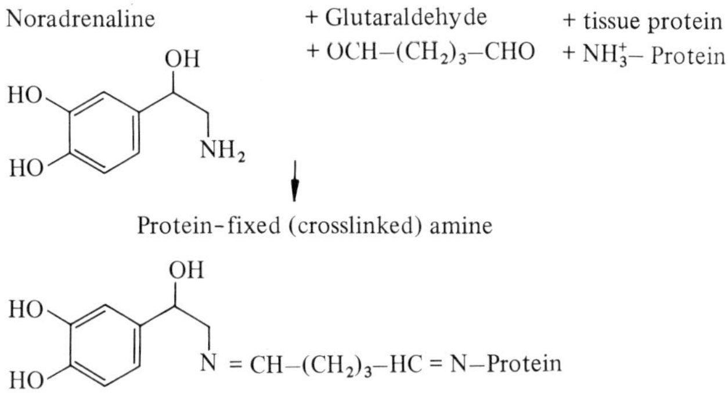

Such covalent bonds cannot be affected by subsequent dehydration and embedding procedures.

2.2 Electron Dense Staining of the Fixed Amine

The two hydroxyl groups of the fixed amine become oxidized by osmium tetroxide giving rise to a highly electron dense, insoluble reaction product, osmium black (a cyclic osmium ester). Osmium tetroxide alone, i.e., without prior crosslinking, is incapable of giving an electron dense reaction product (Fig. 1, 2). "False" transmitters such as 5-hydroxydopamine, with a further hydroxyl group for oxidation, are more osmiophilic and consequently excellent electron histochemical "stains":

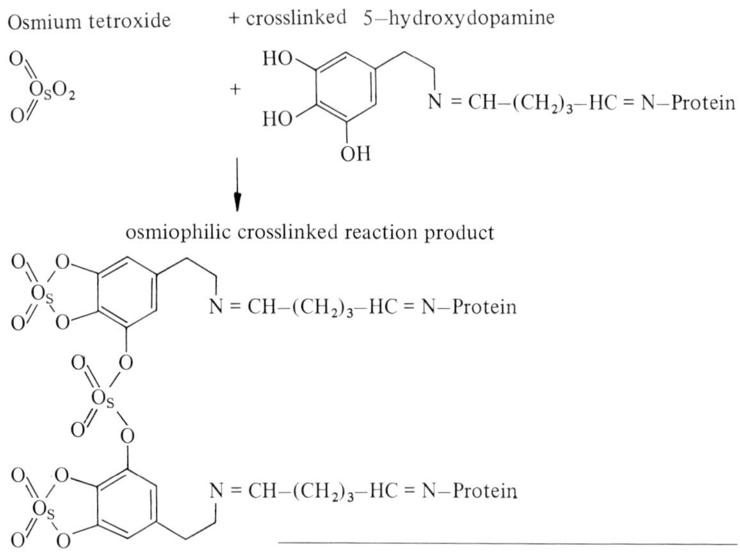

Although the initial reaction outlined above seems likely to occur, the essential feature is the ultimate formation of osmium black. In the process the crosslinked amine becomes oxidized to a quinone and eventually, through a complex series of reactions, to a melanin-like product.

In the chromaffin reaction, the oxidizing agent is the dichromate ion which, in the absence of post-osmication (which, in addition stains proteins and unsaturated lipids), renders the amine storage sites selectively electron dense. In the uranaffin reaction, UO_2^{2+} ions probably interact with phosphate groups of 5′-phosphonucleotides rendering the latter highly electron dense.

3 Chromaffin Reaction

Wood and Barrnett (1964) were the first to show that the century-old chromaffin reaction could be of value for the identification of biogenic amines at the ultrastructural level in adrenomedullary cells (chromaffin cells). These cells yield a brown color when treated with chromium salts. The chromaffin reaction identifies not only adrenaline but also other aromatic compounds such as dihydroxy and polyhydroxy phenols, aminophenols and polyamines (Hopwood [1971]). It does not differentiate between the various neurotransmitter amines such as NA, DA, and 5-HT.

The reaction has recently been developed and adapted for the electron histochemical localization of biogenic amines in various monoaminergic neurons (Tranzer and Richards [1976]). The following is a detailed account of the method as modified and improved in our laboratory.

3.1 Method

3.1.1 Primary Fixation

The primary fixative is composed of 1% glutaraldehyde +0.4% formaldehyde in 0.1 M sodium chromate/potassium dichromate buffer at pH 7.2. This is made up as follows:

4 ml	25% glutaraldehyde solution (Merck-Schuchardt)
0.4 g	paraformaldehyde powder suspended in 10 ml distilled water and heated to 60 °C before adding 1 N NaOH dropwise until the milky solution clears
50 ml	0.2 M sodium chromate/potassium dichromate buffer pH 7.2 (47.5 ml 0.2 M sodium chromate +2.5 ml 0.2 M potassium dichromate)
40 ml	distilled water.

The primary fixation is carried out at 0–4 °C either by immersion with continuous rotation (to improve permeation of the tissue) or by vascular perfusion.

For immersion fixation the tissue is quickly excised from rats under light ether anesthesia and immediately transferred to ice-cold fixative and cut into small (1-mm) cubes. The duration of the primary fixation varies according to the tissue being investigated. Rat vas deferens, heart and pineal are fixed for 10 min whereas rat iris (an extremely thin, almost transparent tissue) requires only 1 min exposure to the fixative. In the last case the eyeball is quickly removed from decapitated anesthetized animals, halved with a razor blade in ice-cold saline, and then the lens and suspensory ligament are removed leaving the iris intact in situ. Using absorbant tissue paper, the saline is quickly removed and ice-cold fixative is added dropwise and continuously for 1 min.

For perfusion fixation animals are lightly anesthetized with ether. Ice-cold fixative, preceded by 5 ml 0.9% NaCl at 19 °C, is perfused via the heart for 10–15 min at a pressure equivalent to the normal blood pressure of the animal. To achieve this in the rat, a bottle containing the fixative is placed 140 cm above the animal.

3.1.2 Storage

The second step in the reaction is a very long (18 h) incubation at 0–4 °C in 0.2 M sodium chromate/potassium dichromate buffer at pH 6.0. The solution is made up as follows:

22.5 ml	0.2 M sodium chromate
75.0 ml	0.2 M potassium dichromate

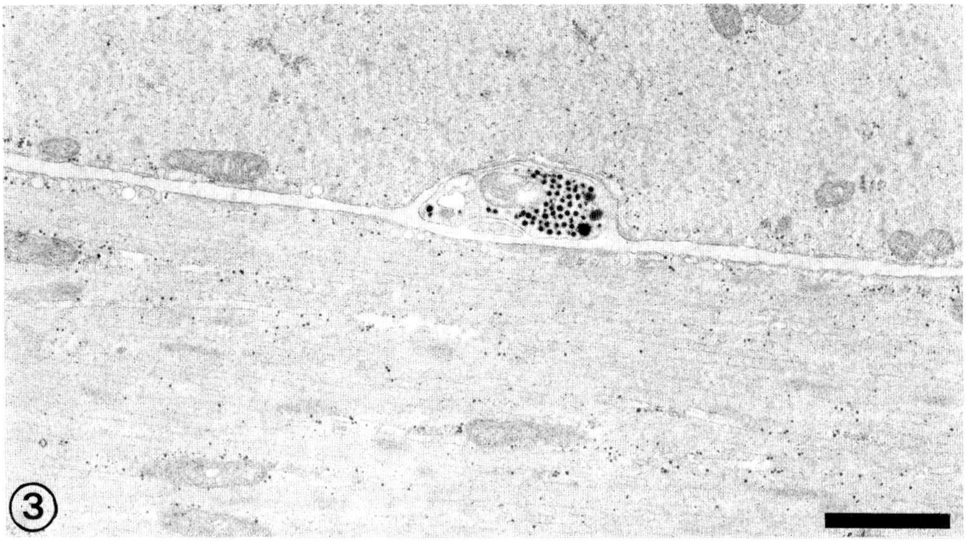

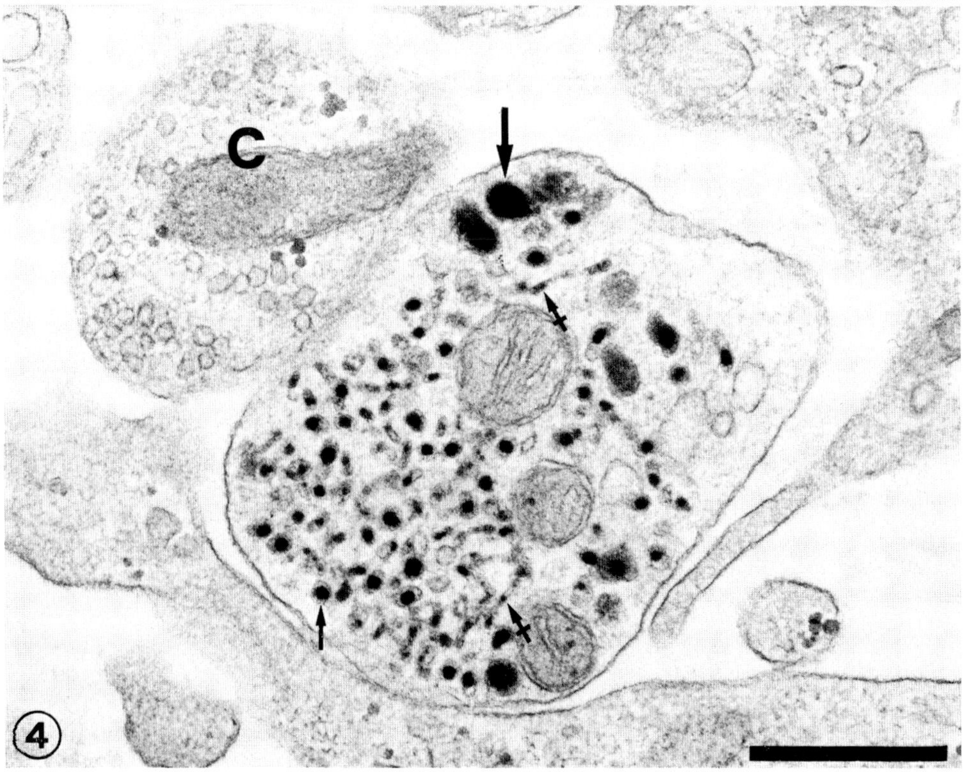

Figs. 3, 4. Rat vas deferens and iris. Chromaffin reaction by perfusion and immersion fixation. **Fig. 3** illustrates the selective reaction product in an adrenergic nerve terminal profile in vas deferens with concomitant good ultrastructural preservation of tissue after perfusion. **Fig. 4** illustrates the chromaffin reaction in an adrenergic nerve terminal of iris after immersion fixation. Note the electron dense reaction product in large (⟶) and small (→) vesicles and in a neuronal tubular reticulum (+→) but its absence in an adjacent (presumably cholinergic) terminal (*c*). Fig. 3: bar = 1 μm, × 17,400; Fig. 4: bar = 0.5 μm, × 57,000

As in the case of the primary fixative, the pH of the buffer can be corrected by varying the relative amounts of the two components. For immersion-fixed tissues the primary fixative is replaced by the slightly acidic buffer (by several changes) and rotated continuously for 18 h. Fixation of irides is continued by removing the primary fixative using absorbant tissue paper and replacing this simultaneously with the acidic buffer initially dropwise with a pasteur pipette. After a few minutes the iris is excised and suitably cut for easy orientation and rotated in the same buffer for 18 h.

Perfusion fixation is continued for 30 min with the acidic buffer after which peripheral organs and brain are removed and the tissue to be investigated is isolated and rotated in the same buffer for 18 h.

3.1.3 Postfixation

The fixative, 2% osmium tetroxide in 0.1 M sodium chromate/potassium dichromate at pH 7.2, is made up as follows:

25 ml 4% osmium tetroxide in distilled water
25 ml 0.2 M sodium chromate/potassium dichromate buffer at pH 7.2 (23.75 ml 0.2 M sodium chromate + 1.25 ml 0.2 M potassium dichromate).

Tissues are transferred to this fixative for 1 h at 0–4 °C (without rotation). Only half of the tissue blocks are postfixed. After fixation all tissues are dehydrated in a graded series of alcohols and embedded in Epon 812. Ultrathin sections (approximately 60 nm) are viewed, poststained or unstained, in the electron microscope. Only lead citrate is used as a section stain.

3.2 Pharmacological Treatments

Drugs which affect the storage or metabolism of biogenic amines can be used to modify the chromaffin reaction and thereby demonstrate its specificity, e.g., reserpine (Serpasil [Ciba], 10 mg/kg i.p. 15–18 h before sacrifice), metaraminol (Aramine [Merck], 2×4 mg/kg i.p. 24 and 4 h), nialamide (Niamid [Pfizer], 300 mg/kg i.p. 6 h), and finally nialamide plus reserpine. Control animals should receive the drug vehicle (0.9% NaCl).

3.3 Critical Evaluation of the Method

The chromaffin reaction modified as above fulfils to a large degree the requirements for an ideal electron histochemical reaction for biogenic amines (see Bloom, 1970 for criteria) since it produces a highly selective and electron dense reaction product in well preserved tissue (Fig. 3). Moreover, the reaction specificity is supported by the observation that:

a) Vesicles in cholinergic nerve terminals, which are often found adjacent to adrenergic nerve terminals in peripheral sympathetically-innervated organs such as iris, do not contain chromaffin-positive electron dense cores (Fig. 4).

b) Although ribosomes, glycogen particles, and mitochondrial granules are highly electron dense in tissues in which the chromaffin reaction is followed by osmica-

Figs. 5, 6. Rat brain. Chromaffin reaction by perfusion fixation. **Fig. 5** illustrates a supra-ependymal nerve terminal profile above the neostriatum, containing large (⟶) and small (⟶) dense-cored vesicles and a tubular reticulum (⟶). That the electron dense (chromaffin) cores in all three organelles are absent in those nerve terminals of rats pretreated with parachlorophenylalanine provides strong evidence for the localization of 5-HT in these nerves. *C*, cilium; *E*, ependyma; *V*, lateral ventricle. In **Fig. 6**, a varicose axon (a) in the periventricular hypothalamus is identified as monoaminergic (probably noradrenergic) by virtue of its chromaffinity (⟶). Fig. 5: bar = 0.5 μm, ×56,000; Fig. 6: bar = 0.5 μm, ×44,000

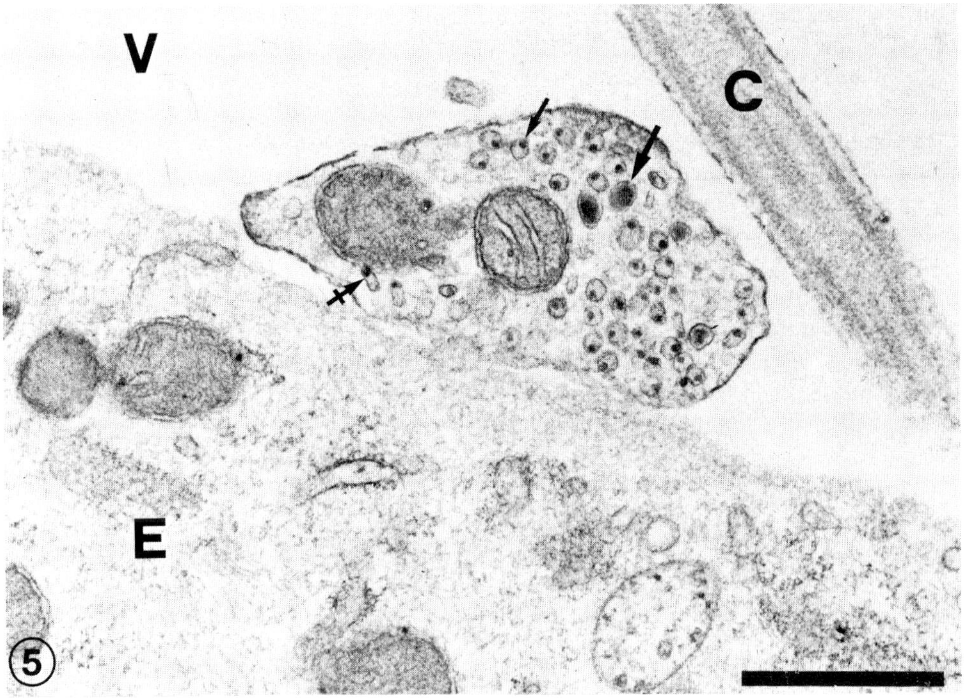
V
C
E
5

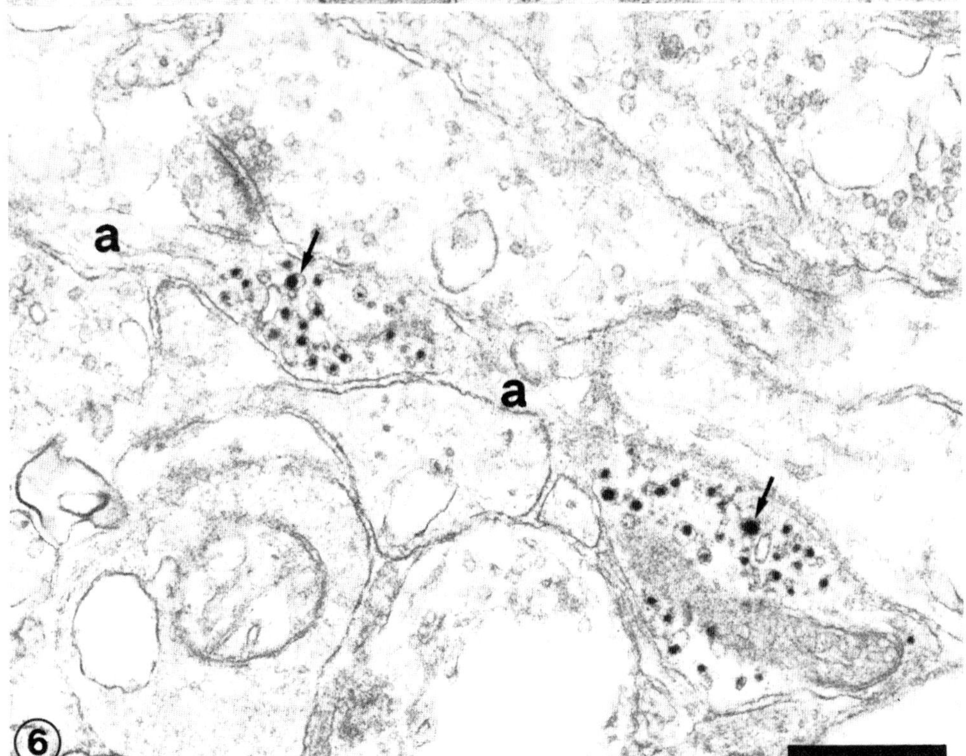
a
a
6

tion, they are absent in nonosmicated tissues. On the other hand, small and large electron dense cores are observed in unstained, nonosmicated tissues indicating that chromium is mainly responsible for the specificity of the reaction in adrenergic nerve terminals and that osmium and lead only increase the contrast of the reaction product.

c) Reserpine, which depletes sympathetically innervated organs of their noradrenaline content, also depletes the small and large vesicles of their chromaffin cores although the large vesicles of both adrenergic and cholinergic nerve terminals contain in addition an electron dense proteinaceous matrix which is not related to the presence of amine.

d) Metaraminol, which behaves as a "false" transmitter, has an effect similar to reserpine by displacing the endogenous NA from the vesicles. Metaraminol is unreactive in the chromaffin reaction probably because only one hydroxyl group is available on the aromatic part of the molecule which restricts the number of sites at which Cr^{6+} can react.

No extravesicular distribution of the precipitate is found after treatment with nialamide or nialamide plus reserpine. The former increases the extravesicular amine pool of that released by reserpine.

A detailed evaluation of the fixation parameters in the chromaffin reaction is described by Tranzer and Richards (1976).

Ultrastructural studies on peripheral adrenergic nerve terminals in various experimental conditions have shown that the bound amines are present in small and large dense-cored vesicles as well as in a tubular reticulum. Recent subcellular fractionation studies of sympathetic nerves from the rat vas deferens confirm this view. Variations in the amount of reaction product, especially in the large vesicles, probably reflect the physiological state of amine loading in these organelles.

In order to differentiate between various amines, specific pharmacological tests must be used. Substances which inhibit the synthesis of specific amines will block the chromaffin reaction for that particular amine. The amine stored in supra-ependymal nerve terminals which occur throughout the rat cerebroventricular system (Fig. 5) has been identified as 5-HT since parachlorophenylalanine (but not α-methylparatyrosine) selectively depletes the nerve terminals of their dense cores. These drugs are known to be potent inhibitors of the enzymes tryptophan hydroxylase and tyrosine hydroxylase respectively which are rate-limiting steps in the synthesis of 5-HT and NA. With a few exceptions (the above described supra-ependymal plexus, median eminence and subependymal paraventricular brain regions (Fig. 6), the chromaffin reaction is unable to detect amine storage sites in the central nervous system. The small size and water-soluble nature of biogenic amines, their release by depolarization during fixation and changes in permeability of the vesicular and/or nerve terminal membrane during fixation might lead to their leakage from the storage sites. Although, these factors also play a role in the localization of noradrenaline in peripheral organs, the compact structure of the brain probably makes it less accessible to the reaction solutions (despite perfusion fixation) and thereby makes it more sensitive to these factors.

4 Uranaffin Reaction

Uranyl ions have an extremely high affinity for amine-storing organelles of sympathetic nerve terminals when the reaction is performed after glutaraldehyde fixation but before dehydration. Recently, the uranaffin reaction has been proposed as a new electron histochemical technique for the localization of adenine nucleotides which are highly concentrated in these organelles (Richards and Da Prada, 1977). The details of the reaction have been worked out using blood platelets of several animal species as models.

In platelets, biogenic amines, mainly 5-HT, are stored in specific subcellular organelles together with nucleotides, e.g., ATP (Da Prada et al., 1978). Electron microscopy reveals that platelet 5-HT is stored in strongly osmiophilic organelles which are frequent in rabbit but much less frequent in man. Biochemical analyses of purified amine-storing organelles isolated from platelets of various species have shown that they contain concentrations of 5-HT and 5′-phosphonucleotides, which are much higher than whole platelets, but contain very little water-soluble protein. As mentioned earlier, in order to account for their osmotic stability, the formation of aggregates between 5-HT and ATP, in the presence of bivalent cations has been proposed. In animal strains with storage pool deficiency (inherited bleeding disorders), abnormally low platelet 5-HT levels seem to be related to a reduced content of nucleotides.

The storage of 5-HT in platelets appears to resemble amine storage in various other cells and tissues, e.g., adrenal medulla, sympathetic neurons and central monoaminergic neurons, in which ATP is also believed to be part of the storage complex.

That the uranaffin reaction reveals ATP and not a biogenic amine is demonstrated by the presence of the reaction in amine-depleted platelets and in megakaryocytes, whose organelles do not contain 5-HT until platelet formation and release into the circulation. On the other hand, the absence of an uranaffin reaction in platelets treated with thrombin, which releases both 5-HT and 5′-phosphonucleotides, is due to the absence of nucleotides. The value of uranyl salts (mainly uranyl acetate) as a stain and a fixative in electron microscopy is well known. Nucleic acid (phosphonucleotide)-containing structures in a variety of tissues are strongly and preferentially stained with uranyl salts. At the very low pH used in the uranaffin reaction, the uranyl acetate probably contains only uncomplexed uranyl ions (UO_2^{2+}). Studies of the infrared spectra of the deoxyribonucleic acid (DNA)-uranyl complex suggest that the uranyl ion is bound at phosphate loci; at pH 3.5 one uranyl ion is attached to every phosphate group in DNA. The complexing of uranyl ions with 5′-phosphonucleotides may arise through interactions similar to those occurring with DNA.

When the phosphate groups are highly concentrated, as is the case for nucleotides in 5-HT organelles, one uranyl ion may crosslink these groups in adjacent molecules leading to their neutralization and stabilization. Indeed, X-ray microanalyses of ultrathin sections of platelets after the uranaffin reaction, reveal the excellent correlation between the highly electron dense reaction product and the presence of high concentrations of phosphorus (Figs. 7 and 8).

4.1 Method

The uranaffin reaction essentially consists of three steps: first, fixation in 3% glutaraldehyde in 0.1 M sodium cacodylate buffer; second, a thorough rinsing in 0.1% NaCl then, third, staining in 4% aqueous uranyl acetate for 18 h.

4.1.1 Fixation

Fixation by immersion is carried out for 90 min at 19 °C with rotation and by perfusion for 30 min at the same temperature followed by 1-h rotation of excised tissue pieces in the same fixative. The fixative is made up as follows:

12 ml 25% glutaraldehyde solution (Merck-Schuchardt)
88 ml 0.1 M sodium cacodylate at pH 7.2 (pH adjusted with 0.1 N HCl).

4.1.2 Rinsing

Tissues are now rinsed several times (three changes of solution every 15 min) in 0.9% NaCl before staining.

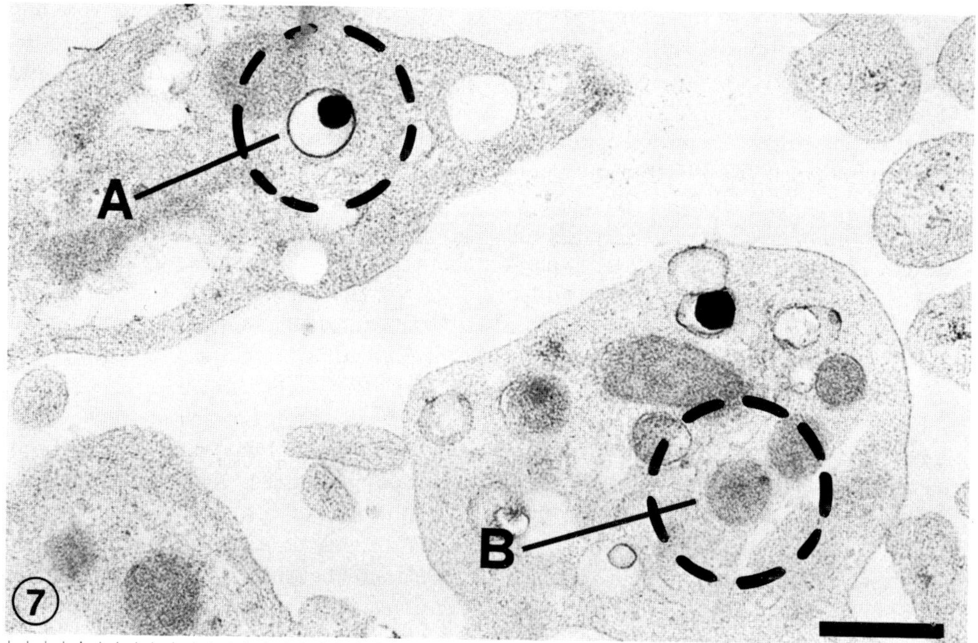

A
B
7

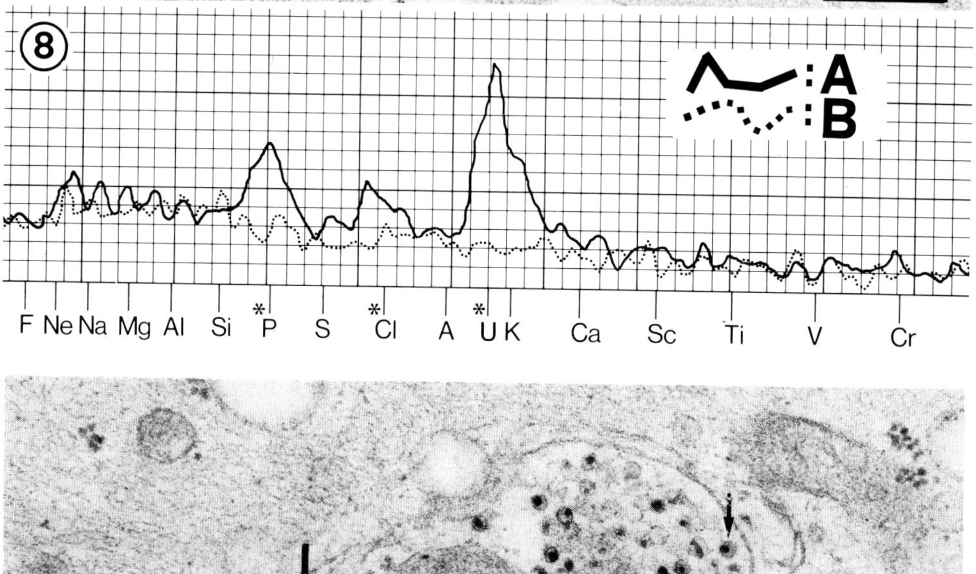

8
A
B
F
Ne
Na
Mg
Al
Si
*
P
S
*
Cl
A
*
U
K
Ca
Sc
Ti
V
Cr

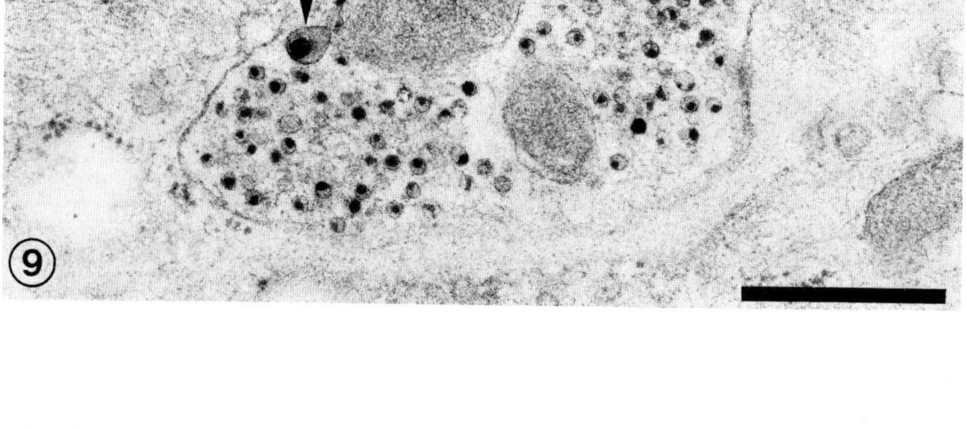

9

4.1.3 Staining

The reaction is carried out in a 4% aqueous uranyl acetate solution at pH 3.9 for 18 h at 4 °C. Since a 4% solution is a saturated solution, the powder will take some time to solubilize even when using a magnetic stirrer. Care should be taken to filter the final solution directly before use.

Step 2 is repeated once more before the tissues are dehydrated in graded alcohols and embedded in Epon. Ultrathin sections are either stained with lead citrate or left unstained.

4.2 Critical Evaluation of the Method

Although uranyl ions are well known to confer contrast to membrane phospholipids throughout cells, the extremely high concentrations of 5′-phosphonucleotides in amine-storing organelles produces an intense reaction which is easily observed in stained and unstained tissues. In platelets and adrenergic nerve terminals both the matrix and membrane of amine storage organelles are uranaffin positive which suggests that ATP is also highly concentrated in the membrane, possible bound to a Mg^{2+}-dependent ATP-ase.

The uranaffinity of adrenomedullary granules and amine storage vesicles of sympathetic neurons, e.g., vas deferens (Fig. 9), confirms the presence of ATP as a component of the storage complex in these tissues.

Biochemical studies on amine storage vesicles isolated from bovine splenic nerve and vas deferens of castrated rats (for details see Richards and Da Prada, 1980) have revealed the presence of ATP (as well as NA) in large and possibly small dense-cored vesicles. Since even purified preparations can be contaminated with ATP from other sources (e.g., smooth muscle cells), biochemical analyses cannot provide reliable supportive evidence for the electron histochemical localization of ATP in amine storage vesicles.

Efforts to date have failed to localize ATP in nerve terminals in brain, even in identified structures such as the supra-ependymal nerve terminals. It is perhaps too soon to conclude that amine storage in the central nervous system does not involve complexing with ATP.

5 The Use of "False" Transmitters as Electron Histochemical Stains

As mentioned earlier, amine storage sites in the peripheral and central nervous system can be selectively "stained" (labelled) with exogenous amines ("false" transmitters) by virtue of the interspecific nature of the high affinity uptake mechanism for terminating the action of endogenous (physiological) transmitters (Fig. 10). Thus, in the brain this approach is an extremely useful alternative to the chromaffin reac-

Fig. 7. Rabbit platelets. Uranaffin reaction by immersion fixation. Both the membrane and matrix of 5-HT organelles (*A*) are highly electron dense. α-granules (*B*) are only moderately reactive. bar = 0.5 μm, ×35,500

Fig. 8. X-ray microanalyses of rabbit platelet profiles after the uranaffin reaction. The graph illustrates that the relative amounts of the elements uranium and phosphorus in regions similar to *A* and *B* (Fig. 7) correlate with the presence or absence of a reaction product. In other words, where the phosphorus content is high the uranaffin reaction is most intense. These analyses were kindly performed by Mr. D. M. Williams, Dept of Metallurgy and Materials Technology, University College of Swansea, Wales

Fig. 9. Rat vas deferens. Uranaffin reaction by perfusion fixation. Note the presence of a reaction product in large (⟶) and small (→) vesicles as well as in the membranes of these vesicles. This uranaffinity is reserpine-resistant. bar = 0.5 μm, ×56,000

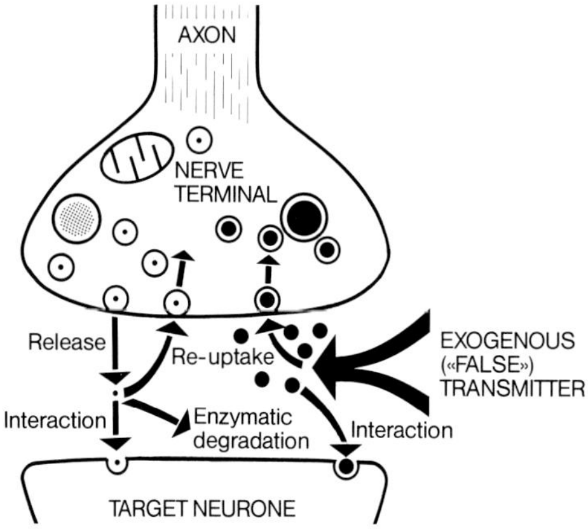

Fig. 10. Schematic illustration of the synaptic events which result in the selective accumulation of osmiophilic "false" transmitters, e.g., 5-OHDA, in monoaminergic nerve terminals. Impulse-induced release of the physiological transmitter (⊙) results in an interaction with the amine receptor on the target neuron. Termination of the transmitter effect is achieved by reuptake and enzymatic degradation. Exogenous osmiophilic transmitters (◉) not only interact with the same receptors but are also incorporated in synaptic vesicles where they displace the endogenous transmitter

tion which generally fails to identify endogenous amines. Moreover, the chromaffin reaction can be used in combination with "false" transmitter labelling in order to optimize the retention and visualization of the exogenous amine.

Although a number of "false" transmitters are known, only a few have the characteristics (strong osmiophily and/or selective chemical neurotoxicity) which lend themselves to the aforementioned approach (Fig. 11). The phenylethylamines 5-hydroxydopamine (5-OHDA) and 6-hydroxydopamine (6-OHDA) have been shown, by direct and indirect evidence, to be transported into aminergic neurons by the same neuronal pump as the physiological transmitter (Thoenen and Tranzer, 1971). For the electron histochemical localization of "false" transmitters the fixation procedure is of crucial importance. Primary fixation with glutaraldehyde is essential for the subsequent identification of an osmiophilic reaction product. Pretreating animals with 5-OHDA or 6-OHDA leads to a depletion of tissue NA in peripheral sympathetically innervated organs, as occurs after reserpine, the difference being that the amine storage sites do not become empty but filled with a highly electron dense reaction product (Fig. 12). There is also a difference between the effects of these two "false" transmitters. Whereas 5-OHDA, after displacing endogenous NA, gradually becomes displaced itself by newly synthesized NA, 6-OHDA, once it has reached a critical concentration in the nerve terminal, is locally toxic, i.e., a chemical lesion is induced (Malmfors and Thoenen, 1971). In brain, both types of "false" transmitters have been widely used to identify the localization and investigate the function of monoaminergic neurons. There is one real disadvantage in this approach: the false transmitters have to be injected into the cerebroventricular system (i.c.v.) to circumvent the blood-brain barrier to monoamines. This limits studies to paraventricular brain regions, due to slow diffusion of the amine through the negligible extracellular space of the brain.

By analogy to 6-OHDA, it is not surprising to find that hydroxylated serotonin, i.e., 5,6-dihydroxytryptamine (5,6-DHT, 6-hydroxyserotonin) and 5,7-dihydroxytryptamine (5,7-DHT, 7-hydroxyserotonin), are both neurotoxic agents which selectively destroy 5-HT nerve terminals (Baumgarten and Björklund 1976). Indeed, if one compares the effects of injecting, intraventricularly, 5,6-DHT with 6-OHDA on the population of supra-ependymal 5-HT nerve terminals, the former has a much higher affinity. As little as 5 μg 5,6-DHT abolishes the formaldehyde-induced fluorescence specific for indoleamines and leads to a degeneration of supra-ependymal nerve terminals, whereas even 50 μg 6-OHDA does not have a marked effect on these nerves (Richards 1978). Paraventricular (subependymal) 5-HT nerve terminals

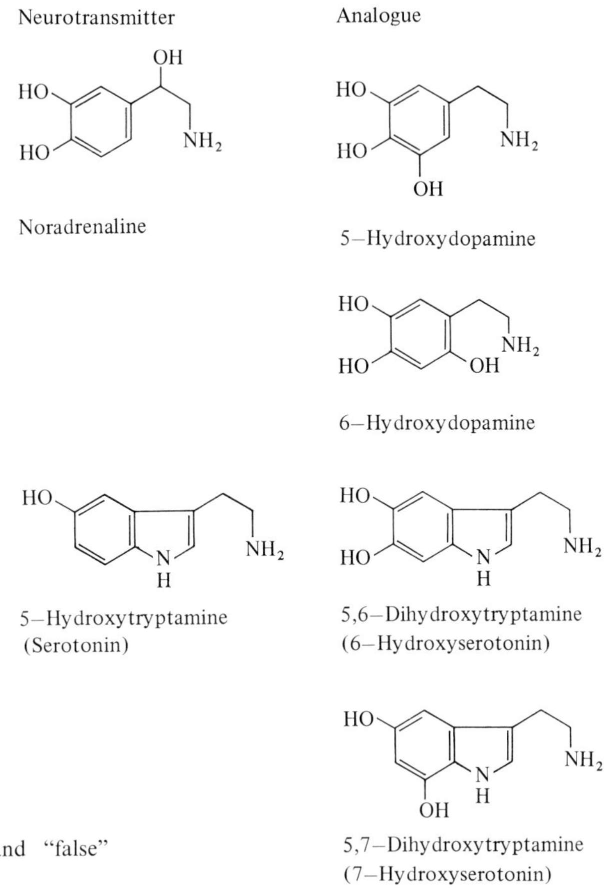

Fig. 11. Neurotransmitter amines and "false" transmitter analogues

are also destroyed by 5,6-DHT (Fig. 13). Since chemical denervation methods are described in detail in Chap. 5, the following account of the methods is restricted to the use of osmiophilic "false" transmitters as electron histochemical stains.

5.1 Method

The dose and route of administration of "false" transmitters will vary according to the tissue under investigation. Table 1 is designed to provide a simple guide to the drug source, dose, time to killing, drug specificity and tissue investigated. In the case of 6-OHDA, 5,6-DHT, and 5,7-DHT, prolonging the time interval between injection and killing results in nerve terminal degeneration.

Since there is no strict chemical specificity, e.g., 5,7-DHT enters both serotoninergic and noradrenergic nerve terminals, animals should be pretreated with selective uptake inhibitors, e.g., dismethyl imipramine, when the effect of 5,7-DHT on 5-HT systems is being investigated. The reason for the neurotoxicity of these compounds (with the exception of 5-OHDA) when they are allowed approximately 24 h to elicit their effects, has been the subject of much discussion (Rotman 1977). Two theories have been proposed for which there is some experimental evidence. Both theories suggest, as the first stage, the non-enzymatic autoxidation to a 1,4-paraquinone.

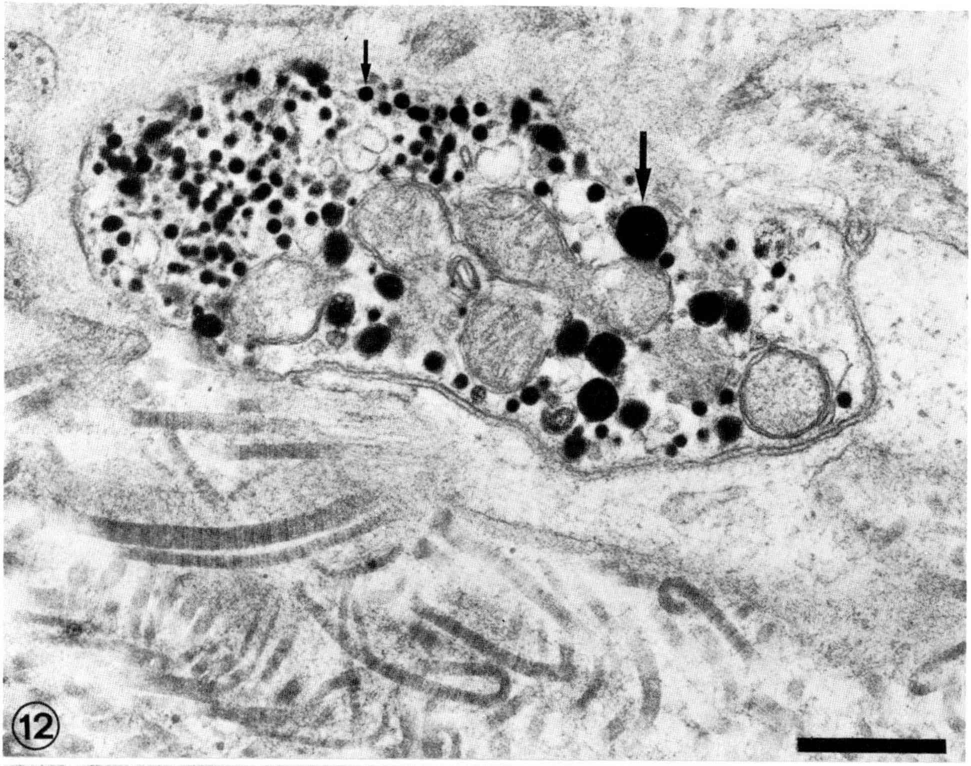
12

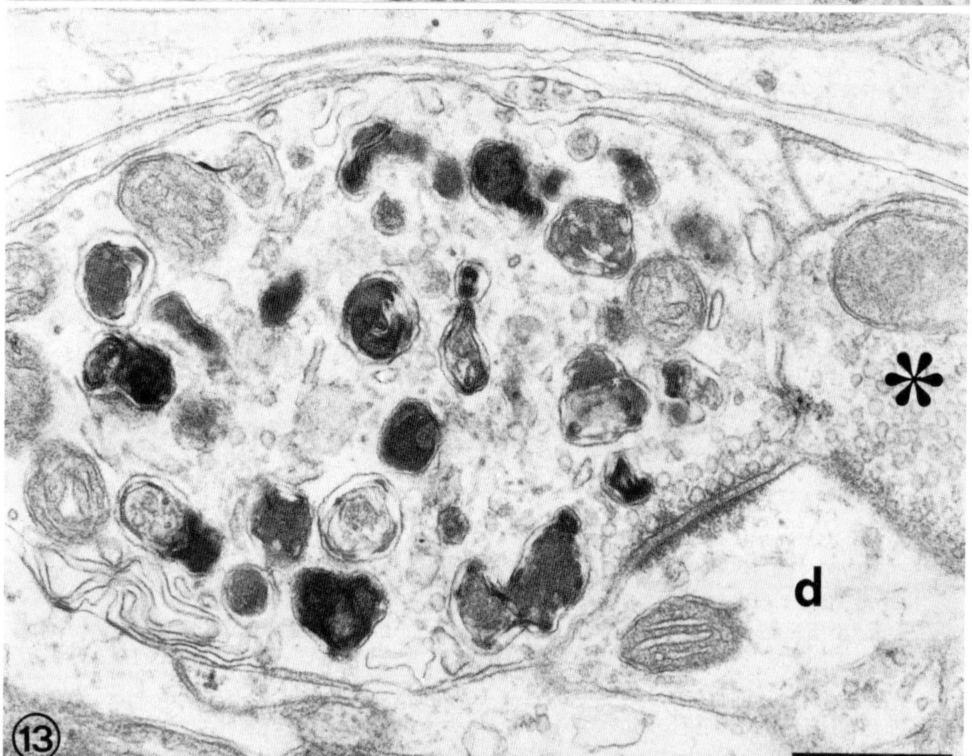
13
*
d

Table 1. Guide to drug source, dose, time to killing, drug specificity and tissue investigated

Drug (source)	Recommended dose	Time of survival after injection	Specificity	Tissues investigated
5-OHDA HCl (Regis)	50 mg/kg i.p. 10 mg/kg i.v. 100 μg i.c.v.	2 h 30 min 1 h	NA, 5-HT	Vas deferens, iris, heart, median eminence Supra-ependymal nerves, neostriatum, periventricular hypothalamus
6-OHDA HCl (Regis)	50 mg/kg i.p. 10 mg/kg i.v. 200 μg i.c.v.	2 h 30 min 1 h	NA, DA	Vas deferens, iris, heart, median eminence Neostriatum, periventricular hypothalamus
5,6-DHT creatinine sulfate monohydrate (Regis)	10 mg/kg i.v. 200 μg i.c.v.	30 min 1 h	5-HT	Median eminence Supra-ependymal nerves, neostriatum
5,7-DHT creatinine sulfate (Regis)	10 mg/kg i.v. 200 μg i.c.v.	30 min 1 h	5-HT, NA	Median eminence Supra-ependymal nerves, neostriatum, periventricular hypothalamus

This either binds covalently to polymerize and denaturate essential cell proteins or it produces a local concentration of peroxides which are highly toxic. Whatever the mode of action of neurotoxic "false" transmitters, they have become valuable tools in the selective labelling and degeneration of catecholaminergic and serotoninergic nerve terminals in the brain.

A further, as yet unexploited, approach for the selective electron histochemical "staining" of monoaminergic nerve terminals in the central nervous system might be to inject the "false" transmitter intravenously to newborn rats in which the blood-brain barrier has not yet developed, and to carry out the chromaffin reaction (by perfusion fixation) on these animals. Dupin et al. (1976) have recently employed this approach for the autoradiographic visualization of central catecholaminergic neurons. By co-injecting an excess of NA, for example, one could study the selective labelling of serotoninergic nerve terminals with 5-OHDA.

All in all, the chromaffin and uranaffin reactions as well as the staining and degeneration induced by osmiophilic "false" transmitters offer a useful repertoire of electron histochemical techniques for the identification of transmitter-specific monoaminergic nerve terminals in neuroanatomical research.

Acknowledgments. The author is indebted to Drs. M. Da Prada, H. P. Lorez, and A. Saner for helpful discussions during preparation of the manuscript.

◄

Figs. 12, 13. Rat vas deferens and subependymal neostriatum. Effects of "false" transmitters. In **Fig. 12**, 5-OHDA has been administered intravenously and renders amine storage vesicles of adrenergic nerve terminals in the vas deferens highly osmiophilic. On the other hand, 24 hours after i.c.v. treatment of animals with 5,6-DHT (**Fig. 13**), 5-HT nerve terminals in the subependymal and supraependymal regions (not illustrated) of the neostriatum show signs of degeneration: osmiophilic myelin figures, reduced number of vesicles and terminal swelling. In **Fig. 13** an adjacent nerve terminal (*), synapsing on the same dendrite (*d*), is unaffected, which demonstrates the selective uptake of the neurotoxic "false" transmitter. Fig. 12: bar = 0.5 μm, ×40,400; Fig. 13: bar = 0.5 μm, ×46,000

6 References

Baumgarten HG, Björklund A (1976) Neurotoxic indoleamines and monoamine neurons. Annu Rev Pharmacol Toxicol 16:101–113

Bloom FE (1970) The fine structural localization of biogenic monoamines in nervous tissue. Int Rev Neurobiol 13:27–66

Da Prada M, Richards JG, Lorez HP (1978) Blood platelets and biogenic monoamines: biochemical, pharmacological, and morphological studies. In: De Gaetano G, Garattini S (eds) Platelets: a multidisciplinary approach. Raven Press, New York, pp 331–353

Dupin J, Descarries L, De Champlain J (1976) Radioautographic visualization of central catecholamine neurons in newborn rat after intravenous administration of tritiated norepinephrine. Brain Res 103:588–597

Hayat MA (1970) Principles and techniques of electron microscopy: biological applications, 1st edn, vol 1. Van Nostrand Reinhold, New York

Hopwood D (1971) The histochemistry and electron histochemistry of chromaffin tissue. Prog Histochem Cytochem 3:1–66

Hopwood D (1972) Theoretical and practical aspects of glutaraldehyde fixation. Histochem J 4:267–303

Malmfors T, Thoenen H (1971) 6-Hydroxydopamine and catecholamine neurons. North-Holland, Amsterdam London

Richards JG (1978) Cytochemistry and autoradiography in the search for transmitter-specific neuronal pathways. In: Coupland RE, Forssmann WG (eds) Peripheral neuroendocrine interaction. Springer, Berlin Heidelberg New York, pp 1–14

Richards GJ, Da Prada M (1977) Uranaffin reaction: a new cytochemical technique for the localization of adenine nucleotides in organelles storing biogenic amines. J Histochem Cytochem 25:1322–1336

Richards JG, Da Prada M (1980) Cytochemical investigations on subcellular organelles storing biogenic amines in peripheral adrenergic neurones. In: Eränkö O, Sonila S, Päivärintä H (eds) Histochemistry and cell biology of autonomic neurons, SIF cells and paraneurons [Adv Biochem Psychopharmacol Vol 25]. Raven Press, New York, pp 269–278

Rotman A (1977) The mechanism of action of neurocytotoxic compounds. Life Sci 21: 891–900

Thoenen H, Tranzer JP (1971) Functional importance of subcellular distribution of false adrenergic transmitters. Prog Brain Res 34: 223–236

Tranzer JP, Richards JG (1976) Ultrastructural cytochemistry of biogenic amines in nervous tissue: methodologic improvements. J Histochem Cytochem 24:1178–1193

Wood JG, Barrnett RJ (1964) Histochemical demonstration of norepinephrine at a fine structural level. J Histochem Cytochem 12: 197–209

Chapter 17

The Zinc Iodide-Osmium Tetroxide (ZIO) Method

M. Reinecke

1 Introduction

As early as 1913, Champy introduced a mixture of osmium tetroxide and sodium iodide as a staining procedure for autonomic nerves. This method was modified by Maillet (1962) who used divalent cations like calcium, cadmium and zinc instead of sodium. Later the solution containing zinc was shown to stain autonomic nerve fibres more selectively than the solution originally used by Champy (Jabonero 1964; Taxi 1965; Maillet 1968). Akert and Sandri (1968) were the first to employ a modification of this technique in electronmicroscopical neurocytology. A distinct improvement of the zinc iodide-osmium tetroxide (ZIO) method was introduced by Martin et al. (1969) who succeeded in carrying out the reaction after prefixation with glutaraldehyde, thus resulting in a better preservation of tissue.

Based on the ZIO-positivity of vesicles in cholinergic nerve endings Akert and Sandri (1968) suggested a transmitter specificity of the reaction. However, it has since been shown that in addition to cholinergic (Akert and Sandri 1968; Martin et al. 1969; Párducz et al. 1971) aminergic (Pellegrino de Iraldi and Geuedet 1968; Pellegrino de Iraldi and Suburo 1971; Pellegrino de Iraldi 1975; Pellegrino de Iraldi and Cardoni, 1979), and glutaminergic (Reinecke and Walther 1978 a, b) vesicles react with ZIO, indicating that the reaction is not specific for a particular transmitter.

In addition to synaptic vesicles other cell organelles can also be stained by ZIO reaction under appropriate conditions, e.g. rough and smooth endoplasmic reticulum, mitochondria, dictyosomes, and lysosomes in a variety of vertebrate and invertebrate tissues (Pellegrino de Iraldi and Geuedet

1968; Niebauer et al. 1969; Clark and Ackerman 1971; Stelzner 1971; Elias et al. 1972; Vrensen and de Groot 1974; Giorgi et al. 1976; Reinecke and Walther 1978 b; Gilloteaux and Naud 1979). The substrate of this cytochemical reaction is, therefore, still under discussion. Nevertheless, for various types of synaptic vesicles it has been shown that ZIO-reactivity is based on the presence of intravesicular SH-groups (Pellegrino de Iraldi 1975; Reinecke and Walther 1978 a, b, Pellegrino de Iraldi and Cardoni 1979).

To describe a method for carrying out the ZIO reaction that can be used with every neurobiological preparation would seem to be impossible at present. However, the recipe given here should enable the reader to obtain reliable results so far as synapses are concerned and, based on these guidelines, it is possible to develop modifications by altering different parameters (cf. Chap. 3).

2 Procedure for the ZIO Reaction

2.1 Preparation of the Solutions

2.1.1 Stock Buffer Solution

Prepare a tris buffer solution with:

66.0 g NaCl
1.6 g $CaCl_2 \cdot 2\,H_2O$
6.2 g $MgCl_2 \cdot 6\,H_2O$
12.1 g tris-(hydroxymethyl-)aminomethane

Solve the substances one after the other in 900 ml of doubly distilled water. Adjust pH to 4.0 with 1 N HCl. Fill up the solution to 1000 ml and control pH. The osmolarity of the buffer is about 2500 mosmol. The buffering capacity of the tris buffer is rather poor in the range required, so that the actual pH must be ascertained immediately before use. If altered bring back to pH 4.0.

2.1.2 Zinc Iodide Solution

Place 6 g zinc powder into an Erlenmeyer flask and add 40 ml of doubly distilled water. Stir the mixture magnetically and add 2 g iodine resublimate in small quantities within 1 min. Exothermic reaction will occur! Allow the mixture to cool by stirring for another 5 min. Filter the mixture immediately after stirring through a hard paper. Mix the solution with the tris buffer in the ratio 1 : 1. The zinc iodide should be prepared shortly (about 30 min) before use. Its color is pale yellow. The osmolarity of the solution is 570 mosmol.

2.1.3 ZIO Reagent

Mix 4 parts of the freshly prepared zinc iodide solution with 1 part of a 2% OsO_4 solution in doubly distilled water 5–10 min before use. Shake gently. The pH of the final ZIO reagent is by 0.3–0.6 pH units more alkaline than that of the tris buffer. The color is yellow-brown.

2.2 Schedule for the ZIO Reaction

1. Rinse specimens in the tris buffer solution four times for 5 min at room temperature whether freshly dissected or prefixed. The thickness of the specimens should not exceed 1 mm to guarantee a complete penetration by the ZIO reagent.
2. Incubate specimens in the dark for 12–16 h at 4 °C in the ZIO reagent.
3. Rinse in tris buffer solution four times for 15 min at room temperature.
4. If required, poststain with aequeous phosphotungstic acid (PTA) (PTA solution: 1% PTA in the tris buffer) for 2 h at room temperature.
5. Dehydration in graded series of ethanol and embedding are carried out as usual. However, dehydration time should be as short as possible to avoid bleaching by alcoholic extraction of the reaction products (Martin et al. 1969; Akert and Sandri 1975).

6. After sectioning, poststaining with lead citrate can be carried out. ZIO seems to impair somewhat the stainability of the membranes, therefore, prolong staining time to 20 min to obtain sufficient contrast.

3 Reaction Properties

The selective staining of nerve terminals as observed in the light microscope (Jabonero 1964; Taxi 1965; Maillet 1968) "is based on its affinity to synaptic vesicles" (Akert and Sandri 1968). In fact, in all systems studied so far ZIO has been found to react almost exclusively with the vesicular matrix (Fig. 1 c) leaving an unstained halo between the stained core and the membrane. Apart from synaptic vesicles only cisternae of the smooth endoplasmic reticulum (Akert et al. 1971; Stelzner, 1971; Akert and Sandri 1975; Reinecke and Walther 1978 b) and multivesicular bodies (Akert et al. 1971) give a positive reaction while mitochondria and neurotubules remain unstained.

While the above staining properties are generally accepted as indicating a specific ZIO reaction the following observations remain to be a matter for discussion:

1. In most preparations only a part of the vesicle population within a given terminal reacts with ZIO (Fig. 1 c), e.g., under nearly identical technical conditions in different systems an average of 50% of the synaptic vesicles were found to be ZIO-positive (Ibata et al. 1972; Reinecke and Walther 1978 b).

2. A small fraction of the ZIO-positive vesicles is only partially stained (Fig. 1 c), in a way that the black deposit is most intense close to the vesicular membrane leaving an unstained core (Kawana et al. 1969; Martin et al. 1969; Akert et al. 1971; Reinecke and Walther 1978 a, b).

For the first phenomenon two possibilities may be considered: technical failure or biochemical alterations of the ZIO-positive substrate (Ibata et al. 1972; Akert and Sandri 1975; Halász et al. 1978). Concerning the second phenomenon it has been proposed that it may be caused by the geometry of the vesicles (Kawana et al. 1969; Akert et al. 1971). However, in locust motor nerve terminals it has recently been suggested that the partially ZIO-positive vesicles represent an intermediate stage of vesicle maturation from ZIO-negative to ZIO-positive (Reinecke and Walther 1978 b).

4 Parameters Influencing ZIO Reaction

4.1 Prefixation

ZIO has been shown to yield good results in staining synaptic vesicles after prefixation with glutaraldehyde (Martin et al. 1969; Reinecke and Walther 1978 a, b), with formaldehyde (Akert and Sandri 1975), with a mixture of both (Párducz et al. 1971; Vrensen and de Groot 1974) and with formaldehyde followed by glutaraldehyde (Ibata et al. 1972). Though prefixation can have an influence on the differential sensitivity of ZIO reaction (Owman and Rüdeberg 1970; Pellegrino de Iraldi and Suburo 1971; Elias et al. 1972; Joó et al. 1973), for locust motor synapses it has been shown that the method given here yields identical results with and without prefixation in glutaraldehyde (Reinecke, unpublished). Since tissue preservation is by far better after prefixation with aldehydes the reader is recommended to test his particular preparation as to the influence of prefixation on the reaction properties.

4.2 pH-Value

As shown for different types of synapses (Pellegrino de Iraldi and Suburo 1971;

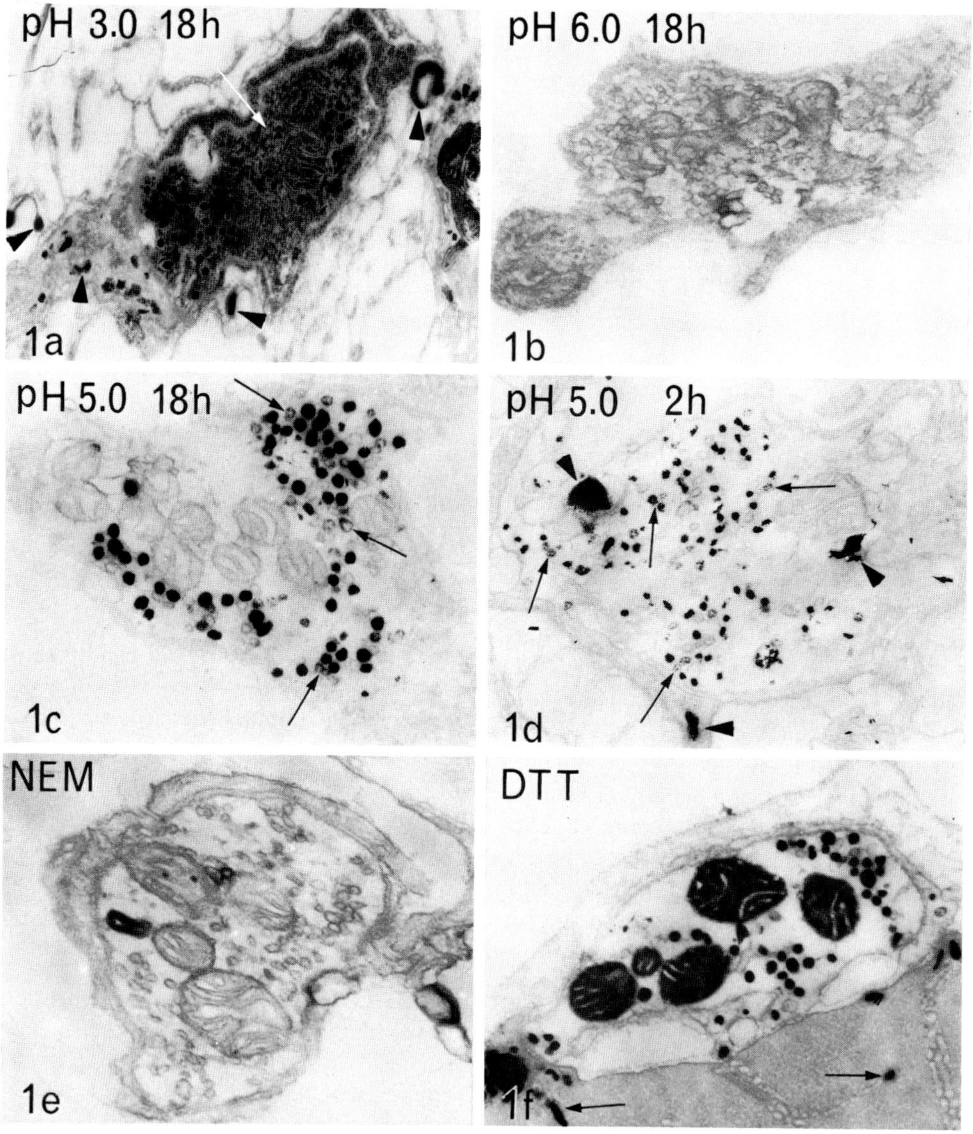

Fig. 1 a–f. Motor nerve terminals in locust nerve muscle preparations. Prefixation in 3% glutaraldehyde. ZIO reaction at 4 °C in the dark under different conditions. **a** ZIO reaction at pH 3.0 for 18 h. The matrices of all synaptic vesicles and of the mitochondria are stained. The interior of the neurotubules is ZIO-positive (*arrow*). Several artifacts are present (*arrowheads*). Unspecific reaction. ×45,000 **b** ZIO reaction at pH 6.0 for 18 h. No subcellular structure is specifically stained. ×39,000 **c** ZIO reaction at pH 5.0 for 18 h. About half of the synaptic vesicles are ZIO-positive, a minority being partially stained (*arrows*). The matrices of the mitochondria are unstained. Specific reaction. ×47,000 **d** ZIO reaction at pH 5.0 for 2 h. The contour of the vesicular matrices stained is irregular. Some vesicles show only spots of black deposits (*arrows*). Several artifacts are present (*arrowheads*). ×39,000 **e, f** Preparations treated with SH-group affecting agents for 30 min before carrying out ZIO reaction at pH 5.0 for 18 h. **e** 1 mM N-ethylmaleimide (NEM) (SH-group blocking agent). No synaptic vesicles are specifically stained. ×45,000 **f** 1 mM dithiotreitol (DTT) (SH-group protecting agent). The majority of the synaptic vesicles are completely stained. The matrices of the mitochondria show a positive reaction. Part of the T-system of the muscle is filled with black deposit (*arrows*). ×39,000

Vrensen and de Groot 1974; Reinecke and Walther 1978 b) the pH of the ZIO incubation medium is of critical importance. Only a small shift of the pH level can have significant effects on reaction properties (Vrensen and de Groot 1974; Reinecke and Walther 1978 b).

While some authors report ZIO to give the most satisfactory results at pH 6.25 (Kawana et al. 1969; Martin et al. 1969; Akert and Sandri 1975) others have obtained equivalent results in a range of pH 4.2–5.0 (Ibata et al. 1972; Vrensen and de Groot 1974; Reinecke and Walther 1978b). This may in part be due to the different preparations used, or may result from differences in the preparation of the ZIO reagent, as obvious for synapses in the rat spinal cord (Kawana et al. 1969; Ibata et al. 1972). It is also assumed that the influence of pH on the reaction properties depends on the type and quality of the prefixation applied (Vrensen and de Groot 1974). Thus, a good deal of the different results obtained in staining subcellular structures by ZIO is probably based on differences in pH.

The influence of different pH levels on reaction properties is shown in Fig. 1 a–c.

At a pH of 3.5 or less almost all synaptic vesicles give a positive reaction and exhibit a completely black matrix (Fig. 1 a). In addition, the matrices of the mitochondria are stained and neurotubules are filled with black precipitate. Often the cytoplasm shows granulated reaction products. Artifacts are present all over the section. However, preparations obtained with ZIO at this extremely low pH can be useful in neuroanatomical research, as shown by Vrensen and de Groot (1974) who recorded a facilitation of counting of synaptic vesicles with these preparations. Also for light microscopical investigations, e.g., study of peripheral innervation, counting of synapses, it is recommended to apply ZIO at a low pH to achieve a better contrast between the stained synapses and the more or less unstained surrounding tissue. At a pH of 5.5 or higher only occasionally are synaptic vesicles ZIO-positive. In most cases no subcellular structure is clearly stained (Fig. 1 b). Some artifacts are visible. A negative result of ZIO reaction with a newly applied preparation may, therefore, be due to a pH too alkaline. It is recommended to make a second attempt at 1.0 pH unit lower before accepting ZIO-negativity.

4.3 Incubation Time

Since there are rather few studies dealing with the effect of incubation time on ZIO reaction (Elias et al. 1972; Ibata et al. 1972) this parameter might be considered of minor importance. ZIO has been applied to different preparations for times ranging from 1 to 60 h. Generally an incubation time of 12–20 h is considered to result in an optimal reaction.

For the method given here the minimal incubation time was found to be about 4 h (Reinecke and Walther 1978 a). At this time the staining results are nearly identical to those obtained after 18 h except for a higher content of artifacts. Reduction of incubation time to 2 h or less results in an incomplete reaction (Reinecke, unpublished): the percentage of ZIO-positive vesicles is decreased. The shape of the vesicular matrices stained is polygonal (Fig. 1 d) and not as round as after sufficient incubation time (Fig. 1 c). Often only spots of black deposits are present within the vesicular matrix (Fig. 1 d). The number of artifacts and of unspecifically "faintly" stained structures (Elias et al. 1972) is increased. Therefore, the effect of incubation time is well to recognize.

4.4 Ion Content of the Buffer

The tris buffer solution as medium for the ZIO reagent given in the recipe has been shown to yield optimal staining properties in various nervous systems (Kawana et al. 1969; Martin et al. 1969; Vrensen and de Groot 1974; Akert and Sandri 1975; Reinecke and Walther 1978 a, b). Two parameters seem to be of importance: the hyperosmolarity of the buffer and the presence of Ca^{2+}- and Mg^{2+}-ions (Vrensen and de Groot 1974).

4.5 Temperature

ZIO seems to react with synaptic vesicles in a closely similar manner whether applied at 4 °C or at room temperature (e.g., Akert and Sandri 1968, 1975), but tissue preservation has been found to be better after incubation at 4 °C (Owman and Rüdeberg 1970). In addition, after incubation at 4 °C the number and extent of artifacts is far lower than at higher temperatures (Reinecke, unpublished). However, in dealing with special pharmacological problems it can be useful to apply ZIO at different temperatures (Pellegrino de Iraldi and Cardoni 1979).

5 Significance of the ZIO Reaction

Maillet (1968) has presumed that ZIO reacts with lipid moieties uncoupled from lipoprotein complexes. Further evidence in favor of this hypothesis has been derived from the failure of ZIO reaction after preincubation of the tissue in lipid solvents (Niebauer et al. 1969; Elias et al. 1972; Giorgi et al. 1976). However, these treatments may also remove non-lipid components and result in conformational changes of proteins.

Recently, based on X-ray microanalysis of ZIO precipitates it has been suggested (Gilloteaux and Naud 1979) that ZIO has an affinity to Ca^{2+}-binding sites associated with macromolecules. In addition, the black deposits have been shown to contain zinc and osmium in a ratio of 1:1, whereas no iodine has been found. Therefore, the ZIO precipitates probably consist of $ZnOsO_4$ (Gilloteaux and Naud 1979).

With different neuronal systems experiments have been carried out applying the ZIO reagent after previous incubation in SH-group blocking (Fig. 1 e) and SH-group protecting (Fig. 1 f) agents both with unfixed (Pellegrino de Iraldi 1975) and with prefixed (Reinecke and Walther 1978 a, b) preparations. These studies indicate that ZIO reacts with intravesicular protein(s) containing sulfhydryl groups. Further evidence has been obtained from the inactivation of ZIO reaction by protein precipitating treatments (Reinecke and Walther 1978 a).

With this in mind it is evident that ZIO reaction is a useful tool which can be applied to all kinds of neuroanatomical research. So far ZIO has been used in neuropharmacology (Pellegrino de Iraldi and Geuedet 1968; Pellegrino de Iraldi and Suburo 1972; Pellegrino de Iraldi and Cardoni 1979), in experimental neuropathology (Nickel and Waser 1969; Snyder 1973; Akert and Sandri 1975), in experimental neurobiology (Párducz et al. 1971; Matsuura et al. 1976; Halász et al. 1978; Reinecke and Walther 1978 b), in neurocytology (Akert and Sandri 1968, 1975; Kawana et al. 1969; Martin et al. 1969; Vrensen and de Groot 1974), and for the study of development of the nervous system (Stelzner 1971).

6 References

Akert K, Kawana E, Sandri C (1971) ZIO-positive and ZIO-negative vesicles in nerve terminals. Prog Brain Res 34:223–240

Akert K, Sandri C (1968) An electronmicroscopical study of zinc iodide-osmium impregnation of neurons. I. Staining of synaptic vesicles at cholinergic junctions. Brain Res 7:286–295

Akert K, Sandri C (1975) Significance of the Maillet method for cytochemical studies of synapses. In: Santini M (ed) Golgi centennial symposium proceedings. Raven Press, New York, pp 387–399

Champy C (1913) Granules et substances réduisant l'ioduré d'osmium. J Anat Physiol Norm Pathol (Paris) 49:323–343

Clark MA, Ackerman GA (1971) Osmium-zinc iodide reactivity in human blood and bone marrow cells. Anat Rec 170:81–96

Elias PM, Park HD, Patterson AE, Lutzner MA, Wetzel BK (1972) Osmium tetroxide-zinc iodide staining of Golgi elements and surface coats of hydras. J Ultrastruct Res 40:87–102

Gilloteaux J, Naud J (1979) The zinc iodide-osmium tetroxide staining-fixative of Maillet. Nature of the precipitate studied by X-ray microanalysis and detection of Ca^{2+}-affinity subcellular sites in a tonic smooth muscle. Histochemistry 63:227–243

Giorgi G, Bucci Innocenti S, Ragghianti M (1976) Osmium zinc-iodide staining of Golgi elements in oocytes of Triturus cristatus. Cell Tissue Res 172:121–131

Halász N, Joó F, Karnushina I (1978) Studies on the fine structural localization of zinc iodide-osmium reaction in the brain. III. Some characteristics of localization in the synaptosomes. J Neurocytol 7:93–105

Ibata Y, Nojyo Y, Matsuura T, Ochi J (1972) A modified zinc iodide-osmium tetroxide staining method for nerve terminals in spinal cords of the rat. Acta Histochem Cytochem 5:97–105

Jabonero V (1964) Über die Brauchbarkeit der Osmiumtetroxyd-Zinkjodid-Methode zur Analyse der vegetativen Peripherie. Acta Neuroveg 26:184–210

Joó F, Halász N, Párducz Á (1973) Studies on the fine structural localization of zinc iodide-osmium reaction in the brain. I. Some characteristics of localization in the perikarya of identified neurons. J Neurocytol 2:393–405

Kawana E, Akert K, Sandri C (1969) Zinc iodide-osmium tetroxide impregnation of nerve terminals in the spinal cord. Brain Res 16:325–331

Maillet M (1962) La technique de Champy à l'osmium-ioduré de potassium et la modification de Maillet à l'osmium-ioduré de zinc. Trab Inst Cajal Invest Biol 54:1–36

Maillet M (1968) Etude critique des fixations au tetraoxyde d'osmium ioduré. Bull Assoc Anat 53:233–394

Martin R, Barlow J, Miralto A (1969) Application of the zinc iodide-osmium tetroxide impregnation of synaptic vesicles in cephalopod nerves. Brain Res 15:1–16

Matsuura T, Ibata Y, Sana Y (1976) The zinc iodide-osmium tetroxide (ZIO) reaction on nerve endings in the median eminence of the rat under normal and experimental conditions. Cell Tissue Res 173:279–286

Nickel E, Waser PG (1969) An electron microscopic study of degenerated motor endplates after zinc iodide-osmium impregnation. Brain Res 13:168–176

Niebauer G, Krawczyk WS, Kidd RL, Wilgram GF (1969) Osmium zinc iodide reactive sites in the epidermal Langerhans cell. J Cell Biol 43:80–89

Owman C, Rüdeberg C (1970) Light, fluorescence, and electron microscopic studies on the pineal organ of the pike, Esox lucius L., with special regard to 5-hydroxytryptamine. Z Zellforsch Mikrosk Anat 107:522–550

Párducz Á, Halász N, Joó F (1971) Lack of correlation between the zinc iodide-osmium positivity of cholinergic terminals and the cholinergic transmission in the sympathetic ganglia of the cat. J Neurochem 18:97–100

Pellegrino de Iraldi A (1975) Localizing SH-groups in monoaminergic synaptic vesicles with the mixture of zinc iodide-osmium tetroxide (ZIO). Brain Res 94:363–367

Pellegrino de Iraldi A, Cardoni R (1979) ZIO staining in synaptic vesicles of the rat pineal nerves after inhibition of serotonin and noradrenaline synthesizing enzymes. Cell Tissue Res 200:91–100

Pellegrino de Iraldi A, Geuedet R (1968) Action of reserpine on the osmium tetroxide-zinc iodide reactive site of synaptic vesicles of the pineal nerves of the rat. Z Zellforsch Mikrosk Anat 91:178–185

Pellegrino de Iraldi A, Suburo AM (1971) Two compartments in the granulated vesicles of the pineal nerves. In: Wolstenholme GE, Knight J (eds) Ciba Foundation symposium on the pineal gland. Churchill, London, pp 177–195

Pellegrino de Iraldi A, Suburo AM (1972) Effect of tyramine on the compartments of the granulated vesicles in rat pineal nerve endings. Eur J Pharmacol 19:251–259

Reinecke M, Walther C (1978a) Zinc iodide-osmium tetroxide reaction: its effect on the synaptic vesicles in locust neuromuscular junctions and its chemical basis. In: Sturgess, J. M. (ed): Electron Microscopy 1978 Vol. II. The Imperial Press Ltd; Ontario, Canada pp 614–615

Reinecke M, Walther C (1978b) Aspects of turnover and biogenesis of synaptic vesicles at locust neuromuscular junctions as revealed by zinc iodide-osmium tetroxide (ZIO) reacting with intravesicular SH-groups. J Cell Biol 78: 839–855

Snyder RL (1973) ZIO staining of degenerating dorsal roots in spinal cords of cats. Anat Rec 175:446

Stelzner DJ (1971) The relationship between synaptic vesicles, Golgi apparatus, and smooth endoplasmic reticulum: a developmental study using the zinc iodide osmium technique. Z Zellforsch Mikrosk Anat 120:332–345

Taxi J (1965) Contribution à l'étude des connexions des neurones moteurs du système nerveux autonome. Ann Sci Nat Zool (Paris) 7:413–674

Vrensen G, de Groot D (1974) Osmium-zinc iodide staining and the quantitative study of central synapses. Brain Res 74:131–142

Chapter 18

Combined Freeze-Fracturing and Autoradiography Techniques: Freeze-Fracture Autoradiography

A. Schiller and R. Taugner

1 Introduction

In the past many efforts have been made to apply classical techniques of fixation and embedding to the autoradiography of soluble material. There is general agreement today that this goal can only be reached by cryotechniques (Amlacher 1974).

Since the introduction of frozen sections to the whole-body autoradiography (Ullberg 1954, 1958) and the light microscopic autoradiography (Oster et al. 1955; Taugner and Wagenmann 1958; Taugner et al. 1961), these methods have been developed to daily practice (Kinter et al. 1960; Appleton 1964; Hammarström et al. 1965; Kinter and Wilson 1965). However, the applicability of frozen-section techniques is considerably limited by several sources of artifacts during the production and handling of the sections, with the exception of the whole-body autoradiography which provides only a low resolution.

Light microscopic autoradiography is substantially hampered in that its resolution is usually not sufficient to analyze soluble compounds at the cellular level on account of the thickness of common cryostat sections and the high ice-crystal damage which is frequently underestimated when examining sections after thawing and staining. Using thin frozen sections (1–2 μm) Stumpf and Roth (1964, 1966) obtained improved resolution which enabled them to localize labelled steroids in cell nuclei (Stumpf 1968).

One additional drawback of applying autoradiography to cryostat sections is the inevitable dislocation of labelled material in the extracellular compartment due to fragmentation and drying of its frozen contents during sectioning and autoradiographic exposure (c.f. Taugner and Iravani 1963; Wedeen 1969; Wedeen and Thier 1971). It is therefore not possible to reliably compare concentrations of substances in the extracellular spaces with those within the cell.

Cryo-ultramicrotomy (Bernhard and Nancy 1964; Appleton 1969, 1972; Christensen 1969; Hodson and Marshall 1969, 1970) was expected to solve some of these problems. However, when combined with autoradiography, this technique presents new problems, and it is doubtful whether cryo-ultramicrotomy avoids the sources of artifacts previously mentioned. Freeze-drying and freeze-substitution are further candidates for a high resolution autoradiography of diffusible substances in frozen tissue (Rogers 1973). Both techniques, however, include the contact of the specimen with fluids, at least with the monomer of the embedding medium. Thereby, soluble compounds may be dissolved, and even insoluble radioactive material may be displaced and redistributed by bulk liquid flow, especially in fluid-filled extracellular spaces.

A first attempt to an autoradiography with improved resolution performed on frozen tissue block surfaces instead of sections, was "freeze-grinding" (Pellerin et al. 1959; Taugner and Iravani 1963). Paul and Bartsch (1972) reported experiments with the autoradiography of polymeric surfaces by using special replication techniques.

The development of the freeze-fracture technique (c.f. Chapt. 12) gave occasion to a new approach to an autoradiography of diffusible compounds performed on replicated surfaces of frozen tissue blocks. As will be shown, the freeze-fracture autoradiography (FFA) is a valuable method for studies of single cells and biomembranes (Fisher and Branton 1976; Rix et al. 1976).

2 Description of the Method

2.1 Preparation of Film Monolayers for Freeze-Fracture Autoradiography

Monolayers which are routinely used for the electron microscopic autoradiography (Caro 1962; Caro and Van Tubergen 1962) are simply made of liquid film emulsion and distilled water. In this composition, they are not suitable for use at low temperature, because they become brittle and fragile when transferred to a cryostat. The properties of the film monolayers are markedly improved when glycerol is added to the emulsion in a concentration of 4%–5%. With higher concentrations of glycerol the flexibility of the film is further enhanced to a surprising degree (even in-vacuo); however, the distribution of the silver halide crystals gradually becomes inhomogenous with increasing concentration, and in the electron microscope the high glycerol content causes "boiling" of the emulsion. In our laboratory the routine emulsion is produced in the following manner:

Two parts of Ilford L 4 emulsion are diluted by three parts of distilled water, and 4% water-free glycerol is added. The mixture is then gently stirred for 10 min at 42 °C. After that, a stainless steel wire loop with a diameter of 3–4 cm is dipped in the emulsion and slowly withdrawn. The loop is stored vertically until the excess water has evaporated. Then the small area of gelled film monolayer shows purple to golden interference colours, and the emulsion is flexible and adhesive. Film monolayers prepared in this way are ready for the coating of the frozen-replicated specimens.

2.2 Freeze-Fracture Procedures

Freeze-fracturing can be performed in different ways. In Chap. 3 the preparation with a Moor-Balzer's apparatus is described. Our experiments, however, were carried out with the EPA 100 freeze-fracture plant produced by Leybold-Heraeus (Cologne, West Germany). After cryoprotective pretreatment, tissue specimens of 6×1×1 mm are inserted in hollow brass rivets (3 cm in length, 1–2 mm in diameter) which are

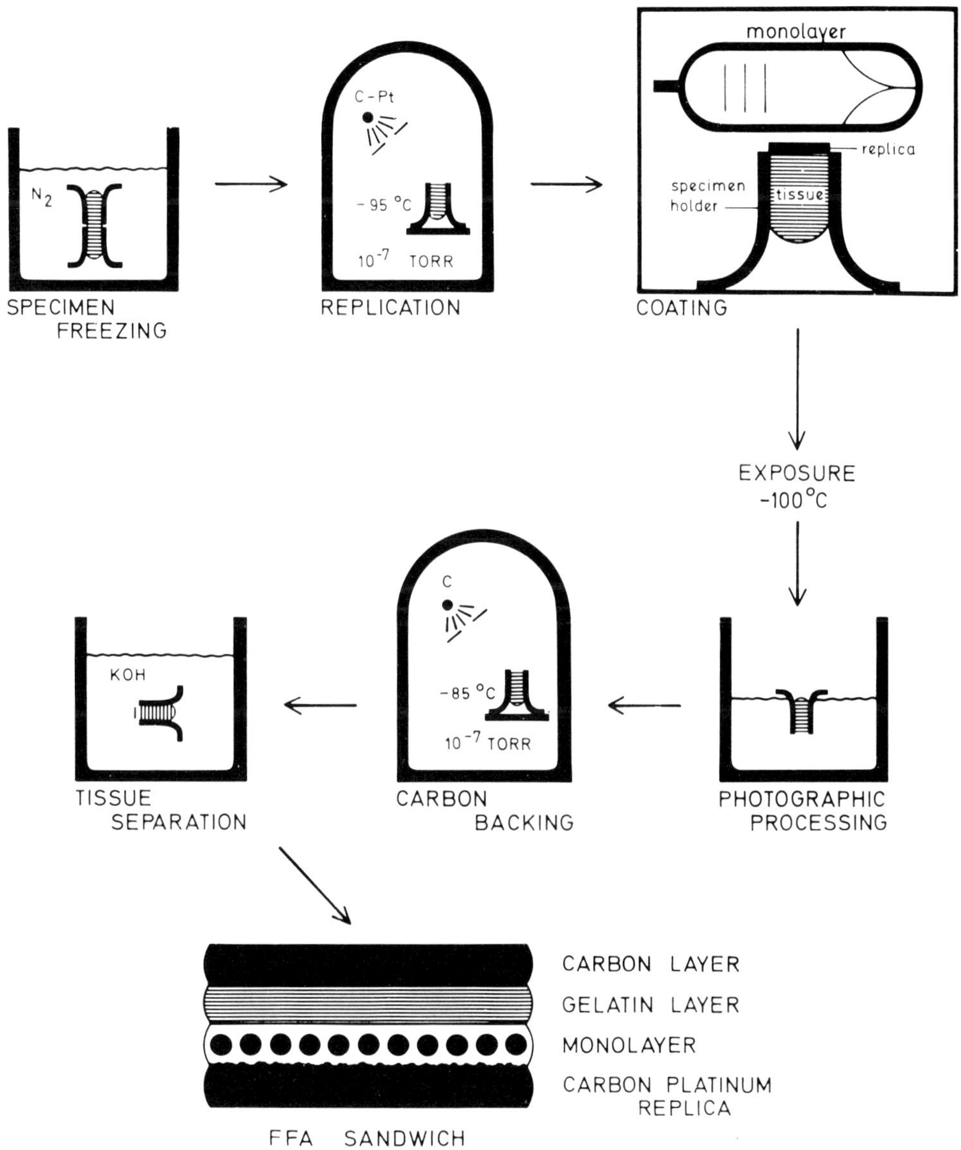

Fig. 1. Schematic representation of the preparatory steps of the FFA-technique with coating at atmospheric pressure

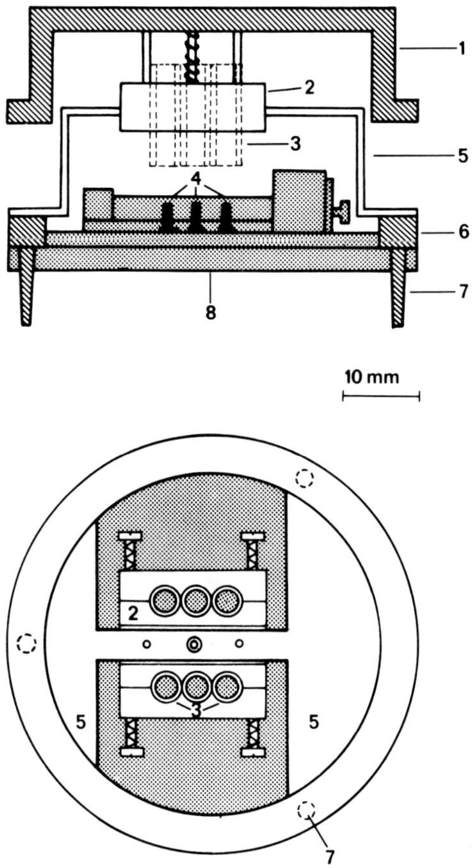

Fig. 2. Device designed for the in-vacuo coating. *Upper diagram.* Vertical section of the coating device adjusted to the sample plate. *Lower diagram.* Horizontal section of the coating device. The lower (metallic) part (5) serves to adjust the device by means of three pivots (7) fitting in corresponding holes of the sample plate (8) which carries the specimen holders (4). For better thermal insulation the ring-shaped area of contact between the sample plate and the device is made of plastic (6). The upper part of the coating apparatus consists of a transparent plastic cylinder (1) which is rigidly connected to the holder (2) for six coating tubes (3). The lower part of the device slides into the upper like a piston in a cylinder with a lift of about 5 mm. This construction enables one to adjust the coating tubes exactly to the specimens, which are thereby kept at a safe distance from the vulnerable monolayers. When the correct adjustment has been obtained, the upper part of the device is pressed down with the transport forceps, and the prepared monolayers are thereby transferred from the coating tubes to the replicated specimens

held top-to-top, and the sample is snap-frozen in melting nitrogen (see Fig. 1). The double-rivet obtained is mounted to the fracture mechanism of the sample plate (c.f. Fig. 2). After the transfer into the EPA 100 unit the specimens are fractured and replicated with platinum and carbon at 10^{-7} torr and −100 °C to −95 °C. The fracturing is carried out by breaking the double rivet with a mirror-image mechanism. In contrast to the freeze-"fracturing" with a microtome this true fracturing produces relatively uneven tissue block surfaces which can be coated only partially, if at all.

Since a microtome device was not available for the freeze-fracture plant used in our experiments, we had to cut the frozen specimens under liquid nitrogen in a Reichert Om P microtome outside the plant (c.f. Fig. 3). For this purpose, tissue samples, suspensions, or emulsions are filled in single hollow rivets and frozen in melting nitrogen. The rivets are then mounted on the microtome, cut with a razor blade under liquid nitrogen, and stored in nitrogen until replication. With this procedure, precautions should be taken to protect the cut specimens from ice contamination during the transfer to the freeze-fracture plant. We obtain satisfactory results by covering each of the specimen holders with a somewhat larger hollow copper rivet which is not removed until replication.

For studies of single cells, cell cultures, or biomembranes the freeze-fracture technique described by Fisher (1975) can be used. For this purpose, cells, e.g., erythrocytes, are spread on polylysine-coated glass disks, covered with a highly-polished copper disk and rapidly frozen. When this sandwich is fractured, the cell bodies mostly adhere to the copper disk, while the external leaflets of the plasmalemma stick to the glass. This can be shown by replicating both sides. A similar method using freshly-cleaved mica instead of glass disks was described by Nermut and Williams

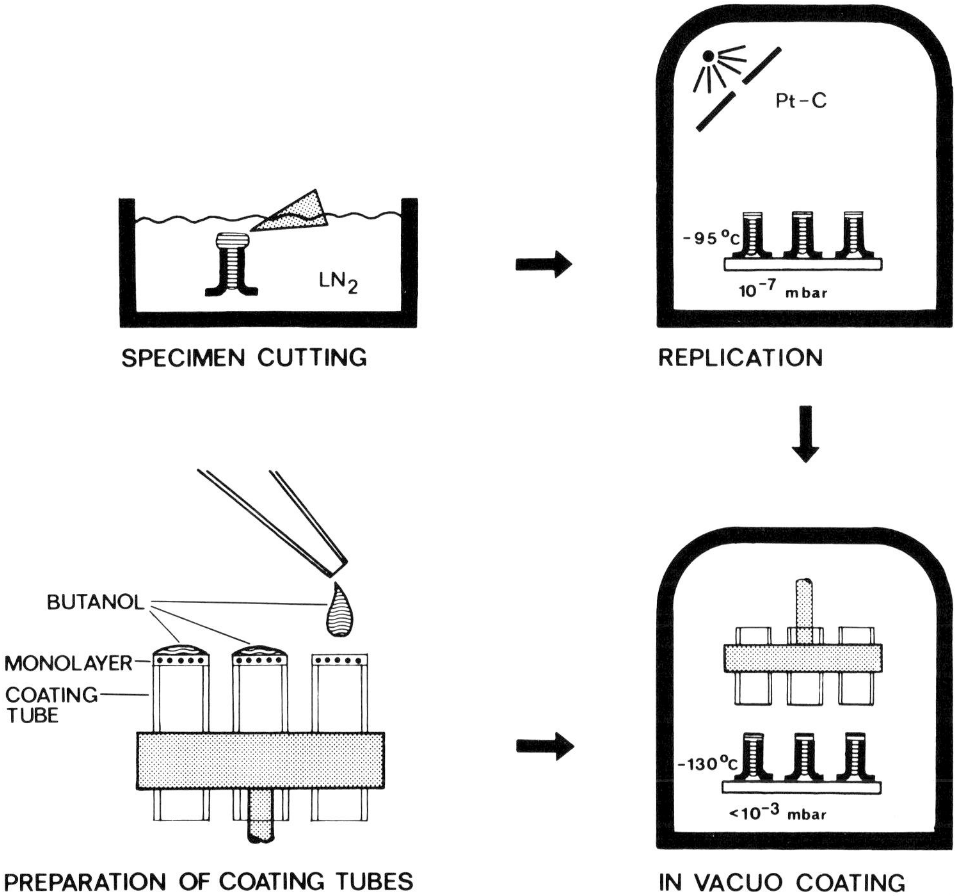

Fig. 3. Schematic representation of the modified FFA-technique used for in-vacuo coating

(1977). In our model experiments a slightly modified technique has been used to demonstrate ^{125}iodine-labelling of the extern leaflet of erythrocytes.

2.3 Coating of the Replicated Freeze-Fracture Specimens

For freeze-fracture autoradiography, the frozen-replicated specimens must be coated with a film monolayer at low temperatures around −100 °C to −130 °C. In the original approaches of Fisher and Branton (1976) and Rix et al. (1976) coating was performed at atmospheric pressure. Using the approach of this laboratory specimens are withdrawn from the freeze-fracture unit and transferred to a cryostat cabinet (temp. −20 °C to −100 °C) in a darkroom illuminated by Ilford F 904 safelights. Since the transfer includes the risk of ice contamination of the replicated fracture plane, it can be tried to "defrost" the replica by flowing dry cold nitrogen gas. Then a monolayer of film emulsion is applied to the replica and fitted to it with a stream of dry cold nitrogen. A strengthening layer of clear gelatin can optionally be applied with a wire loop to the film emulsion. In our experience, uncontrolled ice contamination of the replica occurs frequently during this procedure and the "defrosting" remains incomplete. The layer of ice-crystals between replica and film should thus greatly reduce the autoradiographic resolution.

This problem can be solved in two ways, the first of which appears to be limited to very thin specimens like single cells, cell cultures, and biomembranes. These samples can be easily freeze-dried for several hours in the freeze-fracture unit, replicated in the state of drying desired, and then warmed to room temperature. Immediately afterwards the dry warm specimens are coated at atmospheric pressure or stored in a desiccator until coating. This procedure, however, is not appropriate for the analysis of diffusible compounds in tissue blocks, since freeze-drying of these specimens would introduce unacceptible artifacts, as previously discussed. Therefore, cold replicated tissue blocks can be safely coated with emulsion only in a vacuum, preferably in the freeze-fracture unit.

Although it is possible to apply film emulsions with a wire loop even in-vacuo, we would not recommend this approach because of the difficulties of correctly fitting the small monolayer area of the loop emulsion to the replica when working with manipulators in a vacuum chamber. For better standardization a coating device is advantageous, such as the one used in our experiments which is adapted to the commercially available sample plate of the EPA 100 unit (c.f. Fig. 2). The single-grain area of the emulsion can be safely selected under visual control as usual, and then be transferred to a coating tube. These preselected monolayers can then be introduced into the vacuum chamber following a standardized time course which is requisite due to the short period available for in-vacuo coating. Adjustment of the film to the position of the specimen is easy and the conditions of coating are better reproducible.

For the application of the film monolayers small tubes are used. These coating tubes carrying the monolayers are usually prepared a few minutes prior to use. For this purpose, plastic tubes 13 mm in length, 3 mm inner diameter, and 0.5 mm wall diameter are covered at one end with a monolayer of air-dried Ilford L 4 emulsion using a stainless steel loop (Caro 1962). After fixation of the tubes in the tube holder, the coating device is ready for use.

Earlier attempts to use in-vacuo coating had already revealed that the properties of L 4 film emulsion are considerably altered when transferred from atmospheric pressure to a vacuum. Air-dried film emulsion is not really dry, but contains a certain amount of bound water. When it encounters high vacuum, however, rapid drying of the monolayer causes immediate loss of its flexibility and adhesiveness even in the presence of glycerol. For this reason one is obliged to modify the coating technique.

In our experience, very small amounts of a suitable volatile fluid, when applied to the monolayer, can promote the essential adhesion of the film emulsion to the replica without the risk of autoradiographic artifacts. A spreading substance promoting adhesion of the monolayer to the replica has to fulfill certain conditions. When applying the substance, the film emulsion must remain mechanically intact, with the homogenous distribution of the silver halide crystals undisturbed. At temperatures around −100 °C, which are required for the coating of freeze-fracture specimens, the substance has to remain liquid and volatile in high vacuum. Finally, artifacts due to chemography, thawing, or dislocation should not occur.

Using a mixture of 1-butanol (melting point −79.9 °C) and 2-butanol (melting point −114.7 °C) the following coating procedure can be employed: Labelled specimens are fractured with a microtome and replicated at about −100 °C, as usual, and afterwards further cooled to −130 °C within a cold shroud. At the same time film monolayers and the coating device are prepared. Immediately prior to their introduction into the vacuum chamber, about 1 microliter of a 1-butanol/2-butanol mixture (1 : 1) is applied with a micropipette to the replica side of the monolayer (Fig. 3).

It should be pointed out, that the success of the coating procedure depends on the observance of the standardized time course described here, since butanol evaporates rapidly at room temperature. A further requirement is the availability of an air lock which diminishes the steep pressure gradient from atmosphere to the main vacuum chamber, and thus the risk of high photographic background values of the film emulsion due to rapid drying and mechanical strain. The air lock provides additional advantages in that most of the butanol evaporates within the lock, and the increase in pressure within the main vacuum chamber is relatively low and transitory during the coating.

Directly after butanol application, the coating device is picked up with transport forceps, which are attached to the air lock of the freeze-fracture unit, and the lock is immediately evacuated. After 10–15 s of pumping, the device is locked into the vacuum chamber and adjusted to the sample plate as soon as possible. Then the monolayers together with the unevaporated residues of butanol are transferred to the replicated specimens as delineated previously. After that, the coating device is removed from the vacuum chamber and the air lock sealed. During locking the pressure in the chamber increases to 10^{-5}–10^{-3} torr but falls, after coating, usually within a few seconds to less than 5×10^{-7} torr.

The specimens are then slowly warmed from –130 °C to –100 °C and kept at this temperature. After 45 min or less the butanol is completely evaporated and the monolayers are in close adhesive contact with the replicated specimens. After this time the coated cold specimens are transferred from the freeze-fracture unit into a chamber, cooled, at atmospheric pressure, by liquid nitrogen, and exposed at –120 °C.

Visual control to check the success of the coating procedure in the vacuum chamber is difficult but not impossible, even at safelight illumination, since the monolayer can frequently be recognized as a thin film slightly altering the appearance of the replicated specimen surface. Further information on the success of the coating procedure can be obtained from the appearance of the coating tubes after withdrawal of the device.

2.4 Autoradiographic Exposure of the FFA Specimens

For optimal protection of the specimens from recrystallization during the autoradiographic exposure, the safe temperature range colder than –130 °C is preferred, especially with samples which contain no cryoprotectants. The temperature range between –100 °C and –130 °C appears to be an acceptable compromise particularly for cryoprotected samples, since the velocity of recrystallization is low enough and the sensitivity of the film emulsion not too much reduced at this temperature (Debeauvais-Wack 1963).

In this laboratory, these low temperatures of the FFA specimens are maintained by storing the samples in styrofoam containers floating in liquid nitrogen in large dewar vessels. Within certain limits the temperature can be regulated by variation of the distance between the samples and the level of the liquid nitrogen. The duration of the autoradiographic exposure may range from 1 to 12 weeks.

2.5 Photographic Processing

After exposure, the FFA specimens (replicated tissue with overlying film) are thawed and immediately immersed in Amidol developer at 18 °C. The developer is made up of 0.675 g Amidol, 2.7 g sodium sulphite, and 0.12 g potassium bromide dissolved in

300 ml water. Finally 0.66 g Hostapon (Hoechst) per 100 ml are added. Duration of development is usually 3 min.

Fixation is performed in sodium thiosulphate. With biological specimens approximately tissue-isotonic solutions provide best results, because osmotic volume changes of the tissue and rupturing of the replica-film sandwich are thus minimized. For this purpose, the 30% sodium thiosulphate fixer was diluted to a 5%–10% solution. The fixation should last 6–10 min. Rinsing is performed in isotonic sodium chloride solution and subsequently in distilled water.

2.6 Cleaning of the Replica-film Sandwich

When using cell suspensions or artificial emulsions it is relatively easy to remove the replicated material from the replica by careful rinsing in distilled water and, in case of lipids sticking to the replica, in dilute alcohols.

One is faced with a much more serious problem, when solid tissue blocks have to be digested. Strong acids and bases (e.g., sulfuric acid, sodium hypochlorite) which are used in routine freeze-fracturing (c.f. Chap. 3), would directly attack silver grains of the film emulsion. In our experience, unfixed tissue can be satisfactorily removed from the replica by immersion in 1 M potassium hydroxide solution alternating with distilled water. The duration of the cleaning procedure depends on the properties of the tissue; with frog spinal cord it was found that the immersion in KOH for 6–12 h, several times interrupted by a 30 min rinsing in distilled water, was sufficient to separate the replica-film sandwich from the tissue block. Obviously, this procedure implies a considerable mechanical strain on the replica-film sandwich which occasionally causes a breaking of the replica and even a detaching of the film emulsion.

With crucial tissues it is helpful to stabilize the sample before cleaning by an additional layer of carbon on the film layer (see Fig. 1). For this purpose the specimens (rivets containing the coated freeze-fracture samples) are dried after the photographic processing by storing them for several hours in a desiccator. After that the specimens are rapidly frozen in melting nitrogen, transferred to the freeze-fracture unit, etched for 30 min to remove ice from the film emulsion, and coated with carbon at −85 °C. Then the specimens are thawed and cleaned as described. In our experience the yield is considerably improved with this procedure. After cleaning, the FFA sandwiches are picked up on grids and examined at low beam current in the electron microscope. Figs. 4–6 demonstrate that the film monolayers are intact after photographic processing and treatment with KOH respectively.

2.7 Model Applications of FFA

Several model applications of FFA have so far been tested in this laboratory. Frog spinal cord tissue was used to examine the single preparatory steps which are required for the freeze-fracture autoradiography of diffusible substances performed on tissue blocks. The specimens were prepared as follows: Frogs (Rana esculenta, 50–70 g) were decapitated and the spinal cords dissected in cold Ringer's solution. Pachymeninx and leptomeninx are carefully removed, and the cords incubated at 22 °C in 20 ml Ringer's solution containing ^{3}H-serotonine (10^{-7} M) or ^{3}H-strychnine (10^{-6} M); all solutions are bubbled with a mixture of 95% O_2/5% CO_2 at pH 7.4.

After 2 h the spinal cords are transferred to a Ringer's solution containing 20% of the polymeric cryoprotectant PVP (Polyvinylpyrrolidone, Kollidon K 12 or K 30, BASF, Ludwigshafen, West Germany) which does not penetrate the cells. After varied intervals, tissue samples are dissect-

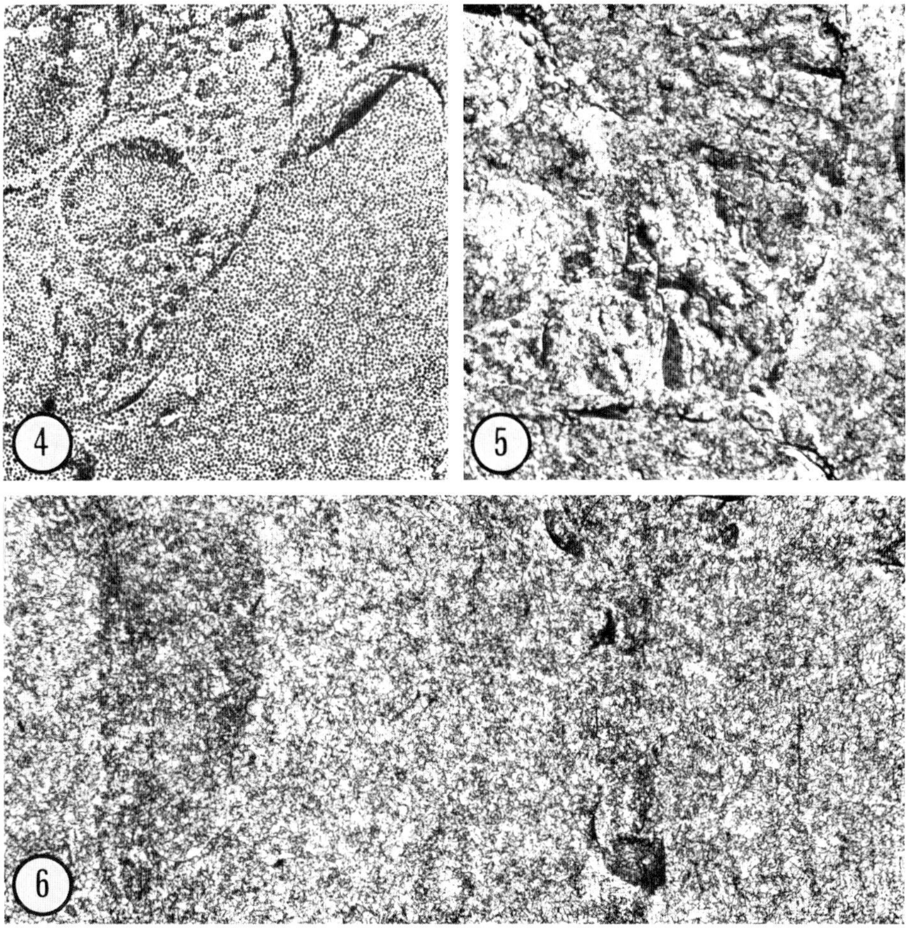

Figs. 4–6. FFA-"sandwiches" after the successive preparatory steps. For these test preparations replicas already cleaned were coated with a monolayer at –20 °C. **Fig. 4.** Before photographic processing. **Fig. 5.** After photographic processing and carbon backing. **Fig. 6.** After immersion in 1 M potassium hydroxide. ×3200

ed, inserted in the sample holders, and snap-frozen in liquid nitrogen. The further processing is performed as described in Sects. 2.2 and 2.3.

The autoradiographs from our first experiments showed no specific distribution of the labelled substances (c.f. Fig. 7). In order to verify that the lack of label accumulation was real, several preparatory uncertainties were ruled out by the following model experiments with the simple, but well-defined, label distribution in an emulsion of ^{3}H-oleic acid in water. The emulsion of ^{3}H-oleic acid is prepared by adding 50 µl (250 µCi) ^{3}H-oleic acid to 1 ml solution containing 40% (W/Vol) glycerol and 20 mg of a detergent (Pril), and shaking the mixture for 45 min. The emulsion is then put into siliconized rivets and shock-frozen in liquid nitrogen slush (Umrath 1974). The further preparation is performed as described in Sect. 2.

The FFAs of the oleic acid emulsions can be evaluated immediately after photographic processing and short rinsing in ethanol. Figure 8 demonstrates an auto-

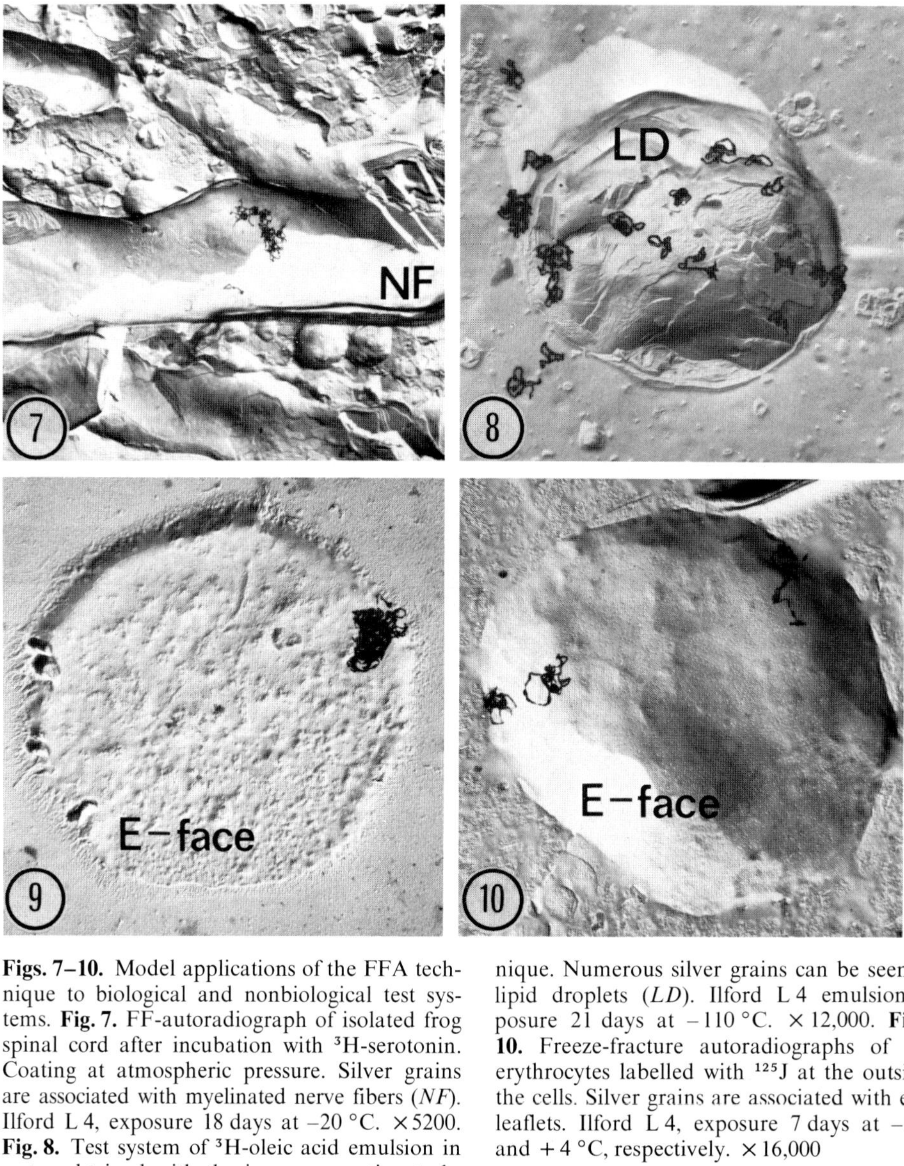

Figs. 7–10. Model applications of the FFA technique to biological and nonbiological test systems. **Fig. 7.** FF-autoradiograph of isolated frog spinal cord after incubation with ^{3}H-serotonin. Coating at atmospheric pressure. Silver grains are associated with myelinated nerve fibers (*NF*). Ilford L 4, exposure 18 days at –20 °C. ×5200. **Fig. 8.** Test system of ^{3}H-oleic acid emulsion in water obtained with the in-vacuo coating technique. Numerous silver grains can be seen over lipid droplets (*LD*). Ilford L 4 emulsion; exposure 21 days at –110 °C. × 12,000. **Figs. 9, 10.** Freeze-fracture autoradiographs of sheep erythrocytes labelled with ^{125}J at the outside of the cells. Silver grains are associated with extern leaflets. Ilford L 4, exposure 7 days at –20 °C and +4 °C, respectively. ×16,000

radiograph from this test system. Silver grains are accumulated over lipid droplets.

To prove the applicability of the FFA to thin layers of single cells and isolated biomembranes sheep erythrocytes are iodinated using a modification of the method according to Phillips and Morrison (1971). The cells are thoroughly washed with a 310 mOsM/liter phosphate buffer according to Dodge et al. (1963) and resuspended to a concentration of 4×10^{9}/ml. A 250 µl cell suspension is incubated at 0 °C–4 °C with 5 µl diluted LPO (Lactoperoxidase, Boehringer) and 250–300 µCi $Na^{125}I$ (Amersham). After repeated washing in 310 DB buffer until the supernatant is free of radioactivity, the cryoprotectant glycerol is gradually added to some of the samples up to a maximum concentration of 15%. The erythrocytes are then spread on polylysine-treated glass disks (Fisher 1975) for 30 min, and washed twice with buffer and glycerol-buffer solution, respectively. Then a copper sample-holder is pressed, with its highly polished surface, upon the cell layer, and the whole sample snap-frozen in melting nitrogen. In the freeze-fracture plant the cells are fractured at −100 °C and 10^{-7} torr and subsequently freeze-dried at −100 °C for 60–90 min. The specimens are then replicated with platinum and a somewhat heavier carbon layer, and slowly heated to room temperature. After withdrawal from the freeze-fracture plant the specimens are stored in a desiccator and subsequently coated, at atmospheric pressure, with a monolayer of Ilford L 4 emulsion. Exposure is performed in a refrigerator. Photographic processing is identical to that described by Rix et al. (1976), and the replicas are cleaned in 1 M KOH. Figures 9 and 10 show autoradiographs of ^{125}J-labelled erythrocytes.

3 Preparatory Problems and Sources of Artifacts

3.1 Deficient Contact

The contact between film and replicated specimen depends on the surface to be coated and the stickiness of the emulsion. Plane surfaces provide better conditions for coating than surfaces with steep fracture steps. Fracturing with a microtome is therefore preferred. Coating of freeze-dried specimens at room temperature is carried out conventionally. Coating at low temperature and atmospheric pressure, however, presents several new problems concerning the film contact. Frequently bubbles of enclosed air prevent the contact between film and replica.

At temperatures around −100 °C ice contamination of the replicated specimen may occur with the consequence of reduced contact and loss of autoradiographic resolution. For this reason, it is preferred to coat the replicated cold specimens in-vacuo and to protect the fractured surfaces during transfers through the atmosphere from contamination by means of devices which surround the entire sample with cold surfaces.

Special precautions must be taken to prevent the rapid drying of the film, when exposed to vacuum, and the subsequent alteration of its mechanical properties. For this purpose volatile stretching substances are applied to the replica side of the film monolayer immediately prior to coating.

3.2 Thawing of the Frozen Specimen

Special attention has to be focused on undesirable effects of the application of butanol as a stretching substance which might eventually cause thawing of the superficial layer of the specimen and thus favor chemographical artifact formation. The volume of butanol applied to the monolayer at room temperature prior to coating should be less than 1 µl. Butanol evaporates continuously during the locking-in of the coating device lasting about 20 s. Thus the butanol volume in contact with the replica is further diminished. The evaporation of the butanol and water residues of the film emulsion during the locking procedure quenches both monolayer and coating tubes which are initially at room temperature. Thus the temperature gradient between film and specimen is lowered. To prevent thawing, the specimen to be coated must be kept at a temperature of −130 °C when the film monolayer is applied. Furthermore, the specimen holder consists of a brass rivet in close contact with the massive copper sample plate. This provides good heat conductivity. Finally, the carbon layer of the replica is assumed to provide some thermal insulation between specimen and the film monolayer moistened with butanol. Moreover, precooled butanol could be used if necessary.

Simulations of the coating procedure were performed under conditions specifically intended to be unfavorable (Schiller et al. 1978). These experiments gave no evidence of melting of the ice phase of the tissue; dislocation due to thawing and histochemigraphy can therefore be excluded for normal FFA specimens.

3.3 Background

With the use of the in-vacuo coating the autoradiographic background was low in our experiments except at places where the film had obviously undergone mechanical strain or where it had come in contact with freshly-treated metal surfaces of the sample holder; the latter increase in background is probably due to luminescence phenomena.

3.4 Film Sensitivity

The reduction of the sensitivity of the film emulsion at temperatures colder than −100 °C, which are required to prevent recrystallization in frozen-hydrated specimens, is expected to be moderate (Debeauvais-Wack 1963) and can be compensated for by increasing the time of exposure.

3.5 Histochemography

Histochemographical artifacts were not seen in our in-vacuo preparations of frozen-hydrated tissue blocks: Insulating effects of the intact replica separating the film from the specimen and the low specimen temperature itself probably play the major role in preventing chemography. In the experiments with freeze-dried erythrocytes chemographical artifacts were occasionally observed at places where the replica had ruptured and the cell layer had come in contact with the film emulsion. These artifacts could be minimized by interposing, with a wire loop, a layer of clear (silver halide-free) gelatin between replica and film emulsion. However, this procedure reduces the autoradiographic resolution and should therefore be omitted if the carbon backing is strong enough to prevent a rupturing of the replica.

3.6 Mechanical Damage

During the photographic processing and subsequent cleaning the FFA specimens should be carefully handled to minimize the mechanical strain of the sample which might cause lateral dislocations of silver grains and rupturing of the replica. Approximately tissue-isotonic developer and fixer solutions provide best results (c.f. Sect. 2.5).

3.7 Problems of Resolution

The autoradiographic resolution of the FFA technique has so far not been systematically investigated. With tissue blocks the resolution is determined by the "infinite thickness" of the sample and the mean range of 1–2 μm of tritium. The loss in resolution due to the intervening thin layer of the replica (2 nm platinum, 20–30 nm carbon) appears to be negligible. Fisher and Branton (1976) estimated the resolution to at least 250 nm (half distance). With very thin sources like membranes or membrane leaflets the resolution should be considerably better (Caro 1962).

3.8 Potential Artifacts of the Freeze-Fracture Technique

Freeze-fracturing, like all cryotechniques, is hampered by artifacts due to freezing of the aqueous phase of the specimen (c.f. Chap. 12). If the distribution of diffusible compounds is studied in unfixed tissue in the presence of cryoprotectants, the influence of the cryoprotectant on the in-vivo state of the structures investigated has to be controlled (c.f. Schiller et al. 1979 a, b). If the application of cryoprotectants is unacceptable, satisfactory cryofixation of a thin tissue layer can be obtained by using quick-freezing techniques (c.f. Chap. 12). One can imagine that freeze-fracture autoradiography could be performed on such small zones of well-cryofixed tissue if a precise in-vacuo cryo-ultramicrotome would be at hand (c.f. Schiller and Taugner 1979).

Recrystallization of frozen aqueous phases can be avoided by working with specimens free of cryoprotectants at safe temperatures colder than −130 °C. With cryoprotected tissue the danger of recrystallization should be minimal even in the temperature range between −80 °C and −130 °C (Luyet 1966).

4 The Applicability of FFA

This has been demonstrated so far with several models of label distribution like emulsions of lipids, erythrocytes, and their leaflets (Fisher and Branton 1976; Schiller et al. 1978, 1979 a, b; Nermut and Williams 1980), resin beads (Fisher and Branton 1976), and, as the first application to nervous tissue, with the frog spinal cord (Rix et al. 1976).

Further studies of the frog spinal cord and of membrane receptors in the CNS are presently in progress in this laboratory with the modified technique of the in-vacuo coating described. Moreover, the freeze-fracture autoradiography, on account of the relatively simple procedure requisite for studies of single cells and "half" membranes might become an attractive technique for immunological and immunocytochemical studies. Finally, it can be imagined that, with improved techniques of cryofixation, FFA studies of concentrations and concentration gradients of soluble substances can be performed on fluid-filled spaces which are not accessible to conventional techniques like micropuncture. Most of these applications are expected to gain interest in neuroanatomical research.

5 References

Amlacher E (1974) Autoradiographie in Histologie und Zytologie. Fischer, Stuttgart

Appleton TC (1964) Autoradiography of soluble-labelled compounds. J R Microsc Soc 83: 277–281

Appleton TC (1969) The possibilities of locating soluble labeled compounds by electron microscope autoradiography. In: Roth LJ, Stumpf WE (eds) Autoradiography of diffusible substances. Academic Press, New York London, pp 301–319

Appleton TC (1972) "Dry" ultra-thin frozen sections for electron microscopy and X-ray microanalysis: the cryostat approach. Micron 3:101

Bernhard W, Nancy MT (1964) Coupes à congélation ultrafines de tissue inclus dans la gélatine. J Microsc (Paris) 3:579

Caro LG (1962) High-resolution autoradiography. II. The problem of resolution. J Cell Biol 15:189–199

Caro LG, Van Tubergen RP (1962) High-resolution autoradiography. I. Methods. J Cell Biol 15:173–188

Christensen AK (1969) A way to prepare frozen thin sections of fresh tissue for electron microscopy. In: Roth LJ, Stumpf WE (eds) Autoradiography of diffusible substances. Academic Press, New York London, pp 349–362

Debeauvais-Wack M (1963) Study of the ionographic emulsions sensitivity as a function of temperature and application to corpusculare physics. Ann Phys 8:41–66

Dodge JT, Mitchel C, Hanahan DJ (1963) The preparation and chemical characteristics of hemoglobin-free ghosts of human erythrocytes. Arch Biochem Biophys 100:119–130

Fisher KA (1975) "Half" membrane enrichment: verification by electron microscopy. Science 190:983–985

Fisher KA, Branton D (1976) Freeze-fracture-autoradiography: feasibility. J Cell Biol 70: 453–458

Hammarström L, Appelgren L-E, Ullberg S (1965) Improved method for light microscopy autoradiography with isotopes in water-soluble form. Exp Cell Res 37:608–613

Hodson ST, Marshall J (1969) A device for trimming frozen biological tissue preparatory to ultra-thin sectioning. J Microsc 89:373–375

Hodson ST, Marshall J (1970) Ultracryotomy: a technique for cutting ultra-thin sections of unfixed frozen biological tissues for electron microscopy. J Microsc 91:105–117

Kinter WB, Leape LL, Cohen JJ (1960) Autoradiographic study of diodrast-J^{131} transport in Necturus kidney. Am J. Physiol 199:931–941

Kinter WB, Wilson TH (1965) Autoradiographic study of sugar and amino acid absorption by everted sacs of hamster intestine. J Cell Biol 25:19–39

Luyet BJ (1966) Anatomy of the freezing process in physical systems. In: Meryman HT (ed) Cryobiology. Academic Press, London New York, pp 115–138

Nermut MV, Williams LD (1977) Freeze-fracturing of monolayers (capillary layers) of cells, membranes and viruses: some technical considerations. J Microsc 110:121–132

Nermut MV, Williams LD (to be published) Freeze-fracture autoradiography of the red blood cell plasma membrane. J Microsc

Oster H, Kundt H-W, Taugner R (1955) Methodische Untersuchungen zur autoradiographischen Darstellung wasserlöslicher Stoffe in der Niere. Naunyn Schmiedebergs Arch Exp Pathol Pharmakol 224:476–482

Paul D, Bartsch D (1972) Electron microscopic autoradiography of surfaces. Mikroskopie 28:274–277

Pellerin P, Fallot P, Laine-Boszormenyi M, Serrel F (1959) Low-temperature autoradiography for the detection of tritium in tissue, with removal of luminescence induced by tritium. Nature 184:1385–1386

Phillips DR, Morrison M (1971) Exposed protein on the intact human erythrocyte. Biochemistry 10:1766–1771

Rix E, Schiller A, Taugner R (1976) Freeze-fracture Autoradiography. Histochemistry 50: 91–101

Rogers AW (1973) Techniques of autoradiography. Elsevier, Amsterdam London New York

Schiller A, Rix E, Taugner R (1978) Freeze fracture autoradiography: the in-vacuo coating technique. Histochemistry 59:9–16

Schiller A, Taugner R (1979) Cryo-ultramicrotomy after coating of the cut surface of the tissue block with carbon and metals before sectioning. Histochemistry 62:153–157

Schiller A, Sonnhof U, Taugner R (1979a) Tissue function-compatible cryoprotectants in cryo-ultramicrotomy and freeze-fracturing. Mikroskopie 35:23–30

Schiller A, Taugner R, Rix E (1979b) Freeze-fracture autoradiography: Progress towards a routine technique. J Histochem Cytochem 27:1514–1515

Stumpf WE (1968) Estradiol-concentrating neurons: Topography in the hypothalamus by dry-mount autoradiography. Science 162: 1001–1003

Stumpf WE, Roth LJ (1964) Vacuum freeze-drying of frozen sections for dry-mounting, high resolution autoradiography. Stain Technol 39:219–223

Stumpf WE, Roth LJ (1966) High resolution autoradiography with dry mounted freeze-dried frozen sections. Comparative study of six methods using two diffusible compounds ^3H estradiol and ^3H mesobilirubinogen. J Histochem Cytochem 14:274–287

Taugner R, Wagenmann U (1958) Serienmäßige Herstellung von Gefrierschnitt-Autoradiogrammen mit optimalem Kontakt. Naunyn Schmiedebergs Arch Exp Pathol Pharmakol 234:336–342

Taugner R, Iravani J, Taugner G, von Egidy H, Braun A (1961) Zur autoradiographischen Lokalisation der Phosphatrückresorption in der Katzenniere. Naunyn Schmiedebergs Arch Exp Pathol Pharmakol 241:393–401

Taugner R, Iravani J (1963) Short-lived radioisotopes and autoradiography of frozen material. IAEA Bull II:187–199

Ullberg S (1954) Studies on the distribution and fate of S^{35}-labelled benzylpenicillin in the body. Acta Radiol [Suppl] (Stockh) 118:1–110

Ullberg S (1958) Autoradiographic studies on the distribution of labelled drugs in the body. Proc 2nd United Nations Int Conf on the Peaceful Uses of Atomic Energy (Geneva) 24: 248–254

Umrath W (1974) Cooling bath for rapid freezing in electron microscopy. J Micros 191: 103–105

Wedeen RP (1969) Autoradiography of freeze-dried section: Studies of concentrative transport in the kidney. In: Roth LJ, Stumpf WE (eds) Autoradiography of diffusible substances. Academic Press, New York London, pp 147–160

Wedeen RP, Thier SO (1971) Intrarenal distribution of nonmetabolized amino acids in vivo. Am J Physiol 220:507–512

Part IV

Investigation of Living Nervous Tissue

Chapter 19

Extracellular Marking and Retrograde Labelling of Neurons

Heinz Wässle and Klaus Hausen

1 Marking the Tip Positions of Recording Microelectrodes

Microelectrodes of different types are used by neurophysiologists to record the electrical activity of single nerve cells or groups of neurons, and it is often desirable to localize the structure producing the physiological response. Ideally the nerve cells whose activity is being monitored should be anatomically characterized. With intracellular recording of a single neuron, a stain can be iontophoretically injected into the neuroplasm, and the cell unambiguously identified. Such recordings, however, are very difficult to achieve in the mammalian brain, and most experimenters still rely on extracellular recordings for their physiological analysis. Although it is not generally possible to identify the recorded structure to the neuronal level using extracellular techniques, the ordered topology of some structures in the brain, such as cerebellum, hippocampus, and retina, may permit cellular identification if the tip position of the microelectrode can be accurately marked.

This first section of this chapter describes a number of methods for anatomically identifying microelectrode recording sites following extracellular monitoring. Short descriptions are given of how to manufacture commonly used microelectrodes, because the marking techniques available depend upon the type of electrode employed.

1.1 Metal Microelectrodes

Metal microelectrodes are wires or needles which are electrolytically sharpened to a very fine tip; the shaft is insulated so that only the tip has electrical contact with the nervous tissue. Suitable metals for microelectrodes are stainless steel, tungsten, and platinum-iridium alloy. Metal microelectrodes are commonly insulated by coating the shaft with lacquer or glass. Detailed reviews of microelectrodes are found in Frank and Becker (1964), Snodderly (1973), Ferris (1974).

1.1.1 Steel Microelectrodes

Stainless steel insect pins (size 000) are electropointed (6 V, a.c.) in concentrated hydrochloride against a carbon electrode (Green 1958). Insulation is obtained by dipping the electrode into lacquer (Insl-X-E33 red), quickly withdrawing it and drying at room temperature with the tip upward. The recording site may be marked by passing a current of about 2 μA for 20 s, electrode positive. The animal is perfused with a solution of 1% potassium ferrocyanide in 10% formalin. Frozen 50 μm sections of the brain are counterstained with nuclear red, mounted, dehydrated in ethanol, and cleared in xylene. The ferric ions deposited from the tip of the electrode are visible as a prussian blue spot.

1.1.2 Tungsten Microelectrodes

Tungsten wire (Φ 100–150 μm), prestraightened and cleaned, is electropointed (6 V, a.c.) in a solution containing 71 g $NaNO_2$ and 34 g KOH in 100 ml distilled water (Levick 1972). The electrode is either insulated with lacquer (Hubel 1957) or with glass. Glass-insulated, tungsten microelectrodes have particularly good recording quality and mechanical strength (Fig. 1 A). Two methods of glass insulation are used: The sharpened tungsten wire can be pushed through a glass micropipette until the point of the wire protrudes some 7 μm beyond the pipette tip (Levick 1972). Alternatively, a glass-coating can be pulled over the point of the tungsten wire with a microelectrode puller and the glass broken away to expose the metal tip (Merill and Ainsworth 1972; Ainsworth et al. 1977). A current of about 2 μA for 5 s, electrode negative causes a lesion in the tissue (Hubel 1959) which can be detected in serial sections (Fig. 3 A). This current does not destroy the electrode tip and therefore several lesions can be made during a single penetration and the electrode track later reconstructed. The animal is perfused with 10% formalin in normal saline, the brain is embedded in paraffin and serial sections of about 15 μm are stained with cresylviolet. The lesions are some 50 μm in diameter with microglia surrounding the focus of degeneration (Fig. 3 A).

The tip position of coarse tungsten microelectrodes can be marked using an alternative method (Pabst 1973). A current of about 20 μA is passed for up to 30 s, electrode positive. After perfusion with 10% formalin, frozen sections are immersed through a solution containing 10 g $SnCl_2$ in 100 ml 3N HCl, which reduces the tungsten ions at the recording site to tungsten blue.

1.1.3 Platinum-Iridium Electrodes

The electrodes are made from 70:30 platinum-iridium wire (Φ 200 μm) which is electro-pointed (6 V, a.c.) in a solution containing 30 g NaOH and 30 g NaCN in 100 ml distilled water (Wolbarsht et al. 1960). The electrode is insulated by passing it through a drop of molten solder-glass (Corning 7570). Marking of the recording site can be achieved by an electrolytic lesion in the tissue as described for tungsten electrodes.

1.2 Glass Microelectrodes

Glass microelectrodes are made by drawing capillary-glass to a fine point. The lumen of the pipette is filled with an electrolyte and a wire is inserted into the stem to form the electrical connection (Fig. 1 B). Reviews of glass electrode-

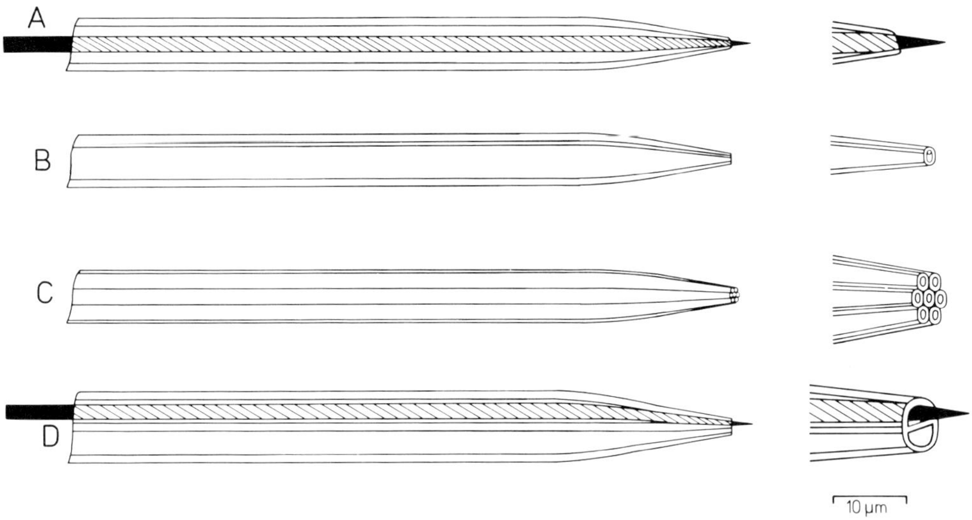

Fig. 1 A–D. Microelectrodes used for extracellular recording from single units in the nervous system. **A** Tungsten-in-glass electrode of the Levick (1972) type. The point of the tungsten wire protrudes 7 µm from the tip of the ensheathing glass. **B** Glass capillary microelectrode. The filament fused to the inner wall of the pipette facilitates filling with electrolyte. **C** Multi-barreled electrode for iontophoretic application of drugs (Curtis 1964). The barrel in the center is used for extracellular recording; the six surrounding capillaries are filled with drugs which can be released by current injection. **D** Double-barreled electrode made from ⊖-profile glass tubing. One shaft contains a sharpened tungsten wire; the other shaft is filled with an electrolyte

making techniques are found in Curtis (1964), Frank and Becker (1964), and La Vallée et al. (1969)

Borosilicate glass tubing between 0.5 and 2 mm in outer diameter is used for making microelectrodes. The glass should have a relatively thin wall to increase the volume of electrolyte, and a glass filament fused to the inner wall aids in filling the micropipette. The glass tubing is drawn on a commercial microelectrode puller to a fine tip between 0.1 and 1 µm diameter. Just before recording, the electrode is filled from the open end with the electrolyte using a syringe and narrow injection needle. Ideally, the filling electrolyte should be a saline solution which is isotonic to the tissue in which the microelectrode is to be used. The following electrolytes and stains have been used for marking the recording site after extracellular recording.

1.2.1 Complex Anions of Copper and Citrate

(Galifret and Szabo 1960)

The electrolyte is prepared by dissolving 81.1 g tripotassium citrate monohydrate and 21.8 g cupric chloride dihydrate in 100 ml water and adjusting the pH to 7 with strong KOH solution. Marking is obtained by passing a continuous 2 µA current for 2 min, microelectrode negative. The specimen is fixed in 10% formalin in saline and frozen sections cut which are then Nissl-stained. A colorless spot of 50–100 µm diameter surrounded by a 500-µm halo marks the position of the electrode tip in the sections.

1.2.2 Fast Green FCF

(Thomas and Wilson 1965)

Fast Green FCF (C.I. No. 42053) is an acid dye which has a high solubility in water and a low solubility in alcohol. Shortly before use the electrolyte containing 2–4 M sodium chloride is heated and saturated with fast-green by adding the dye in small amounts (Fukuda and Stone 1975). A current of 5 μA, electrode negative, is passed for about 5 min to mark the recording site. The tissue is perfused with 10% formalin in saline and sectioned at 50 μm on a freezing microtome. The dye spots in the unstained frozen sections can be seen under a dissecting microscope. The sections can be counterstained with a Nissl stain, dehydrated in alcohol, cleared, and mounted in the usual way. Thomas and Wilson (1966) suggest that methyl blue (C.I. No. 42780) sometimes gives better results than fast green.

1.2.3 Chicago Blue 6 B (Niagara Blue 6 B, Pontamine Sky Blue 6 BX)

Chicago blue 6B (C.I. No. 24410) is an acid dye which is very soluble in water and insoluble in organic solvents. Chicago blue has been successfully used for intracellular filling (Potter et al. 1966; Kaneko and Hashimoto 1967) and for extracellular marking (Hellon 1971). The electrolyte is made up as a 2% solution of the dye in 0.5 M sodium acetate (pH 7.7) and electrodes filled with this solution (Hellon 1971) have resistances in the range of 2–5 MΩ (internal tip diameter 1–2 μm). If a current of 2–10 μA is passed for 1–2 min (electrode negative), the resulting dye spot has a diameter of 10–30 μm and can be seen with a dissecting microscope during sectioning on a freezing microtome. Kaneko and Hashimoto (1967) state that the perfusion fixative in the case of perfusions should be at pH 4 because a neutral fixative might cause the dye spot to disappear. The sections containing the marks can be counterstained with a red dye (e.g., Phloxin or Sudan IV).

1.2.4 Alcian Blue 8 GX (C.I. No. 74240)

The dye is made up as a 3% or 8% solution in 0.5% sodium acetate. With tip diameters ranging from 1 to 4 μm the electrode resistance does not exceed 10 MΩ and good extracellular recordings can be achieved. Blockage of the microelectrode is a problem with Alcian blue, especially with pipettes of small tip diameter. Currents of 0.5–1 μA (electrode positive) passed for 1 min produce dye spots of about 50 μm diameter (Lee et al. 1969). The tissue is perfused with 10% formalin in saline and frozen sections are cut. A variety of counterstaining procedures can be used without causing any deterioration in the color of the spots. Fig. 3 B shows an example of marking the electrode position with an Alcian blue spot.

1.2.5 Multi-barrelled Microelectrodes

Glass microelectrodes made from several fused-glass capillaries (Fig. 1 C) are commonly used for iontophoretic application of drugs such as neurotransmitters (Curtis 1964; Steiner 1971). Double-barrel electrodes made from ⊖ profile tubing are advantageous for marking the recording site. The recording and staining barrels are seperated allowing the use of both an optimum recording electrolyte and a highly concentrated dye solution, which can be iontophoretically or pressure injected. A twin-barrelled tungsten-in-glass electrode (Fig. 1 D) combines the excellent recording stability of the tungsten electrode with the possibility of applying drugs (Fries and Zieglgänsberger 1974) or a marking dye (Donoghue and Kidd 1979).

2 Staining of Neurons with Extracellular Microelectrodes

The previous section was mainly concerned with the localisation of the electrode position by means of a lesion or a dye spot. This section describes procedures whereby ions or dyes are released from the tip of the microelectrode and taken up by neurons surrounding the injection point.

2.1 Silver Staining

Spinelli (1975) describes a method for local silver staining with metal microelectrodes. The tip of a platinum-iridium electrode is plated with silver which is deposited in the tissue by passing a 100 μA current for some 20 s (electrode positive). After perfusing the animal with 10% formalin in saline, thick frozen sections are cut at 80–120 μm. The sections are then carried through a staining sequence comparable to a photographic developing process, and this may result in staining of single cells against a featureless background.

2.2 Local Staining with Horseradish Peroxidase

Horseradish peroxidase (HRP type II SIGMA) released from the tip of a micropipette is taken up by surrounding neurons. Although the mechanism of uptake has not been adequately characterized, it does appear that both the intact cell body membrane and damaged dendrites or axons take up the HRP. At *short survival times*, "Golgi-like" staining can reliably be produced near the injection site (Lynch et al. 1974; Vanegas et al. 1978). With survival times of up to 48 h, "Golgi-like" staining is also found further away from the injection site in areas where the HRP is probably carried by intraaxonal transport. At longer survival times, however, edema around the electrode tends to blur the staining of single elements near the injection site (Keefer 1978). Vanegas et al. (1978) have given a detailed description of the time course of this local HRP labelling and found that survival times of some 30 min gave the best results.

Lynch et al. (1974) use glass microelectrodes with a tip diameter of 1–4 μm which are filled with 0.5%–1% HRP in 2 M NaCl solution and can be used for extracellular, single-unit recording. The enzyme is applied iontophoretically by passing a current of 0.1–2 μA (electrode negative). Alternatively, the HRP solution can be administered by pressure injection. The methods available for visualizing HRP will be described in the following section. Neurons stained by this technique are labelled uniformly with HRP reaction product and the finest tips of their dendrites are filled. This local staining with HRP is a powerful tool allowing neurons in defined areas of the brain to be selected electrophysiologically and reliably stained. The HRP staining procedure is relatively simple and can be performed on frozen sections and the ultrastructure of labelled neurons can be examined electron microscopically (Cullheim and Kellerth 1976). In some cases this local extracellular staining with HRP might be more suitable than the more difficult intracellular filling (Jankowska et al. 1976; Snow et al. 1976).

2.3 Cobalt Labelling of Single Neurons with Extracellular Recording Electrodes

This technique, which was originally described by Rehbein et al. (1974), has been mainly used to impregnate single insect interneurons during extracellular recordings. Glass micropipettes (2–8 MΩ) are backfilled with 2–3 M $CoCl_2$ and used immediately to record the activity of single nerve cells. After the experiment, the tissue is immersed in a solution of ammonium sulphide to precipitate the cobalt and treated according to the procedure described in the following section.

Rehbein et al. (1974) report that their cobalt method results in a single cell impregnation if the recording has been stable for several minutes and if the tip of the electrode has been positioned in direct vicinity of the recorded neuron (indicated by extracellular spike amplitudes of several mV). Since neither pressure injection nor iontophoresis are used in this procedure it is assumed that cobalt ions diffuse passively out of the electrode and are taken up from the extracellular space. In control experiments, stable recordings from physiologically identical units in different preparations led to impregnation of neurons which were anatomically identical.

3 The Use of Retrograde Axonal Transport for Studying Neuronal Connectivity

Retrograde axonal transport of tracers has proved to be an extremely powerful tool for elucidating nervous pathways. Ten years ago Kristensson and Olsson (1971 a, b) and La Vail and La Vail (1972) described retrograde transport of the enzyme horseradish peroxidase (HRP), which can be localized at the cellular level by an enzymatic-histochemical method (Graham and Karnovsky 1966). Since then HRP-labelling has become one of the most widely used techniques in histology of the mammalian brain (La Vail 1975 a, b; Jones and Hartmann 1978). Retrograde filling of neurons using the cobalt technique (Pitman et al. 1972) has been an advance of similar importance for invertebrate neuroanatomy. These techniques are now so widely used that many different refinements on the original methods are to be found in the literature, and a complete review is beyond the capacity of this article. The tracers which will be considered in this section are HRP, cobalt, and fluorescent dyes. The use of radioactive-labelled tracers, including ^{3}H-labelled HRP (Geisert 1976), intracellular injection techniques, anterograde and transneuronal transport are the topic of Chap. 11.

3.1 Retrograde Transport of Horseradish Peroxidase (HRP)

3.1.1 Injection, Uptake, and Transport of HRP

HRP is either injected into the brain with pressure or by microiontophoresis (Graybiel and Devor 1974). The enzyme is positively charged (Bunt et al. 1976) and can be transported out of the electrode tip by applying a current (electrode positive). The HRP solution should be below pH 9.0, the isoelectric point of the enzyme. With iontophoretic application it is possible to physiologically localize the injection area by extracellular recording with the same micropipette. Damage to the tissue is restricted to a small area around the electrode tip and very small volumes of HRP can be injected. Only weak solutions of HRP should be used because the tip of the electrode can easily block. Pressure injection systems allow the administration of more concentrated HRP solutions and also of larger volumes. Systems used range from simply mounting a microliter syringe on a stereotaxic manipulator (Schubert and Holländer 1975) to complicated devices for microinjection (McCaman et al. 1977; Källström and Lindström 1978; Guglielmotti 1979). A simple pressure-injection system is illustrated in Fig. 2.

HRP is taken up at the injection site by neighboring cell bodies, by axons synapsing nearby and by passing axons damaged by the electrode. HRP is taken up by undamaged axons passing the injection site to only a small extent (Krishan and Singer 1973) or not all (La Vail and La Vail 1974; Nauta et al. 1974; La Vail 1975 a, b; Herkenham and Nauta 1977; Oldfield and McLachlan 1977). Several factors facilitate uptake of the injected HRP. The enzyme should be present at the injection site in a high concentration: 0.01–1 μl aqueous solutions 20%–50% HRP are commonly injected. The enzyme should stay as long as possible at the injection site and various

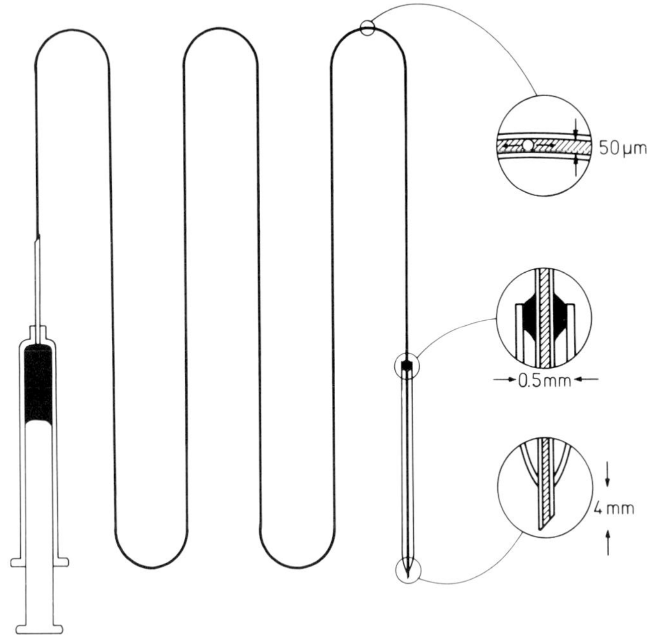

Fig. 2. Simple pressure-injection system for extracellular application of HRP. A long (~ 1 m), thin glass filament is inserted into a pipette and they are cemented together at the wide end of the pipette (De Khotinsky-cement medium, CENCO). The filament is handmade by heating a piece of glass tubing (o.d. 2.5 mm, i.d. 1.3 mm) over a bunsen flame and quickly drawing it after it has melted. The distal end of the filament is cemented into a 26-G needle which is attached to a 1-ml tuberculine syringe with Luer Lok fitting. The inner diameter of the filament (40–50 µm) can be gauged on a microscope and the injected volume measured precisely by watching an air bubble travelling along the filament. A 50 cm length of the filament contains about 1 µl injection solution. The injection site in the brain is first established by single-unit recordings using tungsten-in-glass microelectrodes (Fig. 1 A). The injection pipette has the same outer dimensions as the recording electrode and can therefore replace it accurately within the brain

forms of HRP binding have been tested such as HRP-containing granules (Kawamura et al. 1978), pellets or slow-release gels (Griffin et al. 1979). The uptake of HRP through axonal endings is apparently increased by adding dimethylsulfoxide (Keefer 1978) or poly-L-ornithin (Hadley and Trachtenberg 1978) to the HRP solution. It is often claimed that the use of certain commercially available HRP preparations gives better results than others, but the literature is contradictory.

HRP is transported retrogradely at a rate of 50–80 mm a day but this may vary in different parts of the mammalian nervous system (La Vail 1975 a,b). Survival times of the animals are 1–3 days in general, but the optimal period should be determined for each experimental system, because at long survival times HRP might disappear from the cell bodies.

3.1.2 Fixation of Nervous Tissue for HRP Demonstration

Following the original description of Graham and Karnovsky (1966), which was primarily developed to achieve good tissue preservation for electronmicroscopy, many neuroanatomists use fixatives containing high concentrations of glutaraldehyde (GA) and paraformaldehyde (PA). Several

Table 1. Summary of the characteristics of nine different procedures employed for the demonstration of HRP (modified from Mesulam and Rosene 1979)

Source	Fixative	Chromogen and Incubation Parameters								Additional steps
		Chromogen	Buffer	Alcohol	Temperature	Additives	Time (min)	H_2O_2 (%)	Color	
Mesulam (1978)	1.25% GA, 1% PA in 0.1 M phosphate buffer, pH 7.4	Tetramethyl benzidine 5 mg/100 ml	Acetate 0.01 M pH 3.3	2.5% Ethanol	19 – 23 °C	Sodium nitroferricyanide	20	0.009	Blue	Pre-reaction soak 20 min at room temp stabilization 20 min at 0 °C
Streit and Reubi (1977)	5% GA in 0.16 M phosphate buffer	Diaminobenzidine tetrahydrochloride 10 mg/100 ml	Citric ammonium acetate 0.05 M, pH 5.0	None	19 – 23 °C	P-cresol	60	0.01	Brown	None
Malmgren and Olsson (1978)	1.5% GA in 0.1 M phosphate buffer, pH 7.4	Diaminobenzidine tetrahydrochloride 200 mg/100 ml	Cacodylate 0.1 M, pH 5.1	None	19 – 23 °C	None	30	0.01	Brown	None
De Olmos and Heimer (1977)	1.5% GA, 1% PA, 4% sucrose in 0.1 M phosphate buffer, pH 7.4	Benzidine dihydrochloride 88 mg/10 ml	Acetate 0.01 M, pH 4.3	45% Methanol	–10 °C	DMSO; gelatine; $CoCl_2$; sodium nitroferricyanide	330	Gradual change from 0.004 to 0.028	Blue	Pre-reaction soak 10 min at –10 °C; stabilization 10 min at –10 °C
Mesulam (1976)	1.25% GA, 1% PA in 0.1 M phosphate buffer, pH 7.4	Benzidine dihydrochloride 50 mg/100 ml	Acetate 0.01 M, pH 5.0	30% Ethanol	19 – 23 °C	Sodium nitroferricyanide	25	0.012	Blue	Pre-reaction soak 20 min at room temp; stabilization 20 min at 0 °C
De Olmos et al. (1978)	1.5% GA, 1% PA, 0.2% Chloraldehyde, 4% sucrose in 0.06 M phosphate buffer, pH 7.5	Tetramethyl benzidine 6.5 mg/100 ml	Acetate 0.0009 M, pH 4.3	14% Ethanol	0 °C	DMSO; gelatine; sodium nitroferricyanide	60	Gradual change from 0.009 to 0.018	Blue	Pre-reaction soak in nickel ammonium sulfate 5 min at room temp

La Vail and La Vail (1974)	1.25% GA, 1% PA in 0.05 M phosphate buffer, pH 7.4	Diaminobenzidine tetrahydrochloride 50 mg/100 ml	Phosphate 0.1 M, pH 7.4	None	19 – 23 °C	None	20	0.01	Brown	Pre-reaction soak 20 min at room temp
De Olmos (1977)	1% (4%) GA, 5% sucrose in 0.05 M phosphate buffer, pH 7.2 – 7.4	*o*-Dianisidine 38 mg/100 ml	Acetate 0.012 M, pH 4.3	14% Methanol	−5 °C	DMSO; ethylene glycol, sodium nitroferricyanide	120	Gradual change from 0.02 to 0.06	Green	Pre-reaction soak 10 min at −10 °C, stabilization 10 min at −10 °C
Adams (1977)	GA in 0.1 M phosphate buffer, pH 7.4	Diaminobenzidine tetrahydrochloride 50 mg/100 ml	Phosphate 0.1 M, pH 7.3	None	19 – 23 °C	None	15	0.01	Blue-brown	Pre-reaction soak in $CoCl_2$ and Tris 10 min at room temp

reports now present clear evidence that PA in the fixative reduces HRP activity (Kim and Strick 1976; Malmgren and Olsson 1978).

According to the method of La Vail and La Vail (1974), the animal is perfused with 0.9% NaCl in 0.1 M phosphate buffer (pH 7.4) followed by a fixative containing 1% PA and 1.25% GA in 0.1 M phosphate buffer (pH 7.4). The brain is removed and immersed in the fixative at 4 °C for 6–12 h. The tissue is transferred to phosphate buffer containing 5% sucrose where it is stored overnight at 4 °C and the brain is then sectioned on a freezing microtome at 40 μm.

Malmgren and Olsson (1978) recommend perfusion with 0.9% saline in 0.1 M phosphate buffer (pH 7.4) followed by a fixative containing 1.5% GA in 0.1 M phosphate buffer (pH 7.4). The brain is removed, immersed for 4 h in the fixative and later rinsed for 12 h at room temperature in phosphate buffer containing 5% sucrose (pH 7.4). The brain is then sectioned on a freezing microtome at 40 μm thickness.

3.1.3 Methods to Demonstrate HRP in Nerve Cells

The original procedure of Graham and Karnovsky (1966) for demonstrating HRP-involved incubation in a tris-HCl buffered solution of hydrogen peroxide and 3.3′-diaminobenzidine tetrahydrochloride (DAB) at pH 7.6. La Vail and La Vail (1974) substituted 0.1 M phosphate buffer (pH 7.4) for the tris-HCl buffer. Other chromogens have recently been introduced as an alternative to DAB: Some are more sensitive while the reaction product of others is more easily visualized. A summary of incubation parameters, chromogens, and other additives presently used to demonstrate HRP is given in Table 1. Two of these methods, the DAB method of Malmgren and Olsson (1978) and the benzidine dihydrochloride method of Mesulam (1976) will be discussed in more detail.

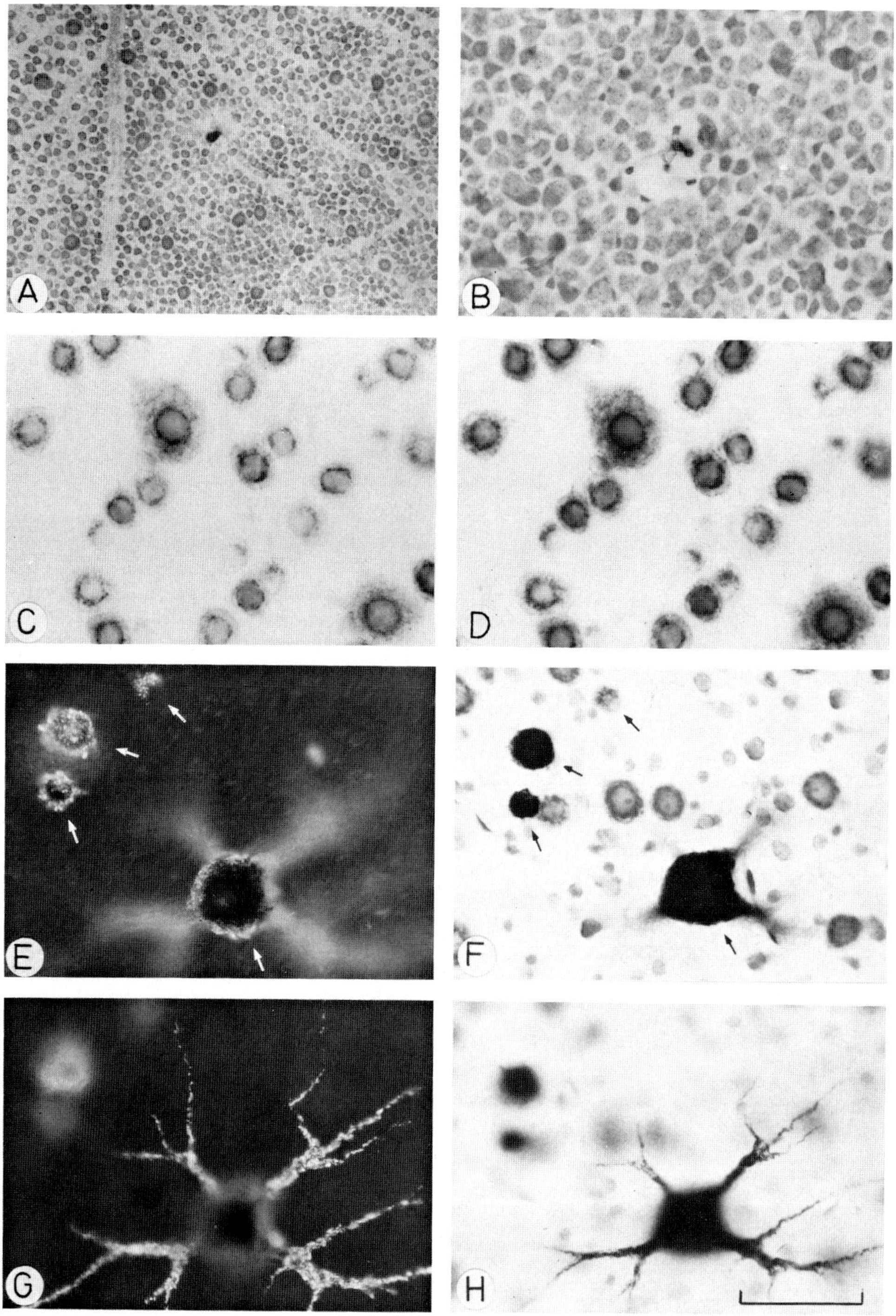
A
B
C
D
E
F
G
H

3.1.3.1 Technique of Malmgren and Olsson (1978)

Their method of fixation has been described above. The frozen sections are reacted for 30 min in the dark at room temperature in an incubation medium made up of 200 mg DAB and 1 ml of 1% H_2O_2 in 100 ml cacodylate buffer (0.1 M, pH 5.1) and agitated during the fraction period. Sections are then washed in buffer, counterstained for 1 min in 0.5% toluidine blue solution, mounted onto gelatinized slides, dried in air, dehydrated in alcohol, cleared in xylene, and mounted in Permount. Labelled neurons contain reddish-brown granules of reaction product (Fig. 3 C, D). Sometimes they contain only a few granules; sometimes they are solidly filled. Adams (1977) has introduced a method for improving the visibility of the DAB reaction product. The sections are preincubated for 10 min in 0.1 M tris-HCl buffer (pH 7.6) containing 0.5% $CoCl_2$, with the result that the reaction product becomes much darker. Some neurons are retrogradely labelled with a "Golgi-like" quality and smooth reaction product fills their dendrites and axons (Adams and Warr 1976; Keefer et al. 1976; Keefer, 1978). There is some evidence that HRP uptake from sectioned or damaged axons may produce their uniform staining (Ferster and Le Vay 1978).

Graham and Karnovsky (1966) have shown that the DAB reaction product is visible at the ultrastructural level and electron microscopy of HRP-filled neurons has proved to be a powerful tool (La Vail and La Vail, 1974). The synaptic contacts of smoothly-labelled cells, in particular, can be analyzed after reembedding and serial sectioning for electron microscopy. The preservation and transparency of HRP-labelled material is superior to that seen in comparable electron micrographs of Golgi-impregnated nerve cells (Cullheim and Kellerth 1976).

3.1.3.2 Technique of Mesulam (1976)

In order to increase the sensitivity of the HRP method and to improve the contrast of the reaction product, Mesulam (1976) has used benzidine dihydrochloride (BDHC) as a chromogen for the HRP reaction: he has adapted a prescription of Straus (1964) for use in the nervous tissue. The fixation method is identical with that of La Vail and La Vail (1974) previously described. The frozen sections are presoaked for 20 min in a solution containing 100 mg sodium nitroferricyanide, 50 mg BDHC, 5 ml acetate buffer (0.2 M; pH 5.0), 65 ml water, and 30 ml absolute ethanol. Four milliliters of 0.3% H_2O_2 are then added to this solution and the sections are incubated for a further 25 min. The sections are

Fig. 3. A Electrolytic lesion in the ganglion cell layer of a cat retina, made after extracellular recordings with a tungsten-in-glass microelectrode (1.5 μA, 7 sec). **B** Dye mark in the ganglion cell layer of a chicken retina (alcian blue, 1 μA, 10min). **C** ganglion cells in a wholemount preparation of the cat retina, retrogradely labelled with HRP from the lateral geniculate body. DAB was used as chromogen for the HRP demonstration. **D** Same field as in C, but photographed through a blue gelatin filter to increase the contrast of the reaction product. **E** Four ganglion cells labelled in the cat retina after HRP injection into the superior colliculus. The preparation is placed between crossed-polarising filters and the crystalline BDHC reaction product lights up. **F** same field as in E, but the retina has been counterstained with cresyl-violet to make possible a comparison between labelled and unlabelled cells. The micrograph is taken using bright field illumination. **G** polarization micrograph of the same field as in E, but the focus is taken at the level of dendritic branching. There is good labelling of the primary dendrites of the large cell in the middle of the field. **H** The same dendritic branching as in G, after counterstaining and under bright field illumination. The scale represents 200 μm for **A** and 50 μm for **B–H**

transferred to a stabilizer (9 g sodium nitroferricyanide, 5 ml 0.2 M acetate buffer pH 5.0, 50 ml absolute ethanol, and 45 ml distilled water) for 20 min and then rinsed in distilled water. They are mounted on chromalum-gelatin coated slides (Macqueen 1978) and air-dried. The sections are then counterstained with 1% neutral red for 2.5 min, differentiated and dehydrated in alcohol, cleared in xylene, and mounted in Permount. The visibility and contrast of the blue BDHC reaction product is superior to the brown reaction product of DAB incubated cells.

Mesulam and Rosene (1979) have attempted to grade the different HRP procedures according to their sensitivity. The methods they judge to be most sensitive are listed at the top of Table 1; less sensitive methods are listed near the bottom. It has to be emphasized that the visibility and stability of the reaction product, the filling of dendrites, the quality of the smooth "Golgi-like" staining, and the possibility of using the material for electronmicroscopy might be more important for some experiments than the absolute sensitivity of the method.

HRP has recently been used as a neuronal marker in the invertebrate nervous system (Muller and McMahan 1976; Coggehall 1978; Eckert and Boschek 1980), but it is not yet as commonly used with invertebrates as the cobalt technique described in the following section.

3.1.3.3 Improvement of the Visibility of the HRP Reaction Product

Malmgren and Olsson (1978) have tested a variety of optical filters in order to enhance the contrast of the reddish-brown DAB reaction product (absorption peak at 465 nm). They found that Kodak Wratten filter No. 46 (transmittance 430–480 nm) increases the contrast very effectively. Inexpensive gelatin filters (Edmund Scientific, No. 841, 842, 843, 846) have been used in our laboratory for the same purpose (Fig. 3 C, D).

The visibility of the DAB reaction product is greatly improved using dark field illumination, especially at low magnification. The visibility of the BDHC reaction product is improved if the specimen is placed between crossed polarizing filters (Illing and Wässle 1979). If the microscope is not equipped for polarisation microscopy, inexpensive polaroids inserted in the condensor and ocular can be used to produce this effect. Figures 3 G and 3 H compare bright field and polarization microscopy on HRP-labelled cells.

3.1.3.4 Safety Precautions

Many of the chemicals used in HRP incubation media are potentially dangerous and benzidine in particular is a potent carcinogen. Safety precautions which prevent skin contact or breathing the dust of these substances should therefore be enforced. The working area and glassware should be treated with sodium hypochlorite to denature the incubation chemicals (Adams 1977).

3.2 Cobalt Sulphide Impregnations

The cobalt technique was introduced by Pitman et al. (1972) and has been substantially improved in recent years by combination with the sulphide-silver reaction (Timm 1958; Tyrer and Bell 1974). The method is based on the filling of living nerve cells with cobalt ions which are subsequently immobilized by sulphide treatment:

$$Co^{2+} + S^{2-} \rightarrow CoS.$$

As a result, a black insoluble cobalt sulphide precipitate is formed intracellularly, which allows the discrimination of filled profiles as grey or black structures when examined under the light microscope.

The contrast of impregnated cells is usually unsatisfactory for detailed structural analyses. It can be strongly enhanced in an intensification procedure, in which silver ions are catalytically reduced and converted into black, amorphous silver which accumulates at the cobalt sulphide containing profiles:

$$Ag^+ \xrightarrow[\text{CoS, Reducer}]{} Ag^\circ.$$

Since large parts of filled neurons and even complete cells very often become visible only after appropriate silver intensification, this procedure should be routinely employed in cobalt histology.

Cobalt methods are widely used to label and identify single neurons after intracellular or extracellular recordings (Burrows 1973; Rehbein 1976; Siegler and Burrows 1979). In addition, various procedures are used to resolve light-microscopically the topography and arborization patterns of neural ensembles in vertebrates (Fuller and Prior 1975; Székely and Gallyas, 1975; Mason et al. 1977; Gallyas et al. 1978) and invertebrates (Godman 1974; O'Shea and Williams 1974; Wine and Hagiwara 1977; Strausfeld and Obermayer 1976; Altman and Tyrer 1977; Strausfeld and Hausen 1977; Hausen and Strausfeld 1980) and to label specific profiles with cobalt and silver as electron-dense markers in electron microscopical investigations (Kirkham et al. 1975; Mason 1975; Mobbs 1976; Székely and Kosaras 1976; Butler et al. 1977; Hausen and Wolburg-Buchholz 1980).

Intracellular cobalt injections are described in Chap. 11. Here, we will discuss two further cobalt techniques, both of which employ in principle identical histological procedures. These will be described in the following sections.

3.2.1 Filling Techniques

3.2.1.1 Mass Impregnations of Neural Ensembles After Cobalt Injections into Neuropil

This technique has been developed by Strausfeld and Hausen (1977) and was used to delineate the structure and arrangements of interneurons in the optic lobes of insects. Fused fiber glass micropipettes, drawn with conventional electrode pullers and broken to tip sizes of 5–50 μm, are backfilled with an aqueous solution of 5% $CoCl_2$. The nervous tissue of a living animal is exposed, and the cobalt filled micropipette is directly implanted into the desired neuropil region by means of a micromanipulator. The micropipette is left in the tissue for a certain "injection" period, during which cobalt ions are allowed to diffuse into the extracellular space around the pipette tip. After the injection period the pipette is removed and the animal is kept alive for an additional diffusion period. Care should be taken that the animal survives the injection and diffusion period in good condition.

Working with insects, short injections may be carried out at room temperature, whereas prolonged injections should be performed at 4 °C. Injections of this kind lead to an impregnation of complete classes of interneurons, whose individual members can be resolved in their entirety. The method thus combines the advantages of reduced silver stainings (resolution of general neuroarchitecture) with the qualities of Golgi impregnations (resolution of structural details of individual neurons) and is highly reliable: the same populations of neurons can be easily impregnated in a large number of preparations. The actual uptake mechanisms of cobalt ions into living neurons during the injection and diffusion phase are unclear and can be treated only hypothetically. A series of methodological experiments has revealed the following:

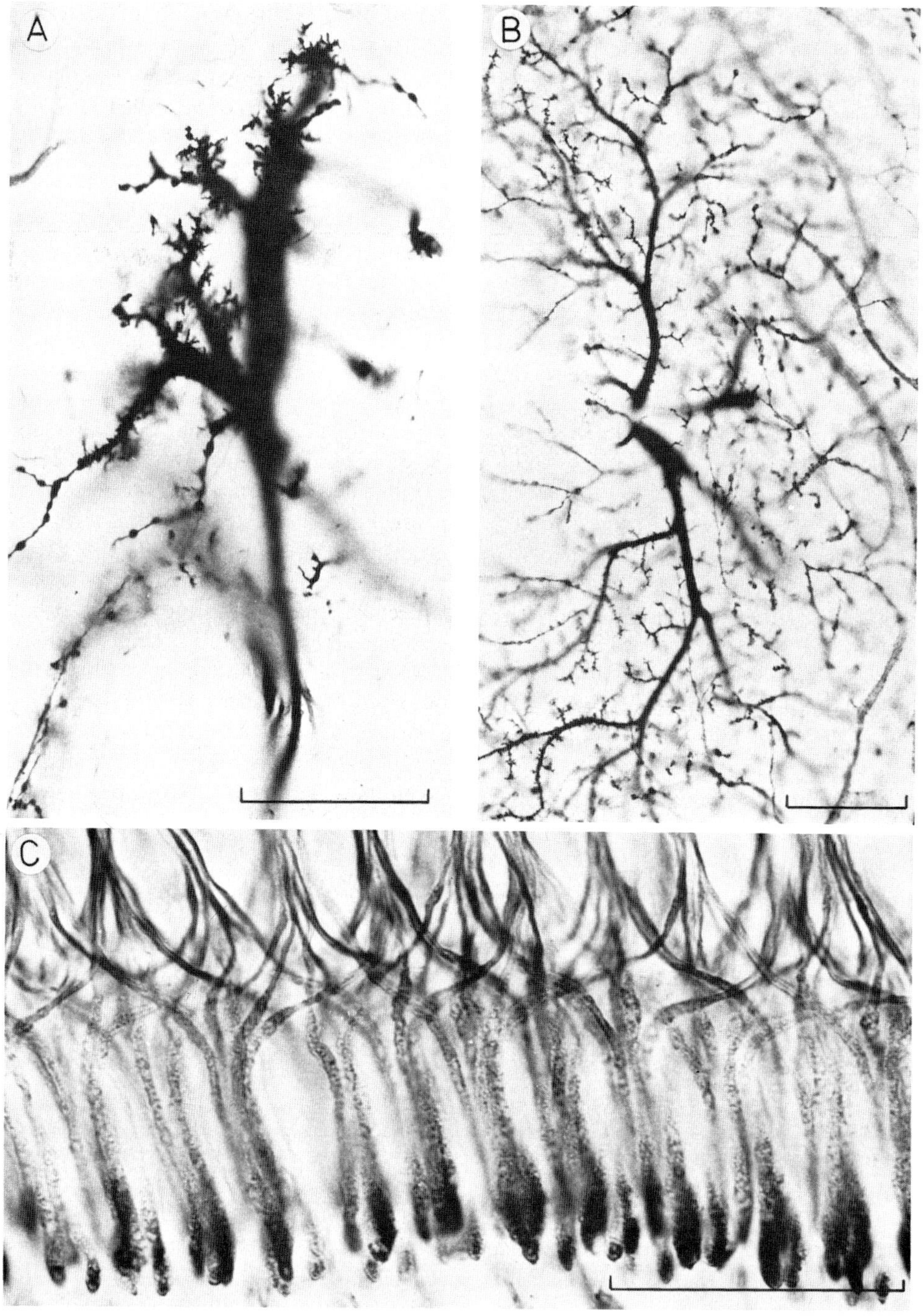

Fig. 4 A–C. Cobalt sulphide impregnated and silver intensified neurons in the visual and central nervous system of the fly (Calliphora erythrocephala). **A** Dendrites of a descending interneuron projecting from the brain to the thoracic ganglion filled by axonal diffusion. **B** Dendritic arborization of a visual interneuron filled by extracellular cobalt injection. **C** Axon endings of receptor cells in the first optic neuropil filled by cobalt-injection into the eye. Scales: 50 μm

a) The number of neurons filled with this technique depends on specific neuro-architecture of the injection site; it increases with the tip diameter of the micropipette and the injection time. In insects, single neurons can be impregnated after injections of several minutes (Fig. 4 B); large populations of cells are delineated after injections of 1–2 h (Fig. 4 C).

b) The quality of impregnation cannot be improved by iontophoretic or pressure-injection; on the contrary, best results are achieved using passive diffusion as described previously.

c) Cobalt ions are taken up from the extracellular space by intact neurons, passing through the vicinity of the electrode tip; hence, membrane damage caused by the micropipette during implantation is not a prerequisite for a successful filling.

d) The uptake takes place preferentially in the telodendritic arborizations and axons of cells; an uptake in the dendritic region was only rarely observed.

e) The question, whether cobalt ions are distributed within the filled cells by active transport mechanisms or by diffusion is unsolved. The latter, however, seems more likely, since high intracellular concentrations of cobalt are strongly poisonous to the cellular metabolism.

Cobalt injections into neuropil very often result in the impregnation of neurons which are located far away from the injection site, and whose arborizations are in close contact with the dendrites of heavily labelled cells, filled directly by the injection. Obviously, these neurons have taken up cobalt ions from the latter. Test experiments in insects have shown that such "second order" uptake occurs preferentially in cells being presynaptic to directly filled profiles. This phenomenon has been termed "transsynaptic migration" of cobalt (Strausfeld and Obermayer 1976). However, the mechanism underlying second-order fillings is unknown and it is not clear if synapses are in fact involved in it.

3.2.1.2 Axonal Diffusion and Iontophoresis

A further technique introduced by Iles and Mulloney (1971) is widely used to fill nerve trunks or single nerve fibers emerging from neuropils. The nerve is cut with a sharp (!) knife or scissors and a drop of distilled water is brought onto the cut for several minutes in order to cause swelling of the dissected axons. The cut end is then placed into a small vaseline cup, which is built up inside the body of the animal using a fine syringe, and which is filled with a 5% CoCl solution. The cup should be carefully sealed against the surrounding hemolymph or blood in order to prevent contamination with cobalt. Special care should be taken to avoid contact between the cut surface and the vaseline. The cup is then closed by a small piece of parafilm to prevent evaporation. Cobalt ions are allowed to diffuse into the cut axons for a certain diffusion period, whose length depends on the specific requirements of the tissue under investigation. In general, diffusion times of 1–2 h should be sufficient for an intracellular diffusion of cobalt ions over a distance of 1000 μm. Fillings of this kind can also be carried out iontophoretically. In this case a current is applied between the cobalt pool (positive) and the surrounding tissue (negative) using silver or platinum wires as electrodes. Again, the optimal duration of the iontophoresis and the amplitude of the applied current are mainly dependent on the preparation investigated. In general, currents of 10–100 μA are applied for several hours. A comparison of fillings achieved by pure diffusion and by iontophoresis demonstrates that, in most cases, as good or even better results are obtained using the diffusion technique.

It should be noted, that the axonal diffusion technique does not allow filling of entire neurons, but rather dendritic or teledendritis endings of the dissected cells (Fig. 4 A).

3.2.2 Histological Processing of Cobalt-Filled Tissue

3.2.2.1 Precipitation and Fixation

After completion of the injection and diffusion phase, the tissue is briefly washed in Ringer solution and subsequently placed for precipitation into a solution of ammonium sulphide. Tissue blocks larger than 3 mm^3 should be cut into smaller pieces and 0.5%–1% solutions of fresh $(NH_4)_2S$ in Ringer solution or distilled water are generally used. Ammonium sulphide penetrates the tissue rapidly and precipitation takes place immediately, indicated by the occurrence of a black coloration at the injection site. Precipitation should be carried out as quickly as possible since ammonium sulphide causes considerable tissue damage. In general, precipitation times of 3–5 min are sufficient. A number of other precipitation media are described in the literature, e.g., Na_2S, H_2S, and H_2S-saturated Ringer solution. However, the alkaline ammonium sulphide seems to be the superior medium for achieving complete and quick precipitation.

The tissue is then thoroughly washed in Ringer solution and fixed in a conventional fixative for light microscopy. AAF, Carnoy, Bouin, and Karnovsky fixatives can be recommended. Further steps in the processing depend on the intensification method applied. There are, in principle, three different possibilities: the fabrication of (1) wholemounts or sections of unintensified material, (2) section-intensified preparations, and (3) block-intensified sections or wholemounts.

3.2.2.2 Unintensified Preparations

The fixed specimens are dehydrated, embedded in paraffin or epoxy resin, sectioned, and mounted for light microscopical examination. All of these steps follow usual histological routine and will not be discussed in detail. Alternatively, the fixed and dehydrated specimens are cleared in styrol, methylbenzoate or methylsalicylate (10–30 min), and placed for microscopic inspection in a depression slide. Such wholemounts are either mounted in the respective clearing medium or in Canada balsam. Storage of the preparations in darkness to prevent fading is recommended by some authors.

As mentioned above, the use of unintensified material can hardly be recommended for detailed anatomical investigations, since weakly-filled profiles may remain invisible. Unintensified wholemounts may show sufficient details, however, to confirm the identity of known neurons recorded and injected in electrophysiological experiments.

After inspection, wholemounts may be embedded and section intensified or rehydrated for block intensification. Both can be done even after storage of the wholemount in the clearing medium for up to several months.

3.2.2.3 Section Intensification

For section intensification (Tyrer and Bell 1974) the specimens are embedded in paraffin or epoxy resin, sectioned, and mounted on slides. The slides are then transferred into a freshly made developer bath, composed of 10 ml 40% gum arabic, 2 ml 10% citric acid, 2 ml 5% hydrochinon, and 1 ml 1% silver-nitrate. This developer has been successfully used for insect nervous tissue. Slightly different developers used for other preparations can be found in the literature previously cited. The intensification is carried out in darkness to prevent light-induced initiation of the silver reduction (developer solutions turn black under illumination due to the formation of reduced silver). The speed of the development depends strongly on temperature. Optimal working temperatures are 40–60 °C; development times range between 15–30 min for these temperatures. The degree of development, that is the amount of silver deposited in cobalt-containing profiles, can be easily observed light microscopically after rinsing the slides in distilled water. Sufficiently intensified profiles turn yellow-brown or black. Insufficient intensifications may be continued until satisfactory contrast is achieved.

Some precautions should be observed in the intensification procedure: (a) All heavy metal sulphides, not only cobalt sulphide, can start the silver reduction. Hence, tissue containing other metals than the injected cobalt may turn black. For this reason sections should not be handled with metal tools before and during intensification. (b) Sectioned-material embedded in epoxy resin is intensified only superficially; hence, cobalt-filled profiles may not be contrasted throughout but rather at the surface of the sections. This problem can be solved by using either thin (1–2 μm) sections or paraffin embedding, since the latter is dissolved from the section before intensification. (c) The intensification process should be carefully terminated: "over-intensified" sections turn completely black due to autocatalytic silver reductions.

3.2.2.4 Block Intensification

This intensification technique (Strausfeld and Obermayer 1976; Bacon and Altman 1977; Strausfeld and Hausen 1977) has been devised to enhance the contrast of cobalt-filled profiles in unsectioned specimens. Since block-intensified material can be examined either as wholemount or after thick or thin sectioning, the method is of particular advantage for tracing neural projections over long distances and for analyzing the arborizations of large cells.

Block intensification is carried out directly after fixation of the tissue. The specimen is first presoaked for 10 min in a solution of 10% gum arabic in distilled water at 21 °C and then placed into three subsequent developer solutions composed as follows: (a) 10 ml 40% gum arabic in aqua dist., 2 ml 10% citric acid, 2 ml 1% hydrochinon; (b) 10 ml 40% gum arabic, 2 ml 10% citric acid, 2 ml 1% hydrochinon, 1 ml 0.1% silver nitrate; (c) 10 ml 40% gum arabic, 2 ml 10% citric acid, 2 ml 5% hydrochinon, 1 ml 1% silver nitrate. These steps are carried out at 40 °C in darkness; development times are 10 min in (a), 10 min in (b), 60–75 min in (c). In solution (c) the surface of the specimen turns green-brown. At this point the intensification should be stopped by transferring the specimen into a stop-bath of low pH, composed of 1 g glucose, 0.5 ml of concentrated acetic acid and 10 ml distilled water. All developer solutions should be prepared directly before use, only gum arabic may be stored as a stock solution at 4 °C for longer periods (months). As mentioned in the previous section, the tissue should not be contaminated during intensification by any metals. Any manipulations of the specimens should be carried out with glas tools.

After intensification, the tissue is dehydrated in a graded-alcohol series, embedded in epoxy resin and sectioned. Appropriately-intensified material should show a clear background and dark-brown or black profiles of high contrast reminiscent of Golgi preparations.

The procedure described above was developed for insect nervous tissue. Working with other preparations the schedule should be adapted to the specific requirements of the respective tissue. Slightly different procedures for other preparations can be found in the literature cited.

3.3 Retrograde Axonal Transport of Fluorescent Tracers

The reliability of fluorescent tracers for demonstrating nervous connections has yet to reach the standard of HRP and problems such as diffusion of the tracer from the injection area, uptake by passing fibers and spilling of the tracer from labelled to neighbouring cells have not been studied sufficiently. However, fluorescent dyes seem to be an excellent tool for double-labelling experiments, where two tracers are required to demonstrate axonal bifurcations.

3.3.1 Evans Blue

Evans Blue (EB) gives a red fluorescence when illuminated with ultraviolet light. It has been used as a retrograde tracer in conjunction with bovine serum albumin (BSA) by Kristensson (1970), Kristensson and Olsson (1971 a, b) and Steward and Scoville (1976). A solution of 5% BSA and 1% EB in physiological saline is injected into the brain, and 24 h later the animal is perfused with 5% or 10% formalin in saline. Frozen sections are dehydrated and mounted in a nonfluorescent medium (Depex). Kuypers et al. (1977) have reported that a solution of 10% EB without BSA is transported better and produces a flaming-red fluorescence in the neurons and their primary dendrites.

3.3.2 Primuline (Eastman 1039)

Kuypers et al. (1977) tested an aqueous solution of 10% Primuline (PI) for retrograde transport and found a characteristic golden fluorescence in the parent cell bodies. For details see Kuypers et al. (1977).

3.3.3 4′-6 diamidino-2-phenylindol 2 HCl, DAPI (Serva, Heidelberg 18860)

A 1-µl injection of an aqueous solution of 1.5% DAPI produced a blue fluorescence in the parent cell bodies (Kuypers et al. 1977). A mixture of 10% Primuline and 2% DAPI in phosphate buffer gave a more striking labelling than DAPI or PI alone: the parent cell bodies contained both the blue DAPI and the golden PI fluorescent granules.

3.3.4 Bisbenzimide (Hoechst 33258)

Kuypers et al. (1979) injected an aqueous solution of 10% Bisbenzimide (Bb) and demonstrated that it can be used as a retrograde tracer. The animal was perfused with 10% formalin, frozen sections were mounted, air dried, but not covered. Retrograde-labelled neurons contained the yellow/green fluorescent Bb. Kuypers et al. (1979) reported that glia near the labelled nerve cells and axons took up tracer which had apparently spilled over.

3.3.5 Propidium Iodide (Sigma P-5264)

Kuypers et al. (1979) showed that Propidium iodide (10% in aqueous solution) is taken up by nerve endings and can be demonstrated as a brilliant orange fluorescence after retrograde transport. The same mounting procedure was used as described for Bisbenzimide.

3.3.6 Fluorescent Substances Binding to Adenine-thymidine Rich DNA

Bentivoglio et al. (1979) recently tested 6 substances related to DAPI and found two of them, True Blue (150/129) and Granular Blue (186/134) suitable as retrograde fluorescent tracers. They give a strong blue fluorescence and are transported over long distances (Björklund and Skagerberg 1979).

3.3.7 Double Labelling of Neurons with Fluorescent Substances

Two new fluorescent retrograde tracers were recently described (Bentivoglio et al. 1980 a, b). One of them, Nuclear Yellow (Hoechst S769121) preferably labels the nucleus of the neuron and is transported more rapidly. The other one, Fast Blue (diamido compound 253/50) has a slower transport rate and is accumulated in the neuronal cytoplasm. A neuron which has taken up both tracers at axon collaterals shows strong blue fluorescence of the cytoplasm and a yellow fluorescent nucleus. At longer survival times, Nuclear Yellow has the tendency to spill out of labelled neurons to surrounding nerve and glia cells (Bentivoglio et al. 1980 a; Illing, 1980). DeOlmos and Heimer (1980) have recently used Granular Blue, Nuclear Yellow and propidium iodide for triple labelling of neurons.

For research purposes small samples of Nuclear Yellow can be obtained from Dr. H. Loewe, Hoechst A.G., Post Box 800320, D-6230 Frankfurt 80, W-Germany, and small samples of Fast Blue can be obtained from Prof. O. Dann, Institut für Pharmazie und Lebensmittelchemie, Universität Erlangen, Post Box 2044, D-8520 Erlangen, W-Germany.

Acknowledgements. We are most grateful to T. Wiegand for technical assistance and to B. Köhler for secretarial help. R.-B. Illing allowed us to use his material for Fig. 3C, D, while G. Rosner provided the material for Fig. 3B. We would like to thank especially D. I. Vaney for carefully reading and correcting the manuscript.

4 References

Adams JC, Warr WB (1976) Origins of axons in the cat's acoustic striae determined by injection of horseradish peroxidase into severed tracts. J Comp Neurol 170:107–122

Adams JC (1977) Technical considerations on the use of horseradish peroxidase as a neuronal marker. Neuroscience 2:141–145

Ainsworth A, Dostrovsky JO, Merrill EG, Millar J (1977) An improved method for insulating tungsten microelectrodes with glass. J Physiol, London 269:4P

Altman J, Tyrer NM (1977) The locust wing hinge receptors. I. Primary sensory neurons with enormous central arborizations. J Comp Neurol 172:409–430

Bacon JP, Altman JS (1977) A silver intensification method for cobalt filled neurons in wholemount preparations. Brain Res 138: 359–363

Bentivoglio M, Kuypers HGJM, Catsman-Berrevoets CE, Dann O (1979) Fluorescent retrograde neuronal-labelling in rat by means of substances binding specifically to adenine-thymine rich DNA. Neurosci Lett 12:235–240

Bentivoglio M, Kuypers HGJM, Catsman-Berrevoets CE (1980 a) Retrograde neuronal labelling by means of bisbenzimide and nuclear yellow (Hoechst S769121). Measures to prevent diffusion of the tracers out of retrogradely labelled neurons. Neurosci Lett 18:19–24

Bentivoglio M, Kuypers HGJM, Catsman-Berrevoets CE, Loewe H, Dann O (1980 b) Two new fluorescent retrograde neuronal tracers which are transported over long distances. Neurosci Lett 18:25–30

Björklund A, Skagerberg G (1979) Evidence for a major spinal cord projection from the diencephalic A11 dopamine cell group in the rat using transmitter-specific fluorescent retrograde tracing. Brain Res 177:170–175

Bunt AH, Haschke RH, Lund RD, Calcins DF (1976) Factors affecting retrograde axonal transport of horseradish peroxidase in the visual system. Brain Res 102:152–155

Burrows M (1973) Physiological and morphological properties of the metathoracic common inhibitory neuron of the locust. J Comp Physiol 82:59–78

Butler AB et al. (1977) Cytochemical affinity of pyramidal cell dendrites for divalent cobalt during initiation and calcium-induced blockade of epileptiform discharge. Exp Neurol 56:386–399

Coggehall JC (1978) Neurons associated with the dorsal longitudinal flight muscles of *Drosophila melanogaster*. J Comp Neurol 177:707–720

Cullheim S, Kellerth J-O (1976) Combined light and electron microscopic tracing of neurons, including axons and synaptic terminals, after intracellular injection of horseradish peroxidase. Neurosci Lett 2:307–313

Curtis DR (1964) Microelectrophoresis. In: Nastuk WL (ed) Physical techniques in biological research, vol 5 A. Academic Press, New York London, pp 144–190

Donoghue S, Kidd C (1979) A twin-barrelled tungsten-glass micro-electrode for extracellular recording from neurons. J Physiol (Lond) 290:8P

Eckert HE, Boschek CB (1980) The use of horseradish peroxidase as a neuronal marker in the arthropod central nervous system. In: Strausfeld NJ, Miller TA (eds) Neuroanatomical Techniques. Insect Nervous System. Springer, New York Heidelberg Berlin, pp 326–338

Ferris CD (1974) Introduction to bioelectrodes. Plenum Press, New York London

Ferster D, Le Vay S (1978) The axonal arborizations of lateral geniculate neurons in the striate cortex of the cat. J Comp Neurol 182: 923–944

Frank K, Becker MC (1964) Microelectrodes for recording and stimulation. In: Nastuk WL (ed) Physical techniques in biological research, vol 5 A. Academic Press, New York London, pp 22–87

Fries W, Zieglgänsberger W (1974) A method of discriminating axonal from cell-body activity and to analyze "silent cells". Exp Brain Res 21:441–445

Fukuda Y, Stone J (1975) Direct identification of the cell bodies of Y-, X-, and W-cells in the cat's retina. Vision Res 15:1034–1036

Fuller PM, Prior DJ (1975) Cobalt iontophoresis technique for tracing afferent and efferent connections in the vertebrate CNS. Brain Res 88:211–220

Galifret X, Szabo T (1960) Locating capillary microelectrode tips within nervous tissue. Nature 188:1033–1034

Gallyas F, Lénárd L, Lázár G (1978) Improvement of cobalt-transport in axons by complexing agents. Neurosci Lett 9:213–216

Geisert EE (1976) The use of tritiated horseradish peroxidase for defining neuronal pathways: a new application. Brain Res 117: 130–135

Goodman C (1974) Anatomy of locust ocellar interneurons: Constancy and variability. J Comp Physiol 95:185–201

Graham RC, Karnovsky MJ (1966) The early stages of absorption of injected horseradish peroxidase in the proximal tubules of mouse kidney: Ultrastructural cytochemistry by a new technique. J Histochem Cytochem 14: 291–302

Graybiel AM, Devor M (1974) A microelectrophoretic delivery technique for use with horseradish peroxidase. Brain Res 68:167–173

Green JD (1958) A simple microelectrode for recording from central nervous system. Nature 182:962

Griffin G, Watkins LR, Mayer DJ (1979) HRP pellets and slow-release gels: two new techniques for greater localization and sensitivity. Brain Res 168:595–601

Guglielmotti V (1979) A thermally-controlled microinjector. Stain Technol 54:151–157

Hadley RT, Trachtenberg MC (1978) Poly-l-ornithine enhances the uptake of horseradish peroxidase. Brain Res 158:1–14

Hausen K, Strausfeld NJ (1980) Sexually dimorphic interneuron arrangements in the fly visual system. Proc R Soc Lond [Biol] 208:57–71

Hausen K, Wolburg-Buchholz K (1980) An improved cobalt sulphide-silver intensification method for electronmicroscopy. Brain Res 187: 462–466

Hellon RF (1971) The marking of electrode tip positions in nervous tissue. J Physiol (Lond) 214:12P

Herkenham M, Nauta HJW (1977) Afferent connections of the habenular nuclei in the rat. A horscradish peroxidase study with a note on the fiber-of-passage problem. J Comp Neurol 173:123–146

Hubel DH (1957) Tungsten microelectrode for recording from single units. Science 125: 549–550

Hubel DH (1959) Single-unit activity in striate cortex of unrestrained cats. J Physiol London 147:226–238

Iles JF, Mulloney B (1971) Procion yellow-staining of cockroach motor neurons without the use of microelectrodes. Brain Res 30: 397–400

Illing R-B (1980) Axonal bifurcation of cat retinal ganglion cells as demonstrated by retrograde double labelling with fluorescent dyes. Neurosci Lett 19:125–130

Illing R-B, Wässle H (1979) Visualization of the HRP reaction product using the polarization microscope. Neurosci Lett 13:7–11

Jankowska E, Rastad J, Westman J (1976) Intracellular application of horseradish peroxidase and its light and electron microscopical appearance in spinocervical tract cells. Brain Res 105:557–562

Jones EG, Hartmann BK (1978) Recent advances in neuroanatomical methodology. Annu Rev Neurosci 1:215–296

Källström Y, Lindström S (1978) A simple device for pressure-injections of horseradish peroxidase into small central neurons. Brain Res 156:102–105

Kaneko A, Hashimoto H (1967) Recording site of the single-cone response determined by an electrode-marking technique. Vision Res 7: 847–851

Kawamura S, Fukushima N, Hattori S, Tashiro T (1978) A ventral lateral geniculate nucleus projection to the dorsal thalamus and the midbrain in the cat. Exp Brain Res 31:95–106

Keefer DA (1978) Horseradish peroxidase as a retrogradely-transported, detailed dendritic marker. Brain Res 140:15–32

Keefer DA, Spatz WB, Misgeld U (1976) Golgi-like staining of neocortical neurons using retrogradely transported horseradish peroxidase. Neurosci Lett 3:233–237

Kim CC, Strick PL (1976) Critical factors involved in the demonstration of horseradish peroxidase retrograde transport. Brain Res 103:356–361

Kirkham JB et al. (1975) Identification of cobalt in processes of stained neurons using X-ray energy spectra in the electron microscope. Brain Res 85:33–37

Krishan N, Singer M (1973) Penetration of peroxidase into peripheral nerve fibers. Am J Anat 136:1–14

Kristensson K (1970) Transport of fluorescent protein tracer in peripheral nerves. Acta Neuropathol (Berl) 16:293–300

Kristensson K, Olsson Y (1971 a) Retrograde axonal transport of protein. Brain Res 29: 363–365

Kristensson K, Olsson Y (1971 b) Axonal uptake and retrograde transport of exogenous proteins in the hypoglossal nerve. Brain Res 32: 399–406

Kuypers HGJM, Bentivoglio M, Van der Kooy D, Catsman-Berrevoets CE (1979) Retrograde transport of bisbenzimide and propidium iodide through axons to their parent cell bodies. Neurosci Lett 12:1–7

Kuypers HGJM, Catsman-Berrevoets CE, Padt RE (1977) Retrograde axonal transport of fluorescent substances in the rat's forebrain. Neurosci Lett 6:127–135

La Vail JH (1975 a) The retrograde transport method. Fed Proc 34:1618–1624

La Vail JH (1975 b) Retrograde cell degeneration and retrograde transport techniques. In: Cowman WM, Cuénod M (eds) The use of axonal transport for studies of neuronal connectivity. Elsevier, Amsterdam Oxford New York, pp 217–248

La Vail JH, La Vail MM (1972) Retrograde axonal transport in the central nervous system. Science 176:1416–1417

La Vail JH, La Vail MM (1974) The retrograde intraaxonal transport of horseradish peroxidase in the chick visual system: a light and electron microscopic study. J Comp Neurol 157:303–358

La Vallée M, Schanne OF, Hebert NC (1969) Glass microelectrodes. Wiley, London

Lee BB, Mandl G, Stean JPB (1969) Microelectrode tip position marking in nervous tissue: a new dye method. Electroencephalogr Clin Neurophysiol 27:610–613

Levick WR (1972) Another Tungsten microelectrode. Med Biol Eng 10:510–515

Lynch G, Deadwyler S, Gall C (1974) Labelling of central nervous system neurons with extracellular recording microelectrodes. Brain Res 66:337–341

Macqueen CL (1978) An improved mounting solution for frozen brain sections. Stain Technol 53:243–244

Malmgren L, Olsson Y (1978) A sensitive method for histochemical demonstration of horseradish peroxidase in neurons following retrograde axonal transport. Brain Res 148: 279–294

Mason CA (1975) Delineation of the rat visual system by the axonal iontophorese – cobalt sulfide precipitation technique. Brain Res 85: 287–293

Mason CA et al. (1977) Structural features of the retinohypothalamic projection in the rat during normal development. Brain Res 132

McCaman RE, McKenna DG, Ono JK (1977) A pressure system for intracellular and extracellular ejections of picoliter volumes. Brain Res 136:141–147

Merill EG, Ainsworth A (1972) Glass-coated platinum-plated tungsten microelectrodes. Med Biol Eng 10:662–672

Mesulam M-M (1976) The blue reaction product in horseradish peroxidase neurohistochemistry: incubation parameters and visibility. J Histochem Cytochem 24:1273–1280

Mesulam M-M (1978) Tetramethyl benzidine for horseradish peroxidase neurohistochemistry: a non-carcinogenic blue reaction-product with superior sensitivity for visualizing neural afferents and efferents. J Histochem Cytochem 26:106–117

Mesulam M-M, Rosene DI (1979) Sensitivity in horseradish peroxidase neurohistochemistry: a comparative and quantitative study of nine methods. J Histochem Cytochem 27:763–773

Mobbs PG (1976) Golgi staining of material containing cobalt-filled profiles in the insect CNS. Brain Res 105:563–566

Muller KJ, McMahan UJ (1976) The shapes of sensory and motor neurons and the distribution of their synapses in the ganglia of the leech: a study using intracellular injection of horseradish peroxidase. Proc R Soc Lond [Biol] 194:481–499

Nauta HJW, Pritz ME, Lasek RJ (1974) Afferents to the rat caudoputamen studied with horseradish peroxidase. An evaluation of a retrograde neuroanatomical research method. Brain Res 67:219–234

Oldfield BJ, McLachlan EM (1977) Uptake and retrograde transport of HRP by axons of intact and damaged peripheral nerve trunks. Neurosci Lett 6:135–141

Olmos J De (1977) An improved HRP-method for the study of central nervous connections. Exp Brain Res 29:541–551

Olmos J De, Heimer L (1977) Mapping of collateral projections with the HRP-method. Neurosci Lett 6:107–114

Olmos J De, Heimer L (1980) Double and triple labelling of neurons with fluorescent substances; the study of collateral pathways in the ascending raphe system. Neurosci Lett 19:7–12

Olmos J De, Hardy H, Heimer L (1978) The afferent connections of the main and the accessory olfactory bulb formations in the rat: an experimental HRP-study. J Comp Neurol 181:213–244

O'Shea M, Williams JLD (1974) The anatomy and output connection of a locust visual interneuron: the lobular giant movement detector (LGMD) neuron. J Comp Physiol 91:257–266

Pabst A (1973) A simple method for use with tungsten microelectrodes for the localization of recording sites. Pflügers Arch 339:355–358

Pitman RM, Tweedle CD, Cohen MJ (1972) Branching of central neurons: intracellular cobalt injection for light and electron microscopy. Science 176:412–414

Potter DD, Furshpan EJ, Lennox ES (1966) Connections between cells of the developing squid as revealed by electrophysiological methods. Proc Natl Acad Sci USA 55: 328–336

Rehbein H et al. (1974) Structure and function of acoustic neurons in the thoracic ventral nerve cord of Locusta migratoria (Acrididae). J Comp Physiol 95:263–280

Rehbein H (1976) Auditory neurons in the ventral cord of the locust: morphological and functional properties. J Comp Physiol 110:233–250

Schubert P, Holländer H (1975) Methods for the delivery of tracers to the central nervous system. In: Cowan WM, Cuénod M (eds) The use of axonal transport for studies of neuronal connectivity. Elsevier, Amsterdam Oxford New York, pp 113–125

Siegler MVS, Burrows M (1979) The morphology of local interneurons in the metathoracic ganglion of the locust. J Comp Neurol 183: 121–148

Snodderly DM (1973) Extracellular single-unit recording. In: Thompson RF, Patterson MM (eds) Bioelectric recording techniques, part A. Academic Press, New York San Francisco London, pp 137–163

Snow PJ, Rose PK, Brown AG (1976) Tracing axons and axon collaterals of spinal neurons using intracellular injection of horseradish peroxidase. Science 191:312–313

Spinelli DN (1975) Silver-tipped metal microelectrodes: a new method for recording and staining single neurons. Brain Res 91:271–275

Steiner FA (1971) Neurotransmitter und Neuromodulatoren. Thieme, Stuttgart

Steward O, Scoville SA (1976) Retrograde-labelling of central nervous pathways with tritiated or Evans-blue-labelled bovine serum albumin. Neurosci Lett 3:191–196

Straus W (1964) Factors affecting the cytochemical reaction of peroxidase with benzidine and the stability of the blue reaction-product. J Histochem Cytochem 12:462–469

Strausfeld NJ, Hausen K (1977) The resolution of neuronal assemblies after cobalt injection into neuropil. Proc R Soc Lond [Biol] 199: 463–476

Strausfeld NJ, Obermayer M (1976) Resolution of intraneuronal and transsynaptic migrations of cobalt in the insect visual and nervous system. J Comp Physiol 11:1–12

Streit P, Reubi JC (1977) A new and sensitive staining method for axonally-transported horseradish peroxidase (HRP) in the pigeon visual system. Brain Res 126:530–537

Székely C, Gallyas F (1975) Intensification of cobaltous sulphide-precipitate in frog nervous tissue. Acta Biol Acad Sci Hung 26:175–188

Székely C, Kosaras B (1976) Dendro-dendritic contacts between frog motoneurons shown with the cobalt-labelling technique. Brain Res 108:194–198

Thomas RC, Wilson VJ (1965) Precise localization of Renshaw cells with a new marking technique. Nature 206:211–213

Thomas RC, Wilson UJ (1966) Marking single neurons by staining with intracellular recording electrodes. Science 151:1538–1539

Timm F (1958) Zur Histochemie der Schwermetalle. Das Sulfid-Silberverfahren. Dtsch Z Gesamte Gerichtl Med 46:706–711

Tyrer NM, Bell EM (1974) The intensification of cobalt-filled neuron profiles using a modification of Timm's sulphide-silver method. Brain Res 73:151–155

Vanegas H, Distel H, Holländer H (1978) Early stages of uptake and transport of horseradish peroxidase by cortical structures, and its use for the study of local neurons and their processes. J Comp Neurol 177:193–212

Wine JF, Hagiwara C (1977) Crayfish escape behavior. I. The structure of efferent and afferent neurons involved in abdominal extension. J Comp Physiol 121:145–172

Wolbarsht ML, Macnichol EF, Wagner HG (1960) Glass-insulated platinum microelectrode. Science 132:1309–1310

Chapter 20

Cell, Tissue, and Organ Culture in Neuroanatomy

Klaus Unsicker

1 Introduction

More than 70 years have elapsed, since R. G. Harrison (1906/07, 1907, 1908) started to maintain nerve cells in vitro and investigated the genesis of the nerve fiber. Over the years, tissue culture of the nervous system has increasingly intrigued the neurobiologists as a tool for unraveling the intricacies of the nervous system and to analyze its constituents and potentialities by morphological, physiological, and biochemical means.

During the pre-World War II era emphasis in nerve tissue culture was particulary on growth. As more refined media and substrates became available in the 1950s, sophisticated organotypic cultures of sensory ganglia, cerebellum, cerebrum, spinal cord, and sympathetic ganglia came into use and their highly organized patterns became accessible to fine structural and electrophysiological analysis. In the late 1960s neurochemical needs prompted the development of cultures of isolated cells from normal and neoplastic tissues and of cell lines. For reviews on the changing uses of nerve tissue culture, see Bunge (1975) and Murray (1977).

Nerve tissue culture has now become an almost indispensable tool for all neurobiological disciplines and the profit it gives to neuroanatomy can hardly be dissected out from that provided for neurophysiology, neurochemistry, and neuropharmacology. Recent advances in our understanding of the regulation of differentiation, synaptic transmission, effects of putative neurotransmitters and neuromodulators, neuronal-glial interactions, mechanisms of actions of neuronal connections, specific neuronal and glial proteins, surface antigens, and neurological mutant disorders would presumably not have been made without the use of nerve tissue cultures. A huge body of literature including a large number of substantial reviews on nerve tissue culture are now available (reviews and recommended texts on tissue culture are separately listed in Sect. 8).

The aim of this chapter is to present some of the principles and techniques of nerve tissue culture. Culture techniques will be described in three parts. Some general features of cell and tissue culture methods will be given in Sect. 2 and 3. The nerve tissue culture techniques which are currently employed in our laboratory and those which we do not routinely use are separately described in Sect. 4 and 5.

2 Establishment and Equipment of a Tissue Culture Laboratory

The design and equipment of a tissue culture laboratory can vary greatly according to the research program carried out. Newcomers to the field of tissue culture should know that even under rather modest circumstances excellent work can be done.

2.1 Rooms

A separate room away from the traffic of other laboratories, equipped with a large sink, a plentiful water supply, about three to four square meters in area, and wall benches is recommended. The arrangement of our tissue culture laboratory is shown in Fig. 1. The room should be equipped with ultraviolet light. Hoods lacking vertical or horizontal laminar air flow or even a clean piece of bench may still be sufficient for some purposes, although specialized hoods with laminar air flow are very convenient for working with the dissection microscope and for the preparation of media. Vertical laminar flow hoods should be used to minimize health risks when cells of established lines are used, which may be associated with oncogenic RNA viruses (Hooks et al. 1972; Lieber et al. 1973). No specialized hoods are required for work with primary cultures if a room is equipped with a positive-pressure system. Optimum conditions for a tissue culture room are achieved if the room is supplied with temperature controlled air, which has passed through a filter calculated to be 96% effective in removing particulate matter and through a precipitation electrostatic filter. The air is delivered into the room under positive pressure in relationship to the surrounding laboratories and exchanged six times an hour. Walls should be coated with epoxy paint, and each morning surfaces, especially benches should be wiped down with 70% and 100%

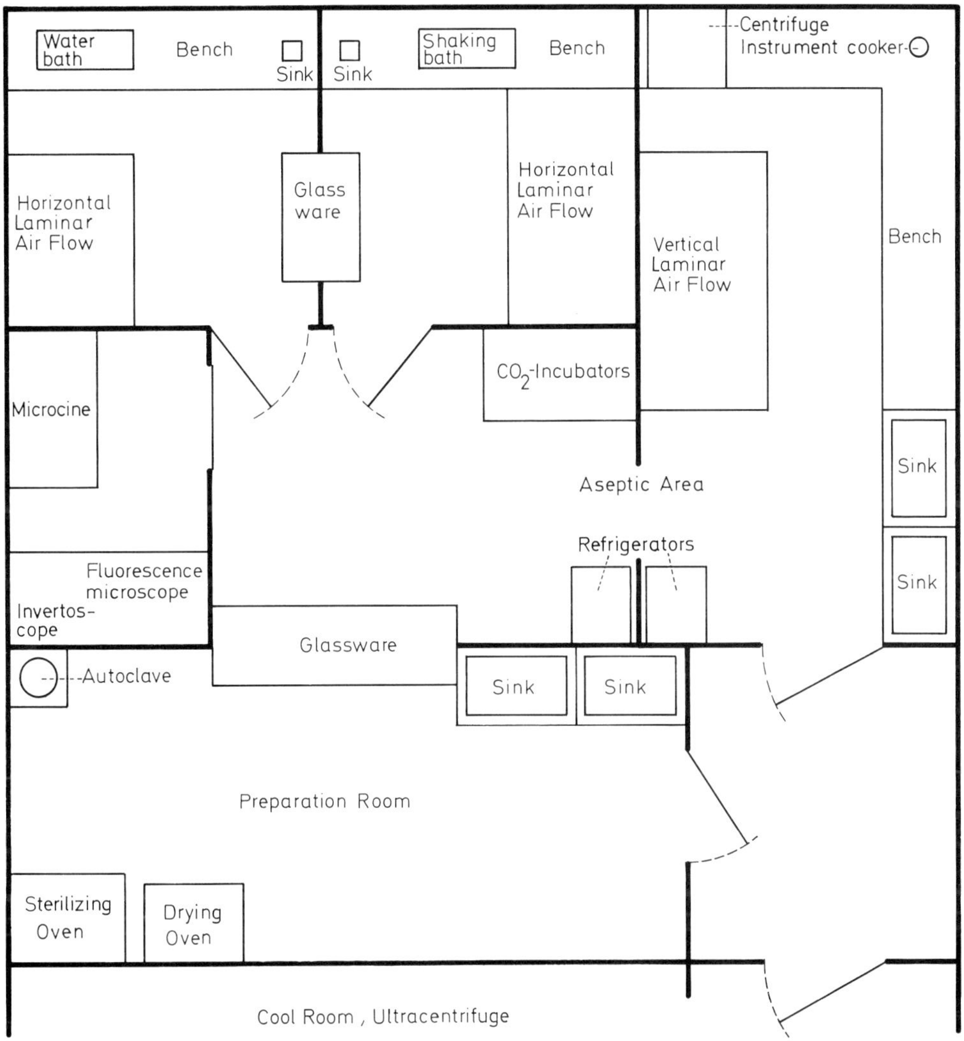

Fig. 1. Arrangement of our tissue culture laboratory. The facilities include separate rooms for washing up, sterilizing, and autoclaving (Preparation Room), microscopy, and an aseptic area with laminar air flow benches.

ethanol. If a laboratory suite is designed for tissue culture work, it should have separate rooms for preparation, sterilization, and microscopy arranged around an incubator room. A hot room with the air temperature at 37 °C is also desirable for a permanent tissue culture suite. For further suggestions for the design of a tissue culture laboratory, see Paul (1972, Chap. X) and Douglas and Dell'Orco (1979).

2.2 Equipment

Equipment usually found in a tissue culture laboratory include a CO_2 incubator, an inverted phase contrast microscope, a sterilizing oven, an autoclave, a refrigerator, a centrifuge, a magnetic stirrer, a rough and a sensitive balance, a deioniser for water, a pipette washer, and buckets for collecting and soaking used glassware.

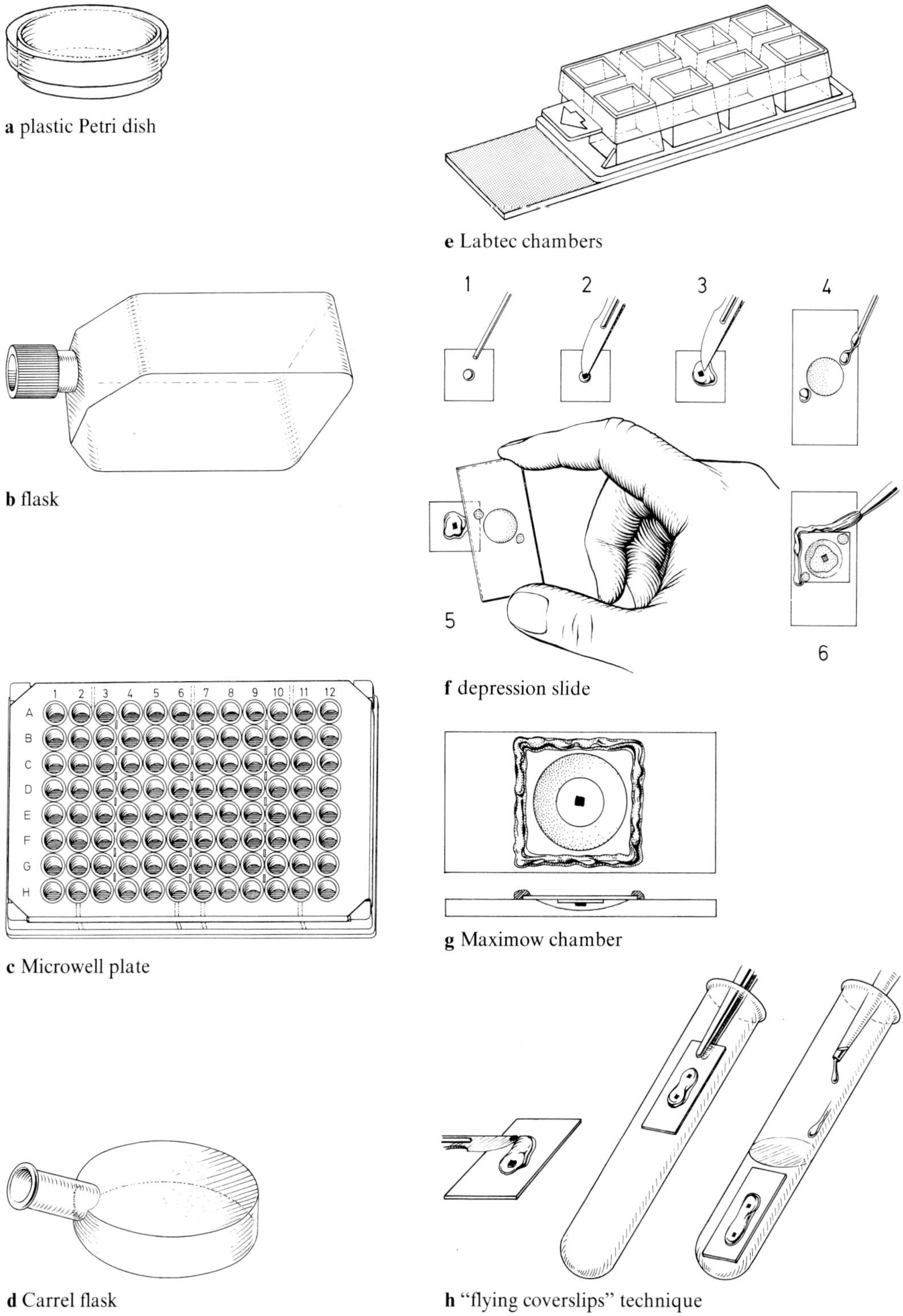

Fig. 2a–h. Vessels used for growing nerve tissue and cells

Instead of using a CO_2 incubator desiccators can be filled with the desired mixture of gas, sealed, and stored in a warm cupboard. A normal phase contrast microscope can be used for working with Rose chambers.

For microcinematography time-lapse studies we use a Zeiss Standard or inverted microscope fitted with a Bolex camera and Paillard-Wild Variotimer.

Requirements for glassware and instruments vary greatly according to the techniques used. A list of initial requirements, which is reasonably representative for most purposes, is given by Paul (1972, pp. 163–165).

2.3 Vessels Used for Growing Nerve Tissue and Cells

(Fig. 2)

A great variety of culture vessels is commercially available. Selecting the most appropriate vessels for a particular application can be a procedure as painstaking as selecting the most appropriate medium.

Many variations of depression slides, (Fig. 2f), Carrel flasks (Fig. 2d), and roller tubes are used for primary explantation techniques of nerve tissues and organs. Slide cultures, e.g., the Maximow double coverslip (Fig. 2g) are simple, relatively inexpensive, and favor differentiation and

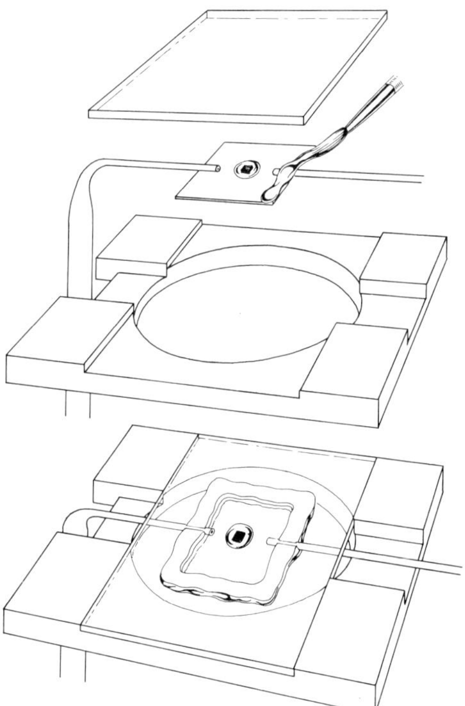

a Pomerat chamber

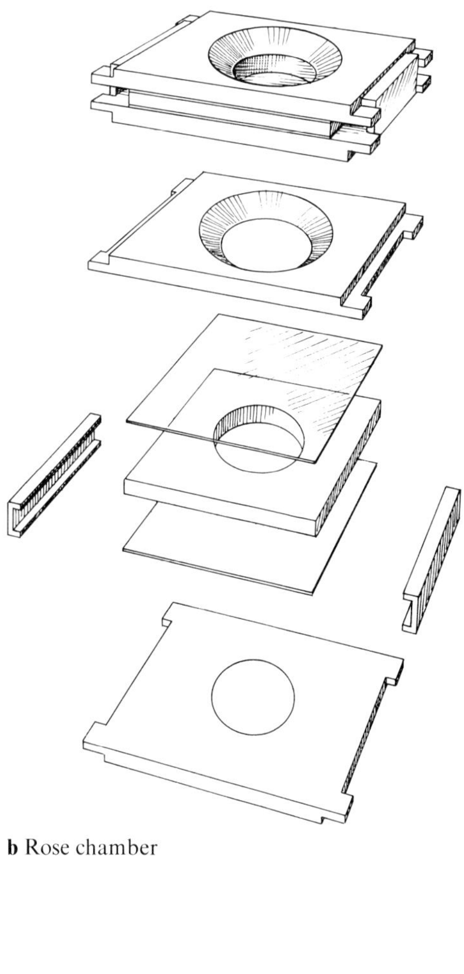

b Rose chamber

Fig. 3a, b. Culture vessels for growing nerve tissue and cells that can also be employed as perfusion chambers

maturation. Microscopic examination and photography is easy. The cells grow directly on the cover-slip and can be easily fixed and stained. Carrel flasks (Fig. 2d) must have excellent optical properties if they are to be favored over plastic flasks (Fig. 2b). Ordinary test tubes can be used as culture vessels and set up either in roller drums or in stationary racks. Coverslips can be slid into test tubes producing so-called flying coverslip cultures (Fig. 2d).

Plastic Petri dishes and microwell plates of various designs (Fig. 2a, c) and from different manufacturers are in use worldwide for nerve cell, tissue, and organ cultures. Although the plastic material is often of good optical quality, conditions for microscopic examinations can be improved by fitting coverslips with nontoxic glue, silicone grease, or wax to the bottom of holes drilled into Petri dishes. Recently a gas-permeable plastic foil (Heraeus-Biofolie) has been developed which can be used as the bottom of culture vessels and which has considerably improved the oxygen supply of cultured cells. Another chamber system (Labtec) for culturing tissues and cells combining the advantages of the slide technique and microwell plates is also new on the market (Fig. 2e).

For providing optimum environmental conditions for nerve tissues and facilitating investigation of the effects of drugs various perfusion chamber models can be used. A simple one is the Pomerat chamber (Fig. 3a). The most widely used is probably the Rose chamber (Rose 1954), which consists of two coverslips sandwiched between a piece of silicone rubber with an aperture in the center to form the culture chamber on one side and two steel plates on the other side (Fig. 3b). More sophisticated perfusion chambers have been designed by Rieske and Kreutzberg (1978) and by Dvorak and Stotler (1971).

A tissue culture chamber fitted with a fixed-array multielectrode system in the floor which allows simultaneous morphological studies and long-term monitoring of single unit extracellular electrical activity of neurons has been designed by Gross et al. (1977).

The culture chamber mostly used in our laboratory is a slightly modified Rose chamber. The reasons for this preference are: optimum conditions for microscopic examinations and microcinematography time-lapse studies, easy handling for micromanipulation and intracellular electrophysiological recording techniques, and easy processing for further ultrastructural and biochemical studies.

3 General Lines of Culture Techniques

3.1 Preparation and Sterilization of Glassware and Other Tissue Culture Accessories

Goldseal coverslips (43×50 mm, thinness I) are used for Rose chambers and Goldseal coverslips (22 mm, round, thinness I, and 40 mm square, thinness III) for Maximow depression slides (plate glass, 75×45 mm and 7–8 mm thick). All other glassware should be borosilicate. When new, coverslips are cleaned by soaking in reagent-grade nitric acid (70%) for 24 h or by boiling them in detergent solution for 10 min. Then they are rinsed in tap water many times, in distilled water twice, once in 70% ethanol, and twice in absolute ethanol. The rack shown in Fig. 4a is convenient for this procedure and for drying the coverslips in the oven. Put 20 coverslips in a Petri dish and sterilize dry (200 °C for 2 h). To reuse coverslips wax and vaseline have to be removed with a chloroform swab.

All new glassware is first soaked in 10% reagent grade HCl overnight. Used glassware is soaked overnight in 2% 160 cc/2 gal R.B.S. 25 or another detergent, brushed in detergent, rinsed 10 times in tap and twice in distilled water. Glassware can also be cleaned by boiling in sodium meta-

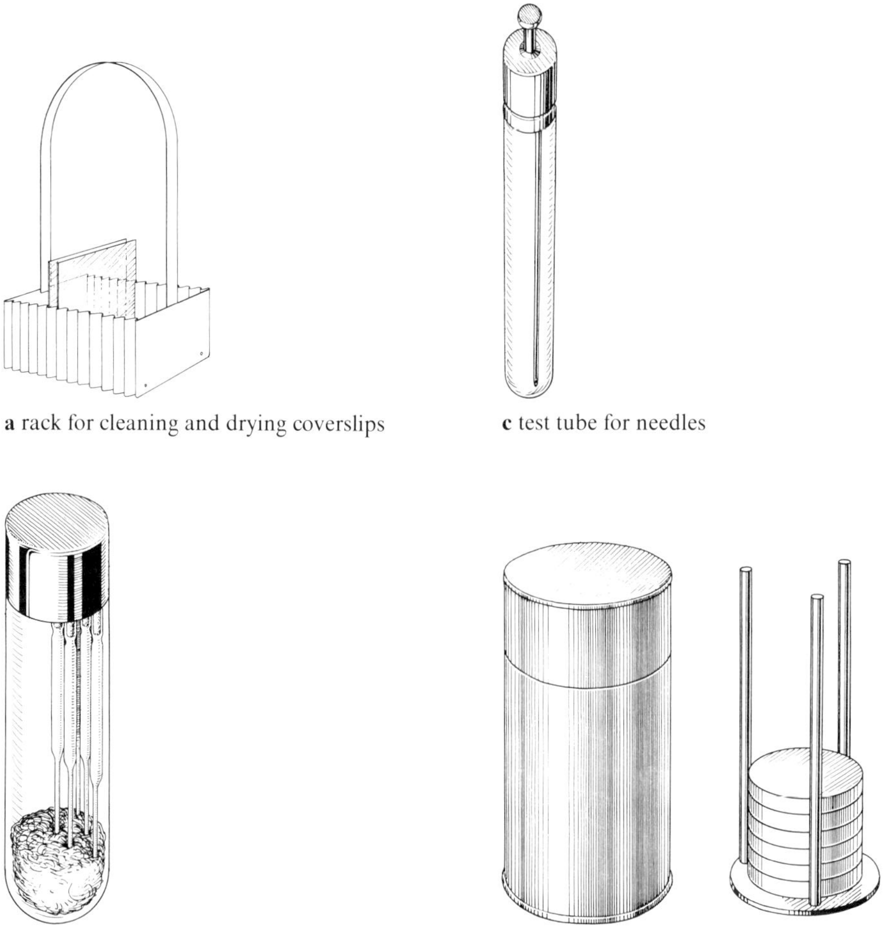

a rack for cleaning and drying coverslips

b pipette holder

c test tube for needles

d Petri dish holders

Fig. 4a–d. Tissue culture accessories

silicate (40 ml of a 20% stock solution are added to 2 liters of distilled water). The glassware is then rinsed once in distilled water and soaked overnight in 1% HCl in distilled water. After repeated rinsing with hot and cold distilled water, it is dried at 250 °C for 2 h. For sterilizing, items are either put into culture dish holders (Fig. 4d) or wrapped in aluminium foil or a heat-resistant paper.

Pipettes may be soaked overnight in 2% R.B.S. 25 in a pipette washer, boiled in R.B.S. for 20 min, rinsed exhaustively in tap and distilled water, plugged with cotton wool, dried, and sterilized in a pipette holder (Fig. 4b).

Silicon rubber gaskets for Rose chambers are boiled in tap and distilled water, dried in Petri dishes and autoclaved for 20 min at 121 °C (15 psi).

Hyponeedles and syringes are boiled in 1% liquinox for 30 min, washed in tap water, and boiled in distilled water before being dried and sterilized. We keep needles in test tubes fitted with metal caps. (Fig. 4c).

For autoclaving we use an autoclave, type Webeco (POLZIN, Kiel, German Fed-

Table 1

Item	Time	Temperature	Pressure
Glassware	20 – 30 min	121 °C	15 psi
Millipore filters and stainless steel filter holders	10 min	121 °C	15 psi
Gelman filters and plastic holders	15 min	121 °C	15 psi

eral Republic). Recommended times and temperatures for autoclaving are given in Table 1.

To avoid rupturing the filters the autoclave should be exhausted slowly. Solutions in flasks up to 250 ml volume should not be autoclaved for more than 10 min.

3.2 Solutions, Media, and Special Culture Surfaces

The media used for growth of tissue and cells in culture contain buffers, carbohydrates, salts, amino acids, and vitamins. It is recommended to use media which have already been found to work with a particular tissue culture system, whenever possible. Most media have a sodium bicarbonate-CO_2 buffering system requiring either 5% CO_2/95% air or 10% CO_2/90% air. Tissue culture media for the use in a normal air environment are also available (e.g., Leibowitz L-15).

Nutritional requirements which are peculiar to the culture of nerve tissue and cells have been reviewed by Silberberg (1972). High glucose concentrations are one such special requirement (Pomerat and Costero 1956). Survival of certain nerve cells in culture is enhanced by nerve growth factor (Levi-Montalcini and Angeletti 1968). Various sera are used to supplement defined culture media. A survey of commercially available tissue culture media has been given by Morton (1970). For a review on media and growth requirements of cell cultures see also Ham and McKeehan (1979). Recently, great efforts have been undertaken to grow cells in serum-free hormone-supplemented media (for review see Bottenstein et al. 1979), among them rat neuroblastoma, melanoma, and C_6 glial cells.

Solutions and media listed in this chapter are those used in our laboratory for culturing explants and isolated cells of adrenal medullae, PC 12 pheochromocytoma cells, and autonomic ganglia and neurons. The preparation and use of special media for culturing other cells and tissues from the central and peripheral nervous system are described in the corresponding chapters. As a rule our media are made up from 10× concentrated stock solutions, which we mostly purchase from Flow Laboratories and Gibco.

3.2.1 Hanks' Balanced Salt Solution (HBSS)

To prepare 100 ml of this solution 10 ml 10× concentrated HBSS (Flow), 89.5 ml autoclaved bi-distilled water, 0.47 ml 7.5% sodium bicarbonate (Flow), and 0.2 ml phenol red are mixed. For some purposes HBSS is supplemented with 10% or 20% fetal calf serum (FCS). For the transport of bovine adrenal medullae from the slaughterhouse to the laboratory gentamycin (20.0 mg/100 ml) is added to HBSS. The pH of all solutions and media is adjusted using 1 or 0.1 N HCl or NaOH, respectively.

3.2.2 Medium 199 (M 199)

For most of our cultures glucose-enriched M 199 supplemented with 20% FCS is used. The medium is prepared with 89.5 ml pyrogene-free distilled water (Ampuwa), 0.47 ml 7.5% sodium bicarbonate, 1.25 ml 200 mM glutamin, and 2.5 ml gentamycin (can be replaced by 1% of Gibco Antibiotic Mixture consisting of 50 units/ml penicillin and 26 μg/ml streptomycin) are added to 10 ml 10× concentrated M 199 (Flow). Then 5 ml of a 10% glucose stock solution is filtered through Millipore 0.45 and 0.2-μm filters and dispensed into the medium, together with 0.2 ml phenol red. Finally, FCS is added to give a final concentration of 20%. The medium is stored in 125-ml Erlenmeyer flasks and refrigerated until use. Media are not stored for more than 1 week. An aliquot of the medium is usually incubated at 37 °C for sterility testing (see Sect. 3.3.3).

3.2.3 Dulbeccos Modified Eagle Medium (DME Medium)

DME medium (Gibco), to which 3.7 g sodium bicarbonate are added per liter, is used in our laboratory for growing PC 12 pheochromocytoma cells. The medium is supplemented with 10% heat-inactivated horse serum (Gibco), 5% FCS (Flow), and 1% of Gibco Antibiotic mixture (optional if a careful technique is used).

3.2.4 Collagenase Solution

For enzymatic dissociation of tissue and softening of explants we use collagenase (Worthington Biochemical Corporation). 100 mg collagenase is dissolved in 100 ml of Eagles Minimum Essential Medium (EMEM) (containing Ca^{2+} and MG^{2+}, since lack of these ions inhibits collagenase) or HBSS, passed through a Millipore 0.45 μm filter, dispersed in 1 ml amounts, and frozen at –25 °C. A combination of 0.5% collagenase and 0.5% elastase (Sigma) can be profitably used for the dissociation of collagenase-resistant tissues.

For the perfusion of bovine adrenal medullae we use a 0.5% solution of collagenase (see Sect. 4.3).

3.2.5 Trypsin Solution

Trypsin digestion occupies a central position among disaggregation methods for the preparation of cell suspensions from fresh tissues. Trypsin is commonly used at 0.1%–0.5%. We dissolve 0.125% Trypsin either in Ca^{2+}- and Mg^{2+}-free phosphate-buffered saline (PBS) or Dulbeccos Balanced Salt Solution supplemented with 2 g/liter of glucose and 1 ml/liter of phenol red, stir it in cold for one hour and filter it through 0.45-μ and 0.2-μ millipore filters. Amounts of 25 cc are stored at –25 °C and thawed just before use.

3.2.6 Preparation of Collagen-Coated Coverslips

Many isolated tissues and cells, in particular neurons, grow better on collagen than on plastic or glass surfaces. Reconstituted rat-tail collagen, as suggested by Ehrmann and Gey (1956), has proved very useful in morphological studies and has been adapted for both coverslip and test tube cultures.

We mostly prepare our collagen according to a recipe given by Bornstein (1973). Freshly obtained tails from two to four 400–500 g rats are soaked with 80% ethanol for 15 min. The tails are fractured successively from the tip to the root into small pieces, the tendons are pulled out and allowed to drop into a Petri dish containing sterile distilled water. The tendons are teased apart into finer filaments, transferred to a sterile 150 ml bottle containing 75–100 ml of 1:1000 acetic acid solution depending on the total mass of tendon. After storage at 4 °C for 24 h, the contents of the bottle is transferred to sterile centrifuge tubes and centrifuged at 6,000–7,000 rpm at 4 °C for 1–2 h. The supernate is removed, stored at 4 °C, and can be used later, if the collagen has the appropriate viscosity to be spread on coverslips. Otherwise, it is stored until dialysis. If the tendons have not separated from the supernate, up to 25 ml of acetic solution can be added and the contents thoroughly shaken. The mixture is spun again and the supernate removed. For dialysing, a section of 7/8-in. dialyzer tubing is tied onto a glass tube which is held in the center hole of a stopper of a 1-liter flask containing 700 ml of distilled water (Fig. 5). The unit is autoclaved for 30 min and, after cooling,

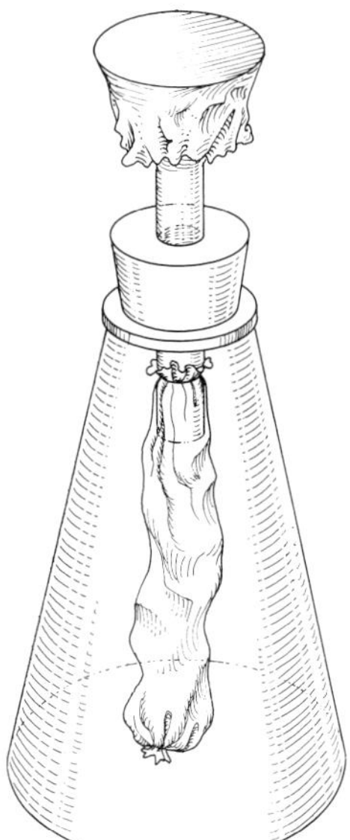

Fig. 5. Unit for dialysing collagen solution

7–10 ml of the supernate is placed into a cellophane bag and dialysed for 24–48 h at 4 °C until the solution has reached an adequate viscosity. The solution can be stored in sterile bottles at 4 °C for up to 6 months.

To prepare collagen-coated coverslips one to two drops of collagen are placed on a coverglass and spread with a glass rod. Then small pieces of filter paper are soaked in strong ammonia for 5 min and the paper is put at the edge of a Petri dish containing the collagen-coated coverslip and left until the collagen gels (up to 10 min). The coverslip is washed in three changes of distilled water (10 min, overnight, and again 10 min) and stored at 4 °C in HBSS plus 10% FCS until use.

For the preparation of collagen-coated coverslips or Petri dishes from acid soluble calf skin collagen powder (Sigma), 50 mg of the powder are dissolved in 0.5 ml of pure acetic acid to give a highly viscous solution. This solution is diluted with distilled water to 100 ml and a small amount put into a Petri dish, swirled around, and poured into another dish, until a number of dishes has been coated. The residue of collagen will dry in a dish within 3–4 h. However, in our experience the quality of reconstituted rat-tail collagen in terms of survival of adrenal chromaffin cells and sympathetic neurons is superior to acid soluble calf-skin collagen surfaces.

As an alternative to the collagen preparation described by Bornstein (1973, as mentioned previously), a clear collagen extract (one adult rat tail per 250 ml of 0.1% v/v acetic acid) can be diluted 1:4 with distilled water and three drops can be placed on a coverslip. The coverslips are dried in a desiccator for 24 h at room temperature and sterilized by ultraviolet irradiation (Hawrot and Patterson 1979).

3.2.7 Preparation of Culture Surfaces Other Than Collagen

Polylysine- and polyornithine-treated coverslips have been successfully used for culturing various neuronal and nonneuronal cell types, although survival of the cells in long-term cultures (7–14 days) is not always optimal (Yavin and Yavin 1974).

Polylysine can be linked to an underlying layer of dried gelatin, which has to be activated by incubation with glutaraldehyde. A few drops of 7.5 mg/ml swine-skin gelatin are dissolved by heating in a hot water bath and applied to the coverslip. After drying 2.5% glutaraldehyde in 0.12 M sodium phosphate buffer, pH 7.4, is added. After 1 h the coverslips are rinsed twice with distilled water and 5 mg/ml polylysine in a solution of 0.15 M sodium borate buffer, pH 8.4, is added to the gelatin. The coverslips are stored at 4 °C overnight, rinsed twice with distilled water and several times with HBSS prior to UV sterilization and use. Finally, pre-existing monolayers of nonneuronal cells can be used as substrata for growing neuronal cell and tissue cultures.

3.3 Preparation of Cultures

3.3.1 General Lines of Preparation

Before dissection starts cupboards and drawers are stocked with sterile supplies and all surfaces are wiped down with 70% and 100% ethanol. Sterile hoods with laminar air flow are turned on 15 min before work starts. Instruments are boiled for 20 min, put into Petri dishes (one pair of forceps and scissors in each dish), and stored under the sterile hood.

3.3.2 Some General Remarks on Dispersion and Disruption of Tissues

Methods used for preparing tissue fragments and isolated cells include mechanical, chemical, and enzymic procedures. Most frequently used techniques are combinations of two or all three categories. Whatever method is chosen, there are a few general points which should be observed in all cases as far as it is possible.

For the preparation of the tissue it is important that it is kept moist. A large choice of balanced salt solutions (e.g., HBSS, Sect. 3.2.1) are available for this purpose (for the composition of commercially available balanced salt solutions see manuals of various suppliers and Bashor 1979, p. 121). They provide the cells with water and inorganic ions, maintain a physiological pH and osmotic pressure. If a salt solution is used at an air atmospheric pressure, it should not be buffered with bicarbonate, since loss of CO_2 will cause the solution to become too alkaline. Phenol red as an indicator of pH should be included.

A minimal amount of time should elapse between extirpation of the tissue and initiation of culture. If transportation and extensive storage is involved glucose should be added to the salt solution and the storage vessels should be chilled with ice. If organs or tissues are prepared for explant or single cell cultures they should be cut into 1–3 mm cubes by passing two very sharp scalpels smoothly in opposite directions through the tissue. Scissors should be avoided. Further mechanical disruption of the fragments include shaking on a gyrorotary shaker, vortexing, triturating with wide-bore and fine-bore pipettes, and passing the mince through a nylon or stainless-steel mesh. Tissues from early embryological stages are more suitable for this type of disrupting fragments than tissues from postnatal animals.

More frequently, however, enzymic and/or chemical disruption methods combined with mild mechanical treatment will be used. Trypsin, collagenase, hyaluronidase, elastase, papain, pronase, and desoxyribonuclease are the most popularly used enzymes. The choice of the most suitable enzyme preparation depends upon its properties, the intended use, and precedents described in the literature. For example, four types of crude collagenase are available from Worthington Biochemical Corporation. Type I has a "normal balance" of enzyme activities, Type II has a high clostridian activity, Type III is low in proteolytic activity, and Type IV has low tryptic activity. One consideration in the choice of an enzyme is the exclusion or inclusion of calcium and magnesium and the addition of chelators such as EDTA or EGTA. Collagenase and DNase require the presence of Ca or Mg ions, respectively, while trypsin has to be dissolved in Ca^{2+}- and Mg^{2+}-free Salt Solutions.
Agitation of tissue fragments for obtaining cell suspensions is either accomplished by

trituration with large- or small-bore pipettes, by special trypsinizing flasks, by shaking, or by gentle vortexing.

Usually the procedure of cell dispersation is concluded by stopping the enzyme action (e.g., serum contains trypsin inhibitors) by filtration through a nylon mesh, brief centrifugation, washing, and inoculation into the culture vessel.

3.3.3 Cell Counting and Viability Testing

Cell counting and viability testing are important steps in cell culturing both before inoculation into culture vessels and for the quantitation of growth and the determination of the viable cell population during culture.

The most commonly used method for counting cells is that employing a hemocytometer (with Neubauer rulings). Cell suspensions are diluted with balanced salt solution to give final concentrations of 300,000–500,000 cells/ml, added to both chamber sides, and cells are counted in a sufficient number of squares using a microscope with 16-mm objective and a 10-power ocular. If 100 total cells are counted in 10 1 mm^2 squares and if the original cell suspension had been diluted 1:10, 100 cells $\times$ 10 (dilution) $\times$ 1000 (mm^3 in 1 cm^3) equals 1×10^6 cells/ml in the original suspension.

When a large number of samples has to be counted blood cells counters can be used (for details see Daly 1973, and Harris 1973). Chemical methods for calculating the growth of cells include protein and DNA determinations (for details see Patterson 1979).

Cell viability can be determined by numerous assay methods, of which the most commonly used are the "dye exclusion" tests. Dyes which have been used for this purpose include erythrocin, nigrosin, alcian blue, trypan blue, and acridine orange. Trypan blue is made up by adding 400 mg to 90 ml water containing 810 mg NaCl, 60 mg K_2HPO_4, and 50 mg methyl *p*-hydroxybenzoate. After boiling the mixture is cooled, adjusted to pH 7.2 and filled up with water to a final volume of 100 ml. 0.9 ml of a cell suspension and 0.1 ml trypan blue are mixed in a test tube and blue-stained cells are counted as nonviable in a hemocytometer.

3.3.4 Contamination in Cultures

Contamination, which may be bacterial, mycoplasmal, fungal, viral, or cellular, is incompatible with the concept of standardized cell and tissues cultures. Generally addition of antibiotics to cultures in order to prevent contamination does not solve the problem, since they can yield false negatives and mask contamination. Instead, certain precautionary measures can be recommended to avoid contamination: (1) all manipulations required for setting up cultures should be routinely conducted with extreme care and under sterile conditions; (2) batches of freshly purchased or mixed media and sera should be incubated at 37 °C and observed for 3–4 days before being used in cultures; (3) a set of various sterility tests for bacteria, fungi, and mycoplasma should be established in the laboratory (for details see McGarrity 1979).

3.3.5 Use of Antibiotics in Cell Culture

Although the growth of cells and tissues in cultures, which are free of antibiotics, must be the ultimate goal in culture technique, the use of antibiotics for preventing and eliminating microbial contaminants from cultures is sometimes unavoidable. For most purposes penicillin G and dihydrostreptomycin for elimination or suppression of bacteria and gentamycin to prevent growth of mycoplasmas can be recommended. If the bacterial contaminations turn out to be resistant to penicillin plus streptomycin, treatment with tetracycline or chloramphenicol should be tried. A list of commercially available antibiotics including their antimicrobial spectrum, the recommended concentration, and the stability in media is found in Perlman (1979).

4 Culture Techniques Currently Employed in Our Laboratory

4.1 Rat Adrenal Medulla – Explants

Newborn and young postnatal animals (up to 12 days) are killed by a blow on the head, soaked in 70% alcohol and transferred to a cork plate covered with aluminum foil, which has previously been sterilized by wiping down with 100% ethanol and flaming. Fetuses are removed from the uterus horns under aseptical conditions. The legs of animals are pinned to the plate with sterile needles, the skin of the abdomen and the thorax is opened and pinned to the plate. With another set of fine forceps and scissors the abdominal cavity is opened and adrenal glands are removed with jeweler's forceps and iridectomy scissors. Care is taken to avoid as much trauma as is possible. Adrenals are stored in a small Petri dish containing HBSS plus 10% FCS, which is chilled on ice, until the dissection has been completed. Then the glands are put onto a glass plate with a rough surface, kept in a Petri dish, and covered with a drop of HBSS to avoid drying of the tissue. Under microscopic control the fat and connective tissue capsule are stripped off and the cortex is carefully removed using iridectomy scissors and scalpel blades. The medulla is cut into small fragments the diameter of which should not exceed 0.3 mm and kept in ice-cold HBSS.

For culturing fragments as a whole, the pieces are incubated in 1% collagenase in HBSS or EMEM or in a mixture of 0.5% collagenase and 0.5% elastase in HBSS (see Sect. 3.2.4) for 10–30 min in a water bath at 37 °C with gentle shaking. The enzyme solutions should be thawed immediately before use. Then the pieces are thoroughly washed in HBSS. To set up the Rose chamber assembly one steel plate is turned upside down in a Petri dish and two small pieces of vaseline are put at two corners bracketing the central hole of the plate. The collagen-coated coverslip is removed from its storage fluid by means of coverglass forceps, drained of excess fluid, and centered face-up on the coverslip. Fragments of tissue are picked up in a drop of HBSS between fine jeweler's forceps and placed on the collagen in a row. Then a strip of dialyzing cellophane, which has been previously cut from dialysis tubing material, autoclaved for 30 min in distilled water, and soaked with respective nutrient medium (e.g., M 199) for 24 h is picked up with two pairs of forceps and placed over the explants. The Rose chamber is then closed by adding the rubber gasket, coverslip, steel plate and two clips, which help to tighten the steel plates together (Fig. 3 b). Parts of the cellophane strip extending over the edge of the chamber are cut off, the rubber surfaces are wiped with 70% and 100% ethanol, and two hypodermic needles are inserted from opposite sides through the rubber into the chamber using a strong pair of forceps and carefully avoiding breaking the coverslip. After having filled the chamber with growth medium, the needles are removed and the rubber surfaces wiped with ethanol again. The procedure of inserting and removing the hypodermic needles is repeated with every medium change.

Adrenal chromaffin cells, nerve cells, satellite, and fibroblast-like cells are clearly discernible in the outgrowth of the explants within 1–4 days in culture (Fig. 7 b). A large number of chromaffin cells form axon-like processes (Figs. 7 b, 8 a, b) and store predominantly primary amines (Unsicker and Chamley 1977). Dibutyrylic cyclic AMP and equimolar amounts of theophylline inhibit axon outgrowth in a dose-dependent fashion (Unsicker and Chamley 1976).

4.2 Rat Adrenal Medulla – Isolated Cells

After removing the cortex (see Sect. 4.1) and incubating small pieces of medullary tissue in 1% collagenase in HBSS for up to 60 min, the collagenase solution is discarded and replaced by 2 ml of 0.125% pre-warmed trypsin solution (see Sect. 3.2.5). Incubation is performed at 37 °C in a water bath under gentle shaking for 5–15 min. The supernatant containing liberated cells is removed with a Pasteur pipette to a centrifuge tube containing 2 ml cold FCS for inhibiting further action of trypsin. Trypsinization is repeated stepwise as often as necessary. Then the cells are centrifuged down at 800 rpm for 4 min, the supernatant carefully removed, and the cell pellet gently resuspended in final medium to the required dilution. Cells are injected into Rose Chambers using a 22-G needle. Enzyme-dispersed rat chromaffin cells extend neurite-like processes, which can grow up to several hundred microns. Formation of processes occurs spontaneously if large amounts of non-neuronal cells are present in the cultures. Nerve growth factor enhances axons outgrowth, while dexamethasone inhibits it (Unsicker et al. 1978 a, b, 1979; unpublished).

4.3 Bovine Adrenal Medulla – Isolated Cells

We produce isolated bovine adrenal medullary cells by a modified version of the method described by Fenwick et al. (1978; see also Livett et al. 1979).

Bovine adrenal glands are stored in HBSS supplemented with 10% FCS, freed from fat and cortical tissue, and perfused for 60–120 min through the cannulated adrenal vein with four 30 ml charges HBSS or PBS containing 0.25 or 0.5% collagenase (Worthington Type I). Perfusion is performed under sterile conditions using either a pump (LKB or Desaga) or a 20-ml syringe. The perfusate is kept at 37 °C. Usually the first perfusate containing mainly erythrocytes and cell debris is discarded, whereas the second and third perfusate containing numerous viable chromaffin cells is kept at 4 °C until washing (see below). In the last 30 ml charge the remaining tissue is finely minced and incubated in a shaking water bath at 37 °C for 30 min before being triturated with wide- and fine-bore pipettes. Cells from all charges (except charge I) are then filtered through a 200 μm nylon mesh, washed twice with HBSS, centrifuged twice at 100 g for 5 min, and resuspended in M 199 containing 20% FCS. The cell suspension obtained still contains a few erythrocytes and cell debris, which can be removed by: (1) centrifuging the cells on Percoll at 20 000 *g* for 30 min (recommended by Livett and associates), or (2) injecting the suspension into Rose chambers of Falcon flasks. Chromaffin cells preferentially attach to the collagen or plastic substratum within 15 min and erythrocytes can be removed by changing the medium. One adrenal gland yields $8–25 \times 10^6$ viable chromaffin cells (Figs. 6 d, 8 c). About 50% of the chromaffin cells kept in Rose chambers extend short, broad processes. These processes rarely grow longer than 60 μm and many of them retract after one week in culture. Nerve growth factor does not promote fiber outgrowth. Thus the capacity of bovine chromaffin cells to form neurite-like processes differs considerably from that which corresponding cells from young rats exhibit in vitro (Unsicker et al. 1978a, b, 1979).

4.4 Sympathetic and Parasympathetic (Ciliary) Ganglia

For the preparation of isolated cells and explants (Fig. 7) from sympathetic and ciliary ganglia (newborn rats and guinea

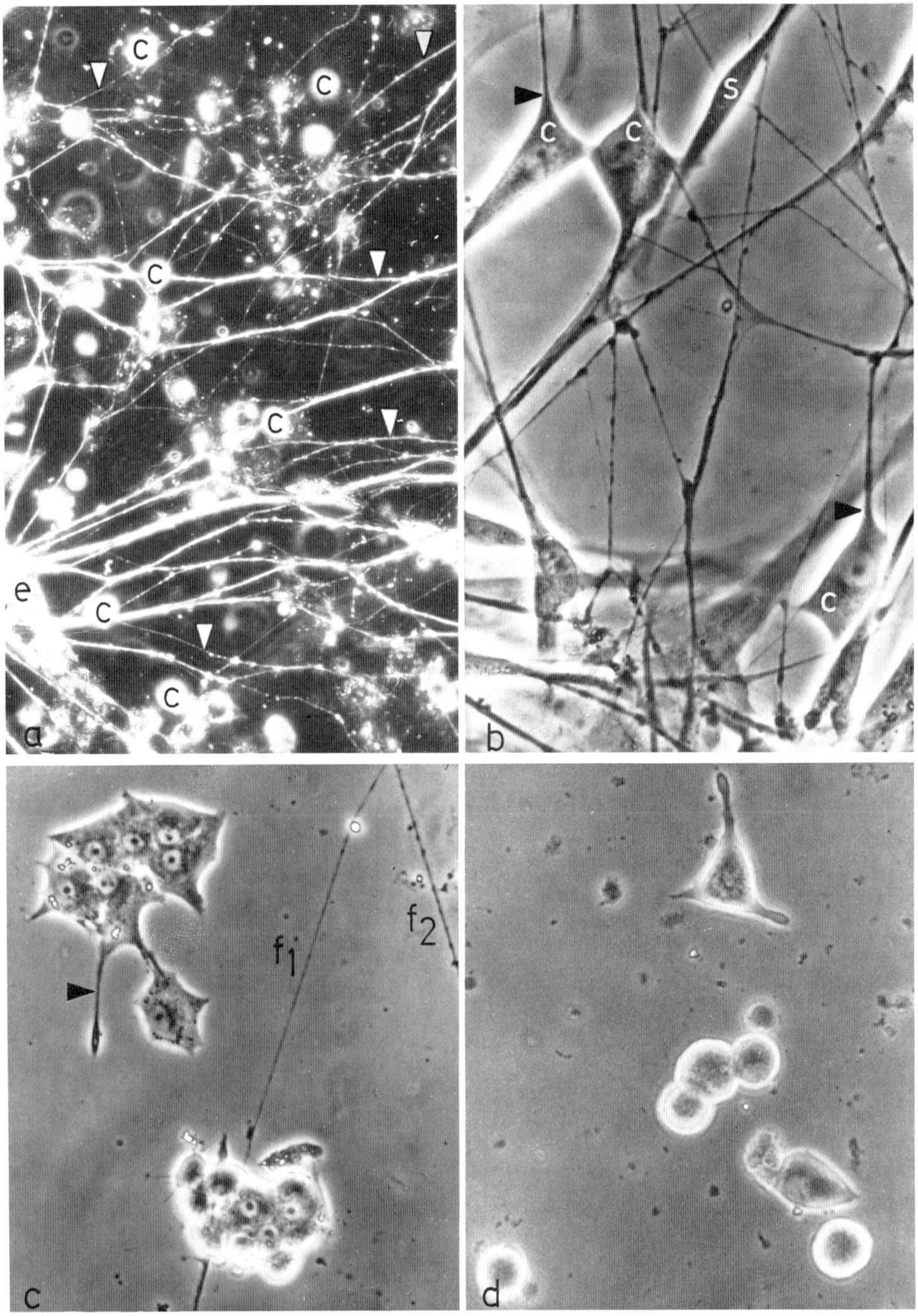

Fig. 6. **a** Dark field micrograph showing a coculture from a sympathetic ganglion explant (*e*) with numerous axonal extensions (*arrow heads*) and enzyme-dispersed single chromaffin cells (*c*). **b** Chromaffin cells (*c*) from a young rat adrenal medulla in culture. Note the dense meshwork of varicose and non-varicose nerve fibers, which, in a few instances (*arrows*), can be seen to originate from chromaffin cells. Schwann cells (*s*). **c** Small clumps of chromaffin cells in various stages of flattening out. One cell has started to extend a neurite-like process (*arrow head*), which ends in a growth cone-like tip. The two long fibres (f_1 and f_2) belong to the outgrowth of a sympathetic ganglion explant. **d** Isolated chromaffin cells from bovine adrenal medulla. **b–d** are phase contrast micrographs. Magnifications: **a** × 140; **b** × 720; **c** × 560; **d** × 500

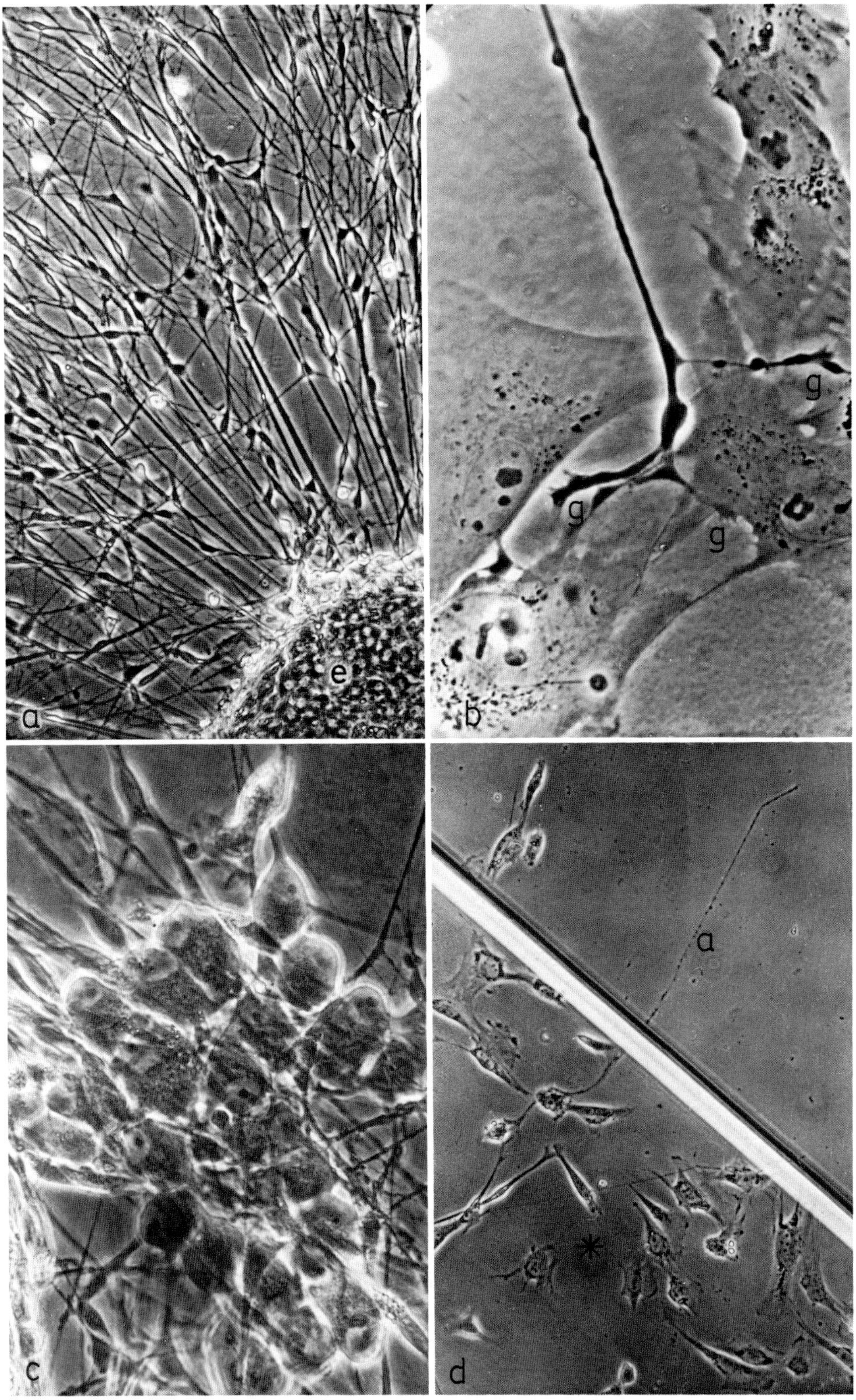
a
e
b
g
g
g
c
d
a
*

pigs) the same methods as described in Sect. 4.1 and 4.2 are routinely used in our laboratory. Alternatively, we also employ the method described by Patterson (cf. Hawrot and Patterson 1979) for obtaining dissociated sympathetic neurons. Ganglia are removed, cleaned from the surrounding tissue and connective tissue capsule, and teased apart using very fine watchmaker's forceps. The chunks obtained are triturated by several passages through a 22 G hypodermic needle using 2- or 5-ml syringes and subsequently with a vortexmixer for 3–5 min to produce standing waves but no swirling vortex. The resulting suspension is filtered through a 20 μm nylon mesh and dissociated cells are centrifuged, resuspended and plated in Rose chambers. Patterson and his group use Falcon Petri dishes, which are modified by affixing a polystyrene coverslip with paraffin to a 1-cm hole in the bottom of the dish.

For the growth of solitary isolated sympathetic neurons Patterson and his group have designed microculture systems using Falcon 3034 Terasaki culture plates (Reichardt and Patterson 1977) or coverslips carrying small collagen islands (Landis 1976).

5 Culture Methods for Neuronal Cells and Tissues (Not Routinely Used in Our Laboratory)

5.1 Organ and Tissue Cultures

Primary cultures consisting of fragments of central nervous system or peripheral ganglia belong to this category. Explant culture is a term which is also frequently applied to this type of culture. Clot techniques and later collagen-coated coverslips in Maximow depression-slide chambers as "lying-drop" preparations (Peterson et al. 1965; Murray 1965, 1971; Peterson and Crain 1970) and the "flying coverslip technique" (Hild and Tasaki 1962, 1964) have been the foundation of the study of organized differentiating nervous tissue in vitro. The Rose chamber (Rose 1954) is also well suited for the study of differentiating nervous tissue. Small plastic Petri dishes are being used more and more extensively.

The preparation procedure includes cutting the tissue (less than 1 mm in each dimension in order to facilitate diffusion) and simultaneously avoiding surgical trauma to the extremely fragile stuctures. Most commonly *embryonic* tissue (brain, spinal, cord, ganglia) is used; culture techniques for CNS tissues from adult mammals have not yet been satisfactorily developed (Crain 1966; cf., Kiernan and Pettit 1971; Drayton and Kiernan 1973). Growth media used for culturing mammalian CNS explants generally contain mammalian serum in a balanced salt solution together with embryo extract or other special nutrients (e.g., 20%–40% human placental serum, 25% Eagle's essential medium and Simm's balanced salt solution supplemented with glucose and insulin). With any explant culture one must be concerned with the viability of the fragments with prolonged culturing. One way to establish the viability of a tissue explant is to assay for certain marker enzymes (cf., Kim et al. 1972; Fry et al. 1973), in particular for enzymes related to the metabolism

◄

Fig. 7. a Sympathetic ganglion explant 5 days in culture. A large number of axons and axon bundles extend from the explant (*e*). Nuclei in the outgrowth belong to Schwann cells. **b** Growth cones (*g*) belonging to axons from a guinea pig ciliary ganglion palpate the surfaces of fibroblast-like cells. **c** Neurons from ciliary ganglion (newborn rat) 18 days in culture. **d** An axon (*a*) has grown out from a ciliary ganglion explant (not shown) cultured in a Rose chamber and has left the area covered with a strip of dialyzing cellophane (*asterisk*). Phase contrast micrographs. Magnifications: **a** ×140; **b** and **c** ×720; **d** ×140

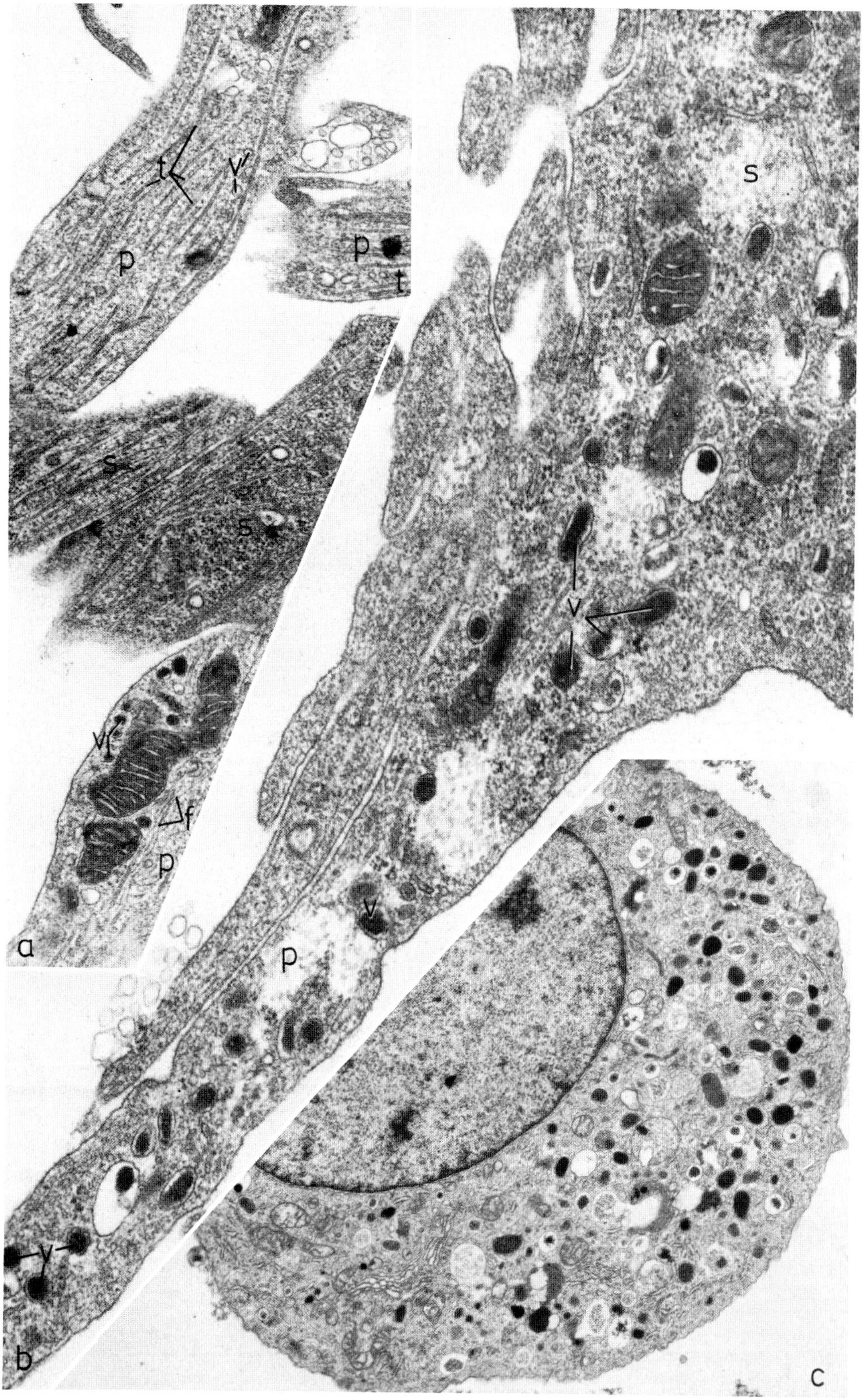

t
v
p
p
t
s
s
v
f
p
a
s
v
v
p
v
b
c

of acetylcholine and catecholamines, or to visualize specific cell products, e.g., catecholamines, by histochemical (Falck-Hillarp method, glyoxylic acid method) or immunocytochemical methods.

5.1.1 Spinal Cord Explants

5.1.1.1 Chick Embryo Spinal Cord (Fisher et al. 1975)

In an attempt to study the effect of osmotic pressure on neuronal differentiation in cultures of chick embryo spinal cord, Fisher et al. (1975) have excised spinal cords from stage 16–19 (2.5–3 days of incubation) or stage 36 (10 days). The embryos are removed, placed in HBSS, and spinal cord segments not longer than 6–7 somites or 0.4 mm are placed on collagen-coated 11×22 mm coverslips. The coverslips are put into test tubes (16×150 mm, Pyrex) and 0.7 ml of culture medium is added. The tubes are sealed with silicone rubber stoppers and, for the first 24 h held in a horizontal position. They are then transferred to a roller drum which revolves at 12 rev/h.

The culture medium consists of 61 ml M 199, 32 ml horse serum, 5 ml 9-day chick embryo extract (1:1 in HBSS), and 3.2 ml of a 20% glucose solution. The pH is adjusted to 7.9 with 1.4% $NaHCO_3$. Cultures are kept for 21 days and then fixed in Cajal's formalin-ammonium bromide fixative and stained by the Bodian Protaryol silver technique (Kim 1971).

5.1.1.2 Mouse and Rat Spinal Cord (13–15 Day Embryo) (Bornstein 1973)

The pregnant animal is anesthetized and soaked in 80% ethanol for 15 min. Skin and peritoneum are opened by two different sets of sterile instruments, the uterus is removed and placed in a sterile Petri dish. Fragments are prepared from the spinal cord of the embryo and kept in the nutrient solution chilled on ice until the dissection has been completed. The Maximow slide assembly is set up and a fragment is placed with a Pasteur pipette on a collagen-coated round coverslip together with a single drop of nutrient medium. Then the Maximow slide is sealed with a paraffin-vaseline mixture and the sealed slide incubated at 34 °C–35 °C in the lying-drop position. The nutrient medium consists of 33% human placental cord serum heat-inactivated at 56 °C for ½ h, 10% 9-day chick embryo extract, 50% Eagle's MEM plus glutamine, 7% Simm's Balanced Salt Solution, 600 mg glucose, and approximately 1.3 µg/ml achromycin.

5.1.1.3 Mouse Spinal Cord Primordia (Juurlink and Fedoroff 1979)

Spinal cord primordia are dissected out from mouse embryos (Theiler stages 14–16, 14–34 somites) by means of tungsten needles at the level of somites 8–12. The primordia are cut into thirds and placed on collagen-coated 11×12 mm coverslips, which in turn are placed into Lux 35 mm Petri dishes. A thin film of growth medium

Fig. 8a–c. Electron micrographs showing portions of rat (**a, b**) and bovine (**c**) chromaffin cells in culture. **a** Axonal profiles belonging to chromaffin cell processes (*p*) contain various kinds of clear- and dense-cored vesicles (*v*), microtubules (*t*) filaments (*f*), and mitochondria. Profiles of Schwann cell processes (*s*). **b** Process (*p*) extending from the soma (*s*) of a chromaffin cell. Both process and cell soma contain the typical chromaffin storage vesicles (*v*). **c** Chromaffin cell immediately after isolation from bovine adrenal medulla. Magnifications: **a** ×24,000; **b** ×36,000; **c** ×6900

is added to the fragments. After 5–10 h of incubation the fragments become firmly attached to the coverslips and growth medium is added to a final volume of 1.5 ml. Growth medium consists of 75 parts of modified Eagle's MEM, 5 parts of fetal mouse extract, and 20 parts of horse serum. The MEM is modified by raising the amino-acid levels five fold and the vitamins four fold. Glutamine is maintained at 2 mM, glucose at 30 mM, $NaHCO_3$ at 25 mM, and NaCl at 120 mM. Fetal mouse extract is prepared by homogenizing Theiler stage 24 mouse fetuses with an equal volume of HBSS. The resulting homogenate is kept for 2 h at 4 °C prior to centrifugation at 800 *g* for 15 min. The supernatant (= extract) is stored at –20 °C until use.

5.1.1.4 Chick Spinal Cord Explants from Neural Tube Stages

(Lyser 1976)

Twelve to 27 somite chick embryos (stages 11–15) are cultured in a fold of vitelline membrane from an unicubated chicken egg (Wolff 1961). Neural tube is freed from other tissues and, together with the vitelline membrane, placed on a millipore filter, which in turn rests upon a stainless steel grid. The grid is maintained in Falcon organ culture dishes.

5.1.1.5 Larval Frog Spinal Cord

(Koves and Pollack 1975)

Cross-sectional explants of early larval Rana pipiens spinal cord are placed on collagen-coated coverslips and sealed into a Maximow slide assembly. Growth medium consists of Eagles's MEM (with Earle's salt and without $NaHCO_3$), 50 µg/ml gentamycin, 100 mg/100 ml glucose, and 10 mM HEPES buffer adjusted to pH 7.4. Explants are incubated at 19 °C at an osmolarity of 260–265 mOsmol and can be maintained up to 4 weeks.

5.1.1.6 Neural Crest

The mechanisms controlling neural crest cell migration and differentiation have been a central issue in developmental neurobiology for many years, mainly because of the broad developmental potential of this tissue (Weston 1970). Neural crest cells usually explanted together with neural tube material have been frequently studied in vitro using avian embryos. The culture technique includes dissection of the region with needles and iris scissors, cleaning the neural tubes from other tissues by brief trypsinization (Cohen 1977), and plating the tubes either on collagen-coated Falcon Petri dishes (Cohen 1977) or, after wrapping it in a piece of vitelline membrane on a milipore filter strip, which is placed on a piece of gel-foam and incubated in a Leighton flask (Bjerre 1973). Growth media used: Bjerre (1973) mixes 3 ml human serum, 3 ml 50% chick embryo extract, and 7 ml Tyrode. Cohen's (1977) medium consists of 10% embryo extract, 15% horse serum, Eagle's MEM, and antibiotics. Maxwell (1976) uses a nutrient medium containing 50 ml H-17 special Ham's F 12 modified (Gibco), 35 ml HBSS, 10 ml FCS, 5 ml embryo extract, 3.0 mg L-glutamine, 1 ml penicillin-streptomycin (Gibco), and 6.3 ml of 5% $NaHCO_3$.

5.1.2 Brain Stem Explants

(Bornstein 1973)

The method for culturing explants of mouse and rat brain stem (13–15 day embryos) is essentially that described for spinal cord explants (see Sect. 5.1.1.2).

5.1.3 Cerebellum Explants

The cerebellum has been intensively investigated in organotypic culture since the 1950s (Pomerat and Castero 1956; Hild 1957; Bornstein and Murray 1958). In vitro studies on the cerebellum, whose cortex has a well-defined specific pattern of organization, illustrate that specific organization as well as differentiation of various neuronal and glial cell types can proceed in vitro. Light and electron microscopic as well as electrophysiological studies have revealed characteristic cerebellar cells and synapses in tissue culture (Wolf 1964, 1970; Kim 1970; Seil and Herndon 1970; Allerand 1971; Privat and Drian 1975; Crain 1976; for review see Hendelmann et al. 1977). In microcinematographic time-lapse studies the dynamic features of migrating cells were established (Privat et al. 1973; Meller et al. 1974).

5.1.3.1 Newborn Mouse and Rat Cerebellum
(Bornstein 1973)

The dissection procedure and culture method in Maximow depression slides is the same as that for spinal cord explants (see Sect. 5.1.1.2). The growth medium contains 40% heat-inactivated FCS, 25% Eagle's MEM with glutamine, 35% Simm's balanced salt solution, 600 mg% glucose, and 0.1 units/ml of low zinc glucagon-free insulin.

5.1.3.2 Embryonic Guinea-pig Cerebellum
(Hauw et al. 1974)

After stripping the leptomeninges, the cerebella (34th day of gestation) are cut into parasagittal sections and placed on collagen-coated coverslips, which are either stored in Leigthon tubes or form part of a Maximow or Rose chamber assembly. Nutrient medium consists of Eagle's MEM supplemented with 20% heat-inactivated calf serum, 5% chick embryo extract, and 50 mg/100 ml glucose.

5.1.3.3 Newborn Mouse Cerebellum
(Hendelmann et al. 1977)

Hendelmann and co-workers favor the Maximow double coverslip assembly. The nutrient medium consists of 50% Eagle's MEM, 25% chick embryo extract, and 25% human cord serum, supplemented with glucose to a final concentration of about 1000 mg%.

5.1.4 Cerebral Neocortex and Hippocampus

Explants of late fetal newborn rodent cerebral cortex show a sequence of morphological and bioelectric changes, which have been monitored and correlated to the in vivo situation in numerous studies (cf., Bornstein 1964; Kim 1972, 1973; LaVail and Wolf 1973; Seil et al. 1974; Crain 1976).

5.1.4.1 Mouse 18-day Embryo to 5-day Postnatal Cerebral Cortex
(Bornstein 1973)

The growth medium is the same as that for cerebellum (see Sect. 5.1.3.1) except that human placental cord serum is used in place of FCS. Explants are grown in the Maximow slide assembly.

5.1.4.2 Fetal Mouse Hippocampus
(Dreyfus et al. 1979)

Hippocampal slices (including the dentate gyrus) are taken from 18-day fetal mice and grown on collagen-coated coverslips in Maximow depression-slide chambers at 34.5 °C as lying-drop preparations. Nutrient medium consists of 33% human placental serum, 53% Eagle's MEM, 10% chick embryo extract, 600 mg% glucose, and achromycin with ascorbic acid (1.2 μg/ml).

5.1.5 Hypothalamus

Studies on organotypic explants of the hypothalamus have mainly emphasized the neurosecretory and bioelectric properties of this tissue (for review see Crain 1976; Pearson 1977).

A large number of processes known to occur in vivo can be observed in the cultured hypothalamus, e.g., the biosynthesis of the classic neurosecretory substances, releasing hormones, and their transport to storage and release sites.

For maintenance of the supraoptic nucleus from neonatal dogs in organotypic culture Sakai et al. (1974) have used coverslips in Leighton tubes and a growth medium consisting of 90% Eagle's MEM and 10% FCS. Explants of adult rat median eminence were cultured by Scott et al. (1974) on nylon nets up to 16 days using M 199.

5.1.6 Pineal Gland

The mammalian and avian gland in explant culture has been demonstrated to retain its in vivo structure and ultramorphological features as well as being able to synthetize melatonin (Klein and Weller 1970; Karasek 1974; Hungerford and Pomerat 1965; Romijn and Gelsema 1976; Nathanson et al. 1977).

Romijn and Gelsema (1976) have cultured fragments of adult rabbit pineals on stainless steel grids in 60×15 mm Falcon organ culture dishes. Nutrient media consisted either of 80% Trowell's T_8 medium plus 20% FCS or of BGJ^b medium supplemented with L-glutamine and insulin (0.001 mM). Nathanson et al. (1977) used Ham's F-12 medium supplemented with 10% FCS and penicillin-streptomycin.

5.1.7 Circumventricular Organs

The reader is referred to a substantial monography on avian circumventricular organs in culture (Moeller 1978) which also includes methodological aspects of the maintenance of choroid plexus, glycogen body, and pineal gland in vitro.

5.1.8 Retina

Although most work on retina cultures has been carried out with dissociated retinal cells, retina explants have also been studied in a few instances. LaVail and Hild (1971) used retinae from 2- and 3-day postnatal rats, which were explanted in plasma clots and grown in vitro with the flying coverslip method.

5.1.9 Organ of Corti

The development of the avian and mammalian otocyst from both embryos and newborn animals have been followed in vitro (Friedmann 1965; Van de Water and Ruben 1971; Orr 1974; Sobkowicz et al. 1975). Sobkowicz et al. (1975) cultured the organ of Corti of newborn mice in Maximow slides, on collagen-coated coverslips and in roller tubes for up to 27 days. The nutrient medium was composed of 40% fresh horse serum, 50% of a mixture containing equal amounts of modified Simm's balanced salt solution and Eagle's MEM, HEPES buffer added to achieve a concentration of 2×10^{-2} M, L-glutamine to achieve a concentration of 2×10^{-3} M, 7% of a modified Simm's balanced salt solution, and 3% of a solution of 20 g glucose in 100 ml modified Simm's salt solution.

5.1.10 Taste Buds

Taste buds require a nervous input for their normal development. An in vitro model for studying nerve-epithelial interactions has been devised by Farbman (1972). He explanted tongue slices including the cirumvallate or foliate areas together with the IX and X cranial ganglia on Millipore filters, which were then placed on stainless steel grids in glass culture dishes. The medium consisted of 50% Weymouth's Medium 752/1 plus 50% newborn calf or human cord serum enriched by 15 mg% ascorbic acid, 750 mg% glucose, 2 units/ml NGF, and 50 units/ml penicillin.

5.1.11 Peripheral Ganglia

A multitude of reports on cultured dorsal root (DRG), sympathetic and parasympathetic ganglia are available, using a large variety of culture techniques, which renders it difficult to make an appropriate selection. Standard methods for culturing DRG include those used by Peterson and Murray (1955) and M. B. Bunge et al. (1967). One standard procedure for DRG explant cultures (mouse and rat 15–18-day embryos) is certainly that recommended by Bornstein (1973). She uses a nutrient medium, which is also employed for growing spinal cord (see Sect. 5.1.1.2). A method for culturing adult DRG has been described by Scott (1977).

Following the discovery that nerve growth factor (NGF) initiates the outgrowth of a dense halo of nerve fibers from DRG isolated from 7–12 day-old chick embryos (Levi-Montalcini and Angeletti 1968) explant cultures of chick DRG have become a useful tool for studying the effects of NGF and for estimating its biological activity (Fenton 1970). A simple culture system for chick DRG has been described by Mizel and Bamburg (1976). The spinal cord with attached DRG is exposed and transferred to F 12 medium. The ganglia are then isolated from the cord by removing the meninges. Falcon dishes (60 mm) are overlayered with 3–5 ml FCS for approx. 1 min. The excess medium is removed, ganglia are transferred to the dishes with a Pasteur pipette, and each ganglion is separately covered with a very thin film of FCS. Ganglia are preincubated at 25 °C for 1 h prior to the addition of 5 ml medium, which consists of F 12, 10% FCS, 100 μg/ml streptomycin sulfate, 100 units/ml penicillin, and 2 μg/ml cytosine arabinonucleoside.

Methods for culturing explants of sympathetic ganglia (chick, rat, and guinea pig) have been described by Chamley et al. (1972a, b) and Benitez et al. (1974) among others. For details of the method employed in our laboratory for culturing sympathetic and ciliary ganglia see Sect. 4.4.

5.1.12 Evertebrate Ganglia

Explants of evertebrate ganglia can be successfully maintained in vitro. As an example a culture system for corpora cardiaca and corpora allata of *Periplaneta americana* (Seshan and Levi-Montalcini 1971) will be described.

Nymphal and adult specimens are anesthetized with carbon dioxide. The dorsal cervical sclerite is sterilized with cotton moistened with 95% ethanol. A slit is made in this region, the corpora allata and cardiaca are removed with watchmaker's forceps and transferred to sterilized insect Ringer solution. The organs or fragments of organs are made to adhere by gentle pressure to small glass coverslips, which in turn are placed in a Petri dish. Tissue culture medium consists of five parts of Schneider insect solution, four parts Eagle's basal medium, 100 units/ml penicillin, 100 μg/ml streptomycin, and 125 μg/ml fungizone.

5.2 Dissociated Cells

Primary cultures of cells dissociated from neural tissue are now extensively used in many neurobiological disciplines. Most current techniques are based on Moscona's (1952) method for the dissociation of chick retinae. Dissociation techniques were further developed by Levi-Montalcini (see also Levi-Montalcini and Angeletti 1963) and then applied by Nakai (1956) to grow isolated chick embryo DRG neurons. In general the procedure involves enzymatic (pronase, trypsin) or mechanical (nylon sieve, Pasteur pipette, syringe) dissociation or a combination of the two (see also Sect. 3.3.2). The dissociated cells can be successfully cultivated either on a collagen substrate in various culture chambers (Maximow depression slides, Rose chambers, plastic flasks, Petri dishes, roller tubes) or directly on plastic surfaces. Due to the enormously expanded literature in this field, I can only present what I think are typical examples for the application of various dissociation techniques.

5.2.1 Spinal Cord

Work with dissociated cells from spinal cord has been carried out by Cavanaugh (1955), Meller et al. (1969), Scott et al. (1969), Bornstein (1972), Bornstein and Model (1972), Kim (1972), Bird and James (1973, 1975 a, b), Contestabile et al. (1973), Fischbach and Dichter (1974), Ransom et al. (1977), Berg (1978), and others. The culture procedure as described by Ransom et al. (1977) is given in detail:

Spinal cords are taken from 12–14 day-old mouse embryos. The pregnant mice are killed by placing them in a CO_2 atmosphere for 2 or 3 min and then fracturing their necks in order to avoid possible damage to tissue due to chloroform or ether anesthesia. The embryos are removed and placed in a culture dish containing a solution, which is made up from 50 ml of 20× concentrated Puck's Dl salt solution, 6 g glucose, 15 g sucrose/liter, and 10 mM HEPES buffer pH 7.3. The complete solution is adjusted to 330 mosM with water. Spinal cords are removed within 1 min, minced with iridectomy scissors, and the equivalent of five spinal cords is transferred to a 15-ml centrifuge tube containing 1.5 ml of nutrient medium. This medium consists of 80% Eagle's MEM, 600 mg/100 ml glucose, 10% heat-inactivated horse serum, 10% FCS, and 1.5 g/liter $NaHCO_3$. No antibiotics are used. The tissue fragments in the centrifuge tube are gently triturated (five to ten times) using a Pasteur pipette. The suspension is allowed to settle for a few minutes and the supernatant is removed and saved. After adding another 1 ml of nutrient medium to the centrifuge tube trituration is repeated using a Pasteur pipette with a slightly narrowed orifice. Then the suspension is again allowed to settle. This cycle of trituration is repeated until the supernatant volume reaches about 4–5 ml. This final suspension is plated on collagen-coated 35 mm Falcon Petri dishes by adding 0.5 ml of the suspension (about 1.5×10^6 cells) to plates containing 1 ml of medium which has been preincubated for about an hour. The first medium change is not performed until day 3–5. With the second medium change 15 μg/ml 5′-fluoro-2′-deoxyuridine (FdU) and 35 μg/ml uridine are added and FCS is deleted in order to control the rapid division of nonneuronal cells. The medium containing FdU and uridine is replaced after 2 days by normal medium.

5.2.2 Brain

The conditions for culturing dissociated brain cells have been systematically explored by Sensenbrenner and co-workers (for review see Sensenbrenner 1977). Dissociated cells from cerebellum have been studied by Lasher and Zagon (1972), Contestabile et al. (1973), Nelson and Peacock (1973), Burry and Lasher (1975, 1978 a, b), Messer (1977), Trenkner and Sidman (1977), and Kása and Bánsághi (1979). A recipe for dissociating *cerebellar cells* from postnatal mice has also been communicated by Barkley et al. (1973). This procedure has been closely followed by Trenkner and Sidman (1977): Cerebella are dissected out from 7-day-old mice, immersed in a Ca^{2+}- and Mg^{2+}-free salt solution, washed three times in this solution, and incubated in 1% trypsin for 14 min at room temperature (20 °C). After washing the tissue is transferred into a medium, which consists of Eagle's basal medium supplemented with 0.25% glucose and 0.05% DNase, where it is triturated with fire-polished long-tip Pasteur pipettes with decreasing pore sizes. The supernate is transferred to a centrifuge tube and centrifuged at 600 rpm for 8–10 min at 4 °C. The pellet is resuspended in culture medium containing Eagle's basal medium supplemented with 0.25% glucose, 2 mM glutamine, 25 U/ml penicillin, 25 U/ml streptomycin, and 10% horse serum. Trenkner and Sidman (1977) plate their single-cell suspension in Falcon microtiter plates at a concentration of 5×10^4–1×10^5 cells per 1 µl medium per well.

Reports on cultures with *cerebral dissociated cells* are numerous and include those by Sensenbrenner et al. (1971 a, b), Booher and Sensenbrenner (1972), Grosse and Lindner (1972, 1974, 1975), Rosenberg (1973), Shapiro and Schrier (1973), Breen and De Vellis (1974), Goodfrey et al. (1975), Yavin and Yavin (1974), Wiesmann et al. (1975), Bonkowski and Dryden (1976), Honegger and Richelson (1976), Bird and James (1977), Dichter (1978) and Peacock et al. (1979).

Dichter (1978) uses a tissue culture technique for growing cortical neurons which is similar to one described by Fischbach (1972) for growing dissociated chick nerve cells. He minces cortices into small pieces and collects them in 0.7 ml of 0.027% trypsin in MEM. Then the tissue is incubated at 37 °C for 2 h and 4.5 ml MEM plus 5% FCS is added. The tissue is triturated 10 times with a Pasteur pipette, once with a narrow-bored pipette and then diluted to 10 ml with FCS. The suspension is filtered through sterilized lens paper and cells plated at 1.2–1.6×10^5 cells on 35-mm Falcon Petri dishes, which have been previously covered with a layer of nonneuronal cells from 15 day rat embryos. Growth medium consists of Eagle's MEM plus 5% rat serum, 100 mg% glucose, 2 mM glutamine, and 20 U/ml penicillin plus streptomycin. Cytosine arabinoside (10^{-5} M for 24 h) is used to inhibit the proliferation of nonneuronal cells.

5.2.3 Pineal Gland

A method for obtaining primary cell cultures from pineal glands of 2-day-old rats and their co-culture with sympathetic neurons has been described by Rowe et al. (1977). Pineal glands are removed and collected in 2 ml of solution containing 137 mM NaCl, 5.4 mM KCl, 0.17 mM Na_2HPO_4, 0.22 mM KH_2PO_4, 5.5 mM glucose, and 59 mM sucrose. Then glands from six litters are incubated in 10 ml of this solution with 0.25% crude trypsin for 30 min at 36 °C and triturated for obtaining single cells. 2 ml FCS are added to the suspension, which is then centrifuged at 500 g for 2 min at room temperature. Cell pellets are resuspended in 11 ml l-15 medium and plated at 0.5 ml portions on Falcon dishes with 7 cm² surface area, to which 1 ml of the same medium is added. After incubation for 48–72 h the medium is changed to either MEM or Dulbecco's MEM, each of which contains 10% FCS.

Cells in these cultures display typical ultrastructural features of pinealocytes from neonatal rats and respond to dibutyryl-cyclic AMP treatment by an increase in the activity of serotonin *N*-acetyltransferase.

5.2.4 Retina

Retina is a relatively simple neuronal system, which contains no mesenchymal cells and whose differentiation can be conveniently studied in vitro (e.g., Sheffield and Moscona 1970; Vogel et al. Combes et al. 1977). A standard recipe for the dissociation of chick (8-day-old) retina (Vogel et al. 1976) is as follows: In Eagle's basal medium dissected retinae are incubated in Ca^{2+}- and Mg^{2+}-free Tyrode for 15 min at 36 °C in an atmosphere of 5% CO_2–95% air. Trypsin and DNase I are added to give final concentrations of 2.5 and 0.05 mg of protein per ml, respectively. After another 15 min incubation. 0.5 ml of cold growth medium (80% Eagle's basal medium with 2 mM glutamine and 20% FCS) are added per retina and the tissue is sedimented by low-speed centrifugation. The pellet is mixed with 0.3 ml of culture medium per retina and triturated with a fire-polished Pasteur pipette. Then 9×10^6 cells in 1.5 ml of growth medium are added to a 35-mm Falcon collagen-coated Petri dish. The cells synthetize synapses which resemble those of the intact retina and are capable of nicotinic acetylcholine receptor synthesis as judged by their α-bungarotoxin binding capacity.

5.2.5 Dorsal Root Ganglia

Dissociated dorsal root ganglia (DRG) neurons have been maintained in short- and long-term cultures for morphological, electrophysiological, and biochemical studies (Nakai 1956; Levi-Montalcini and Angeletti 1963; Scott et al. 1969; Sensenbrenner et al. 1969, 1971 a, b; Lodin et al. 1970, 1973; Miller et al. 1970; Varon and Raiborn 1971; Okun 1972; Varon et al. 1973; Meller 1974; Obata 1974; Bird and Lieberman 1976; Rieske and Kreutzberg 1977; Waxman et al. 1977; Skaper and Varon 1979).

General features of the dissociation technique include the use of trypsin and gentle aspiration of the ganglia fragments with a micropipette. After centrifugation and resuspension the cells are plated into Petri dishes or onto collagen-coated coverslips. Eagle's minimal essential medium with 10% heat-inactivated horse serum and 2% chick embryo extract may be considered to be a useful nutrient medium. Omission of nerve growth factor results in massive degeneration of nerve cells within 48 h.

5.2.6 Sympathetic and Parasympathetic Ganglia

Our method for obtaining dissociated sympathetic neurons has been described in Sect. 4.4. A large amount of literature is available on isolated sympathetic neurons grown in vitro (Burdman 1968; England and Goldstein 1969; Bray 1970; Varon and Raiborn 1972; M. B. Bunge 1973; Mains and Patterson (1973 a, b, c; Jacobowitz and Greene 1974; Obata 1974; Patterson and Chun 1974; Rees and Bunge 1974; O'Lague et al. 1975; Patterson et al. 1975; Chun and Patterson 1977 a, b, c; Patterson and Chun 1977 a, b; Reichardt and Patterson 1977; Walicke et al. 1977; Estridge and Bunge 1978; Greene and Rein 1978; Helfand et al. 1978; Landis 1978; Wakshull et al. 1978; Kim et al. 1979). The main emphasis in these studies has been on the differentiation of the sympathetic neuron and on the determination of neurotransmitter function.

Recently increasing attention has been paid to parasympathetic (ciliary ganglia) neurons kept in vitro. These studies have aimed at obtaining information on principles of axon formation and elongation (Collins 1978; Essells and Nuttall 1978; Nuttall and Wessells 1979), conditions for survival (Bennett and Nurcombe 1979; Bennett and White 1979) and cholinergic neuronotropic factors (Varon et al. 1979). Bennett and associates dissociate ciliary ganglia from 9-day chick embryos in Ca^{2+}- and Mg^{2+}-free HBSS and 0.25% trypsin fo 30 min. Then the ganglia are washed three times in a medium containing 80% Eagle's basal medium, 10% FCS, 10% HBSS supplemented with 1000 U/ml benzyl penicillin and 2 mM glutamine and are disrupted into single cells by gentle aspiration with a fire-polished Pasteur pipette. The cells are grown on polyornithine-coated plastic Petri dishes.

5.2.7 Evertebrate Ganglia

Dissociated neurons from evertebrate ganglia have been successfully grown in vitro (Chen and Levi-Montalcini 1970; Ready and Nicholls 1979). The cells may survive for several weeks, maintain their morphological characteristics and membrane properties, sprout, and form selective connections. Ready and Nicholls (1979) use Leibowitz L-15 medium supplemented with 2% FCS, 6 mg/ml glucose, and 0.1 mg/ml gentamycin. The cells grow on polylysine- and collagen-coated plastic Petri dishes.

5.3 Pure Cultures of Neuronal and Nonneuronal (Glial) Cells

Heterogeneity of cell populations is a characteristic feature of the nervous system, but may be a serious obstacle for studies which want to investigate neuronal or glial properties separately. A large variety of techniques has been developed to obtain purified cell fractions using such divergent features as neuronal resistance against antimitotic agents and γ-irradiation, differential attachment to substrata or differential affinity binding via special cell surface constituents (for review see Varon 1977).

5.3.1 Differential Destruction

Selective destruction of nonneuronal cells by antimitotic agents is presumably one of the most popular techniques for obtaining pure neuronal cultures. Frequently used drugs are 5-fluorodeoxyuridine (FdU), cytosine arabinoside (ara-C), and aminopterin. FdU is a structural analog of deoxyuridine and it inhibits mitosis by inhibition of thymidine synthesis (Cohen et al. 1958; Heidelberger 1963) without being incorporated into DNA. Ara-C is a synthetic structural analog of cytidine and deoxycytidine, whose mode of action in killing dividing cells is not completely understood at present. Possibly its principal effects is on replicative and DNA polymerases (Stenstrom et al. 1974). Various schedules for treatment of cultures with FdU and ara-C have been designed.

A convenient dose for both FdU and ara-C is 10^{-5} M and it should be applied twice on two consecutive days. Longer treatments have also been applied (see Lazarus et al. 1976) (e.g., days 2 and 3 and days 6 and 7). A method for separation of Schwann cells and neurons from DRG using FdU and ara-C has been communicated by Wood (1976). Withholding nerve growth factor from DRG and sympathetic neuron cultures may lead to neuron-free nonneuronal subpopulations (Mains and Patterson 1973a, b; Varon et al. 1973). Omitting the HCO_3^-/CO_2 buffer system from the medium may be a tool for eliminating nonneuronal, fibroblast-like cells from rat superior cervical ganglia cultures (Mains and Patterson 1973a). Irradiation is another means for producing largely pure neuronal cultures. For obtaining chromaffin cell cultures which are virtually free from nonneuronal cells we use γ-irradiation from a cobalt source (6000 rad, 20–30 min, 50 cm distance).

5.3.2 Differential Attachment

Varon and Raiborn (1969) were the first to exploit the higher affinity of nonneuronal cells for glass in order to obtain essentially pure cultures of neurons. The approach has been successfully applied to cerebral (Varon and Raiborn 1969), DRG (Okun et al. 1972; Varon et al. 1973), and sympathetic ganglia cultures (Varon and Raiborn 1972; McCarthy and Partlow 1976). McCarthy's and Partlow's (1976) method involves periodic bursts of vertical vibrations, which are administered to the cultures during the first 4 h and prevent attachment of neurons but not of nonneuronal cells. Differential attachment of dissociated brain cells to plastic surfaces has been exploited to develop pure glial cell populations. Neuronal cells degenerate during the first 2 days and some oligodendroblasts survive for about 1 week, while astrocyte precursor cells survive longer and can even be induced to become mature astrocytes under dbcAMP treatment or after the addition of brain extract (Booher and Sensenbrenner 1972; Lim et al. 1973; Shapiro 1973; Sensenbrenner et al. 1977).

5.3.3 Cell Sorting with Flow Systems

Fluorescence-activated cell sorting is being applied increasingly to biological problems that require the manipulation of fractionated viable cells (Kreth and Herzenberg 1974; Arndt-Jovin and Jovin 1978). Campbell et al. (1977) have applied this approach to dissociated cerebellar cells.

5.3.4 Differential Sedimentation

Many bulk isolation procedures for obtaining cell fractions for biochemical analyses exploit different sedimentation properties, which depend on both size and density of cells. However, many of the solutions currently used (sucrose gradients, Ficoll gradients) have osmotic or toxic properties, which are harmful to neuronal cells. Percoll seems to be tolerated and has been used, e.g., to obtain relatively pure populations of bovine chromaffin cells (Livett, personal communication).

5.3.5 Selection of Cells by Affinity Binding

This cell separation technique exploits cell surface constituents such as hormonal receptors, lectin binding sites, and other cell surface antigens to bind specifically to ligands anchored to an insoluble substratum. Au and Varon (1979) have described an immunoaffinity chromatography system in which chick spinal cord cells are retained on columns containing immune globulin against spinal cord cells, while they pass through when the globulin used is not immunocompetent.

5.3.6 Other Methods for Separating Neuronal and Nonneuronal Cells

An entirely different approach for ganglionic cell separation has been used by Wood and Bunge (1975). DRG from perinatal rats is explanted and grown in nerve growth factor (NGF)-enriched medium, which allows both axon and nonneuronal cell outgrowth. The NGF-enriched medium is used alternatively every other day with a medium containing both NGF and antimitotic drugs, which destroys fibroblasts but allows Schwann cells to survice. After transferring the explants to a new dish a pure population of Schwann cells develops in the outgrowth left behind, while neurites unaccompanied by any other cells grow out from the explants.

5.4 Neuronal and Glial Cell Lines

The disadvantage of primary cell cultures, which do not continue to divide indefinitely, can be overcome by creating cell lines. Cell lines are capable of indefinite cell division and may exhibit interesting neuronal and glial properties. With established cell lines it is possible to select a single cell, which may continue to divide and form a population of cells that is called a clone. For generating new cell lines with a variety of genotypes and for analyzing mechanisms regulating the expression of various phenotypes the genetic material from two parental lines can be incorporated into a single "hybrid" cell (Amano et al. 1974; Hamprecht 1974).

Neuronal cell lines come from several sources. First, mouse neuroblastoma (C-1300) has found widespread use in neurobiology research, since it was established in cell culture in 1969 (Augusti-Tocco and Sato 1969; Schubert et al. 1969). Second, nitroso-urea compounds have been found to induce a large number of CNS tumors, which can be established in culture (Schubert et al. 1974). Glial cell lines available today probably far outnumber neuronal cell lines. Clonal glial cultures may be powerful tools for dissecting glial cell influences on neuronal differentiation. Among all glial cell lines studied, the rat C_6 line has been the most studied. There are excellent reviews available, among which are those by Mandel et al. (1976), Richelson (1976), Nelson (1977), Pfeiffer et al. (1977), and Schubert and Carlisle (1979). As a rule culturing cell lines require less sophisticated techniques than primary cultures do.

Neuronal cell lines are less dependent than primary cells on collagen substrate. The cells can be grown as monolayers on glass or plastic surfaces or even in suspension. Dulbecco's modified Eagle's medium with 10% FCS and high glucose is a widely used nutrient medium for neuroblastoma cells. Serum-free media, where serum is replaced by 5 μg insulin, 100 μg transferrin, 20 mM progesterone, 100 μM putrescine, and 30 nm selenium (all per ml), have also been designed (Bottenstein and Sato 1979).

For subculturing cells are removed with a low concentration of trypsin or with divalent cation-free medium, diluted with medium, and inoculated into fresh flasks or dishes. Subculturing 2–3 times per week maintains the cells in log phase, in which they have one mitotic division every 18–20 h. For culturing the rat pheochromocytoma PC 12 line, see Sect. 3.2.2.3. An important point in studying neuronal and glial cell lines is to ascertain the true nature of the cell in question. This can be achieved by demonstrating a cell to possess one or more characteristic features which are undoubtedly neuronal or glial. Such "markers" may be a distinctive morphology, electrical excitability, action potential formation and propagation, the capacity to produce neurotransmitters and neurotransmitter enzymes, ganglioside patterns, specific intracellular proteins, and cell surface antigens (see Bock 1977; Rosenberg et al. 1977). A serious obstacle for demonstrating the true nature of a certain cell line is the fact that rapidly dividing cells do not in general exhibit a full range of differentiated properties. Thus methods have to be applied which inhibit mitosis and induce differentiation (for review see Prasad 1975). This can be achieved by the administration of bromodeoxyuridine (Schubert and Jacob 1970), serum-deficient medium (Seeds et al. 1970), addition of cyclic AMP (Schubert 1974), or nerve growth factor (Greene and Tischler 1976).

Although the use of cloned cell lines has brought about major breakthroughs in many fields of neurobiology it should be realized that problems of heterogeneity are not completely resolved by the cloning methodology. Many cell lines are not diploid and, hence, a wide range of chromosomal numbers can be found when cloned lines are karyotyped. Moreover, continued propagation of a clone leads to some degree of instability in the karyotype. Therefore, early-passage cells should be kept frozen in growth medium containing 5% or 10% dimethylsulfoxide (DMSO) and should be stored in liquid nitrogen. Then, after working with a particular clone for 1–2 months the cells of high passage can be discarded and early-passage cells are thawed and plated (Mazur 1970).

5.5 Neuroneuronal and Neuromuscular Cocultures

Neuronal tissue cultures can provide valuable model systems for analyses of the mechanisms underlying directed growth of neurites, synapse formation, maturation, and maintenance of synaptic junctions as well as neurotrophic effects of nerve and muscle. As a rule setting up cocultures does not pose technical problems beyond those that exist in culturing explants and dissociated cells. It is for this reason that no detailed account on cocultures will be given here.

5.5.1 Neuromuscular Cocultures

Tissue culture models of neuromuscular relationships using spinal cord and peripheral ganglia in explants and isolated motoneurons, sympathetic and parasympathetic neurons, neuroblastoma cells, and hybrids in dissociated cell cultures have been the subject of intensive investigations. A number of extensive reviews and papers are available (Murray 1965, 1972; Shimada and Fischman 1973; Fischbach 1974; Fischbach et al. 1974; Harris 1974; Nelson

1975; Crain 1976; Fursphan et al. 1976; Landis 1976; Nelson et al 1976; Fischbach and Nelson 1977; Slaaf et al. 1979).

The first indirect evidence for the development of neuromuscular junctions in culture came from Harrison's (1907) work, who explanted frog embryo spinal cord together with attached myotomes. Crain (1964) and Bornstein et al. (1968) produced electrophysiological and morphological evidence that mammalian spinal cord neurons retain the capacity in vitro to form neuromuscular junctions with skeletal muscle. They explanted cross sections of 12–13 day mouse embryos containing spinal cord with attached DRG and paravertebral myoblasts.

The next step in the art of coculturing nerve and muscle was to let motoneurons in explanted fetal rodent spinal cord establish innervation with isolated skeletal muscle explants positioned at a distance of 1 mm from the spinal cord (Peterson and Crain 1970, 1972). Ultrastructurally the newly formed neuromuscular junctions resembled typical motor endplates (Pappas et al. 1971 a, b). Motoneurons dissociated from spinal cord and cocultured with striated muscle may also establish functional contacts (Fischbach 1970, 1974; Nelson 1975; Fischbach and Nelson 1977). Functional cholinergic synapses were also observed in vitro between sympathetic (Crain and Peterson 1974; Nurse and O'Lague 1975) and parasympathetic (Slaaf et al. 1979) neurons and skeletal muscle fibers or myotubes, respectively. Even neuroblastoma×glioma hybrid cells have been documented to form cholinergic synapses on embryonic mouse myotubes (Nelson et al. 1976). Despite the difficulties involved in producing evidence for a functional innervation of smooth muscle in vitro and its "trophic" dependence on autonomic nerves, a number of reports have described the formation of synaptic contacts upon smooth muscle cells and their development in culture in the presence and absence of sympathetic neurons (Chamley et al. 1973; Mark et al. 1973; Purves et al. 1974; Chamley and Campbell 1976).

5.5.2 Neuroneuronal Cocultures

In 1967, Crain and Peterson produced electrophysiologic evidence that DRG with attached cross-sectioned spinal cord from 13–14-day old rats matures in vitro and becomes synaptically coupled. Axons from DRG detached from spinal cord and explanted in close proximity to the cord may invade the CNS explant and form characteristic functional connections (Crain and Peterson 1975; see, however, Bunge and Wood 1973). In vitro experiments have also shown that nerve growth factor-stimulated axons from DRG explants can grow *through* adjacent spinal cord tissue and *onto* brainstem explants, where they establish characteristic functional synapses in the dorsal region, i.e., where dorsal column sensory fibers normally terminate (for review see Crain 1976).

When dissociated sympathetic nerve cells are injected into chambers, where spinal cord has been previously explanted, cholinergic nicotinic synapses form de novo upon sympathetic neurons (Bunge et al. 1974; Bunge 1976; Ko et al. 1976). Specific synaptic connections are also formed between co-cultured explants of spinal cord and sympathetic ganglia (Olson and Bunge 1973). The capacity of dissociated sympathetic neurons in vitro to form both cholinergic and adrenergic synapses upon each other has been clearly documented (O'Lague et al. 1974). Synapses, which according to their capacity to take up 5-hydroxydopamine may be both adrenergic and nonadrenergic (=cholinergic) are also found in explant cultures of sympathetic and ciliary ganglia, to which dissociated adrenal chromaffin cells had been added (Unsicker et al. 1976).

The retinotectal system, a classic model in neurobiology for studying directed axonal outgrowth and specificity of synapse formation (Jacobson 1978), has been adopted for in vitro studies. Data available so far indicate that functional retinotectal connections develop after growth of retina axons into the tectal explants (for review see Crain 1977).

6 Transplantation Techniques for Culturing Nerve Tissue in vivo

Differentiation of neuronal tissues including specific synapse formation have been successfully studied using several auto- and heterograft techniques. These studies are based on the assumption that the best alternatives to a cell's normal environment are similar environments either located in the same animal or in another host. For example, by transplanting immature CNS tissue into the anterior chamber of the eye one may dissect CNS-specific influences upon differention from those that are provided by body fluids in general.

6.1 Transplants to the Chorioallantoic Membrane of the Chick Embryo

(Fig. 9)

Fertile hen's eggs which have been incubated for 9 days are placed in a dark room. The eggs are illuminated with a strong lamp from underneath in order to locate the major blood vessels and the respective area is marked with a pencil. The tissue to be implanted is prepared under sterile conditions. Then the eggshell is wiped with 70% ethanol and a window is drilled into

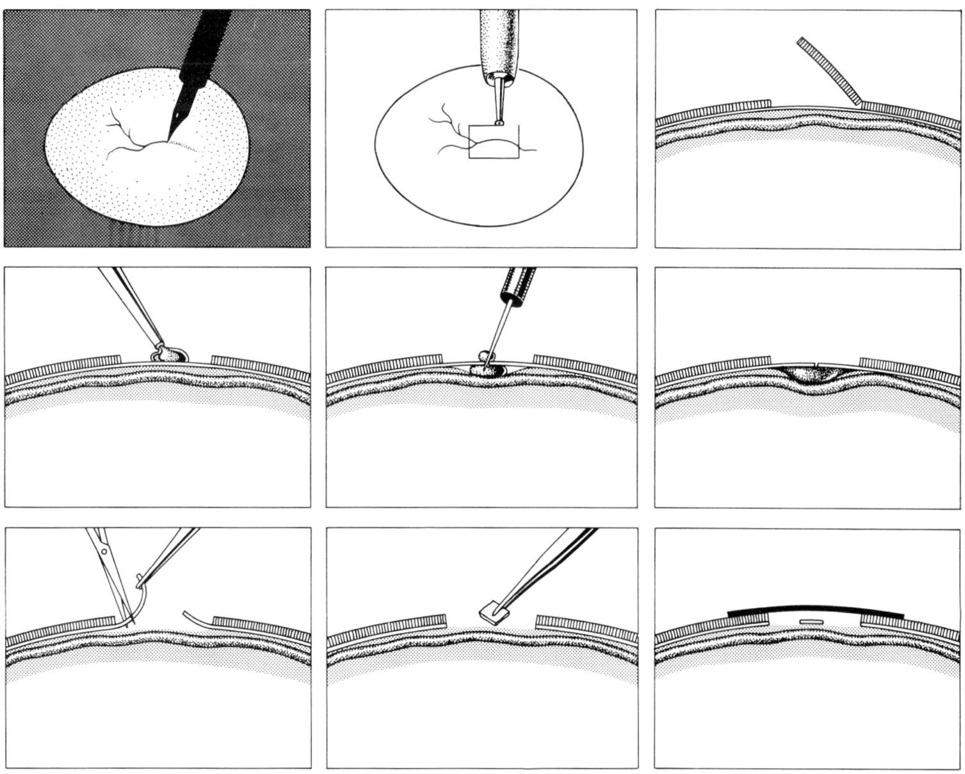

Fig. 9. Technique for transplanting tissue to the chorioallantoic membrane. For description see text

the shell using a dentist's drill. After cutting out the window over the airspace of the egg the shell membrane, which should not be penetrated, is exposed. A drop of salt solution is placed on the membrane. After rupturing the membrane with a sharp scalpel knife or a needle, the fluid passes on to the chorioallantoic membrane. Then the shell membrane is removed leaving the chorioallantoic membrane exposed. The transplant is placed over a large blood vessel and the window is sealed with transparent adhesive tape. The tape can be removed for examining the implanted tissue. The differentiation of chick neural crest (Cohen 1972; Allan 1979) and adrenal chromaffin cells (Unsicker, unpublished results) can be advantageously studied by this system.

6.2 Isotopic and Heterotopic Transplantations in Interspecific Chimeras

This technique, first described by LeDouarin (1971), exploits differences in the structure of the interphase nucleus between two species of birds, the Japanese quail (Coturnix coturnix japonica T. and S.) and the chick (Gallus gallus C.). In the quail a great part of the chromatin is condensed during interphase, whereas in the chick the chromatin is dispersed in a fine network. When quail cells are transplanted into chick embryos, the cells retain their characteristic "nuclear marker" and can be identified in the chimera. Thus, the migration and eventual fate of cells of various origins, as, for example, those of the neural crest, can be studied (LeDouarin et al. 1975, 1978; Fontaine et al. 1977; Teillet 1978). As a first step the neural tube and crest cells of the chick are removed. Then the selected quail portion (e.g., neural primordium) is isolated from the surrounding tissue by incubating it in 0.1% trypsin in Ca^{2+}- and Mg^{2+}-free Tyrode solution. As a second step the quail tissue is grafted into the host chick embryo.

6.3 Transplants to the Anterior Chamber of the Eye

The method for transplanting various peripheral and CNS tissues into the anterior chamber of the eye has been worked out in detail (for references see Olson and Malmfors 1970; Olson 1970; Olson and Seiger 1972, 1973, 1974, 1975, 1976a, b; Hoffer et al. 1974, 1975; Seiger and Olson 1975, 1977a, b, 1978; Seiger et al. 1976; Olson et al. 1977, 1978; Taylor et al. 1978; B. Tschechne 1978; D. Tschechne 1978; Unsicker et al. 1978a, b).

The tissue from the donor animal is removed under sterile conditions, trimmed to adequate size (approx. 1 mm^3) under a binocular microscope, and stored in a sterile salt solution (Ringer, HBSS, Tyrode) at 4 °C until transplantation. The recipient animal is anesthetized with ether and the eye(s) atropinized by local application of one drop of a 1% atropine solution a few minutes before transplantation in order to cause maximal dilation of the iris. A slit is made in the cornea using a sharp scalpel blade. Damage to the iris must be avoided. The transplant is sucked up in a Pasteur pipette and introduced into the anterior chamber through the slit. Then the transplant can be placed in the irido-corneal angle by applying gentle pressure to the cornea from outside with a pair of forceps. Alternatively, the tissue can be put through the slit using a pair of very fine watchmaker's forceps. The transplants establish vascular contact with the irides within a few days and may become reinnervated, if appropriate tissues are used (e.g., Unsicker et al. 1978a–c; Kondo 1978, and papers by Olson and his group, mentioned previously). Rejection of transplants may occur, if allo- or heterografts are used. In order to avoid this complication we have recently transplanted heterografts (bovine adrenal medullary tissue) into the anterior eye chamber of Nunu-mice (Unsicker et al. 1980).

6.4 Transplants Under the Kidney Capsule

The space between the connective tissue capsule and the kidney parenchyma is a particularly convenient space to study regeneration, reinnervation, and plasticity of nerve cells, since it has a rich blood supply and is almost devoid of nerve fibers. This location has been used for the transplantation of iris, superior cervical ganglia, and adrenal medulla (Carruba et al. 1974; Unsicker et al. 1977). The technique is simple; under ether anesthesia the kidneys are exposed and a small incision, 2–3 mm wide, is made in the capsule. Small pieces (1–2 mm^3) dissected under sterile conditions, are then carefully introduced in the space between capsule and parenchyma using watchmaker's forceps. The slit is covered with tissue glue.

6.5 Cerebral Implants

The transplantation of peripheral and CNS target tissues in the brain is a classic and useful approach to study plasticity phenomena in the CNS (for references see Björklund and Stenevi 1971, 1977, 1979; Stenevi et al. 1976; Björklund et al. 1979a, b). Various recipient sites for transplants into the brain can be chosen. For details of the method, see Stenevi et al. (1976).

7 Conclusion: What Tissue Culture Has to Say About Reality

This chapter has demonstrated that a multitude of cell and tissue culture systems is available for studying the structure and function of nervous tissue, neurons, and glial cells. The choice of a certain culture system largely depends on the objectives of the scientist and the design he wishes to make for his experiments.

Organ cultures of brain and spinal cord require considerable skill in order to obtain reproducible results. The advantage of these cultures rests upon their model character and on the accessability of the tissue for direct experimental manipulation. Interdisciplinary morphologic, physiologic, and biochemical studies provide us with valuable insights into cooperative cellular mechanisms underlying the fundamental aspects of spatial relationships in CNS neuronal networks. Cultures of mouse cerebellum are particularly well suited to underline the validity of nerve tissue culture as a model for the in vivo situation. However, significant cytologic and molecular deficits may also develop in complex cultures of CNS tissues.

Primary monolayer cultures of central and peripheral nerve and glial cells may be regarded as useful models for studies at the cellular level and for the evaluation of the basic nature of the synapse.

Established cell lines are relatively easy to culture and ensure a high degree of reproducibility. They represent the least complex system and play a dominant role in elucidating the factors which govern neuronal differentiation. Clonal cells provide more opportunities for genetic analysis, hybridization, and gene regulation than normal cells can. People using these cells certainly do not look at "normal" cells, but other investigators using primary cell cultures should not forget that they are not looking at the real thing either.

In vitro experiments aim at simplification as in vivo experiments do. With simplification normality gets lost, but instead of arguing about it we should rather try to work out how much is lost. Neuronal cell cultures certainly very often prove what neurons can do, not what they do in the intact organism. However, clean answers from clean systems are always a prerequisite for studying more complex systems. Therefore nerve tissue culture will continue to provide new insights into the structure and function of the nervous system.

Acknowledgements. Our work on peripheral nerve tissue cultures described in this article was supported by the Deutsche Forschungsgemeinschaft (Un 34/6). Thanks are due to Carmen Riehl for typing the manuscript and to Christian Fiebiger and Heidi Schneider for help with the illustrations.

8 Recommended Texts on Nerve Tissue Culture

Bunge PR (1975) Changing uses of nerve tissue culture 1950–1975. In: Tower DB (ed) The nervous system: vol 1, The basic neurosciences. Raven Press, New York, pp 31–42

Crain SM (1976) Neurophysiologic studies in tissue culture. Raven Press, New York

Fedoroff S, Hertz L (eds) (1977) Cell, tissue and organ culture in neurobiology. Academic Press, New York

Fischbach GD, Nelson PG (1977) Cell culture in neurobiology. In: Handbook of physiology, section 1: The nervous system, vol I/2. American Physiological Society, pp 719–774

Jacoby WB, Pastan IH (1979) Cell culture. In: Methods in enzymology, (S. P. Colowick and N. O. Kaplan eds). Vol LVIII. Academic Press New York

Kruse PF Jr, Patterson MK Jr (eds) (1973) Tissue culture. Methods and applications. Academic Press, New York

Lumsden CE (1968) Nervous tissue in culture. In: Bourne GH (ed) The structure and function of nervous tissue, vol I. Academic Press, New York, pp 67–140

Mandel P, Ciesielski-Treska J, Sensenbrenner M (1976) Neurons in vitro. In: Gispen WH (ed) Molecular and functional neurobiology. Elsevier, Amsterdam, pp 111–157

Murray MR (1965) Nervous tissue in vitro. In: Willmer EN (ed) The biology of cells and tissues in culture, vol II. Academic Press, New York, pp 373–455

Murray MR (1971) Nervous tissues isolated in culture. In: Lajtha A (ed) Handbook of neurochemistry, vol 5/A. Plenum Press, New York, pp 373–438

Murray MR, Kopech G (1953) A bibliography of the research in tissue culture 1884–1950. Academic Press, New York

Nelson PG (1975) Nerve and muscle in culture. Physiol Rev 55: 1–61

Paul J (1972) Cell and tissue culture, 4th ed. Williams & Wilkins, Baltimore

Pomerat CM, Hendelman CJ, Raiborn CW Jr, Massay JF (1967) Dynamic activities of nervous tissue in vitro. In: Hydén H (ed) The neuron. Elsevier, New York, pp 119–178

Richelson E (1975) Tissue culture of the nervous system: applications in neurochemistry and psychopharmacology. In: Iversen LL, Iversen SD, Snyder SH (eds) Handbook of psychopharmacology. Plenum Press, New York, pp 101–135

Richelson E (1976) Use of tissue culture to study cholinergic function. In: Goldberg AM, Hanin I (eds) Biology of cholinergic function. Raven Press, New York, pp 451–484

Sato G (1973) Tissue culture of the nervous system. Plenum Press, New York

Varon S (1975) Neurons and glia in neural cultures. Exp Neurol 48:93–134

Weiss P (1955) Nervous system. In: Willier B, Weiss P, Hamburger V (eds) Analysis of development. Saunders, Philadelphia, pp 346–401

Willmer EN (ed) (1966) Cells and tissues in culture: methods, biology and physiology I–III. Academic Press, London

Wilt FH, Wessells NK (1967) Methods in developmental biology. Crowell, New York

9 References

Allan I (1979) Experimental studies in the development of the avian peripheral autonomic nervous system. PhD dissertation, University of Melbourne

Allerand CD (1971) Patterns of neuronal differentiation in developing cultures of neonatal mouse cerebellum: a living and silver impregnation study. J Comp Neurol 142:167–204

Amano T, Hamprecht B, Kemper M (1974) High activity of choline acetyltransferase induced in neuroblastoma × glia hybrid cells. Exp Cell Res 84:391–408

Arndt-Jovin DJ, Jovin TM (1978) Automated cell sorting with flow systems. Annu Rev Biophys Bioeng 7:527–588

Au AM-J, Varon S (1979) Neural cell sequestration on immunoaffinity columns. Exp Cell Res 120:269–276

Augusti-Tocco G, Sato G (1969) Establishment of functioning clonal lines of neurons from mouse neuroblastoma. Proc Natl Acad Sci USA 64:311–315

Barkley DS, Rakic LL, Chaffee JK, Wong DL (1973) Cell separation by velocity sedimentation of postnatal mouse cerebellum. J Cell Physiol 81:271–280

Bashor MM (1979) Dispersion and disruption of tissues. Methods Enzymol 58:119–131

Benitez HH, Masurovski EB, Murray MR (1974) Interneurons of the sympathetic ganglia in organotypic culture: a suggestion as to their function, based on three types of study. J Neurocytol 3:363–384

Bennett MR, Nurcombe V (1979) The survival and development of cholinergic neurons in skeletal muscle conditioned media. Brain Res 173:543–548

Bennett MR, White W (1979) The survival and development of cholinergic neurons in potassium-enriched media. Brain Res 173:549–553

Berg DK (1978) Acetylcholine synthesis by chick spinal cord neurons in dissociated cell culture. Dev Biol 66:500–512

Bird MM (1973) The development of synapses in vitro between previously dissociated chick spinal cord neurons. Z Zellforsch 140:203–216

Bird MM, James DW (1975a) The culture of previously dissociated embryonic chick spinal cord cells on feeder layers of liver and kidney, and the development of paraformaldehyde induced fluorescence upon the former. J Neurocytol 4:633–646

Bird MM, James DW (1975b) Myelin formation in cultures of previously dissociated mouse spinal cord. Cell Tissue Res 162:93–105

Bird MM, James DW (1977) The development and ultrastructure of previously dissociated fetal human cerebral cortical cells in vitro. Cell Tissue Res 183:403–417

Bird MM, Lieberman AR (1976) Microtubule fascicles in the stem processes of cultured sensory ganglion cells. Cell Tissue Res 169: 41–47

Bjerre B (1973) The production of catecholamine-containing cells in vitro by young chick embryos studied by the histochemical fluorescence method. J Anat 115:119–131

Björklund A, Kromer LF, Stenevi U (1979a) Cholinergic reinnervation of the rat hippocampus by septal implants is stimulated by perforant path lesions. Brain Res 173:57–64

Björklund A, Segal M, Stenevi U (1979b) Functional reinnervation of rat hippocampus by locus coeruleus implants. Brain Res 170: 409–426

Björklund A, Stenevi U (1971) Growth of central catecholamine neurons into smooth muscle grafts in the rat mesencephalon. Brain Res 31:1–20

Björklund A, Stenevi U (1977) Experimental reinnervation of the rat hippocampus by grafted sympathetic ganglia. I. Axonal regeneration along the hippocampal fimbria. Brain Res 138:259–270

Björklund A, Stenevi U (1979) Regeneration of monoaminergic and cholinergic neurons in the mammalian central nervous system. Physiol Rev 59:62–100

Bock E (1977) Immunochemical markers in primary cultures and in cell lines. In: Fedoroff S, Hertz L (eds) Cell, tissue, and organ cultures in neurobiology. Academic Press, New York, pp 407–422

Bonkowski L, Dryden WF (1976) The effects of putative neurotransmitters on the resting membrane potential of dissociated brain neurons in culture. Brain Res 107:69–84

Booher J, Sensenbrenner M (1972) Growth and cultivation of dissociated neurons and glial cells from embryonic chick, rat, and human brain in flask cultures. Neurobiol 2:97–105

Bornstein MB (1964) Morphological development of neonatal mouse cerebral neocortex in tissue culture. In: Kellaway P, Petersen I (eds) Neurological and electroencephalographic correlative studies in infancy. Grune & Stratton, New York, pp 1–11

Bornstein MB (1972) Development of synapses and myelin in cultures of dissociated embryonic mouse spinal cord, medulla, and cerebrum. Brain Res 37:287–293

Bornstein MB (1973) Organotypic mammalian central and peripheral nerve tissue. In: Kruse PF Jr, Patterson MK Jr (eds) Tissue culture. Methods and applications. Academic Press, New York, pp 86–92

Bornstein MB, Iwanami H, Lehrer GM, Breitbart M (1968) Observations on the appearance of neuromuscular relationships in cultured mouse tissues. Z Zellforsch 92:197–206

Bornstein MB, Model PG (1972) Development of synapses and myelin in cultures of dissociated embryonic mouse spinal cord medulla and cerebrum. Brain Res 37:287–293

Bornstein MB, Murray MR (1958) Serial observation on patterns of growth, myelin formation, maintenance, and degeneration in cultures of newborn rat and kitten cerebellum. J Biophys Biochem 4:499–504

Bottenstein J, Hayashi I, Hutchings S, Masui H, Mather J, McClure DB, Ohasha S, Rizzino A, Sato G, Serrero G, Wolfe R, Wu R (1979) The growth of cells in serum-free hormone-supplemented media. Methods Enzymol 58:94–109

Bottenstein JE, Sato GH (1979) Growth of a rat neuroblastoma cell line in serum-free supplemented medium. Proc Natl Acad Sci USA 76: 514–517

Bray D (1970) Surface movements during the growth of single explanted neurons. Proc Natl Acad Sci USA 65:905–910

Breen GAM, De Vellis J (1974) Regulation of glycerol phosphate dehydrogenase by hydrocortisone in dissociated rat cerebrum cultures. Dev Biol 41:255–266

Bunge MB (1973) Fine structure of nerve fibers and growth cones of isolated sympathetic neurons in culture. J Cell Biol 56:713–735

Bunge MB, Bunge RP, Peterson ER, Murray MR (1967) A light and electron microscope study of long-termed organized cultures of rat dorsal root ganglia. J Cell Biol 32:439–466

Bunge RP (1976) The expression of neuronal specificity in tissue culture. In: Barondes SH (ed) Neuronal recognition. Plenum Press, New York, pp 109–128
Bunge RP, Rees R, Wood P, Burton H, Ko CP (1974) Anatomical and physiological observations on synapses formed on isolated autonomic neurons in tissue culture. Brain Res 66: 401–412
Bunge RP, Wood P (1973) Studies on the transplantation of spinal cord tissue in the rat. I. The development of a culture system for hemisections of embryonic spinal cord. Brain Res 57:261–276
Burdman JA (1968) Uptake of [^{3}H]catecholamines by chick embryo sympathetic ganglia in tissue culture. J Neurochem 15:1321–1323
Burry RW, Lasher RS (1975) Uptake of GABA in dispersed cell cultures of postnatal rat cerebellum: an electron microscope autoradiographic study. Brain Res 88:502–507
Burry RW, Lasher RS (1978a) Electron microscopic autoradiography of the uptake of [^{3}H] GABA in dispersed cell cultures of rat cerebellums. I. The morphology of the GABA synapse. Brain Res 151:1–17
Burry RW, Lasher RS (1978b) Electron microscopic autoradiography of the uptake of [^{3}H] GABA in dispersed cell cultures of rat cerebellums. II. The development of GABA ergic synapses. Brain Res 151:19–29
Campbell F, Le M, Schachner M, Sharrow S (1977) Isolation of glial cell-enriched and -depleted populations from mouse cerebellum by density gradient centrifugation and electronic cell sorting. Brain Res 127:69–86
Carruba M, Ceccarelli B, Clementi F, Mantegazza P (1974) Selectivity in the reinnervation of iris and adrenal medulla by superior cervical ganglion after transplantation under the kidney capsule. Brain Res 77:39–53
Cavanaugh MW (1955) Neuron development from trypsin dissociated cells of differentiated spinal cord of the chick embryo. Exp Cell Res 9:42–48
Chamley JH, Campbell GR (1976) Tissue culture: interaction between sympathetic nerves and vascular smooth muscle. In: Bevan JA (ed) Vascular neuroeffector mechanisms. Karger, Basel, pp 10–18
Chamley JH, Campbell GR, Burnstock G (1973) An analysis of the interactions between sympathetic nerve fibers and smooth muscle cells in tissue culture. Dev Biol 33:344–361
Chamley JH, Mark GE, Burnstock G (1972a) Sympathetic ganglia in culture. I. Neurons. Z Zellforsch 135:287–314
Chamley JH, Mark GE, Campbell GR, Burnstock G (1972b) Sympathetic ganglia in culture. II. Accessory cells. Z Zellforsch 135:315–327
Chen JS, Levi-Montalcini R (1970) Long term culture of dissociated nerve cells from the embryonic nervous system of the cockroach Periplaneta americana. Arch Ital Biol 108: 503–537
Chun LLY, Patterson PH (1977a) Role of nerve growth factor in the development of rat sympathetic neurons in vitro. I. Survival, growth, and differentiation of catecholamine production. J Cell Biol 75:694–704
Chun LLY, Patterson PH (1977b) Role of nerve growth factor in the development of rat sympathetic neurons in vitro. II. Developmental studies. J Cell Biol 75:705–711
Chun LLY, Patterson PH (1977c) Role of nerve growth factor in the development of rat sympathetic neurons in vitro. III. Effects of acetylcholine production. J Cell Biol 75:712–718
Cohen AM (1972) Factors directing the expression of sympathetic nerve traits in cells of neural crest origin. J exp Zool 179:167–182
Cohen AM (1977) Independent expression of the adrenergic phenotype by neural crest cells in vitro. Proc Natl Acad Sci USA 74:2899–2903
Cohen SS, Flaks JG, Barner HD, Loeb MR, Lichtenstein J (1958) The mode of action of 5-fluorouracil and its derivatives. Proc Natl Acad Sci USA 44:1004–1012
Collins F (1978) Axon initiation by ciliary neurons in culture. Dev Biol 65:50–57
Combes PC, Privat A, Pessac B, Calothy G (1977) Differentiation of chick embryo neuroretina cells in monolayer cultures. An ultrastructural study. I. Seven-day retina. Cell Tissue Res 185:159–173
Contestabile A, Minelli G, Ciani F (1973) Enzymic activities in dissociated neurons differentiated in cultures in vitro. J Neurochem 20: 691–698
Crain SM (1964) Electrophysiological studies of cord-innervated skeletal muscle in long-term tissue cultures of mouse embryo myotomes. Anat Rec 148:273
Crain SM (1966) Development of "organotypic" biolectric activities in central nervous tissues during maturation in culture. Int Rev Neurobiol 9:1–43
Crain SM (1977) Synapse formation in neural tissue cultures. In: Fedoroff S, Hertz L (eds) Cell, tissue, and organ cultures in neurobiology. Academic Press, New York, pp 147–190
Crain SM, Peterson ER (1967) Onset and development of functional interneural connections in explants of rat spinal cord-ganglia during maturation in culture. Brain Res 6:750–762
Crain SM, Peterson ER (1974) Development of neural connections in culture. Ann NY Acad Sci 228:6–34
Crain SM, Peterson ER (1975) Selective innervation of target tissues in spinal cord and

medulla explants by isolated dorsal root ganglia. Society of Neuroscience, 5th Annual Meeting, New York, p 751
Daly WF (1973) Electronic enumeration and sizing of cells. In: Kruse PF Jr, Patterson MK Jr (eds) Tissue culture, methods, and applications. Academic Press, New York, pp 398–399
Dichter MA (1978) Rat cortical neurons in cell culture: culture methods, cell morphology, electrophysiology, and synapse formation. Brain Res 149:279–293
Douglas WHJ, Dell'Orco RT (1979) Physical aspects of a tissue culture laboratory. Methods Enzymol 58:3–17
Drayton MR, Kiernan JA (1973) Effects of aprotinin on organ cultures of the cerebellum of the rat. Exp Neurol 39:381–388
Dreyfus ChF, Gershon MD, Crain SM (1979) Innervation of hippocampal explants. Brain Res 161:431–445
Dvorak JA, Stotler WF (1971) A controlled-environment culture system for high resolution light microscopy. Exp Cell Res 68: 144–148
Ehrmann RL, Gey GO (1956) The growth of cells on a transparent gel of reconstituted rat-tail collagen. J Natl Cancer Inst 16:1375
England JM, Goldstein MN (1969) The uptake and localization of catecholamines in chick embryo sympathetic neurons in tissue culture. J Cell Sci 4:677–691
Estridge M, Bunge R (1978) Compositional analysis of growing axons from rat sympathetic neurons. J Cell Biol 79:138–155
Farbman AI (1972) Development of taste buds in organ culture. Anat Rec 172:308
Fenton EL (1970) Tissue culture assay of nerve growth factor and of the specific antiserum. Exp Cell Res 59:383–392
Fenwick EM, Fajdiga PB, Howe NBS, Livett BG (1978) Functional and morphological characterization of isolated bovine adrenal medullary cells. J Cell Biol 76:12–30
Fischbach GD (1970) Synaptic potentials recorded in cell cultures of nerve and muscle. Science 169:1331–1333
Fischbach GD (1972) Synapse formation between dissociated nerve and muscle cells in low-density cultures. Dev Biol 28:407–427
Fischbach GD (1974) Some aspects of neuromuscular junction formation In: Cox RP (ed) Cell communication. Wiley, New York, pp 43–66
Fischbach GD, Cohen SA, Henkart MP (1974) Some observations on trophic interaction between neurons and muscle fibers in cell culture. Ann NY Acad Sci 228:35–46
Fischbach GD, Dichter MA (1974) Electrophysiologic and morphologic properties of neurons in dissociated chick spinal cord cell cultures. Dev Biol 37:100–116
Fisher KRS, Federoff S, Wenger EL (1975) Effect of osmotic pressure on neurogenesis in cultures of chick embryo spinal cords. In Vitro 11:329–337
Fontaine J, LeLièvre C, LeDouarin NM (1977) What is the developmental fate of the neural crest cells which migrate into the pancreas in the avian embryo? Gen Comp Endocrinol 33: 394–404
Friedmann I (1965) The ear. In: Willmer EN (ed) Cells and tissues in culture. Academic Press, New York, pp 521–547
Fry JM, Lehrer GM, Bornstein MB (1973) Experimental inhibition of myelination in spinal cord tissue cultures: enzyme assays. J Neurobiol 4:453–459
Furshpan EJ, MacLeish PR, O'Lague PH, Potter DD (1976) Chemical transmission between rat sympathetic neurons and cardiac myocytes developing in microcultures: evidence for cholinergic, adrenergic, and dual-function neurons. Proc Natl Acad Sci USA 73:4225–4229
Goodfrey L, Massarelli R, Sensenbrenner M, Mandel P (1974) Guanyl cyclase in chick embryo brain cell cultures: evidence of neuronal localization. J Neurochem 23:135–138
Greene LA, Rein G (1978) Release of norepinephrine from neurons in dissociated cell cultures of chick sympathetic ganglia via stimulation of nicotinic and muscarinic acetylcholine receptors. J Neurochem 30:579–586
Greene LA, Tischler A (1976) Establishment of a noradrenergic clonal line of rat adrenal pheochromocytoma cells which respond to nerve growth factor. Proc Natl. Acad Sci USA 73:2424–2428
Grosse GW, Rieske E, Kreutzberg GW, Meyer A (1977) A new fixed-array multi-electrode system for long-term monitoring of extracellular single unit neuronal activity in vitro. Neurosci Lett 6:101–105
Grosse GW, Lindner G (1972) Untersuchungen zur Differenzierung disaggregierter Zellen des Telencephalon vom Hühnerembryo in Langzeit-Zellkulturen. Z Mikrosk Anat Forsch 85: 438–448
Grosse GW, Lindner G (1974) Zytodifferenzierung des Hippocampus fetaler Ratten in der Zellkultur. Z Mikrosk Anat Forsch 88:705–712
Grosse GW, Lindner G (1975) Morphologische Untersuchungen der Entwicklung des Hippocampus in der Zell- und Explantat-Kultur. J Hirnforsch 16:451–456
Ham RG, McKeehan WL (1979) Media and Growth Requirements. Methods Enzymol 58:44–93
Hamprecht B (1974) Cell cultures as model system for studying the biochemistry of differ-

entiated functions of nerve cells. In: Jaenicke L (ed) 25. Kolloquium der Gesellschaft für Biologische Chemie. Springer, Berlin Heidelberg New York pp 391–423
Harris AJ (1974) Inductive functions of the nervous system. Ann Rev Physiol 36:251–305
Harris M (1973) Electronic enumeration and sizing of cells. In: Kruse PF Jr, Patterson MK Jr (eds) Tissue culture. (Methods and applications.) Academic Press, New York, pp 400–405
Harrison RG (1906/07) Observation on the living developing nerve fiber. Proc Soc Exp Biol Med 4:140–143
Harrison RG (1907) Observation on the living developing nerve fiber. Anat Rec 1:116–118
Harrison RG (1908) Embryonic transplantation and development of the nervous system. Anat Rec 2:385–410
Hauw J-J, Bontry J-M, Crosnier-Suttin N, Robineaux R (1974) Morphology of cultured guinea-pig cerebellum. I. Pattern of development. Comparison of phase contrast cinematography and silver impregnations of various cell types. Cell Tissue Res 152:141–164
Hawrot E, Patterson PH (1979) Long-term culture of dissociated sympathetic neurons. Methods Enzymol 58:574–584
Heidelberger C (1963) Biochemical mechanisms of action of fluorinated pyrimidines. Exp Cell Res [Suppl] 9:462–471
Helfand SL, Riopelle RJ, Wessells NK (1978) Non-equivalence of conditioned medium and nerve growth factor for sympathetic, parasympathetic, and sensory neurons. Exp Cell Res 113:39–45
Hendelman WJ, Marshall KC, Aggerwal AS, Wojtowicz JM (1977) Organization of pathways in cultures of mouse cerebellum. In: Federoff S, Hertz L (eds) Cell, tissue, and organ cultures in neurobiology. Academic Press, New York, pp 539–554
Hild W (1957) Myelinogenesis in cultures of mammalian central nervous tissue. Z Zellforsch 46:71–95
Hild W, Tasaki I (1962) Morphological and physiological properties of neurons and glial cell in tissue culture. J Neurophysiol 25: 277–304
Hild W, Tasaki I (1964) The use of tissue cultures in neurophysiological research. In: Methods in medical research, vol 10, section IV. Year Book, Chicago, pp 327–334
Hoffer B, Olson L, Seiger A, Bloom F (1975) Formation of a functional adrenergic input to intraocular cerebellar grafts: ingrowth of inhibitory sympathetic fibers. J Neurobiol 6: 565–585
Hoffer B, Seiger A, Ljungberg T, Olson L (1974) Electrophysiological and cytobiological studies of brain homografts in the anterior chamber of the eye: maturation of cerebellar cortex in oculo. Brain Res 79:165–184
Honegger P, Richelson E (1976) Biochemical differentiation of mechanically dissociated mammalian brain in aggregating cell culture. Brain Res 109:335–354
Hooks J, Gibbs CJ Jr, Chopra H, Lewis M, Gajdusek DC (1972) Spontaneous transformation of human brain cells grown in vitro and description of associated virus particles. Science 176:1420–1422
Jacobowitz DM, Greene LA (1974) Histofluorescence study of chromaffin cells in dissociated-cell cultures of chick embryo sympathetic ganglia. J Neurobiol 5:65–83
Jacobson M (1978) Developmental neurobiology, 2nd edn. Plenum Press, New York
Juurlink BHJ, Fedoroff S (1979) The development of mouse spinal cord in tissue culture. I. Cultures of whole mouse embryos and spinal cord primordia. In Vitro 15:86–94
Karasek M (1974) Ultrastructure of rat pineal gland in organ culture: influence of norepinephrine, dibutyryl cyclic adenosine 3′ 5′-monophosphate and adenophypophysis. Endocrinologie 64:106–114
Kása P, Bánsághi K (1979) Development of neurons containing acetylcholinesterase and cholinacetyltransferase in dispersed cell culture of rat cerebellum. Histochemistry 61: 263–270
Kiernan JA, Pettit DR (1971) Organ culture of the central nervous system of the adult rat. Exp Neurol 32:111–120
Kim SU (1970) Observations on cerebellar granule cells in tissue culture. A silver and electron microscopic study. Z Zellforsch 107:454–465
Kim SU (1971) Demonstration of neurofibrillary degeneration induced by anoxia on spinal motor neurons in vitro. Experienta 27: 264–265
Kim SU (1972) Light and electron microscopy study of mouse cerebral neocortex in tissue culture. Exp Neurol 35:305–321
Kim SU (1973) Morphological development of neonatal mouse hippocampus cultured in vitro. Exp Neurol 41:150–162
Kim SU, Hague-Angeletti R, Gonatas NK (1979) Localization of nerve growth factor receptors in sympathetic neurons cultured in vitro. Brain Res 168:602–608
Kim SU, Oh TH, Johnson DD (1972) Developmental changes of acetylcholinesterase and pseudocholinesterase in organotypic cultures of spinal cord. Exp Neurol 35:274–281
Klein DC, Weller J (1970) Input and output signals in a model neural system: the regulation of melatonin production in the pineal gland. In Vitro 6:197–204

Ko CP, Burton H, Bunge RP (1976) Synaptic transmission between rat spinal cord explants and dissociated superior cervical ganglion neurons in tissue culture. Brain Res 117: 437–460

Kondo H (1978) Reinnervation of the adrenal medulla transplanted in the anterior eye chamber. J Anat 127:323–331

Koves J, Pollack ED (1975) Development of an in vitro model of larval frog spinal cord. J Cell Biol 67:222 A

Kreth HW, Herzenberg LA (1974) Fluorescence-activated sorting of human T and B lymphocytes. I. Direct evidence that lymphocytes with a high density of membrane-bound immunoglobulin are precursors of plasmacytes. Cell Immunol 12:396–406

Landis SC (1976) Rat sympathetic neurons and cardiac myocytes developing in microcultures: correlation of the fine structure of endings with neurotransmitter function in single neurons. Proc Natl Acad Sci USA 73:4220–4224

Landis SC (1978) Growth cones of cultured sympathetic neurons contain adrenergic vesicles. J Cell Biol 78:R8–R14

Lasher RS, Zagon IS (1972) The effect of potassium on neuronal differentiation in cultures of dissociated newborn rat cerebellum. Brain Res 41:482–488

La Vail MM, Hild W (1971) Histotypic organization of the rat retina in-vitro. Z. Zellforsch. 114:557–579

La Vail JH, Wolf MK (1973) Postnatal development of the mouse dentate gyrus in organotypic cultures of the hippocampal formation. Am J Anat 137:47–66

Lazarus KJ, Bradshaw RA, West NR, Bunge RP (1976) Adaptive survival of rat sympathetic neurons cultured without supporting cells or exogenous nerve growth factor. Brain Res 113:159–164

LeDouarin NM (1971) Charactéristiques ultrastructurales du noyau interphasique chez le caille et chez le poulet et utilisation des cellules de caille comme «marqueurs biologiques» en embryologie experimentale. Ann Embryol Morphol 4:125–135

LeDouarin NM, Renaud D, Teillet MA, LeDouarin GH (1975) Cholinergic differentiation of presumptive adrenergic neuroblasts in interspecific chimeras after heterotopic transplantations. Proc Natl Acad Sci USA 72: 728–732

Le Douarin NM, Teillet MA, Ziller C, Smith J (1978) Adrenergic differentiation of cells of the colinergic ciliary and Remak ganglia in avian embryo after in vivo transplantation. Proc Natl Acad Sci USA 75:2030–2034

Levi-Montalcini R, Angeletti PU (1963) Essential role of the nerve growth factor in the survival and maintenance of dissociated sensory and sympathetic embryonic nerve cells in vitro. Dev Biol 7:653–659

Levi-Montalcini R, Angeletti PU (1968) Nerve growth factor. Physiol Rev 48:534–569

Lieber MM, Benveniste RE, Livingston DM, Todaro GJ (1973) Mammalian cells in culture frequently release type C viruses. Science 182: 56–59

Lim R, Mitsunobu K, Li WKP (1973) Maturation-stimulating effect of brain extract and dibutyryl cyclic AMP on dissociated embryonic brain cells in culture. Exp Cell Res 79:243–246

Livett BG, Kozcusek K, Mizobe F, Dean DM (1979) Substance P inhibits nicotinic activation of chromaffin cells. Nature 278:256–257

Lodin Z, Booher J, Kasten FH (1970) Long-term cultivation of dissociated neurons from embryonic chick dorsal root ganglia in the Rose chamber. Exp Cell Res 59:291–298

Lodin Z, Faltin J, Booher J, Hartman J, Sensenbrenner M (1973) Fiber formation and myelinization of cultivated dissociated neurons from chicken dorsal root ganglia. Neurobiology 3:66–87

Lyser KM (1976) Organotypic culture of early embryonic nervous system. In: Evans VJ, Perry VP, Vincent MM (eds) Tissue culture association manual, vol I. pp 121–126

Mains RE, Patterson PH (1973a) Primary cultures of dissociated sympathetic neurons. I. Establishment of long-term growth in culture and studies of differentiated properties. J Cell Biol 59:329–345

Mains RE, Patterson PH (1973b) Primary cultures of dissociated sympathetic neurons. II. Initial studies on catecholamine metabolism. J Cell Biol 59:346–360

Mains RE, Patterson PH (1973c) Primary cultures of dissociated sympathetic neurons. III. Changes in metabolism with age in culture. J Cell Biol 59:361–366

Mark GE, Chamley JH, Burnstock G (1973) Interactions between autonomic nerves and smooth and cardiac muscle cells in tissue culture. Dev Biol 32:194–200

Maxwell GD (1976) Substrate dependence of cell migration from explanted neural tubes in vitro. Cell Tissue Res 172:325–330

Mazur P (1970) Cryobiology: the freezing of biological systems. Science 168:939–949

McCarthy KD, Partlow LM (1976) Preparation of pure neuronal and non-neuronal cultures from embryonic chick sympathetic ganglia: a new method based on both differential cell adhesiveness and the formation of homotypic neuronal aggregates. Brain Res 114:391–414

McGarrity GJ (1979) Detection of contamination. Methods Enzymol 58:18–29

Meller K (1974) The reaggregation of neurons and their satellite cells in cultures of trypsin-dissociated spinal ganglia. Cell Tissue Res 152: 175–183

Meller K, Breipohl W, Wagner HH, Knuth A (1969) Die Differenzierung isolierter Nerven- und Gliazellen aus trypsinisiertem Rückenmark von Hühnerembryonen in Gewebekulturen. Z Zellforsch 101: 135–151

Meller K, Mestres P, Breipohl W, Waelsch M (1974) Time-lapse cinematographic studies on the inhibition of cell motility by puromycin in cultured nervous tissue. Cell Tissue Res 148: 227–235

Messer A (1977) The maintenance and identification of mouse cerebellar granule cells in monolayer culture. Brain Res 130: 1–12

Miller R, Varon S, Kruger L, Coates PW, Orkand PM (1970) Formation of synaptic contacts on dissociated chick embryo sensory ganglion cells in vitro. Brain Res 24: 356–358

Mizel SB, Bamburg JR (1976) Studies on the action of nerve growth factor. I. Characterization of a simplified in vitro culture system for dorsal root and sympathetic ganglia. Dev Biol 49: 11–19

Moeller W (1978) Circumventrikuläre Organe in der Gewebekultur. Adv Anat Embryol 54: 3–95

Morton HJ (1970) A survey of commercially available tissue culture media. In Vitro 6: 89

Moscona A (1952) Cell suspensions from organ rudiments of chick embryos. Exp Cell Res 3: 535–539

Murray MR (1965) Muscle tissues in vitro. In: Willmer EN (ed) Cells and tissues in culture, vol 2. Academic Press, New York, 311–372

Murray MR (1972) Skeletal muscle in culture. In: Bourne GH (ed) Structure and function of the nervous system, vol 1. Academic Press, New York, pp 237–299

Murray MR (1977) Introduction. In: Fedoroff S, Hertz L (eds) Cell, tissue and organ culture in neurobiology. Academic Press, New York, pp 1–8

Nakai J (1956) Dissociated dorsal root ganglia in tissue culture. Am J Anat 99: 81–130

Nathanson MA, Binkley S, Hilfer SR (1977) Cultivation of mammalian pineal cells: retention of organization and function in tissue culture. In Vitro 13: 843–848

Nelson PG (1977) Neuronal cell lines. In: Fedoroff S, Hertz L (eds) Cell tissue and organ culture in neurobiology. Academic Press, New York, pp 347–365

Nelson PG, Christian CN, Nirenberg MW (1976) Synapse formation between clonal neuroblastoma × glioma hybrid cells and striated muscle cells. Proc Natl Acad Sci USA 73: 123–127

Nelson PG, Peacock JH (1973) Electrical activity in dissociated cell cultures from fetal mouse cerebellum. Brain Res 61: 163–174

Nurse CA, O'Lague PH (1975) Formation of cholinergic synapses between dissociated sympathetic neurons and skeletal myotubes of the rat in cell culture. Proc Natl Acad Sci USA 72: 1955–1959

Nuttall RP, Wessells NK (1979) Veils, mounds, and vesicle aggregates in neurons elongating in vitro. Exp Cell Res 119: 163–174

Obata K (1974) Transmitter sensitivities of some nerve and muscle cells in culture. Brain Res 73: 71–88

Okun LM (1972) Isolated dorsal root ganglion neurons in culture: cytological maturation and extension of electrically active processes. J Neurobiol 3: 111–115

Okun LM, Outkean FK, Thomas CA (1972) Removal of nonneuronal cells from suspensions of dissociated embryonic dorsal root ganglia. Exp Cell Res 73: 226–229

O'Lague PH, MacLeish PR, Nurse CA, Claude P, Furshpan EJ, Potter DD (1975) Physiological and morphological studies on developing sympathetic neurons in dissociated cell culture. Cold Spring Harbor Symp Quant Biol 40: 399–407

O'Lague PH, Obata K, Claude P, Furshpan EJ, Potter DD (1974) Evidence for cholinergic synapses between dissociated rat sympathetic neurons in cell culture. Proc Natl Acad Sci USA 71: 3602–3603

Olson L (1970) Fluorescence histochemical evidence for axonal growth and secretion from transplanted adrenal medullary tissue. Histochemie 22: 1–7

Olson L, Freedman R, Seiger Å, Hoffer B (1977) Electrophysiology and cytology of hippocampal formation transplants in the anterior chamber of the eye. I. Intrinsic organization. Brain Res 119: 87–106

Olson L, Malmfors T (1970) Growth characteristics of adrenergic nerves in the adult rat. Fluorescence histochemical and ^{3}H noradrenaline uptake studies using tissue transplantations to the anterior chamber of the eye. Acta Physiol Scand [Suppl] 348: 1–112

Olson L, Seiger Å (1972) Brain tissue transplanted to the anterior chamber of the eye. 1. Fluorescence histochemistry of immature catecholamine and 5-hydroxytryptamine neurons reinnervating the rat iris. Z Zellforsch 175–194

Olson L, Seiger Å (1973) Development and growth of immature monoamine neurons in rat and man in situ and following intraocular transplantation in the rat. Brain Res 62: 353–360

Olson L, Seiger Å (1974) Nerve growth specificity and regulation as revealed by intraocular brain tissue transplants. In: Fuxe K, Olson L, Zottermann Y (eds) Dynamics of degeneration and growth in neurons. Pergamon Press, Oxford New York, pp 499–508

Olson L, Seiger Å (1975) Brain tissue transplanted to the anterior chamber of the eye. 2. Fluorescence histochemistry of immature catecholamine and 5-hydroxytryptamine neurons innervating the rat vas deferens. Cell Tissue Res 158:141–150

Olson L, Seiger Å (1976a) Locus coeruleus: fiber growth regulation in oculo. Med Biol 54:142–145

Olson L, Seiger Å (1976b) Beating intraocular hearts: light-controlled rate by autonomic innervation from host iris. J Neurobiol 7: 193–203

Olson L, Seiger Å, Ålund M (1978) Locus coeruleus fiber growth in oculo-induced by trigeminotomy. Med Biol 56:23–27

Olson MJ, Bunge RP (1973) Anatomical observations on the specificity of synapse formation in tissue culture. Brain Res 59:19–33

Orr MF (1974) The development of the sensory membranes of the inner ear of the embryonic chick. In Vitro 9:361

Pappas GD, Peterson ER, Masurovsky EB, Crain SM (1971a) The fine structure of developing neuromuscular synapses in vitro. Ann NY Acad Sci 183:33–45

Pappas GD, Peterson ER, Masurovsky EB, Crain SM (1971b) The fine structure of developing neuromuscular synapses in vitro. Anat Rec 169:395–396

Patterson MK Jr (1979) Measurement of growth and viability of cells in culture. Methods Enzymol 58:141–152

Patterson PH, Chun LLY (1974) The influence of non-neuronal cells on catecholamine and acetylcholine synthesis and accumulation in cultures of dissociated sympathetic neurons. Proc Natl Acad Sci USA 71:3607–3610

Patterson PH, Chun LLY (1977a) The induction of acetylcholine synthesis in primary cultures of dissociated rat sympathetic neurons. I. Effects of conditioned medium. Dev Biol 56: 263–280

Patterson PH, Chun LLY (1977b) The induction of acetylcholine synthesis in primary cultures of dissociated rat sympathetic neurons. II. Developmental aspects. Dev Biol 60:473–481

Patterson PH, Reichardt LF, Chun LLY (1975) Biochemical studies on the development of primary sympathetic neurons in cell culture. Cold Spring Harbor Symp Quant Biol 40: 389–397

Peacock JH, Rush DF, Mathers LH (1979) Morphology of dissociated hippocampal cultures from fetal mice. Brain Res 169:231–246

Pearson D (1977) Neurosecretion in cultured systems. In: Fedoroff S, Hertz L (eds) Cell, tissue and organ culture in neurobiology. Academic Press, New York, pp 573–587

Perlman D (1979) Use of antibiotics in cell culture media. Methods Enzymol 58:110–116

Peterson ER, Crain SM (1970) Innervation in cultures of fetal rodent skeletal muscle by organotypic explants of spinal cord from different animals. Z Zellforsch 106:1–21

Peterson ER, Crain SM (1972) Regeneration and innervation in cultures of adult mammalian muscle coupled with fetal rodent spinal cord. Exp Neurol 36:136–159

Peterson ER, Murray MR (1955) Myelin sheath formation in cultures of avian spinal ganglia. Am J Anat 96:319–355

Peterson ER, Crain SM, Murray MR (1965) Differentiation and prolonged maintenance of bioelectrically active spinal cord cultures (rat, chick, and human). Z Zellforsch 66:130–154

Pfeiffer SE, Betschart B, Cook J, Mancini P, Morris R (1977) Glial cell lines. In: Fedoroff S, Hertz L (eds) Cell, tissue, and organ cultures in neurobiology. Academic Press, New York, pp 287–346

Pomerat CM, Castero I (1956) Tissue cultures of cat cerebellum. Am J Anat 99:211–247

Prasad KN (1975) Differentiation of neuroblastoma cells in culture. Biol Rev 50:129–265

Privat A, Drian MJ (1975) Specificity of the formation of the mossy fiber-granule cell synapsis in the rat cerebellum. An in vitro study. Brain Res 88:518–524

Privat A, Drian MJ, Manden P (1973) The outgrowth of rat cerebellum in organized culture. Z Zellforsch 146:45–68

Purves RD, Hill CE, Chamley JH, Mark GE, Fry DM, Burnstock G (1974) Functional autonomic neuromuscular junctions in tissue culture. Pflügers Arch 350:1–7

Ransom BR, Neale E, Henkart M, Bullock PN, Nelson PG (1977) Mouse spinal cord in cell culture. I. Morphology and intrinsic neuronal electrophysiologic properties. J Neurophysiol 40:1132–1150

Ready DF, Nicholls J (1979) Identified neurons isolated from leech CNS make selective connections in culture. Nature 281:67–68

Rees R, Bunge RP (1974) Morphological and cytochemical studies of synapses formed in culture between isolated rat superior cervical ganglion neurons. J Comp Neurol 157:1–12

Reichardt LF, Patterson PH (1977) Neurotransmitter synthesis and uptake by isolated sympathetic neurones in microcultures. Nature 270:147–151

Rieske E, Kreutzberg GW (1977) Long-term culture of electrically active sensory neurons free of glial cells. Neurosci Lett 5:153–157

Rieske E, Kreutzberg GW (1978) Neurite regeneration after cell surgery with laser microbeam irradiation. Brain Res 148:478–483

Romijn HJ, Gelsema AJ (1976) Electron microscopy of the rabbit pineal organ in vitro. Evidence of norepinephrine-stimulated secretory activity of the Golgi apparatus. Cell Tissue Res 172:365–377

Rose G (1954) A separable and multipurpose tissue culture chamber. Tex Rep Biol Med 12: 1074–1083

Rosenberg RN (1973) Neuronal and glial enzyme studies in cell culture. In Vitro 8: 194–206

Rosenberg RN, Vance CK, Prashad N, Baskin F (1977) Specific protein species expressed by differentiating neuroblastoma, glioma, and hybrid cells in culture. Evidence for neuroblast-glioblast reciprocal genetic regulation. In: Fedoroff S, Hertz L (eds) Cell, tissue, and organ cultures in neurobiology. Academic Press, New York, pp 393–406

Rowe N, Neale EA, Alvins L, Guroff G, Schrier BK (1977) Pineal gland cells in culture. Morphology, biochemistry, differentiation, and coculture with sympathetic neurons. Exp Cell Res 104:345–356

Sakai KK, Marks BH, George JM, Koestner A (1974) The isolated organ-cultured supraoptic nucleus as a neuropharmacological test system. J Pharmacol Exp Ther 190:482–491

Schubert D (1974) Induced differentiation of clonal rat nerve and glial cells. Neurobiology 4:376–387

Schubert D, Carlisle W (1979) Neuronal cells from rodent neoplams. Methods Enzymol 58: 584–590

Schubert D, Jacob F (1970) 5-bromodeoxyuridine-induced differentiation of a neuroblastoma. Proc Natl Acad Sci USA 67: 247–254

Schubert D, Humphreys S, Baroni C, Cohn M (1969) In vitro differentiation of a mouse neuroblastoma. Proc Natl Acad Sci USA 64: 316–323

Schubert D, Heinemann S, Carlisle W, Tarikas H, Kimes B, Patrick J, Steinbach SH, Culp W, Brandt BL (1974) Clonal cell lines from the rat central nervous system. Nature 249: 224–227

Scott BS (1977) Adult mouse dorsal root ganglia neurons in cell culture. J Neurobiol 8: 417–427

Scott BS, Engelbert VE, Fisher KC (1969) Morphological and electrophysiological characteristics of dissociated chick embryo spinal ganglion cells in culture. Exp Neurol 23:230–248

Scott D, Dudley GK, Hockfield SJ (1974) Ultrastructural analysis of organ cultured median eminence. Anat Rec 178:459–460

Seeds NW, Gilman AG, Amano T, Nirenberg M (1970) Regulation of axon formation by clonal lines of a neural tumor. Proc Natl Acad Sci USA 66:160–167

Seiger Å, Olson L (1975) Brain tissue transplanted to the anterior chamber of the eye. 3. Substitution of lacking central noradrenaline input by host iris sympathetic fibers in the isolated cerebral cortex development in oculo. Cell Tissue Res 159:225–238

Seiger Å, Olson L (1977a) Reinitiation of directed fiber growth central monoamine neurons after intraocular maturation. Exp Brain Res 29:15–44

Seiger Å, Olson L (1977b) Quantitation of fiber growth in transplanted central monoamine neurons. Cell Tissue Res 179:285–316

Seiger Å, Olson L (1978) Innervation of peripheral tissue grafts by locus coeruleus in oculo: only partial correspondence with degree of sympathetic innervation. Brain Res 139: 233–247

Seiger Å, Olson L, Farnebo L-O (1976) Brain tissue transplanted to the anterior chamber of the eye. 4. Drug-modulated transmitter release in central monoamine nerve terminals lacking normal postsynaptic receptors. Cell Tissue Res 165:157–170

Seil FJ, Herndon RM (1970) Cerebellar granule cells in vitro. A light and electron microscope study. J Cell Biol 45:212–220

Seil FJ, Kelly JM, Leiman A (1974) Anatomical organization of cerebral neocortex in tissue culture. Exp Neurol 45:435–450

Sensenbrenner M (1977) Dissociated brain cells in primary cultures. In: Fedoroff S, Hertz L, (eds) Cell, tissue, and organ cultures in neurobiology. Academic Press, New York, pp 191–213

Sensenbrenner M, Lodin Z, Treska J, Jacob M, Kage MP, Mandel P (1969) The cultivation of isolated neurons from spinal ganglia of chick embryo. Z Zellforsch 98:538–549

Sensenbrenner M, Booher J, Mandel P (1971a) Cultivation and growth of dissociated neurons from chick embryo cerebral cortex in the presence of different substrates. Z Zellforsch 117:559–569

Sensenbrenner M, Ciesielski-Treska J, Hermetet JC (1971b) Cultures de neurones isolés. CR Soc Biol (Paris) 165:506–509

Sensenbrenner M, Moonen G, Delaunoy JP, Bock E, Poindron P, Mandel P (1977) Morphological and biochemical differentiation of rat astroblasts in primary culture. Trans Am Soc Neurochem 8:43

Seshan KR, Levi-Montalcini R (1971) In vitro analysis of corpora cardiaca and corpora allata from nymphal and adult specimens of

Periplaneta americana. Arch Ital Biol 109: 81–109
Shapiro DL (1973) Morphological and biochemical alterations in fetal rat brain cells cultured in the presence of monobutyryl cyclic AMP. Nature 241:203–204
Shapiro DL, Schrier BK (1973) Cell cultures of fetal rat brain. Growth and marker enzyme development. Exp Cell Res 77:239–247
Sheffield JB, Moscona AA (1970) Electron microscopic analysis of aggregation of embryonic cells: the structure and differentiation of aggregates of neural retina cells. Develop. Biol 23:36
Shimada Y, Fischman DA (1973) Morphological and physiological evidence for the development of functional neuromuscular junctions in vitro. Dev Biol 31:200–225
Silberberg DH (1972) Cultivation of nerve tissue. In: Rothblat GH, Cristofalo VJ (eds) Growth nutrition and metabolism of cells in culture, vol II. Academic Press, New York, pp 131–167
Skaper SD, Varon S (1979) Sodium dependence of the nerve growth factor-regulated hexose uptake in chick embryo ganglionic cells. Brain Res 172:303–313
Slaaf DW, Hooisma J, Meeter E, Stevens WF (1979) Effects of innervation by ciliary ganglia on developing muscle in vitro. Brain Res 175: 87–107
Sobkowicz HM, Bereman B, Rose JE (1975) Organotypic development of the organ of Corti in culture. J Neurocytol 4:543–572
Stenevi U, Björklund A, Svendgaard NA (1976) Transplantation of central and peripheral monoamine neurons of the adult rat brain: techniques and conditions for survival. Brain Res 114:1–20
Stenstrom ML, Edelstein M, Grisham JW (1974) Effect of ara-CTP on DNA replication and repair in isolated hepatocyte nuclei. Exp Cell Res 89:439–442
Taylor D, Seiger Å, Freedman R, Olson L, Hoffer B (1978) Electrophysiological analysis of reinnervation of transplants in the anterior chamber of the eye by the autonomic ground plexus of the iris. Proc Natl Acad Sci USA 75:1009–1012
Teillet MA (1978) Evolution of the lumbo-sacral neural crest in the avain embryo: Origin and differentiation of the ganglionated nerve of Remak studied in interspecific quail-chick chimerae. Wilhelm Roux Arch Entwicklungsmech Org 184:251–268
Trenkner E, Sidman RL (1977) Histogenesis of mouse cerebellum in microwell cultures. Cell reaggregation and migration, fiber and synapse formation. J Cell Biol 75:915–940
Tschechne B (1978) Ultramorphologische, histo- und biochemische Untersuchungen zur Differenzierung adrenaler chromaffiner Zellen des Meerschweinchens in Transplantaten in die vordere Augenkammer und in der Gewebekultur. Dissertation, Philipps-Universität Marburg
Tschechne D (1978) Neuronale Transformation und Reinnervation von adrenalen chromaffinen Zellen in Transplantaten in der vorderen Augenkammer des Meerschweinchens. Dissertation, Philipps-Universität Marburg
Unsicker K, Chamley JH (1976) Effects of dbcAMP and theophylline on rat adrenal medulla grown in tissue culture. Histochemistry 46:197–201
Unsicker K, Chamley JH (1977) Growth characteristics of postnatal rat adrenal medulla in culture. Cell Tissue Res 177:247–268
Unsicker K, Chamley JH, Burnstock G (1976) Studies on the interactions between nerve fibers from para- and orthosympathetic ganglia and adreno-cortical and -medullary cells in joint culture. Cell Tissue Res 178: 533–549
Unsicker K, Zwarg U, Habura O (1977) Electron microscopic evidence for the formation of synapses and synaptoid contacts in adrenal medullary grafts. Brain Res 120:533–539
Unsicker K, Tschechne B, Tschechne D (1978a) Formation of cholinergic synapses on adrenal chromaffin cells in anterior eye chamber transplants. Brain Res 152:334–340
Unsicker K, Krisch B, Otten U, Thoenen H (1978b) Nerve growth factor-induced fiber outgrowth from isolated rat adrenal chromaffin cells: impairment by glucocorticoids. Proc Natl Acad Sci USA 75:3498–3502
Unsicker K, Tschechne B, Tschechne D, Löffelholz K, Lindmar R, Wolf U (1979) Neuronale Transformation von adrenalen chromaffinen Zellen in Transplantaten in die Vordere Augenkammer. Verh Anat Ges 73:963–970
Unsicker K, Griesser GH, Müller Th, Ziegler W (in press) Isolierung, Langzeit-Kulturen und Augenkammertransplantate chromaffiner Zellen aus Rindernebennierenmark (abstr). Verh Anat Ges 75
Unsicker K, Rieffert B, Ziegler W (to be published) Effects of the cell culture conditions, nerve growth factor, dexamethasone, and cyclic AMP on adrenal chromaffin cells in vitro. Proceedings of the IIIrd International Symposium on Nervous Transmission, Helsinki, September 2–6, 1979. Raven Press, New York
Van de Water TR, Ruben RJ (1971) Organ culture of the mammalian inner ear. Acta Otolaryngol (Stockh) 71:303–312

Varon S (1977) Neural cell isolation and identification. In: Fedoroff S, Hertz L (eds) Cell, tissue, and organ cultures in neurobiology. Academic Press, New York, pp 237–261

Varon S, Manthorpe M, Adler R (1979) Cholinergic neuronotropic factors. I. Survival, neurite outgrowth, and choline acetyltransferase activity in monolayer cultures from chick embryo ciliary ganglia. Brain Res 173:29–45

Varon S, Raiborn C (1969) Dissociation, fractionation and culture of embryonic brain cells. Brain Res 12:180–199

Varon S, Raiborn C (1971) Excitability and conduction in neurons of dissociated ganglion cell cultures. Brain Res 30:83–98

Varon S, Raiborn C (1972) Dissociation, fractionation, and culture of chick embryo sympathetic ganglionic cells. J Neurocytol 1: 211–221

Varon S, Raiborn C, Tyszka E (1973) In vitro studies of dissociated cells from newborn mouse dorsal root ganglia. Brain Res 54: 51–63

Vogel Z, Daniels MP, Nirenberg M (1976) Synapse and acetylcholine receptor synthesis by neurons dissociated from retina. Proc Natl Acad Sci USA 73:2370–2374

Wakshull E, Johnson MI, Burton H (1978) Persistence of an amine uptake system in cultured rat sympathetic neurons which use acetylcholine as their transmitter. J Cell Biol 79:121–131

Walicke PA, Campenot RB, Patterson PH (1977) Determination of transmitter function by neuronal activity. Proc Natl Acad Sci USA 74: 5767–5771

Waxman SG, Dichter MA, Hartwieg EA, Matheson JK (1977) Recapitulation of normal neuro-glial relations in dissociated cell cultures of dorsal root ganglia. Brain Res 122: 344–350

Wessells NK, Nuttall RP (1978) Normal branching, induced branching, and steering of cultured parasympathetic motor neurons. Exp Cell Res 115:111–122

Weston JA (1970) The migration and differentiation of neural crest cells. Adv Morphog 8:41–114

Wiesmann UN, Hofmann K, Burkhart T, Herschkowitz N (1975) Dissociated cultures of newborn mouse brain. I. Metabolism of sulfated lipids and mucopolysaccharides. Neurobiology 5:305–315

Wolf MK (1964) Differentiation of neuronal types and synapses in myelinating cultures of mouse cerebellum. J Cell Biol 22:259–279

Wolf MK (1970) Anatomy of cultured mouse cerebellum. II. Organotypic migration of granule cells demonstrated by silver impregnation of normal and mutant cultures. J Comp Neurol 140:281–298

Wolff E (1961) Utilisation de la membrane vitelline de l'œuf de poule en culture organotypique. I. Technique et possibilités. Dev Biol 3:767–786

Wood PM (1976) Separation of functional Schwann cells and neurons from normal peripheral nerve tissue. Brain Res 115:361–375

Wood PM, Bunge RP (1975) Evidence that sensory axons are mitogenic for Schwann cells. Nature 256:662–664

Yavin E, Yavin Z (1974) Attachment and culture of dissociated cells from rat embryo cerebral hemispheres on polylysine-coated surface. J Cell Biol 62:540–546

Subject Index

V. Chan-Palay

Cerebellar Dentate Nucleus

Organization, Cytology and Transmitters

1977. 293 figures including 79 plates, some in color.
XXI, 548 pages
ISBN 3-540-07958-0

The product of more than four years of intensive research, this book is a compendium of experiments on the largest and most highly developed of the deep cerebellar nuclei, the dentate nucleus, in the laboratory rat and the rhesus monkey. It includes a detailed cytological and quantitative analysis of the neurons and neuroglial cells and synapses in this nucleus on the basis of Golgi preparations and electron micrographs. Several chapters are devoted to the most complex analysis to date of the relations of this nucleus – both afferent and efferent – with other centers in the medulla, midbrain, and thalamus. The tract tracing methods that have been employed include not only experimental degeneration but also the transport of horseradish peroxidase and of protein labelled with radioactive amino acids. Extensive work is reported on the serotoninergic and catecholaminergic nerve fiber supply to this nucleus. A theoretical treatment is given of the roles of the dentate in the coordination of sensory and volitional input with motor output. The book contains a large number of new findings not previously and it is illustrated by superb drawings and photomicrographs of light microscope preparations, electron micrographs, autoradiographs at the light and electron microscopic levels, diagrams, and charts which contribute to making this volume the definitive work on the subject.